AF479184

THE RED CELL

PROGRESS IN CLINICAL AND BIOLOGICAL RESEARCH

THE RED CELL

Proceedings of the Fourth International Conference
on Red Cell Metabolism and Function held at the
University of Michigan, Ann Arbor, September 14–17, 1977

Editor

GEORGE J. BREWER

Departments of Human Genetics and Internal
Medicine, University of Michigan
Ann Arbor, Michigan

ALAN R. LISS, INC. • NEW YORK • 1978

Library of Congress Cataloging in Publication Data

International Conference on Red Cell Metabolism
    and Function, 4th, University of Michigan,
    1977.
    The red cell.

    (Progress in clinical and biological research;
v. 21)
    Includes bibliographies.
    1. Erythrocyte disorders – Congresses.
2. Hemoglobinopathy – Congresses. 3. Erythrocytes
– Congresses. 4. Hemoglobin – Congresses.
I. Brewer, George J., 1930– II. Title.
III. Series. [DNLM: 1. Erythrocytes – Congresses.
2. Cell membrane – Congresses. 3. Hemoglobins –
Congresses. 4. Hemoglobinopathies – Congresses.
W1 PR668E v. 21 / WH150 I57 1977r]
RC64.I57 1977   612'.111   78-71
ISBN 0-8451-0021-1

Acknowledgments

We gratefully acknowledge the generous support of:

Department of the Navy
Office of Naval Research
Arlington, Virginia 22217

Meyer Laboratories, Inc.
1900 West Commercial Boulevard
Ft. Lauderdale, Florida 33309

Dow Chemical U.S.A.
Midland, Michigan 48640

Warner Lambert/Parke-Davis
Pharmaceutical Research Division
2800 Plymouth Road
Ann Arbor, Michigan 48105

Transidyne General Corp.
903 Airport Road
Ann Arbor, Michigan 48104

American Instrument Co.
8030 Georgia Avenue
Silver Spring, Maryland 20910

Contents

PARTICIPANTS

John A. Black, Department of Biochemistry, University of Oregon Health Sciences Center, Portland, Oregon.

George J. Brewer, Department of Human Genetics, University of Michigan Medical School, Ann Arbor, Michigan.

Olen R. Brown, John M. Dalton Research Center, University of Missouri, Columbia, Missouri.

Robin Carrell, University Department of Clinical Biochemistry, Addenbrooke's Hospital, Cambridge, England.

Anthony Cerami, The Rockefeller University, New York, New York.

John A. Collins, Department of Surgery, Stanford Medical Center, Stanford, California.

R. Ben Dawson, School of Medicine, University of Maryland, Baltimore, Maryland.

Jochen Duhm, Physiologisches Institut, Universität München, München, Germany.

Thomas Gilroy, Department of Pediatrics, Baylor College of Medicine, Houston, Texas.

Samuel Goldstein, Departments of Medicine and Biochemistry, McMaster University Medical Center, Hamilton, Ontario, Canada.

Donald R. Harkness, Veterans Administration Hospital, Miami, Florida.

Robert P. Hebbel, Division of Hematology, Univ. of Minnesota, Minneapolis, Minnesota.

Paul Hochstein, Department of Pharmacology, U.S.C. School of Medicine, Los Angeles, California.

Titus H.J. Huisman, Department of Cell and Molecular Biology, Medical College of Georgia, Augusta, Georgia.

Donald E. Hultquist, Department of Biological Chemistry, University of Michigan, Ann Arbor, Michigan.

Harry Jacob, University of Minnesota Medical School, Minneapolis, Minnesota

Hermann Lehmann, Department of Clinical Biochemistry, Addenbrooke's Hospital, Cambridge, England.

Lawrence S. Lessin, George Washington University Clinic, Washington, D.C.

Orville A. Levander, Nutrition Institute, Agricultural Research Center, Beltsville, Maryland.

Elaine Mansfield, Department of Genetics, University of California, Berkeley, Berkeley, California.

W. Lawrence Marsh, New York Blood Center, New York, New York.

Donald Miller, Molecular Hematology Branch, National Heart and Lung Institute, Bethesda, Maryland.

Hiroshi Mizukami, Department of Biology, Wayne State University, Detroit, Michigan.

David G. Nathan, Children's Hospital Medical Center, Boston, Massachusetts.

Donald E. Paglia, Center for the Health Sciences, University of California, Los Angeles, Los Angeles, California.

Ananda S. Prasad, Veterans Administration Hospital, Allen Park, Michigan.

Jean Rosa, Unité INSERM U91, Hopital Henri Mondor, Creteil, France.

Allen D. Roses, Division of Neurology, Duke University Medical Center, Durham, North Carolina.

Donald Rucknagel, Department of Human Genetics, University of Michigan Medical School, Ann Arbor, Michigan.

Elizabeth S. Russell, The Jackson Laboratory, Bar Harbor, Maine.

Eric B. Schoomaker, Duke University Medical Center, Durham, North **Carolina.**

Graham R. Serjeant, MRC Laboratories, University of the West Indies, Kingston, Jamaica, West Indies.

Michael P. Sheetz, Department of Physiology, University of Connecticut Heath Center, Farmington, Connecticut.

Stephen B. Shohet, Cancer Research Institute, University of California, San Francisco, San Francisco, California.

Ernest R. Simon, Bureau of Biologics, Bethesda, Maryland.

Charles F. Sing, Department of Human Genetics, University of Michigan, Ann Arbor, Michigan.

Theodore L. Steck, Department of Biochemistry, University of Chicago, Chicago, Illinois.

Douglas MacN. Surgenor, Northeast Regional Red Cross Blood Program, Boston, Massachusetts.

Philip W. Tucker, Department of Genetics, University of Wisconsin, Madison, Wisconsin.

C. Robert Valeri, Naval Blood Research Laboratory, **Bos**ton, Massachusetts.

Ronald S. Weinstein, Rush-Presbyterian-St. Luke's Medical Center, Rush Medical College, Chicago, Illinois.

Edward W. Westhead, Department of Biochemistry, University of Massachusetts, Amherst, Massachusetts.

Darryl Williams, Division of Medicine, Louisiana State University, Shreveport, Louisiana.

Dr. Christine Winterbourn, Department of Clinical Biochemistry, Christchurch Hospital, Christchurch, New Zealand.

Michael L. Baird, The University of Chicago, Chicago, Illinois.

David Bartnick, Biology Department, Wayne State University, Detroit, Michigan.

A. Gerald Beaudoin, Biology Department, Wayne State University, Detroit, Michigan.

Ann Bell, University of Tennessee Center for Health Sciences, Memphis, Tennessee.

Elaine M. Berger, Department of Medicine, University of Minnesota, Minneapolis, Minnesota.

Shelly C. Bernstein, Comprehensive Sickle Cell Center, The University of Chicago, Chicago, Illinois.

Yves Beuzard, Unité Inserm U 91, Hopital Henri Mondor, Creteil, France.

Nirmala Bhoopalam, 273 East Madison, Elmhurst, Illinois.

Michael C. Brain, Department of Medicine, McMaster University, Hamilton, Ontario, Canada.

Effie M. Brosious, Hematology Division, Center for Disease Control, Atlanta, Georgia.

Timothy W. Brotherton, McMaster University Medical Center, Hamilton, Ontario, Canada.

Lawrence N. Button, Children's Hospital Medical Center, Boston, Massachusetts

Bruce Cameron, Papanicolaou Cancer Research Institute, Miami, Florida.

Earl W. Campbell, Jr., Department of Medicine, Michigan State University, East Lansing, Michigan.

Robert T. Card, Department of Medicine, University Hospital, Saskatoon, Saskatchewan, Canada.

Oswaldo Castro, Center for Sickle Cell Disease, Howard
University, Washington, D.C.

Jack C. Chaffin, 6315 Barton Mill, San Antonio, Texas.

Robert R. Chilcote, Division of Pediatric Hematology, The
University of Chicago, Chicago, Illinois.

David H.K. Chui, McMaster University Medical Center, Hamilton, Ontario, Canada.

Margaret R. Clark, Cancer Research Institute, University
of California, San Francisco, San Francisco, California.

Beth Dover, Department of Biology, Wayne State University,
Detroit, Michigan.

John W. Eaton, Department of Medicine, University of Minnesota, Minneapolis, Minnesota.

Grant Fairbanks, Worcester Foundation for Experimental
Biology, Shrewsbury, Massachusetts.

Robert E. Ferrell, Center for Population Genetics, The
University of Texas Health Science Center at Houston,
Houston, Texas.

Steve Forman, Department of Pharmacology, USC School of Medicine, Los Angeles, California.

Shlomo Friedman, 414 Country Club Drive, Cherry Hill,
New Jersey.

Leslie Wo-Mei Fung, Department of Chemistry, Wayne State
University, Detroit, Michigan.

Alfred C. Greenquist, Cancer Research Institute, University of California, San Francisco, San Francisco, California.

Bo Hedlund, Department of Laboratory Medicine and Pathology,
University of Minnesota, Minneapolis, Minnesota.

John Hercules, Sickle Cell Disease Branch, National Institute of Health, Bethesda, Maryland.

William L. Horvath, 3161 North Republic Blvd., Toledo, Ohio.

Kathleen Jewett, Fenwal Laboratories, Division of Travenol
    Laboratories, Inc., Round Lake, Illinois.

Denise P. Kalm, Department of Human Genetics, University
    of Michigan, Ann Arbor, Michigan.

Mitchell T. Kamlay, Department of Biology, Wayne State
    University, Detroit, Michigan.

Lawrence Kass, Simpson Memorial Institute, University of
    Michigan, Ann Arbor, Michigan.

Kinichi Kidoguchi, Medical University of South Carolina,
    Charleston, South Carolina.

Alan Keitt, Department of Pathology, University of Florida,
    Gainesville, Florida.

Helen Kosmidis, Children's Hospital, Wayne State University,
    Detroit, Michigan.

Lorraine M. Kraus, Department of Biochemistry, The Univer-
    sity of Tennessee Center for the Health Sciences,
    Memphis, Tennessee.

Martha Kreimer-Birnbaum, Department of Medicine, Medical
    College of Ohio, Toledo, Ohio.

William Krivit, Department of Pediatrics, University of
    Minnesota, Minneapolis, Minnesota.

Joe Kurantsin-Mills, Division of Hematology, George
    Washington University Medical Center, Washington, D.C.

Dominique Labie, Institut de Pathologie Moléculaire,
    Universite de Paris, Paris, France.

Irving M. London, Program in Health Sciences and Technology,
    Massachusetts Institute of Technology, Cambridge, Massa-
    chusetts.

Alan Lubin, The Mt. Sinai Hospital of Cleveland, Cleveland,
    Ohio.

Roseanne Leipzig, Department of Human Genetics, University
of Michigan, Ann Arbor, Michigan.

Donna Lusczakowski, Wayne State University, Detroit, Michigan.

Ali Mansouri, Veterans Administration, Little Rock Hospital
Division, Little Rock, Arkansas.

Paul R. McCurdy, Washington Regional Red Cross Blood Program,
Washington, D.C.

LaVerne McElroy, Department of Pathology, Univ. of Texas,
Dallas, Texas.

Nydia Meyers, Department of Human Genetics, University of
Michigan, Ann Arbor, Michigan.

Naomi Meyerstein, Ben Gurion University of the Negev,
Beer Sheva, Israel.

Paul F. Milner, Sickle Cell Center, Medical College of
Georgia, Augusta, Georgia.

Lorna Moore, Cardiovascular Pulmonary Lab, University of
Colorado, Denver, Colorado.

Mary Jane Moore, Department of Anthropology, University of
Kansas, Lawrence, Kansas.

Philip D. Morse, II, Department of Biology, Wayne State
University, Detroit, Michigan.

Paul A. Mueggler, Department of Biochemistry, University
of Oregon Health Sciences Center, Portland, Oregon.

Edmund P. Naccash, 3321 Sydenham Street, Fairfax, Virginia.

Nancy Noble, Harbor General Hospital, Torrance, California.

Sue O'Dorisio, Department of Medicine, Ohio State University, Columbus, Ohio.

Fred J. Oelshlegel, Department of Preventive Medicine,
University of Mississippi Medical Center, Jackson,
Mississippi.

Martin H. Steinberg, Veterans Administration Hospital,
    Jackson, Mississippi.

Richard Tashian, Department of Human Genetics, University
    of Michigan, Ann Arbor, Michigan.

Basil Tatis, Queens Hospital Center-Hematology, Jamaica,
    New York.

Malcolm Vye, Evanston Hospital, Evanston, Illinois.

Yeu-ming Wang, The University of Texas System-Cancer Center,
    M.D. Anderson Hospital, Houston, Texas.

Gail D. Wenger, Department of Medicine, Ohio State University,
    Columbus, Ohio.

S.C. Wong, Hemoglobinopathy Laboratory, St. Joseph's
    Hospital, Hamilton, Ontario, Canada.

Patricia A. Wood, Department of Microbiology, University
    of Minnesota, Minneapolis, Minnesota.

Harold Zarkowsky, Department of Pediatrics, St. Louis
    Children's Hospital, St. Louis, Missouri.

Charles G. Zaroulis, Memorial-Sloan Kettering Cancer Center,
    New York, New York.

Carolyn Gruber, The Upjohn Co., Kalamazoo, Michigan.

Roshni Kulkarni, Great Lakes Regional Red Cross Blood
    Program, Lansing, Michigan.

Rosalie Baine, 2779 Meadow Drive, Marietta, Georgia.

Alice Maniatis, St. Luke's Hospital Center, New York, New York.

Yannis Missirlis, Engineering Physics Department, McMaster
    University, Hamilton, Ontario, Canada.

William P. Winter, 2121 Georgia Avenue, N.W., Washington,
    D.C.

Alex Felice, Comprehensive Sickle Center, Medical College
    of Georgia, Augusta, Georgia.

Makio Ogawa, Medical University of South Carolina, Charleston, South Carolina.

Eugene P. Orringer, Department of Medicine, University of North Carolina, Chapel Hill, North Carolina.

Robert M. Petitt, Mayo Clinic, Rochester, Minnesota.

Robert L. Phyliky, Mayo Clinic, Rochester, Minnesota.

Daniel C. Plunket, Department of Pediatrics, The University of Oklahoma Tulsa Medical College, Tulsa Oklahoma.

Y. Ravi, Wayne State University, Detroit, Michigan.

Raymonde Rosa, Unité INSERM U91, Hopital Henri Mondor, Creteil, France.

S. Sarniak, Wayne State University, Detroit, Michigan.

Ian Shine, The Thomas Hunt Morgan Institute of Genetics, Inc., Lexington, Kentucky.

Gerald E. Siefring, Northwestern University, Evanston, Illinois.

N. Simard-Duquesne, 1025 Laurentien, Montreal, Quebec, Canada.

David Simpson, Wayne State University, Detroit, Michigan.

Paulette Smariga, Papanicolaou Cancer Research Institute, Miami, Florida.

Clark M. Smith, Department of Pediatrics, University of Minnesota, Minneapolis, Minnesota.

Robert C. Smith, Animal Science Department, Auburn University, Auburn, Alabama.

Joseph T. Sobota, The Upjohn Company, Kalamazoo, Michigan.

Dushyant T. Soorya, Wayne State University, Detroit, Michigan.

E. C. Abraham, Medical College of Georgia, Augusta, Georgia.

PREFACE

The purposes of the Fourth International Conference on
Red Cell Metabolism and Function are essentially the same as
the first three. The Conference is an opportunity for a mix
of investigators with common interests in blood and the red
blood cell, but with divergent interests in specific research
areas, to come together and share information formally and
informally. Thus, on September 14-17, 1977, researchers and
clinicians from a variety of red cell-related disciplines
met in the Towsley Center for Continuing Medical Education
at the University of Michigan in Ann Arbor to share their
newest work and insights. The meeting was dedicated to Max
Perutz, Nobel Laureate, of Cambridge University, England, in
recognition of his major (and continuing) contributions to
an understanding of the structure and function of hemoglobin.

The red cell membrane continues to be a focus for intensive research. This work can be thought of as comprising
two types of efforts. One involves very basic studies of
membrane structure and function, with the red cell membrane
serving as a convenient and accessible source. Work in this
area is critical to an eventual understanding of biological
membranes, and was amply represented at the Conference. The
second type of work involves the clinical applicability of
discovered abnormalities. Studies of red cell membranes are
beginning to shed light on diseases of membranes of other tissues. For example, one paper dealt with the red cell membrane
abnormalities in muscular dystrophy. Other papers dealt with
clinical abnormalities affecting other tissues in addition to
the red cell, or with abnormalities primarily involving the
red cell.

Red cell metabolism was, as usual, covered in depth.
The possible functional role of acid phosphatase was presented in one paper. A special session dealt with the control
and the genetics of red cell metabolism. This session ranged
from single gene effects to complex multivariate analyses of
polygenic effects. The genetics of red cell metabolism may
emerge as a model for helping to understand the genetics of

complex diseases.

The topics in the hemoglobin and hemoglobinopathy sessions were quite broad, ranging from basic structural studies, to studies of sickling and interaction with thalassemia. to growth characteristics of marrow cells, to the number of alpha globin structural loci, and to hemoglobin A_{1c} levels in diabetes. The latter paper elicited a considerable amount of interest and discussion, and is another example of the use of the red cell to study systemic diseases.

The Conference has always featured some of the recent developments in blood storage and this one was no exception. For example, the recent addition to the blood banker's armamentarium, adenine, to allow longer storage, was discussed. The effects of hypoxia, hyperoxia, and oxidant stress was also important interdisciplinary features of the Conference. One session dealt with the increasingly apparent important function of trace metals in blood cell function.

This volume contains the proceedings of this fourth Conference. It includes the formal papers and much of the informal discussion after the papers. As with the previous three conferences, it represents a compilation of the present state of the art and the status of current thinking in the various areas covered.

The editor owes a debt of gratitude to a number of people who made the conference possible. Most important was the work of my wife, Lucia Feitler Brewer, who worked very hard on all aspects of conference organization. I wish to thank Dr. Walter C. Kruckeberg and Dr. David Leichtman for help with program development. Ms. Virginia Crews, Mr. Conrad Knutsen and Mr. Robert Snyder also contributed much assistance. Ms. Ruth Ann Lewis stepped into a very difficult secretarial situation and accomplished miracles with the typing of the discussion tapes. Financial support from the Office of Naval Research; Meyer Laboratories, Inc., Fort Lauderdale, Florida; Dow Chemical U.S.A., Midland, Michigan; Warner Lambert/Parke-Davis, Ann Arbor,and Detroit, Michigan; Transidyne General Corp., Ann Arbor, Michigan; and American Instrument Co., Silver Spring, Maryland made the conference possible.

THE EDITOR

October 21, 1977

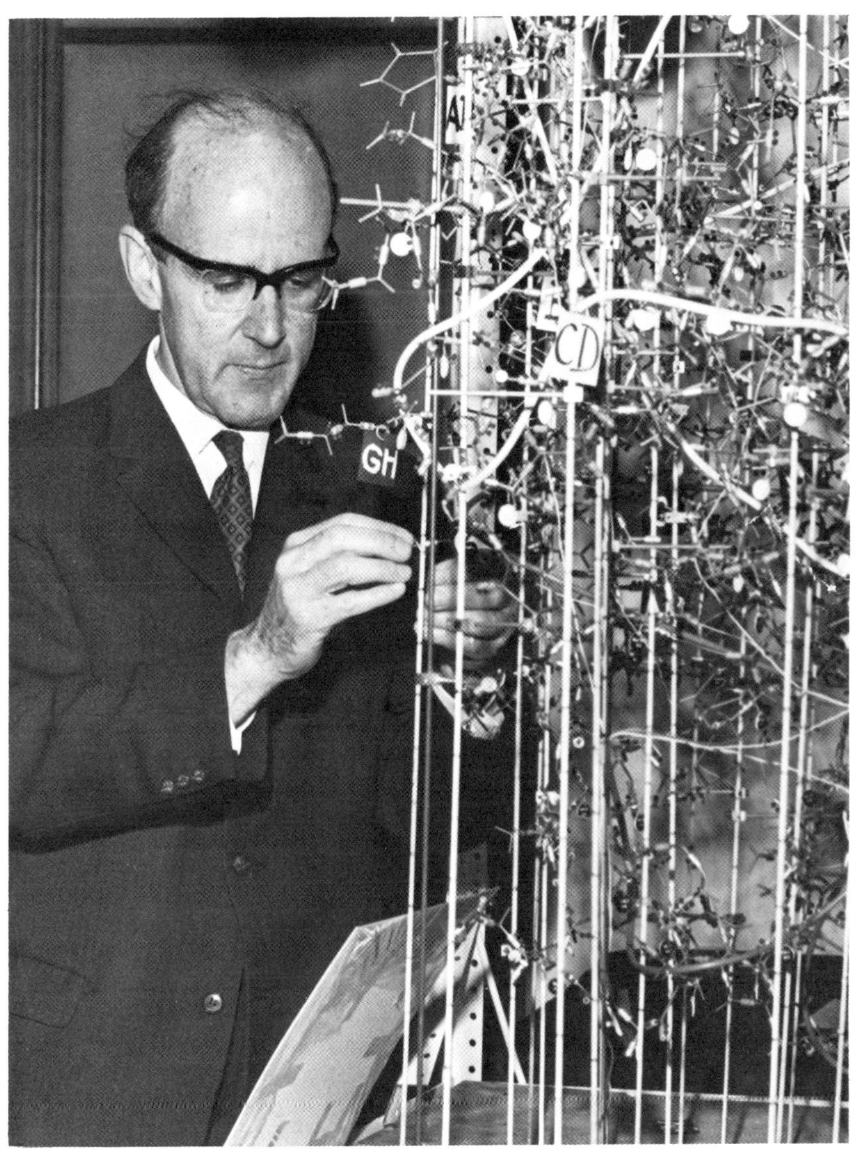

Dr. Max Perutz

DEDICATION
OF THE FOURTH INTERNATIONAL CONFERENCE ON
RED CELL METABOLISM AND FUNCTION TO
DR. MAX PERUTZ
CAMBRIDGE, ENGLAND

Max Perutz is the name written on the flag which
flutters above this meeting.

In dedicating this gathering to Max we are anxious
that this should not resemble a testimonial dinner given
to the distinguished member of a group on his departure
from the active scene. On associating our conference with
his name, and its proceedings with his photograph, we wish
to pay him honour and at the same time we want to catch for
each one of us some inspiration from his charisma and carry
it home afterwards as a driving force in our own research.

Max Perutz' influence is active in work on hemoglobin
in many aspects of this vital pigment. Wherever any of
its functions meets its link with structure, Max is the
foremost oracle. Consequently there is virtually no feature of the hemoglobin molecule which he has not enlight-
ened.

I met Max first in 1938 when the then Master of
Christ's College, Cambridge, a descendant and namesake of
Charles Darwin, invited us to lunch. He wanted us to
meet because he felt that "we might have interests in common". Max was then a glaciologist and I worked on phosphate metabolism, but looking back over forty years, I wonder whether the Master could have said a truer word.

This introduction to our conference is not supposed
to be an eulogy listing Max Perutz' many honours, but one
cannot omit that he was made a Fellow of the Royal Society

at the age of 40, and as we are in the United States, that
he is a Foreign Associate of the National Academy of Sciences. Two of the greatest honours a scientist can receive,
the Nobel Prize and the Royal Medal of the Royal Society
also have come his way. He is the first Director of the
Medical Research Council's Laboratory of Molecular Biology
in Cambridge, an institution of singular repute.

Max has taught us the basic features of the sickling
process beginning with the differences between the solubil-
ities of deoxygenated normal and sickle-cell hemoglobin and
culminating in recent years in important contributions to
the structure of sickled hemoglobin fibres. The problem
of the position of the heme in the globin moiety was solved
when Kendrew and Perutz solved the structure of myoglobin
and hemoglobin:- not four flat plates on the outside of a
rubber ball, not a heme molecule rattling within a shell,
rather like one of those Chinese ivory carvings where one
ball moves within another, and the protein shell having selective pores admitting ligands of a certain size only; the
answer was that the heme plate was pushed into the globin
like a coin into a doughnut.

There was of course the tertiary structure of the
molecule and the differences between the oxy- and the de-
oxyconformation. The recognition of subunit contacts, the
dimeric contacts gluing one α-chain to one β-chain, and the
tetrameric contacts between the α-chain of one dimer with
the β-chain of the other. The involvement of these tetrameric contacts in the transition from the deoxy T-state
into the oxy R-state led further to the recognition of the
changes involved in this process in the environment of the
heme and at the salt bridges maintaining the T-state.

I have to be careful not to produce too much of a
list of achievements, otherwise I shall end up with an address of the style given at a testimonial dinner which we
want to avoid. But don't we remember that exciting finding
that in the primary sequence of the globin chains about
every fourth residue pointing into the interior was hydrophobic so that the interior was kept free of water to allow
its cohesion by Van der Waals forces. The perfect fit of
2:3 diphosphoglyceric acid within the cleft of the two
β-chains of deoxyhemoglobin is another example where the
function of normal and variant hemoglobins found its explanation in structural repercussions shown up by x-ray

crystallography.

In recent years Max and his colleagues have been much concerned with the Bohr effect. We have come a long way from the triumphant statement that the Bohr effect could alas _not_ be associated with the heme-linked histidines, because these were present in myoglobin, which does not show a Bohr effect. Bit by bit, and step by step more percentages of the Bohr effect have found their explanation over the last years, Max Perutz being in the forefront of the contributors to the assembly of this jigsaw puzzle. His final explanation of the alkaline Bohr effect and much of the difference between the acid Bohr effects of Hemoglobins A and F are only a few weeks old. Max Perutz has taught us to understand the heat resistance of Hemoglobin A_2, the alkali resistance of Hemoglobin F, and what is of practical importance for our understanding of the role of this hemoglobin in sickle-cell anemia, the high solubility of Hemoglobin F when in the deoxy form.

The number of collaborators involved is considerable and all have carried away from Cambridge exciting intellectual memories as well as affection and admiration for their guru. Max Perutz is no longer a glaciologist but he skis and climbs without that excuse. All of us who know him realize how much we owe to his wife Gisela for her support. A happy family life may not be essential for a man's scientific output but it helps. I noticed that the paper submitted to this conference acknowledges the advice of his son Robin.

H. Lehmann
University of Cambridge
Cambridge, England

HEMOGLOBIN

Chairman: H. Lehmann

STRUCTURE OF HAEMOGLOBINS ZÜRICH (His E7(63)β→Arg) AND
SYDNEY (Val E11(67)β→Ala) AND THE ROLE OF THE DISTAL
RESIDUES IN LIGAND BINDING

P.W. Tucker[*†], S.E.V. Phillips[*], M.F. Perutz[*],
R. Houtchens[§] and W.S. Caughey[§]

[*] MRC Laboratory of Molecular Biology,
Cambridge, England.
[§] Department of Biochemistry, Colorado State
University, Fort Collins, Colorado 80523, USA.

The iron atom in haemoglobin (Hb) is bonded to a
histidine on the proximal side of the haem; on the distal
side of the haem it is faced by another histidine (E7) and
a valine (E11). Two atoms of the histidine C_ϵ and N_ϵ, are
in van der Waals contact with the porphyrin in both deoxyhb
and oxyhb and N_ϵ is also in contact with haem ligands.
The histidine side chain also acts as a gate to the haem
pocket, not allowing ligands to enter or leave unless it
swings out of the way. The role of Val E11 is more
selective: its methyl γ_2 is in van der Waals contact with
the porphyrin only in the β subunit of deoxyhb where it
overlaps the van der Waals radii of haem ligands, so that
the haem pocket must widen before ligands can bind; this
restriction either does not apply, or applies only to a
much smaller extent, to the α subunit. There, on the
other hand, access to the ligand site is blocked by a water
molecule hydrogen-bonded to His E7 (Perutz, 1970; Bolton
and Perutz, 1970; Fermi, 1975; Ladner *et al*, 1977). What
role do these distal residues play in ligand binding and
cooperativity? We have approached this question by an
X-ray and spectroscopic study of two abnormal Hbs in which
either the histidine or the valine has been replaced by
another residue, leaving behind an empty space in the haem
pocket.

[†] Present address: Laboratory of Genetics, 406 Genetics
Building, University of Wisconsin, Madison, Wis 53706, USA

The Red Cell, pages 3—14

Hb Zürich (His E7(63)β→Arg) causes haemolytic inclusion body anaemia on treatment of its heterozygous carriers with sulphanilamides (Muller and Kingma, 1961; Hitzig *et al*, 1960; Frick *et al*, 1962); it has an abnormally high oxygen affinity, low cooperativity and normal Bohr effect (Winterhalter *et al*, 1969); *in vitro*, but normally not *in vivo*, its β haems•are autoxidized more easily than those of Hb A (Jacob and Winterhalter, 1970). CO is displaced by oxygen more slowly than in Hb A (Wallace *et al*, 1976). Perutz and Lehmann pointed out that the side chain of Arg E7 could not be accommodated in the haem pocket, but would protrude at the surface, leaving a large cavity by the ligand site of the iron (Perutz and Lehmann, 1968).

Hb Sydney (Val E11(67)β→Ala) causes haemolytic anaemia in heterozygous carriers; it is easily autoxidized, and is unstable and loses haem on heating to $50^{\circ}C$ (Carrell *et al*, 1967). Seeing that the replacement of the distal valine by alanine removes an obstruction to ligand binding one would have expected the oxygen affinity of Hb Sydney to be abnormally high, but, in fact, Lehmann and his colleagues found its mean affinity (p_{50}) to be normal. The oxygen equilibrium curve of a mixture of Hb A + Hb Sydney crosses that of Hb A, showing that the mixture has an abnormally low affinity at low and abnormally high affinity at high partial pressures of O_2 (Casey *et al*, 1977). This unexpected behaviour made us suspect that the vacant space left by the removal of the methyl groups of the valine might be filled by a water molecule bonded to the distal histidine.

EXPERIMENTAL

Hb Zürich was purified from haemolysates on a DEAE-cellulose 52 column by a linear gradient of 0.01 M potassium phosphate pH 7.1 vs 0.1 M potassium phosphate pH 7.6 at $4^{\circ}C$. Crystals of its deoxy form were isomorphous with deoxyhb A (Perutz, 1968), but gave disordered X-ray photographs; crystals of HbCO grown by a vapour diffusion modification of the method described for crystallizing HbCO A (Perutz, 1968) gàve small tetragonal bipyramids isomorphous with HbCO A (Perutz *et al*, 1951). a = b = 53.7 Å, c = 193 Å; space group $P4_12_12$ with one αβ dimer in the asymmetric unit. X-ray intensities were recorded on an Arndt-Wonacott rotation camera (Arndt *et al*, 1973) using graphite monochromatized CuKα radiation. A complete set of reflexions within a limiting sphere of 2.7 $\overset{\circ}{A}$ was obtained from one crystal at 20 - 25°C without appreciable degradation. The intensities were measured and processed (Mallett *et al*, 1977) to give 7,500 unique reflexions with an overall film scaling standard deviation in $|F|$ of 8.6%. A difference Fourier synthesis was calculated using $(|F_{CO\ Zürich}| - |F_{CO\ A}|)$ as coefficients together with the phase angles of HbCO A derived from J.M. Baldwin's recent real space and energy refined structure (unpublished). The mean isomorphous difference was 9.7% of the mean $|F_{CO\ A}|$ and the overall rms difference density 0.038 e/$\overset{\circ}{A}^3$.

Hb Sydney cannot be separated from Hb A. A mixture of the two deoxyhbs was crystallized (Perutz, 1968) giving crystals isomorphous with Hb A, with a = 63.2 $\overset{\circ}{A}$, b = 83.6 $\overset{\circ}{A}$, c = 53.8 $\overset{\circ}{A}$, β = 99.34°; space group $P2_1$ with one tetramer in the asymmetric unit. Reflexions within a limiting sphere of 2.73 $\overset{\circ}{A}^{-1}$ were measured on a diffractometer (Tucker and Perutz, 1977) to give 13,764 independent reflexions with an overall standard deviation in $|F|$ of 4.1%; these were matched with the observed amplitudes of deoxyhb A (Ten Eyck and Arnone, 1976). A difference Fourier synthesis was calculated using $(|F_{Sydney\ +\ A}| - |F_A|)$ as coefficients together with the phase angles calculated from the real space refined structure of deoxyhb A (Fermi, 1975). The mean isomorphous difference was 5.7% of the mean F_A and the overall rms difference density was 0.029 e/$\overset{\circ}{A}^3$, much smaller than for Hb Zürich.

RESULTS

The difference map of Hb Zürich shows a large negative peak covering part of the imidazole of His E7 and a dominant positive peak flanking the propionate side chain IV of the haem (Figure 1). This peak clearly represents the side chain of Arg E7. There is also a negative peak by the side chain of Phe CD4 suggesting that it has been pushed upwards, and there are some negative peaks to the left of the bottom edge of the haem, suggesting that this edge has moved to the distal side, so that the haem as seen in the figure has turned anticlockwise. To determine the position of the arginine side chain we fitted a model of it and of the haem to the difference density in a miniature Richards box (Richards, 1968). We kept the α and β carbons as in deoxyhb A, since no difference density is associated with

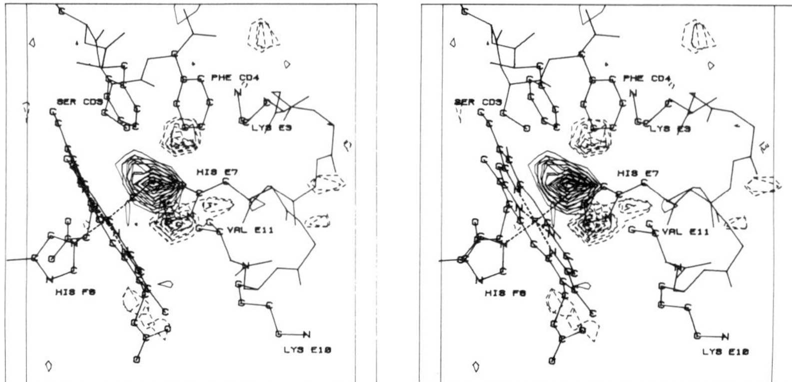

Figure 1.   Difference Fourier synthesis of HbCO Zürich minus HbCO A at 2.76 Å resolution superimposed on the structure of HbCO A. Section intervals are 0.75 Å, contour intervals are 0.025 e/Å^3 (zero level omitted), and negative contours are broken. Shown are sections +17 to +37, cut perpendicular to the crystallographic c axis; ie, the β haem ligand pocket is seen from the 'bottom' according to the conventional view in Figures 3b and 17 of Perutz (1969).

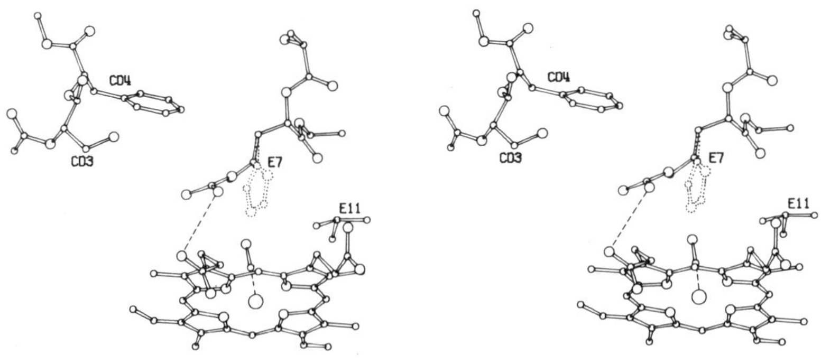

Figure 2.   Orientation of Arg E7 in the β ligand pocket of HbCO Zürich. The position of the replaced distal His E7 is denoted with dotted lines. The view is similar to that of Figure 1.

them, and fitted the rest of the side chain to the difference
peak. We then measured its coordinates and matched them to
the remainder of the HbCO A structure. This placed one of
the guanidinium nitrogens within 2.9 Å of one of the propionate
oxygens, suggesting that the two groups are linked by a salt
bridge (Figure 2). There may also be a very weak hydrogen
bond to Ser CD3. We could find no difference density on the
haem-linked CO, but a slight change in its angle of tilt
would not be detectable at our resolution. Note that the
removal of His E7 not only leaves an empty space in the haem
pocket but leaves the entrance to the pocket wide open. We
next built a model of sulphanilamide and found that it can
enter the haem pocket without distortion of the protein.
Its sulphonamide could form a hydrogen bond with the haem
propionate III, the one that does not interact with Arg E7;
its amino group then comes to lie opposite the iron atom.

The electronic absorption spectra of Hb Zürich closely
resemble those of Hb A. Oxyhb Zürich has its Soret band
red-shifted by $\sim$3 nm and the α and β bands blue-shifted by
$\sim$3 nm. Deoxyhb Zürich has its Soret and visible bands blue-
shifted by $\sim$2 nm. So the bands of the abnormal β subunit
must be shifted by twice these amounts. The CO stretching
frequency in that subunit is raised from its normal value of
1,951 cm^{-1} to 1,958 cm^{-1} (Wallace *et al*, 1976).

Despite the mixed crystals used for the X-ray analysis
the difference map of deoxyhb Sydney + A is quite clear.
The γ carbons of the replaced valine are covered by two
well resolved lobes of negative density (Figure 3). The
only other prominent feature is a large positive peak
extending from N_ϵ of His E7 towards the centre of the haem
pocket; this is most readily interpreted as a water molecule
hydrogen bonded to His E7 and filling part of the gap left by
the replacement of Val E11 by Ala. One naturally suspects
that its presence might signify the oxidation of the haem
iron and formation of aquomethb, but this is unlikely for
three reasons: the α haems are entirely clear of difference
density; the centroid of the difference peak lies at 3.4 Å
from the iron atom, compared to a separation of only 2.1 Å
in methaemoglobin; absorption spectra of crystals measured
before and after exposure to X-rays showed no evidence of
oxidation. The peak seems to represent a water molecule
in contact with the porphyrin but not the iron atom, as in
the α subunits of deoxyhb A and in deoxymyoglobin (Fermi,
1975; Takano, 1977). We next transformed the coordinates

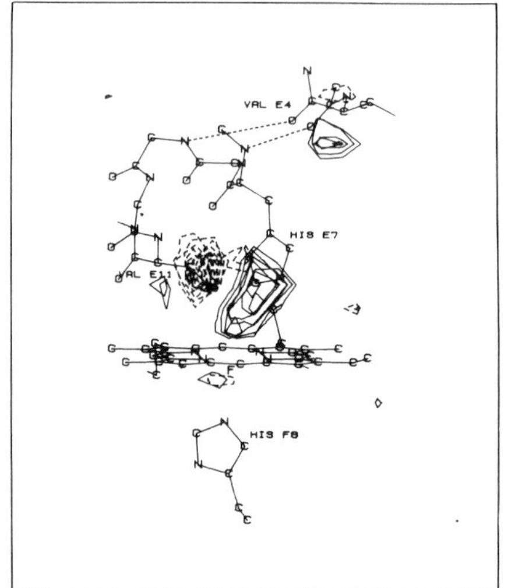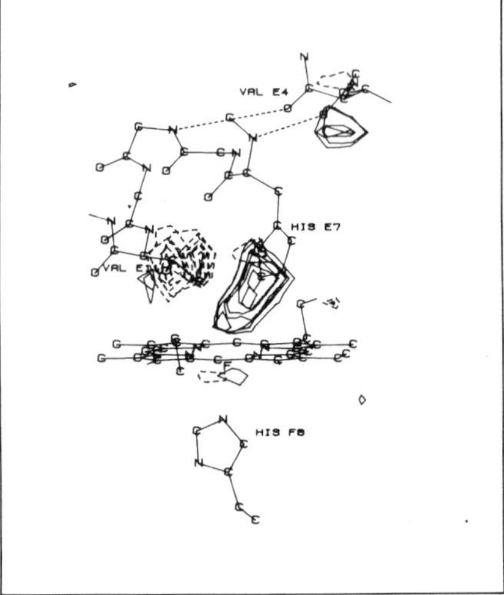

Figure 3. Difference Fourier synthesis of deoxyhb Sydney minus deoxyhb A at 2.73 Å resolution superimposed on the refined atomic positions of the β haem and associated residues of deoxyhb A. Section intervals are 0.75 Å and each section is contoured at 0.018 e/Å^3 with zero levels omitted. Negative contours are broken lines. The figure shows sections −6 to +6 cut approximately perpendicular to the β haem plane. The view is from the top of the molecule down according to the convention in Figures 3b and 17 of Perutz (1969).

of the α and β haems to an identical orientation and superimposed them. Figure 4 shows that the water molecules in the two haem pockets occupy similar positions. The N_ϵ − H_2O distance is too short for a hydrogen bond (2.2 Å), but this could be relieved by turning the imidazole about the C_β − C_γ bond as indicated in the figure. The rotation would make the $N_{porphyrin}$-H_2O-N_ϵ angle more nearly tetrahedral and would explain why the positive peak contains 9% more density than it should if it represented only a water molecule, compared to the two negative peaks representing methyls. The small negative peak near N_ϵ also favours such a rotation. Figure 4 also shows that C_β of Ala E11β occupies roughly the same position relative to the haem as does $C_{\gamma 2}$ of Val E11α, so that the replacement in

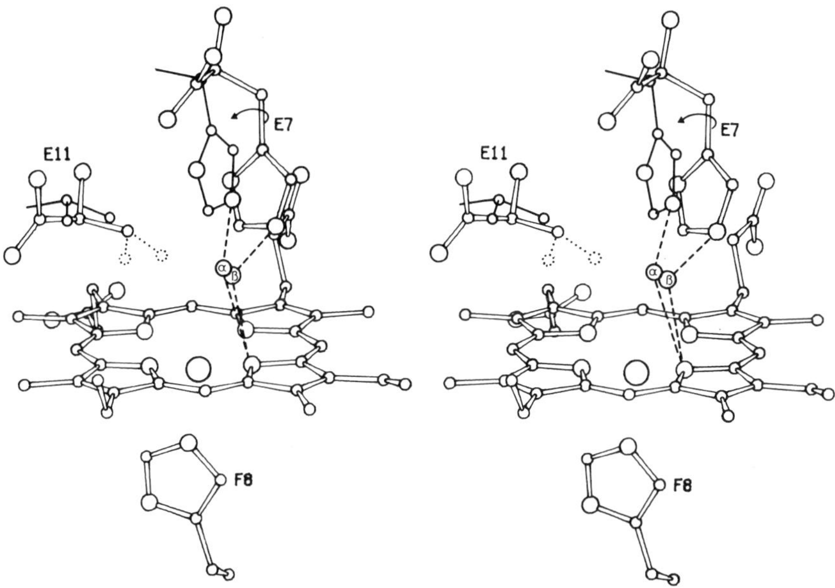

Figure 4.   Comparison of the β haem ligand pockets of deoxyhbs A and Sydney with the α haem ligand pocket of deoxyhb A.   The orientation is similar to that of Figure 3. The structure of the Hb Sydney β pocket is drawn with open perspective bonds;   the replaced γ carbons of Val E11 are denoted in dotted outline.   The structure of the α haem of deoxyhb A is superimposed on that of the β haem and the resulting positions of Val E11α and His E7α are shown as black stick bonds.   The coordination of the water molecules of the Hb Sydney β pocket (β) and native α pocket (α) are shown with broken lines.   The arrow represents the proposed rotation of the distal histidine of Hb Sydney.

Hb Sydney makes the abnormal β haem pocket somewhat similar to that of the normal α haem pocket.   The valine methyls are further from His E7 in the α than in the β subunits of Hb A, so that they allow space for a water molecule bound to the histidine in the former but not in the latter.   The infrared spectra of CO-saturated red cells from the same patient as those used for crystallization showed only the normal CO

stretching frequency at 1,951 cm^{-1}, with a just detectable
satellite at 1,968 cm^{-1}.

DISCUSSION

The replacement of the distal histidine by arginine in
Hb Zürich leaves a gap at the entrance to the haem pocket
which allows sulphanilamides and other small reactive
compounds easy access to the haem iron. Once there, its
amide could act as a one-electron donor to the bound oxygen.
If a second electron were donated by the iron atom, the
oxygen would be reduced to peroxide ion and the β haem
oxidized to the met form. This reaction could initiate the
denaturation of the Hb, formation of Heinz bodies and
haemolysis (Itano, 1970; Wallace and Caughey, 1975). The
high oxygen affinity of Hb Zürich does not appear to be due
to a low allosteric constant L, since its Bohr effect is
normal (Winterhalter *et al*, 1969) and the NMR spectrum of
its deoxy form shows the exchangeable proton resonance at
-9.4 ppm from HDO diagnostic of the quaternary deoxy (T)
structure (Drs G. Pifat and C. Ho, private communication).
Hence these properties must be due to the oxygen affinity of
the β subunits being much higher than that of the α subunits.
Why should that affinity be so high? The structure of
deoxyhb and methb show that steric hindrance to oxygen
binding by His E7 is not an important factor (Fermi, 1975;
Heidner *et al*, 1976; Ladner *et al*, 1977). The electron
density map and the NMR spectrum of Hb Zürich suggest one
mechanism which may contribute to the high affinity.
Figure 1 shows small negative peaks at the bottom of the β
haem which indicate that in Hb Zürich this haem is turned
anticlockwise relative to Hb A. Normally the bottom half of
the haem is in contact with N_ϵ and C_ϵ of the distal histidine.
The difference map suggests that these two atoms help to
clamp the haem in its correct orientation so that their
removal allows it to turn anticlockwise, ie to tilt further
from the vertical. What does this tilt signify in terms of
ligand affinity? Normally ligand binding and shortening of
the Fe - N bonds is accompanied by an anticlockwise, ligand
dissociation and lengthening of the Fe - N bonds by a
clockwise rotation (Perutz and Ten Eyck, 1971; Anderson,
1973). The tilt in Hb Zürich is in the direction normally
associated with shortening of the Fe N bonds. If this
tilt were present also in deoxyhb Zürich it would relax
the restraint on the globin that normally opposes the

shortening of the Fe - N bonds associated with ligand binding and thus make the oxygen affinity of the β haems in the T structure abnormally high. The NMR spectrum of deoxyhb Zürich is consistent with this concept. Deoxyhb A shows a paramagnetically shifted proton resonance from the β haems at -17.6 ppm from HDO, but in deoxyhb Kempsey and others which have the quaternary oxy (R) structure, this resonance lies at -15.3 ppm (Perutz et al, 1974). In deoxyhb Zürich it lies at -15.4 ppm, ie in the same position as in the deoxyhbs in the R structure, even though it has the T structure (Davis et al, 1970). In HbCO Zürich the ring-current shifted resonance of one of the γ methyls of Val E11β is shifted further upfield than in HbCO A by 0.07 ppm (Lindstrom et al, 1972), consistent with a closer approach of the methyl to the porphyrin brought about by the increased tilt. Taken together, these observations suggest that the β haems in the T structure of Hb Zürich may be relaxed and therefore have as high a ligand affinity as they normally have in the R structure.

Another mechanism contributing to their high affinity may be the absence of direct interaction between the distal histidine and the ligand itself. Evidence for such interaction is provided by the CO stretching frequencies which are 1,951 cm^{-1} in Hbs A and Sydney, and 1,958 cm^{-1} in Hb Zürich (Wallace et al, 1976). This tells us that the steric interaction with Val E11 which pushes the CO off the haem axis in Hb A, and presumably also in Hb Zürich, has no effect on the stretching frequency, but that interaction with His E7 does reduce that frequency. N_ϵ of the distal histidine is in contact with the CO carbon, so that the sp^2 orbital of N_ϵ overlaps the π^* antibonding orbital of the carbon. $sp^2{\to}\pi^*$ donation would weaken the CO bond and reduce the CO stretching frequency. It would also oppose $d\pi{\to}\pi^*$ donation from the iron to the CO, thus weakening the Fe - C bond, but this is a second order effect and may therefore make only a small contribution to the lowering of the affinity for CO and other ligands. Accurate oxygen equilibria can decide between the relative importance of the direct effect of the distal histidine on the iron oxygen bond and its indirect effect in relaxing the tilt of the haem. If the indirect effect is dominant then K_T, the equilibrium constant of the T structure, should be abnormally high, while K_R should be near normal. On the other hand, if direct interaction between the distal histidine and the bound oxygen were decisive, then both K_T and K_R should be abnormally high. In fact, it has been

found that in 0.05 M bisTris + NaCl, pH 7.4 and $25^{\circ}C$,
K_R of Hb Zürich is close to K_R of Hb A, while K_T is about 10
times larger than K_T of Hb A (M. Ikeda-Saito, private communication). Hence the high oxygen affinity of Hb Zurich
is due entirely to relaxation of the β haems in the T
structure, and the distal histidine has no significant direct influence on the strength of the Fe - O_2 bond. It
would also be useful to know the partition coefficient of
CO/O_2 in the R structure. In vitro Hb Zürich is autoxidized
more easily than Hb A (Jacob and Winterhalter, 1970), probably because the haem pocket is more accessible to water.

We now come to Hb Sydney. The paradox of its normal
oxygen affinity can now be explained by the water molecule
bound to the distal histidine in deoxyhb Sydney, replacing
the steric hindrance to ligand binding offered by Val Ell
in deoxyhb A. Let us assume that in the absence of haem
ligands this water molecule is present in both quaternary
structures. In the T structure steric hindrance by the
water replaces that normally offered by Val Ell which may
be stronger, so that the oxygen affinity may be higher than
that of Hb A. In the R structure of Hb A Val Ell β offers
little steric hindrance, while that of the water molecule
Hb Sydney would remain as strong as in the T structure.
Therefore Hb Sydney in the R structure may have a lower
oxygen affinity than Hb A. This may be the explanation for
the crossing of the equilibrium curves of Hbs A and Sydney
+ A mentioned in the introduction (Casey et al, 1977).
Though the presence of the water molecule compensates for
the absence of Val Ell, the price paid for this is readier
autoxidation. Moreover, the gap left in the haem pocket
must also be responsible for the instability of Hb Sydney
which leads to haemolytic anaemia. We now come to the
binding of CO. In the 'picket fence' complex CO lies normal to the porphyrin plane and the combination with CO is
irreversible (Collman et al, 1976). In Hb and myoglobin
steric hindrance with His E7 and Val Ell forces the CO off
the haem axis into an inclined orientation, which has been
suggested as the reason why the CO affinity is much lower
than in the picket fence complex (Collman et al , 1976). On
the basis of this argument we would have expected Hb Sydney
to have an abnormally high CO affinity, but in fact it's on
constant appears to be normal (J.A. Sirs, private communication).

ACKNOWLEDGEMENTS

We thank Professor K.H. Winterhalter and Dr S. Charache for gifts of Hb Zürich, Professor H. Lehmann for travelling to Hamburg to bring us some Hb Sydney, and him and Professor Chien Ho for allowing us to mention their unpublished data; Dr R.N. Perutz for advice concerning interaction between the haem ligand and the distal histidine; and Mrs J.M. Baldwin for allowing us to use her unpublished coordinates for phase determination and model building.

REFERENCES

Anderson L (1973) *J Mol Biol* 79:495.

Arndt UW, Champness JN, Phizackerley RP, Wonacott AJ (1973) *J Appl Crystallogr* 6:457.

Bolton W, Perutz MF (1970) *Nature* 228:551.

Carrell RW, Lehmann H, Lorkin PA, Raik E, Hunter E (1967) *Nature* 215:626.

Casey R, Kynoch, PAM, Lang A, Lehmann H, Nozari G, Shinton NK (1977) *Brit J Haem* In press

Collman JP, Brauman JI, Halbert TR, Suslick KS (1976) *Proc Natl Acad Sci USA* 73:3333.

Davis DG, Mock NH, Lindstrom TR, Charache S, Ho C (1970) *Biochem Biophys Res Comm* 40:343.

Fermi G (1975) *J Mol Biol* 97:237.

Frick PG, Hitzig WH, Betke K (1962) *Blood* 20:261.

Heidner EJ, Ladner RC, Perutz MF (1976) *J Mol Biol* 104:707.

Hitzig WH, Frick PG, Betke K, Huisman THJ (1960) *Helv Paediat Acta* 6:499.

Itano H (1970) *Proc Natl Acad Sci USA* 67:485.

Jacob H, Winterhalter KH (1970) *Proc Natl Acad Sci USA* 65:697.

Ladner RC, Heidner EJ, Perutz MF (1977) *J Mol Biol* 114:385.

Lindstrom TR, Norén IBE, Charache S, Lehmann H, Ho C (1972) *Biochemistry* 11:1677.

Mallett JFW, Champness JN, Faruqi AR, Gossling TH (1977) *J Phys E* 10:351.

Muller CJ, Kingma A (1961) *Biochim Biophys Acta* 50:595.

Perutz MF (1968) *J Cryst Growth* 2:54.

Perutz MF (1969) *Proc Roy Soc B* 173:113.

Perutz MF (1970) *Nature* 228:726.

Perutz MF, Liquori AM, Eirich F (1951) *Nature* 167:929.

Perutz MF, Lehmann H (1968) *Nature* 219:902.

Perutz MF, Ten Eyck LF (1971) *Cold Spring Harb Symp Quant Biol* 36:295.

Perutz MF, Ladner JE, Simon SR, Ho C (1974) *Biochemistry* 13: 2163.
Richards FM (1968) *J Mol Biol* 37:225.
Takano T (1977) *J Mol Biol* 110:569.
Ten Eyck LF, Arnone A (1976) *J Mol Biol* 100:3.
Tucker PW, Perutz MF (1977) *J Mol Biol* 114:415.
Wallace WJ, Caughey WS (1975) *Biochem Biophys Res Comm* 62:561.
Wallace WJ, Volpe JA, Maxwell JC, Caughey WS, Charache S (1976) *Biochem Biophys Res Comm* 68:1379.
Winterhalter KH, Anderson NM, Amiconi G, Antonini E Brunori M (1969) *Eur J Biochem* 11:435.

POSTSCRIPT

Since this manuscript was written further data on the oxygen equilibrium curves of Hb Zürich have been sent to us by Dr M. Ikeda-Saito, and infrared spectra have been obtained from a sample of fresh red cells containing Hb A Sydney. Dr Ikeda-Saito writes that in 0.05 M bis-tris, 2 mM DPG, 0.1 M C^-, pH 7.4 and $25^{\circ}C$, $k_1 = 0.105$ and $k_4 = 4.0$ for Hb Zürich, compared to $k_1 = 0.014$ and $k_4 = 8.0$ for Hb A. This confirms the much higher oxygen affinity of Hb Zürich in the T structure, but shows that its oxygen affinity in the R structure is only half that of Hb A, and suggests that His E7 does stabilize the $Fe - O_2$ bond.

The infrared spectra of HbCO A + Sydney showed an absorption band at $1,951$ cm^{-1}, the same as that found for the CO stretching frequency of HbCO A, but its band width was greater by 0.5 ± 0.1 cm^{-1} than that of pure HbCO A. The difference spectrum of the HbCO A + Sydney mixture minus pure HbCO A has its positive maximum at $\sim$.,957 cm^{-1} and its zero at $1,953.8$ cm^{-1}. Its negative peak overlaps with the main positive peak of the spectrum. Since the normal β subunit has its peak at $1,952$ cm^{-1}, these findings suggest that the abnormal β of Hb Sydney has its peak at $1,955$ cm^{-1}. Thus the substitution of Ala for Val in position E11 causes about half the shift caused by the substitution of Arg for His in position E7.

DISCUSSION

<u>Dr. Carrell</u>: I want to make just one additional comment
about the normal carbon monoxide stretch frequency of Hemoglobin Sydney. This didn't come as such a surprise because
Dr. J. Sirs, Department of Biophysics, St. Mary's Hospital,
London, had carried out a carbon monoxide affinity curve
on the same mixture of hemoglobin and obtained a normal result.
This indicates that although valine E11 has been lost and
therefore axial binding should be possible, the affinity for
carbon monoxide is unchanged. This is not published as yet.

<u>Dr. Rucknagel</u>: The chemistry here and the mechanics of the
molecule are fascinating and I am intrigued by what you
say. My colleagues Bill Winter and Ruth Abrahamson and I* have
been measuring heat stability as a continuous variable using
an attachment on the Gilford spectrophotometer that allows
one to monitor absorbance continuously while the temperature
is increased linearly. At acid pH as one increases temperature, absorbance decreases in a sigmoid fashion. The change
in absorbance is reversible; if midway the temperature is
lowered, the absorbance increases to that at ambient temperature. At alkaline pH absorbance increases sigmoidally with
increasing temperature as a consequence of precipitation.
This change is irreversible. With unstable variants these
changes occur at lower temperatures; that is to say, the
curves are displaced to the left. In contrast to what you have
shown us, where amino acid substitutions more or less make
the molecule unstable by disrupting attractive forces, we
have found two stable abnormal hemoglobins in which the denaturation curves are displaced to the right. Hb Ann Arbor,
which is a very unstable one, is displaced far to the left.
Our interpretation of these changes is that they are due to
the formation of new salt bridges within the molecule as a
consequence of the amino acid substitution. One is Hb
Haceteppi. β127 (H12) Gln$\longrightarrow$Glu. This might form a salt
bridge with the arginine residue at B12 of the αchain of the
α_1 β_1 interface. Heterozygotes in the family that we have
studied also possess 50-60 per cent of abnormal hemoglobin
and we wonder whether the two observations are related. The
second variant is Hb Agenogi, β90(F8) Glu$\longrightarrow$Lys. We think
that this lysine forms a salt bridge with the carboxyl group
of the C-terminal amino acid of the same β-chain.

*Winter, W.P., Abramson, R.K. and Rucknagel, D.L. Reversible
heat denaturation: A new method for studying heat unstable
hemoglobin variants. Clin. Chim. Acta. Submitted.

The Red Cell, pages 15—16
© 1978 Alan R. Liss, Inc., New York, New York

Dr. Mansouri: I have studied the autoxidation of hemoglobin
Zurich some time ago, and I would like to mention that the
autoxidation reaction of hemoglobin A is as follows. When
you go from acid pH to an alkaline pH, the rate of oxidation
decreases obviously because the affinity for oxygen increases.
In hemoglobin Zurich the problem is the same, except that
the first part of the reaction is made by the β chains. In
other words, the β chains autoxidize faster than the alpha
chains in that hemoglobin. But the phenomenon that I observed
is that when you go from PH8 to PH9 the autoxidation rate
increases, and this is not the case in hemoglobin A. I have
not interpreted this problem satisfactorily and I have not
been able to study the Bohr effect of hemoglobin Zurich. I
wonder if at the extreme alkaline PH the Bohr effect of hemoglobin Zurich is the same as that of hemoglobin A or if it
is just drastically different which might explain this problem.

Dr. Tucker: In regard to hemoglobin Zurich it occurred to
me that a water molecule, or more probably at high pH,
an hydroxyl ion could be associated with the Arg E7 guanidinium. As the guanidino pK_a is approached at extreme alkaline
conditions this molecule could dissociate and could attack
the iron more readily. Furthermore, the entrance to the
β haem pocket is wide open in Zurich and would be more accessible to external water or nucleophiles--of course the former
would be independent of pH.

Dr. Winterbourn: The structure of hemoglobin Zurich that you
have presented suggests a reason why it has increased accessa-
bility to the heme pocket and an increased autoxidation rate,
yet is not really classified as an unstable hemoglobin. With
most unstable hemoglobins in addition to an increased autoxidation rate there is a greater tendency to form a hemichrome
in which the distal histidine is liganded to the iron. This
seems likely to be one of the main determinants of instability, and it is interesting that in the absence of this histidine, this hemichrome is unlikely to be formed, and the stability is almost normal.

Dr. Lehmann: This is a question of semantics. It depends on
how one determines whether an unstable hemoglobin is one
that causes an inclusion body formation or whether it is one
that causes hemichrome formation.

Structure of the Globin Gene in Differentiating
Erythroid Cells

Donald M. Miller, David Axelrod, Richard Croissant and
Arthur Nienhuis
Clinical Hematology Branch,
National Heart, Lung, and Blood Institute,
National Institutes of Health, Bethesda, Maryland   20014

Introduction:

Several lines of evidence point towards a "beads on a
string" or nucleosomal model for chromatin structure (1-3).
In this model the basic component is the nucleosome, comprised of the histone octamer core (two molecules each of
H2A, H2B, H3, and H4) about which is wrapped a 140 base pair
strand of DNA (4-6). Both transcriptionally active and inactive segments of the total cellular DNA appear to be
present in nucleosomes (7), although active genes have a
somewhat different configuration as implied by their exquisite sensitivity to digestion by pancreatic DNAse I (8,9).

The sensitivity of actively transcribed genes to digestion by DNAse I (8,9) provides a means of investigating
globin gene structure in various cells. We have studied the
sensitivity of globin genes in nuclei of normally differentiating erythroid cells and dimethylsulfoxide (Me$_2$SO) induced Friend mouse erythroleukemia (MEL) cells. These
studies shed light on the evolution of globin gene structure
during normal erythroid differentiation as well as during
induction of globin messenger RNA (mRNA) synthesis in the
virally transformed MEL cells.

Materials and Methods:

Cellular Isolation

Rabbit bone marrow cells from animals previously injected with phenylhydrazine were prepared as previously
described (10). After trituration and suspension in a 2%
solution of bovine serum albumin in Delbecco's phosphate

The Red Cell, pages 17–30

buffered saline (PBS) they were fractionated on a continuous
Ficoll Paque (Pharmacia) gradient. Linear 12.5 ml gradients
were generated by mixing Delbecco's PBS with Ficoll Paque;
8×10^8 cells were loaded on each gradient and centrifugation
at 15° was for 15 min at 6000 rpm in a Spinco SW41 rotor.
Pelletted cells were discarded; the entire supernatent was
further fractionated by 1 g sedimentation in a Sta-put appa-
ratus (11). The cells were characterized morphologically
after staining with Giemsa benzidine. The size distribution
of cells in the early and late fractions was also determined
by Coulter counter analysis.

Hepatoma cells were isolated from C57L/J mice bearing
BW7756 hepatomas which were purchased from Jackson Laboratory.
The hepatomas were removed and suspended in MEM (Modified
Eagles Medium) prior to preparation of nuclei. Adult mouse
livers were removed from 4-5 week DBA mice, minced and tritu-
rated in MEM. Fetal liver cells were obtained from 13-15
day DBA mouse fetuses.

MEL cells were grown by methods described in detail elsewhere (12). The C19 and GM979 lines provided examples of inducible MEL lines. The E5-1B line is a fusion product of MEL
cell line 5000 and enucleated mouse fibroblast line L816-4
(13) which in these experiments demonstrated 40% of benzidine
positive cells after induction with Me_2SO.

Nuclear Isolation

Nuclei were prepared by the method of Marzluff (15).
After one centrifugation through the high sucrose cushion,
the nuclei were free of cytoplasmic tags as revealed by
microscopic examination after staining with methylene blue.

Pancreatic DNAse I Digestion

Pancreatic DNAse I digestion was performed by the method
of Weintraub and Groudine (8) with the following exceptions:
The DNAse I concentration in the digestion mixture was 10 µg
per ml. Digestion was carried out for 1-2 min, until 8-12%
of the DNA was soluble in 10% perchloric acid. Following
digestion the solution was made 5 mm EDTA and 100 µg per ml
proteinase K (Beckman) was added. After 3-4 hr the solution
was made 0.5 M NaCl, and the digestion allowed to proceed
for 6-8 hr at which time the solution was made 0.5% SDS. The
solution was then extracted with phenol:chloroform (1:1) and
chloroform:isoamyl alcohol (24:1). The DNA was recovered by
addition of 2 volumes of ethanol, storage at -20° for 8-16

hr, and subsequent centrifugation. The resulting pellet was
resuspended in 1 x SSC (standard saline citrate; 0.15 M NaCl
and 0.015 M sodium citrate, pH 7.0) and digested for 1 hr
with 100 µg/ml RNAse previously boiled for 10 min. Following
phenol extraction, the DNA was recovered by precipitation
with ethanol as above, desalted on a pad of Sephadex G25, and
appropriate aliquots were annealed to globin complementary
DNA (cDNA).

Hybridization

The cDNA hybridizations were carried out by the method
of Williamson, et al. (15,16). Annealings were performed at
a DNA concentration of 6 mg per ml in 50% formamide, 3X SSC
at 50°. The reaction reached completion by 24 hrs. The DNA
concentration was adjusted to give 25% maximal hybridization
at the cDNA concentration used.

Globin cDNA was made as previously described (17).
Partially purified immunoglobulin messenger RNA from mouse
myeloma cells was a generous gift of Dr. Ru Chi Huang, Johns
Hopkins University.

Results

The validity of cDNA excess hybridization as a quantitative measure of globin gene sequence concentration was tested
by the DNA mixing experiment as shown in Fig. 1. In this
experiment, control mouse hepatoma DNA was annealed to globin
cDNA at a concentration of 6 mg/ml (our routine concentration
is described in Methods), 3 mg/ml, and 0 mg/ml with E. coli
DNA being added to make the final concentrations 6 mg/ml in
each reaction mixture. The cDNA protected by annealing was
directly proportional to the quantity of DNA containing mouse
globin gene sequences added in the individual hybridization
mixtures. This allows use of this method to quantitate the
concentration of globin gene sequences remaining in DNA from
nuclei exposed to DNAse I and thereby to estimate the degree
of sensitivity of globin genes in each nuclear preparation
to nuclease digestion.

Exposure of rabbit spleen nuclei to DNAse I demonstrated
the absence of globin gene digestion in a non-erythroid
tissue (Fig. 2). Insensitivity of globin genes to DNAse I
was also demonstrated in rabbit brain nuclei (data not shown).
Spleen nuclei from rabbits injected for 5 days with phenylhydrazine (10) (70-80% erythroid cells morphologically) were
characterized by partial sensitivity of the globin genes to

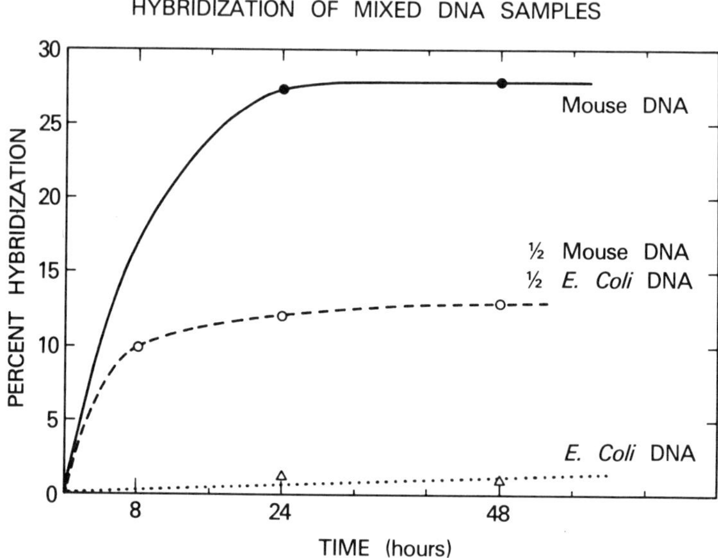

Fig. 1. Hybridization of mouse globin cDNA to mouse hepatoma DNA and E. coli DNA in varying proportions. Hybridizations were performed at 6 mg/ml total DNA in varying proportions. Hybridizations were performed at 6 mg/ml total DNA concentration. The hepatoma DNA concentration was 6 mg/ml, 3 mg/ml, and 0 mg/ml for the three curves with corresponding amounts of E. coli DNA being added to give a constant final DNA concentration. The annealing reactions were performed in cDNA excess and the duplexes were quantitated by S_1 nuclease digestion.

DNAse I as shown in Fig. 2. The remaining fraction of globin genes were thought to be derived from non-erythroid cells present in the spleen cell suspension. However, the globin genes in nuclei from rabbit bone marrow containing only 10-15% myeloid cells were only 50% sensitive to DNAse I digestion as shown in Fig. 2. This result suggested the possibility that globin genes in nuclei from erythroid cells at various stages of maturation might differ in their sensitivity to DNAse I digestion.

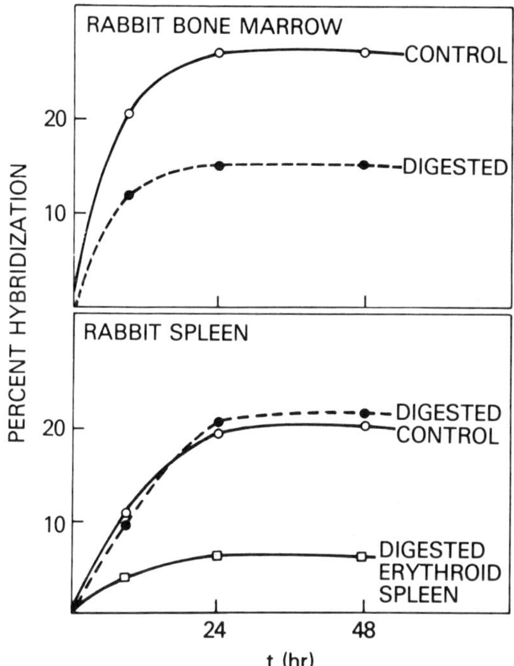

Fig. 2. DNAse I sensitivity of globin genes in rabbit bone
marrow and spleen. Nuclei were prepared from bone marrow
and spleen of rabbits injected with phenylhydrazine and from
spleen of untreated animals as described in Methods. Following exposure to DNAse I the purified DNA samples were
annealed to rabbit globin cDNA. The control samples represent equivalent aliquots of each nuclear sample which were
not exposed to DNAse I but which were treated the same in
every other respect.

Globin Gene Structure in "Early" and "Late" Cells from
Rabbit Bone Marrow:

Bone marrow cells from animals injected with phenylhydrazine were fractionated into "early" and "late" erythroid
cells by a combination of isopynic Ficoll Paque centrifugation
and 1 g sedimentation as described in the Methods. The "early"
fraction was composed of large, rapidly sedimenting cells

which morphologically were predominantly pro- and basophilic
erythroblasts with approximately 10% myeloid contamination.
The "late" fraction was predominantly small, slowly sedimenting poly- and orthochromatophilic erythroblasts with 2-3%
myeloid contamination. The globin genes in nuclei from the
late fraction of bone marrow cells were quite sensitive to
digestion by DNAse in that 80% of gene sequences were destroyed (Fig. 3); the concentration of globin genes remaining
in DNA from digested nuclei was considerably less than that
obtained from nuclei of unfractionated bone marrow.

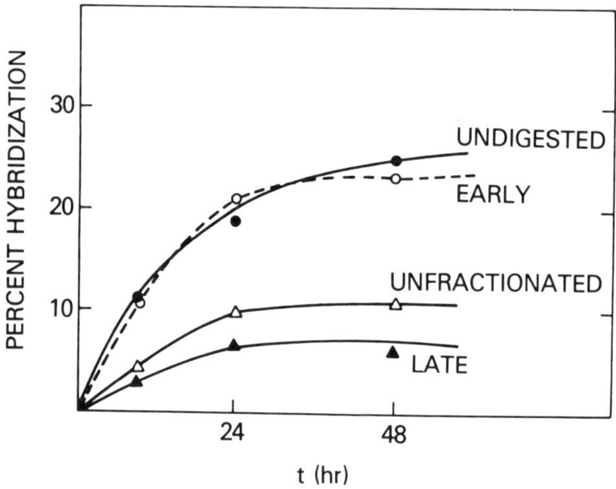

Fig. 3. Annealing of DNA from nuclei of "early" and "late"
rabbit bone marrow cells to globin cDNA. Rabbit bone marrow
cells were fractionated as described in Methods. Nuclei prepared from each fraction were divided into two aliquots, one
was incubated with DNAse I; the other providing non-digested
DNA as a control. The three control curves were identical.

The globin genes in nuclei from the "early" fraction exhibited complete resistance to DNAse I digestion. Thus, although these cells presumably are synthesizing globin mRNA (18), the globin gene structure as revealed by the DNAse I probe, resembled that found in non-erythroid cells. That these cells are committed to the erythroid pathway is indicated by their obvious erythroid morphology. Furthermore, 90% of the cells capable of generating erythroid colonies in plasma clot culture (11) were found in this fraction (data not shown).

Comparison of Globin Gene Structure in Adult and Fetal
Mouse Liver:

Fig. 4 demonstrates the complete sensitivity of the globin genes in nuclei from fetal liver to DNAse I digestion. Conversely, globin genes in nuclei from adult liver were not digested by DNAse I. The 14-15 day fetal livers we utilized were comprised of 90% benzidine-positive cells, and of these 95-99% were late erythroid cells as defined above. The complete sensitivity of the globin genes in nuclei from fetal liver apparently reflects the presence of a homogenous population of cells at the stage corresponding to the late erythroid fraction of rabbit bone marrow.

Globin Gene Structure During Induced Maturation of MEL Cells:

Two MEL cell lines were induced to undergo erythroid maturation by exposure to Me_2SO. Total cellular RNA was isolated from both induced and non-induced cells of each line (19) and annealed to globin cDNA to quantitate the concentration of globin mRNA present. Globin genes in nuclei from induced and uninduced cells of the GM979 line were almost completely sensitive to DNAse I as shown in Fig. 5. As is seen in Fig. 5, this MEL cell line contains almost no globin mRNA prior to induction with Me_2SO despite the apparent sensitivity of the globin genes to DNAse I. Exposure to Me_2SO resulted in a 50-fold increase in globin mRNA concentration. Although the DNA from nuclei exposed to DNAse I did not anneal to globin cDNA, these DNA samples demonstrated significant annealing to mouse immunoglobulin cDNA (data not shown).

The C19 MEL cell line provided a contrast in that there was a higher level of globin mRNA in the non-induced cell population (Fig. 6). However the structure of the globin genes as revealed by their sensitivity to DNAse I in nuclei

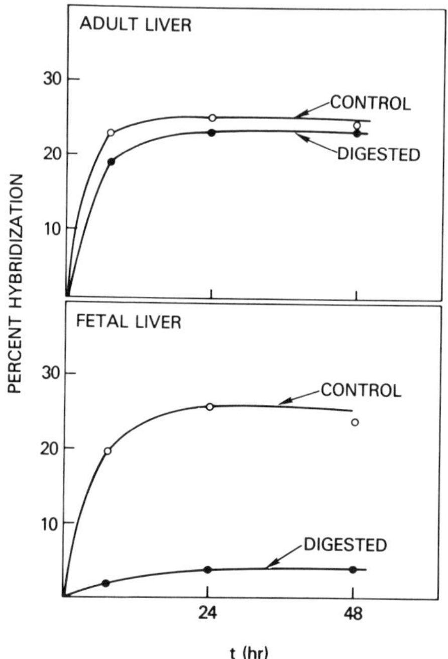

Fig. 4. Annealing of fetal and adult mouse liver DNA to
mouse globin cDNA. Fetal erythroid and adult non-erythroid
liver cells were prepared as described in Methods. Nuclei
from these cells were then exposed to DNAse I.

isolated from these cells was the same both prior to and
after exposure to Me$_2$SO. This implied that the enhanced
globin mRNA synthesis in MEL cells does not derive from a
change in the gene structure in chromatin.

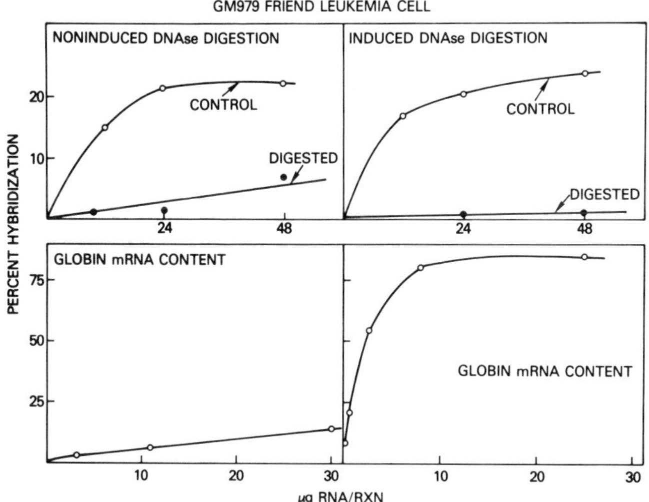

Fig. 5. DNAse I sensitivity of the globin gene and globin mRNA content of GM979 MEL cells. The upper panels show the results of hybridizations performed between globin cDNA and DNA from nuclei exposed to DNAse I from induced and non-induced cells. The cDNA-RNA annealings were performed at constant cDNA concentration and varying RNA input (17).

A third MEL cell line was analyzed; the E5-1B cells were originally derived by fusion of C19 cells with a nucleated fibroblast cytoplasm (13). Only 40% of these cells became benzidine-positive after 4 days of growth in 2% Me$_2$SO. Globin mRNA was present in low concentration in un-induced cells and increased 50 fold after growth of the cells in the inducer. The globin genes in nuclei from the induced and uninduced population were only partially destroyed

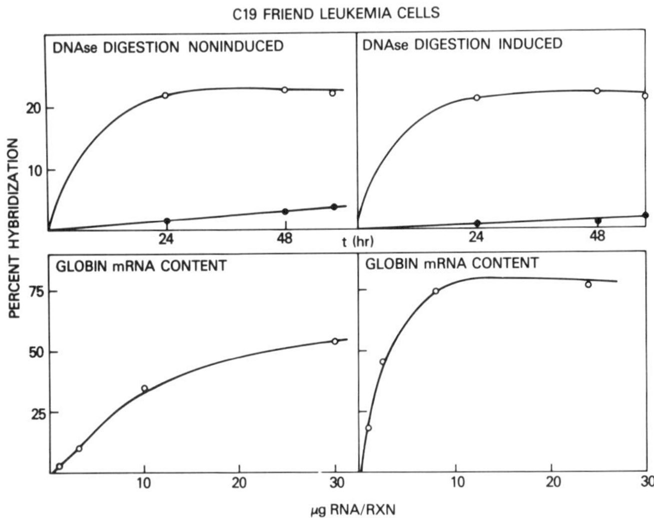

Fig. 6. DNAse I sensitivity of the globin gene and globin mRNA content of C-19 Friend leukemia cells.

by exposure to DNAse I. The most obvious interpretation of these results is that only a fraction of the cells in the uninduced population had 1) globin genes sensitive to DNAse I ("active") and, 2) were inducible as reflected by their benzidine-positive state after growth in Me_2SO. The other cells in the population presumably had both "inactive" genes as revealed by the DNAse I assay and could not be induced to undergo erythroid maturation.

To determine whether the open globin gene might be characteristic of all neoplastic cell types we examined the pancreatic DNAse sensitivity of the globin gene in mouse hepatoma cells. These genes demonstrated complete resistance

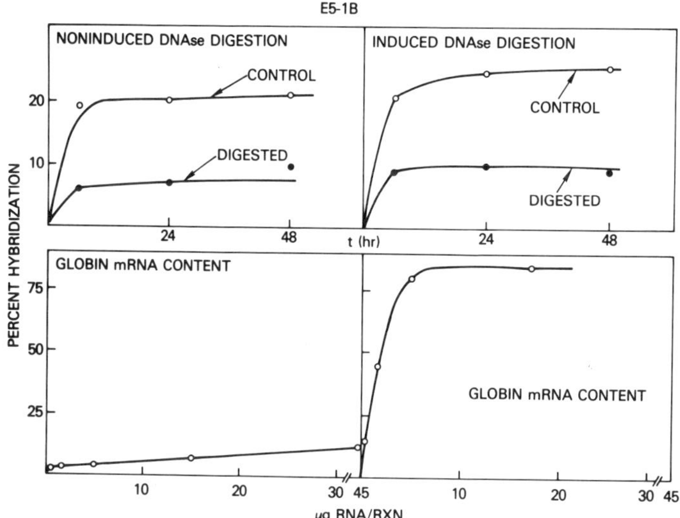

Fig. 7. DNAse I sensitivity of the globin gene and globin mRNA content of E5-1B mouse cybrid line.

to digestion as is shown in Fig. 8. This result indicated that neoplastic transformation of non-erythroid cells does not invariably result in structural changes in the globin gene detectable by this method.

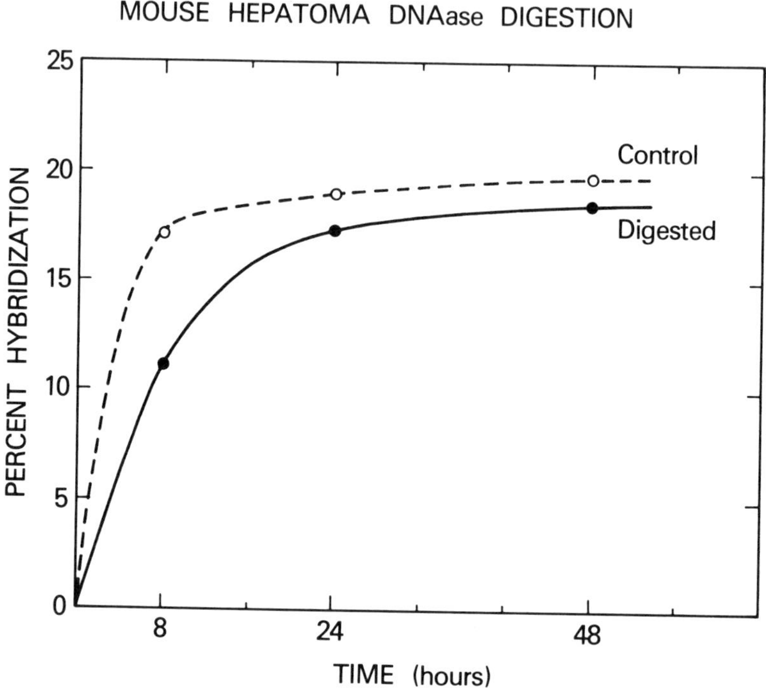

Fig. 8. DNAse I sensitivity of globin genes in BW776 mouse hepatoma cells. Nuclei prepared from BW776 mouse hepatoma were subjected to partial DNAse I digestion. Results are displayed as for previous experiments.

Discussion:

Our studies appear to imply that normal erythroid differentiation involves an erythroid commitment before the chromatin structural changes which render the globin gene transcriptionally active can be detected by the DNAse I probe. Similar results have been obtained in early avian yolk sac cells (80% erythroid by morphological criteria) in which the globin genes were also insensitive to DNAse I digestion (8). That the globin genes in cells which appear to have small amounts of globin mRNA (18) are not DNAse I sensitive lends itself to several explanations. Possibly the globin mRNA is restricted to only a few cells in the population; in these cells the genes might be DNAse I sensitive but in the majority of the cells the genes would be insensitive to digestion. Alternatively, the property of DNAse I sensitivity may be unstable with an equilibrium between the sensitive and insensitive chromatin configuration possibly related to the stage of the cell in cell cycle. Alternatively, some property of the nucleus or nuclear membrane from early erythroid cells might affect the accessibility of DNAse I to chromatin, although we observed release of DNA from these early nuclei during the digestion procedure. Our "late" fraction of erythroid cells is predominantly orthochromatophilic erythroblasts which no longer undergo cell division. Possibly the DNAse I sensitive configuration of the globin genes is permanently established only after cell division ceases.

In contrast to normal erythroid differentiation, transformed MEL cells are arrested in some phase of the maturation sequence which normally leads to a mature erythrocyte. Our results suggest that this arrest occurs after the chromatin structural changes necessary for globin mRNA synthesis. The chemical induction of globin and globin mRNA synthesis in these cells appears to involve a release of this developmental arrest although our results appear to imply that there are no marked changes in the configuration of the globin genes in chromatin during induction. Our results are not in disagreement with nuclear transcription studies (20) which implicate transcriptional control of globin mRNA synthesis during induction of MEL cells. We would infer that the globin genes in the uninduced cells are in a configuration potentially accessible for transcription. Induction then might be accompanied by an increased rate of transcription of these "active" genes.

REFERENCES

1. Olins, A.L. and Olins, D.E. (1974) Science 183: 330-332.
2. Oudet, P., Gross-Bellard, M. and Chambon, P. (1975) Cell 4: 281-300.
3. Clark, R. and Felsenfeld, G. (1971) Nature 229: 101-106.
4. Hewish, D.R. and Bourgoyne, L.A. (1973) Biochem. Biophys. Res. Commun. 52: 504-410.
5. Kornberg, R.D. (1979) Science 184: 868-871.
6. Weintraub, H., Worcel, A., and Alberts, B. (1976) Cell 409-417.
7. Axel, R., Cedar, H., and Felsenfeld, G. (1975) Biochemistry 14: 2989-2995.

8. Weintraub, H., and Groudine, M. (1976) Science 93: 848-858.

9. Garel, A. and Axel, R. (1976) Proc. Nat. Acad. Sci. 73: 3966-3970.

10. Wilson, G.N., Steggles, A.W., and Nienhuis, A.W. (1975) Proc. Nat. Acad. Sci. 72:4835-4839.

11. Barker, J.E., Anderson, W.F., and Nienhuis, A.W. (1975) J. Cell Biol. 69:515-529.

12. Axelrod, D., Gopalakrishnan, P.V., and Anderson, W.F. Submitted to Somatic Cell Genetics.

13. Gopalakrishnan, T.V., Thompson, E.B., and Anderson, W.F. (1977) Proc. Nat. Acad. Sci. 74: 1642-1646.

14. Marzluff, W.F., Murphy, E.C., and Huang, R.C.C. (1973) Biochemistry 12: 3470-3476.

15. Old, J., Clegg, J.B., Weatherall, D.J., Ottolenghi, S., Comi, P., Gillioni, B., Mitchell, J., Tostoshev, P. and Williamson, R. (1976) Cell 7, 13-16.

16. Ottolenghi, S., Lanyon, W.G., Williamson, R., Weatherall, D.J., Clegg, J.B. and Pitcher, C.S. (1975) Proc. Nat. Acad. Sci. 72: 2294-2299.

17. Benz, E.J., Geist, C.E., Steggles, A.W., Barker, J.E. and Nienhuis, A.W. (1977) J. Biol. Chem. 252: 1908-1915.

18. Clissold, P.M., Arnstein, H.R.U., and Chesterton, C.J. (1977) Cell 353-361.

19. Nienhuis, A.W., Falvey, A.K., and Anderson, W.F. (1974) Meth. Enzymol. 30: 621-630.

20. Orkin, S.H., and Swerdlow, P.S. (1977) Proc. Nat. Acad. Sci. 74: 2475-2479.

DISCUSSION

<u>Dr. Winter</u>: There's been a paper just recently in the
journal <u>Cell</u> that describes the production or evidence for
the production of large, short-lived mRNA in early erythroid
cells and proposes that the processing of that mRNA into
10 S pieces for alpha and beta chain synthesis might be the
important step in selecting the particular gene to be transcribed. I wonder if there's room for this thought in your
findings or if it is even possible that the **opening** and
closing of the DNA is relatively incidental to post-transcriptional processing of messenger RNA which might be the
active control site?

<u>Dr. Miller</u>: I think the processing area is a very exciting
one and I think the two mechanisms of control of gene expression are not incompatible. It is not possible at this
time to sort out which is operable in specific cases. Our
results demonstrating that late cells have open genes certainly does not rule out the fact that they might be controlled in terms of the messenger RNA which enters the cyto-
plasma by processing events. I think particularly in the
MEL cells, our results would tend to substantiate that mechanism as one of the possible explanations for the lack of
structural changes during induction.

THE FORMATION OF HB A$_{Ic}$ AS A BIOCHEMICAL MODEL FOR THE
SEQUELAE OF DIABETES.

Anthony Cerami, Ronald J. Koenig, Charles M. Peterson
and Victor J. Stevens
The Laboratory of Medical Biochemistry
The Rockefeller University
New York, New York 10021

Although insulin has been used for over fifty years for
the treatment of diabetes mellitus, these patients continue
to suffer serious and life-threatening complications (e.g.
cataracts, neuropathy, retinopathy, nephropathy and coronary
artery disease) at a relatively early age. As a result of
these complications the life span of diabetics is reduced by
approximately one-third (Dept. H.E.W., 1964). The biochemical
basis for the development of these complications is unknown
and much discussion has taken place regarding the relationship
between the degree of control of blood sugar and the development
of the sequelae. One of the major hypotheses to explain the
pathophysiology of the complications is that they arise from
the thickening of the basement membrane of the capillaries
(Bloodworth, 1963). This thickening is thought to occur from
an increased deposition of glycoproteins (Klein et al., 1975;
Beisswenger et al., 1973) following the onset of the diabetic
state (Williamson et al., 1973). Unfortunately the biochemical
events underlying this process have been difficult to study,
in part, because of the technical problems of obtaining representative tissue samples over the long periods of time it
takes for the complications to arise.

In order to circumvent this problem we suggested (Koenig
et al., 1975) that the glycosylation of hemoglobin A$_{Ic}$ might
be a model reaction for the increased glycosylation that is
purported to occur in diabetes. These studies have revealed
a possible unifying biochemical model for the sequelae of
diabetes and in addition have led to the development of a
practical clinical test to monitor the degree of carbohydrate
control of patients.

The Red Cell, pages 33—40

BIOSYNTHESIS

The basis for choosing hemoglobin A_{Ic} as a model arose from the report of (Trivelli et al., 1971) who found that diabetics have 6-12% of their total hemoglobin as hemoglobin A_{Ic} compared to 3-6% in normal individuals. The ability to quantitate this glycohemoglobin and the lack of protein synthe-sis in the mature erythrocyte offered a unique opportunity to study the time of protein glycosylation. The presence of a glycohemoglobin in the mouse (Koenig and Cerami, 1975; Koenig et al., 1976a) similar to human hemoglobin A_{Ic} allowed the comparison of rate of glycosylation of the normal red cell in the normal and diabetic state. The infusion of ^{59}Fe-labeled reticulocytes isolated from a normal donor into both normal and diabetic mice revealed that the glycosylation of hemoglo-bin A to form hemoglobin A_{Ic} occurs throughout the life of the red cell and that the rate of modification is 2.7 times faster when the donor cells circulate in diabetic recipients than when cells circulate in normal recipients, (Figure 1) (Koenig et al., 1975). A linear post-translational synthesis of hemoglobin A_{Ic} in human red cells has also been noted (Bunn et al., 1976). The postsynthetic addition of the glyco group to form hemoglobin A_{Ic} is very slowly reversible hence the steady state value of hemoglobin A_{Ic} measured in the peripher-al blood for the most part reflects a balance between destruc-tion of old cells laden with hemoglobin A_{Ic} and the production of new cells with little hemoglobin A_{Ic}.

The glyco group of hemoglobin A_{Ic} has been shown to be 1-amino, 1-deoxyfructose which is attached to the amino term-inal valine of the β-chain, (Bunn et al., 1975; Koenig et al., 1977), (Figure 2). This structure was first proposed by Bunn et al., 1975 and was based on the observation that hemoglobin A_{Ic} liberated 0.25 moles of hexose (consisting of glucose and manose in a 3:1 ratio) per mole of hemoglobin dimer and that periodite oxidation of NaB^3H_4 reduced hemoglobin A_{Ic} liberated primarily ^3H formic acid rather than ^3H formaldehyde. This structure has subsequently been confirmed and definitively assigned (Koenig et al., 1977). The assignment was made pos-sible by the isolation of the β-chain amino terminal glycodi-peptides of NaB^3H_4 reduced hemoglobin A_{Ic} and comparison of these naturally derived products with synthetic standards using thin layer chromatography, gas chromatography and proton magnetic resonance spectroscopy.

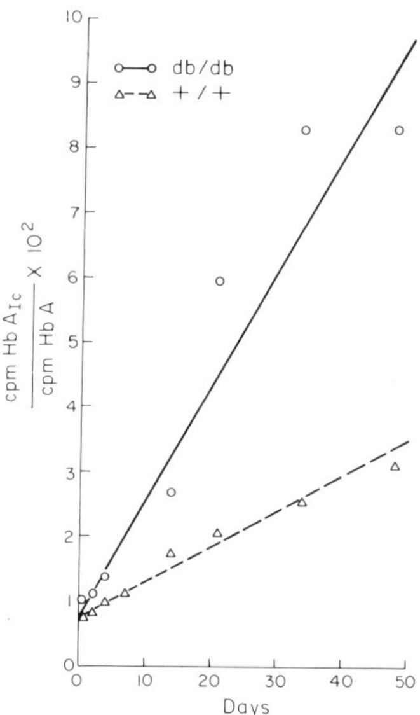

Fig. 1.   The ratio of total cpm of **Hb A$_{Ic}$** **to that of** Hb A
as a function of time in +/+ (△) and db/db (0) mice which
received radio-labeled blood from a +/+ donor.   Reprinted
with permission of Proc Nat Acad Sci 72:3687-3691, 1975.

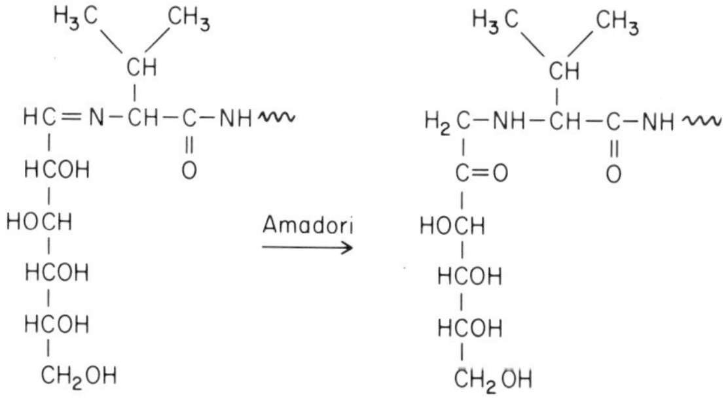

Fig. 2.   The Schiff base adduct between valine and glucose
undergoes an Amadori rearrangement to form 1-deoxy-1(N-valyl-
(fructose).

At present there are two hypotheses to account for the biosynthesis *in vivo* of hemoglobin A_{Ic}. The first (Fluckiger and Winterhalter, 1976) is the direct addition of glucose to hemoglobin A while the second (Haney et al., 1976; Stevens et al., 1977a) proposes that glucose-6-phosphate reacts to form an adduct, possibly hemoglobin A_{Ib} which is then dephosphorylated to form hemoglobin A_{Ic}. In both cases it is proposed that the reaction is nonenzymatic and that the aldehyde of the carbohydrate first forms a Schiff base with the amino terminal valine of the β-chain which subsequently undergoes an Amadori rearrangement (Hodge, 1955). This Amadori rearrangement product is relatively stable and accounts for the accumulation of the glycohemoglobin of the red cell. Although glucose has been shown to react with hemoglobin directly the reaction is not as rapid or specific as that with glucose-6-phosphate with hemoglobin. In addition the reaction of glucose-6-phosphate with hemoglobin is an especially attractive mechanism since the phosphate group would allow the orientation and stabilization of the sugar in the "DPG pocket" of the hemoglobin molecule and accounts for the specificity of the reaction with the amino terminus of the β-chain. It is possible, in fact, to form hemoglobin adducts with a number of glycolytic intermediates (G6P; F6P; $F1,6P_2$; G3P) (Stevens et al., 1977a). The two prerequisites of the glycolytic intermediates for adduct formation are a phosphate and an aldehyde or ketone functionality. No significant adduct formation occurred with glycolytic intermediates which had a blocked aldehyde (G1P; $G1,6P_2$: UDPG). The increased intracellular concentration of G6P in the red cells of diabetics is in accord with this pathway. However, the much higher intracellular concentration of glucose may still account for hemoglobin A_{Ic} synthesis *in vivo*. Further work is needed to define the mechanism *in vivo* for hemoglobin A_{Ic} biosynthesis and its relationship to the other minor hemoglobins-hemoglobin A_{Ia} and hemoglobin A_{Ib}.

CLINICAL RELEVANCE

The quantification of hemoglobin A_{Ic} is proving to be a useful means of identifying diabetics and assessing the degree of carbohydrate control of diabetic patients. A linear relationship of hemoglobin A_{Ic} concentration with the response to an oral glucose tolerance test was observed in a series of juvenile and maturity onset diabetics (Koenig et al., 1976b), (Figure 3). The measurement of hemoglobin A_{Ic} should make it

possible to easily screen for individuals in the general population who do not know that they have diabetes. It is estimated that there are 3 million people in this category in the
United States. The correlation of hemoglobin A$_{Ic}$ concentration
with the degree of carbohydrate control was shown by institut-
ing strict carbohydrate control in a series of diabetic
patients in a hospital setting (Koenig et al., 1976c). Three
to four weeks after the initiation of strict control the
hemoglobin A$_{Ic}$ concentration decreased, (Figure 4). The hemoglobin A$_{Ic}$ concentration does not reflect the instantaneous
glucose concentration nor is it influenced by short term fluctuations of glucose but rather hemoglobin A$_{Ic}$ is an indicator
molecule that integrates the patients blood glucose concentration for the several weeks prior to the measurement. A single
hemoglobin A$_{Ic}$ measurement, therefore, reflects the mean blood
glucose concentration of the patient for the previous month, a
feature unique to this measurement. Periodic monitoring of
hemoglobin A$_{Ic}$ concentrations should allow the measurement of
carbohydrate control in a more objective manner than is now
possible and enable one to evaluate various forms of therapy
and the relationship between carbohydrate control and the
progression of the sequelae of diabetes.

One of the major problems of utilizing hemoglobin A$_{Ic}$
quantification as a means of monitoring patients, has been the
lack of a simple rapid assay. The column chromatographic
method (Trivelli et al., 1971) is slow and tedious. Recently
a high pressure liquid chromatographic system, (Cole et al.,
1977) a colorimetric method (Fluckiger and Winterhalter, 1976)
and a radioimmunoassay (Javid et al., 1977) have been described. The introduction of these new methods should simplify
the quantification of hemoglobin A$_{Ic}$ and allow more widespread
use of this measurement to monitor the control of diabetic
patients .

CONCLUSION

The mechanism of hemoglobin A$_{Ic}$ synthesis may provide a
conceptual framework for the pathogenesis of the sequelae of
diabetes. Just as the postsynthetic glycosylation of hemoglobin to form hemoglobin A$_{Ic}$ alters certain functional properties of the protein (e.g. oxygen affinity), (Bunn et al., 1970)
similar modifications could alter the properties (e.g. enzymatic activity, solubility, half-life) of proteins of other
cells. This glycosylation would be particularly evident in

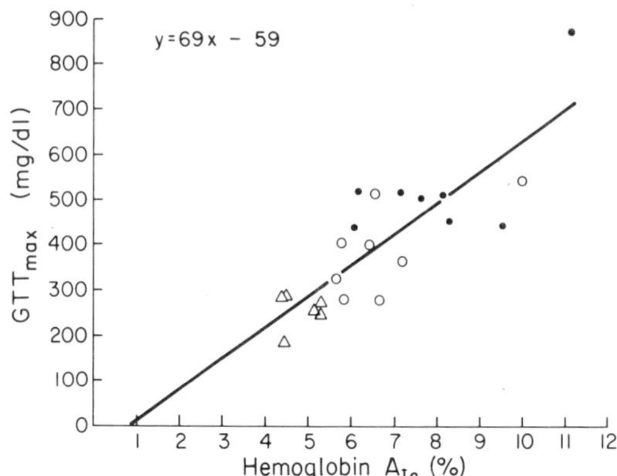

Fig. 3. Correlation between hemoglobin A_{Ic} concentration and maximal response to an oral glucose tolerance test in 22 diabetics (• patients treated with insulin, o patients treated with oral hypoglycemic agents, Δ patients treated with diet alone.) Reprinted with permission from Diabetes 25:230-232, 1976.

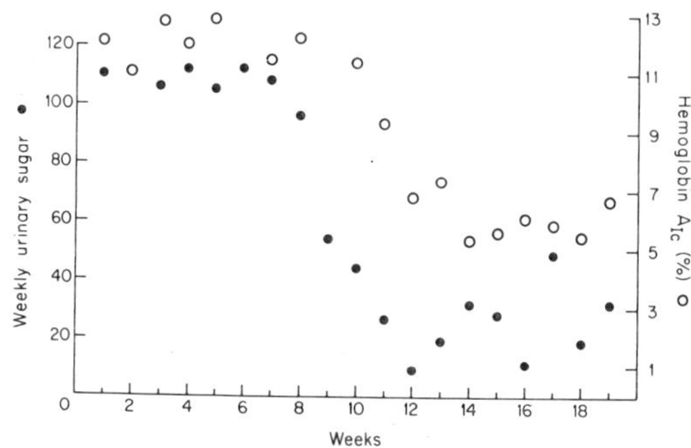

Fig. 4. Temporal relation between weekly urinary sugar (•) and hemoglobin A_{Ic} (o) levels in a patient with diabetes. Semiquantitative (0 to 4+) estimates of urinary sugar levels performed four times per day, were summed over consecutive seven-day periods to obtain weekly urinary sugar values. Reprinted with permission from New Engl J Med 295:417-420, 1976.

cell types independent of insulin for glucose uptake. The red cells like several other types of tissues such as lens and nerve do not require insulin for glucose uptake. In these tissues the concentration of intracellular glucose and glycolytic intermediates probably reflect the extracellular glucose concentration. This relationship is in strong contrast to tissues such as muscle or adipose where insulin is required for glucose entry. As has been noted, (Spiro, 1976) many of the sequelae of diabetes occur in tissues that are insulin independent for glucose uptake.

Further studies are needed to evaluate the glycosylation hypothesis as the basis for the development of the sequelae of diabetes mellitus. We have recently extended our studies form the red cell to a biochemically similar tissue-the lens (Stevens et al., 1977). We have found that a high glucose environment *in vitro* or *in vivo* leads to glycosylation of α-crystallin lens protein and subsequent opacity of the protein matrix mimicking that seen in diabetic cataracts. Hopefully these studies will give insights into the pathogenesis of the disease and ways to prevent these sequelae from occurring.

REFERENCES

Beisswenger PJ, Spiro RG (1973). Studies on the glomerular basement membrane. Composition nature of the carbohydrate units and chemical changes in diabetes mellitus. Diabetes 22:180.

Bloodworth JMB (1963). Diabetic microangiopathy. Diabetes 12:99.

Bunn HG, Briehl RW (1970). The interaction of 2,3-diphosphoglycerate with various human hemoglobins. J Clin Invest 49:1088.

Bunn HG, Haney DN, Gabbay KH, Gallop PM (1975). Further identification of the nature and linkage of the carbohydrate in hemoglobin A$_{Ic}$. Biochem Biophys Res Commun 67:103.

Bunn HG, Haney DN, Kamin S, Gabbay KH, Gallop PM (1976). The biosynthesis of human hemoglobin A$_{Ic}$. J Clin Invest 57:1652.

Cole RA, Bunn HG, Soeldner JS (1977). Diabetes 26 Supl:392

Department of Health, Education and Welfare, Public Health Service (1964). "Diabetes Source Book," Washington, D.C.: publication no. 1168.

Fluckiger R, Winterhalter KH (1976). In vitro synthesis of hemoglobin A$_{Ic}$. FEBS Letters 71:356.

Haney DN, Bunn HG (1976). Glycosylation of hemoglobin in
  vitro: Affinity labeling of hemoglobin by glucose-6-phos-
  phate. Proc Natl Acad Sci USA 73:3534.
Hodge JE (1955). The Amadori rearrangement. Adv Carb Chem
  10:169.
Javid J, Pettis P, Koenig R, Cerami A (submitted, 1977). Immunologic characteristics and quantifiaation of Hb A_{Ic}.
  Brit J of Haematol
Klein L, Butcher DL, Sudilovsky D, Kikkawa R, Miller M, (1975).
  Quantification of collagen in renal glomeruli isolated
  from human nondiabetic and diabetic kidneys. Diabetes 24:
  1057.
Koenig RJ, Cerami A (1975). Synthesis of hemoglobin A_{Ic} in
  normal and diabetic mice: A potential model of basement
  membrane thickening. Proc Natl Acad Sci USA 72:3697.
Koenig RJ, Araujo DC, Cerami A (1976a). Increased hemoglobin
  A_{Ic} in diabetic mice. Diabetes 25:1.
Koenig RJ, Peterson CM, Kilo C, Cerami A, Williamson J (1976b).
  Hemoglobin A_{Ic} as an indicator of the degree of glucose
  intolerance in diabetes. Diabetes 25:230.
Koenig RJ, Peterson CM, Jones RL, Saudek C, Lehrman M, Cerami
  A (1976c). Correlation of glucose regulation and hemoglobin
  A_{Ic} in diabetes mellitus. New Eng J of Med 295:417.
Koenig RJ, Blobstein SH, Cerami A (1977). Structure of the
  carbohydrate of hemoglobin A_{Ic}. J Biol Chem 252:2992.
Spiro RG (1976). Search for a biochemical basis fo diabetic
  microangiopathy. Diabetologia 12:1
Stevens VJ, Vlassara H, Abati A, Cerami A (1977). Nonenzymatic glycosylation of hemoglobin. J Biol chem 252:2998.
Stevens VJ, Rouzer C, Cerami A (manuscript in preparation
  1977).
Trivelli LA, Ranney HM, Lai HT (1971). Hemoglobin components
  in patients with diabetes mellitus. New Eng J Med 284:353.
Williamson JR, Vogler N, Kilo C (1973). The natural history
  of basement membrane diseases in diabetes mellitus. Proceedings of the Eighth Congress of the International Diabetes Federation, Excerpta Medica 424.

DISCUSSION

<u>Dr. Goldstein</u>: Just a note from the practical point of view. You've shown a very nice correlation between Hb A_{1c} and weekly urinary sugar output. So, why not stick to the old fashioned urinary sugar to measure control, if that's what you're after. It's infinitely easier, cheaper and no needle pricks are needed.

<u>Dr. Cerami</u>: Well, I think the only way to answer that is to remind you that clinical experience over many years has shown that that isn't reliable. What is needed is an objective measurement that does not depend on patient compliance.

<u>Dr. Goldstein</u>: The patient could bring the urine to your lab and then you can measure it.

<u>Dr. Cerami</u>: Well, I can argue many reasons why it can't be done. The only thing I can tell you is that people have been trying for the last 30–40 years and have not been very successful in doing this.

<u>Dr. Lehmann</u>: Perhaps, if I may say, the answer is that the urine sugar tells you what happened today and the estimate of Hb A_{1c} tells you what happened over a recent period. The two tests answer different questions. Would that be of some help?

<u>Dr. Cerami</u>: Yes, we also look at it this way. The hemoglobin A_{1c} is an effective integrator of the plasma glucose over a preceding month.

<u>Dr. Schoomaker</u>: This may be anecdotal, but have you in fact observed patients who have profoundly complicated courses seemingly out of proportion to their degree of glucose intolerance who had high Hb A_{1c} levels?

<u>Dr. Cerami</u>: We have not tried to correlate complications with Hb A_{1c}. We did at one point look at basement membrane thickening and tried to correlate this with Hb A_{1c} concentrations. The problem is that like a random blood sugar one concentration only tells you what happened for the preceding month. You have no idea of what happened over the preceding years. That's why it is really important to do prospective studies. The problem is that in the field of

The Red Cell, pages 41—45

diabetes, there are a large number of anecdotal statements, but is has been very difficult to quantitate these impressions. I'm hoping that by monitoring Hb A_{1c} we're going to be able to have an objective measurement which we've not had in the past.

Dr. Harkness: Both your work and Bunn's work suggest that glucose-6-phophate is probably the immediate precursor in A_{1c} formation. If this is so, and it does seem to be so from the data, then you require a method of getting the phosphate off. Have you done any experiments on this? I think Frank Bunn has been able to take it off with alkaline phosphatase. That would not be likely in the cell, of course. Dr. Williams Awad at our institution has made the suggestion that since there is a histidine next door, it might be auto-catalytic. What do you think?

Dr. Cerami: We have not been successful in removing the phosphate. Frank Bunn has reported that he can do this in vitro. I think the possibility you suggest is very interesting.

Dr. Cameron: You showed the falling Hb A_{1c} delayed after the control of the diabetes and mentioned that A_{1c} formation is a reversible reaction, so A_{1c} can be reduced by reversal of formation as well as cell destruction. Are there experiments where you've examined density separated cells to try to quantitate how much of the A_{1c} loss is removal of cells and how much is reversal of the formation? What I mean is, density separation of the erythrocyte during treatment and during reduction of A_{1c} after control of the diabetes, and examination of the separated cells for A_{1c}, you could see if A_{1c} is reduced by removal of old A_{1c} containing cells, or if it is reduced in all cells by reversal of formation.

Dr. Cerami: We have not done studies to look at that directly. Other people have and I don't remember what their data were. Basically there are two phenomena - one is removal of cells and the second is that the slow reversible dissociation of the sugar. The half-life in vitro, in dilute solutions is about 150 hours. I don't know what it is in vivo. This is the kind of thing that has to be done in the future.

Dr. Labie: We have worked on Hb A_{1b}. It is prepared and controlled by isoelectrofocusing. We could differentiate it very clearly from G6P-Hb by several criteria. It has not the same isoelectric pH, its NH_2 terminal valine is free, it does not contain a sizeable amount of either glucose or phosphate. We have strong arguments to think it is a deamidated fraction.

Dr. Cerami: As you noticed I was a bit cautious in mentioning Hb A_{1b} since I've heard of your work. By the methods we used it appeared to have same chromatographic properties as Hb A_{1b}.

Dr. Labie: It has the same chromatographic properties but not the same isoelectric pH. I can show you slides if you want later.

Dr. Cerami: It is not really clear what the structures of Hb A_{1a} or Hb A_{1b} are. This really has to be done. Unfortunately, definitive structure assignments are difficult to do.

Dr. Labie: From the last experiments, we think we know even in which part of the molecule it is.

Dr. Shlomo Friedman: What bothers me and probably many clinicians is when you quantitate A_{1c} levels and all the other studies that we've read about in the literature are that every diabetic has an elevated A_{1c}, except for a few patients that you've kept in the intensive care unit and monitored carefully their glucose levels. It looks like all the diabetics in the world have elevated A_{1c}s and how then are we going to correlate all the complications of diabetes with their elevated A_{1c} levels?

Dr. Cerami: If you look in the average diabetic clinic, most of the patients are poorly controlled as evidenced by elevated Hb A_{1c}. However, if you can convince the patients to properly use insulin and watch their diet on an outpatient basis, you can get their Hb A_{1c} levels down to the normal range. We have had diabetic patients who have been able to achieve this on an outpatient basis. The thing that has impressed us in dealing with diabetics is the social nature of the disease. You have to get people to take care of themselves. It is apparent that insulin is really a great drug which is not used properly.

Dr. Steinberg: Are other hemoglobins, specifically hemoglobin S, glycosylated to the same degree as hemoglobin A and is there any information available on the levels of these altered hemoglobins in sickle cell anemia or in patients with sickle cell trait?

Dr. Cerami: I believe Bunn has measured hemoglobin S_{1c} in a number of patients and finds less.

Dr. Steinberg: Do you know if the colorimetric method of detecting A_{1c} also measures S_{1c}?

Dr. Cerami: I would think it would, since the method is based on the acid hydrolysis in the liberation of an aldehyde which then reacts with thiobarbituric acid. It shouldn't matter whether it comes from Hb S. The method was developed originally for the food industry.

Dr. Vye: Have you studied juvenile labile diabetics in contrast to adult, more benign diabetes?

Dr. Cerami: Yes, we have studied both juvenile and maturity onset diabetics.

Dr. Vye: Are they different significantly?

Dr. Cerami: No, not really. I think on the average, the Hb A_{1c}s when we first see them are a little bit higher.

Dr. Mansouri: If you study the basement membrane of a diabetic and compare it to normal, it has more sugar and it has been shown that the activity of the glucosyl and galactosyl transferases are increased in the basement membrane and insulin has an inhibitory effect on these reactions. Obviously the formation of Hb A_{1c} is a non-enzymatic reaction and its not inhibited by insulin and then there is so much written about aldol reaction and the formation of cataracts in diabetics. So, I think as a word of caution, probably insulin by its presence does something else. It's not that the complications of diabetes are all due to increased glucose and I think we cannot put all these reactions such as cataract formation and Hb A_{1c} formation and thickening of the basement membrane in the same category.

Dr. Cerami: I would agree. I think that the mechanisms for each complication might be different. In both cases,

however, it is the concept that there is a hyperglycemia
in the cells that do not require insulin for glucose uptake
which accounts for the development of the abnormalities.

Studies of Erythropoiesis in Culture

David G. Nathan and Diane G. Hillman

Children's Hospital Medical Center

300 Longwood Avenue, Boston, MA

Introduction: Congenital Hypoplastic Anemia (CHA) is characterized by reticulocytopenia and decreased numbers of bone marrow erythroid cells that are more mature than proerythroblasts. A return of marrow erythroid cellularity and partial remission of the anemia is often achieved by glucocorticoid treatment. To explore the molecular basis of CHA we have compared the number or function of BFU-E (1) and CFU-E (2) in the marrow and peripheral blood of normal individuals and patients with this disorder. These two morphologically undifferentiated erythroid precursor cells can be identified by in vitro cultivation techniques. They differ with respect to size and proliferative capacity. Since BFU-E colonies appear later in marrow cultures than do CFU-E and because BFU-E produce multiple CFU-E-like subcolonies, BFU-E are thought to represent the first identifiable erythroid commitment of the totipotential hematopoietic stem cell. The CFU-E is considered a product of BFU-E differentiation and, therefore, represents a later stage of erythroid development. The proliferation and differentiation of both precursors are influenced by erythropoietin. Tepperman and co-workers showed that both CFU-E and BFU-E could be observed in human marrow cultures (3). Clarke and Housman (4) and Ogawa and co-workers (5) noted BFU-E colonies in culture of human blood mononuclear cells. Gregory also observed BFU-E in normal human marrow (6). Papayannopoulou and Stamatoyannopoulos have shown that the multiple subcolonies characteristic of BFU-E are derived from a single cell (7).

Our methods of culture of human BFU-E and CFU-E in bone

The Red Cell, pages 47—60

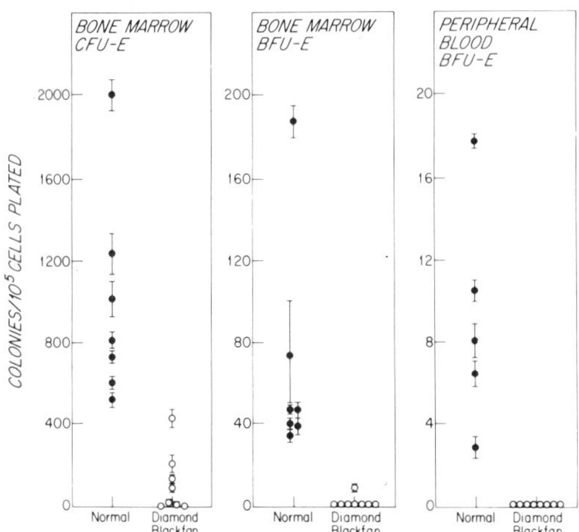

Figure 1: Comparison of the means and standard errors of the means of erythroid precursors in normal individuals (●) and patients with Diamond Blackfan Anemia (O) at 4 I.U. of erythropoietin per ml of clot. Each point represents the mean of a single study. A normal control was studied with each patient.

marrow and BFU-E in blood have been described (4,8). In brief, nucleated cells are prepared by Ficoll-Hypaque centrifugation. Appropriate cell numbers are added in 0.1 ml of suspension to 0.8 ml of the erythropoietin dependent plasma clot incubation system described by McLeod and co-workers (9) as modified by Clarke and Housman (4). Clotting is achieved by the addition of 0.1 ml of NCTC 109 containing 1 unit of Grade I bovine thrombin. One tenth ml aliquots of the clotting mixture are then dispensed in 0.2 ml micro-titer culture wells and incubated for up to 14 days. CFU-E are enumerated on day 7, and BFU-E on day 14.

RESULTS AND DISCUSSION

Figure 1 shows the results of enumeration of bone marrow CFU-E and BFU-E in normal individuals and in patients with CHA. The marked reduction of functioning BFU-E and CFU-E in patients with CHA and the absence of BFU-E in their blood samples is evident. Previously, Freedman and Saunders had also found evidence of CFU-E reduction in CHA marrow (10).

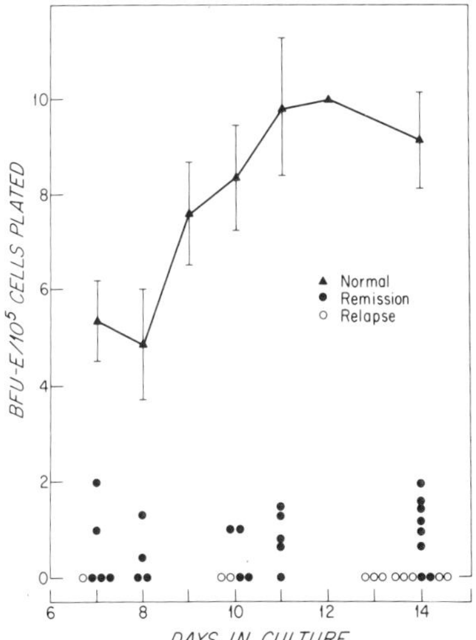

Figure 2: Rate of appearance of BFU-E during culture of
peripheral blood mononuclear cells from normals (▲) and
from patients with CHA in relapse (O) and in remission (●).
For clarity, the standard errors of the means of the CHA
studies are not shown. They range from 10 to 25 percent of
the mean.

Figure 2 shows results of studies of peripheral blood
BFU-E in normals and in patients with CHA in both relapse
and in remission. In patients in relapse, no peripheral
blood BFU-E are noted at any time during culture; and the
values are extremely low even during remission. Hence,
there is clearly a reduction of either the number or
function of both types of erythroid precursor units in the
Diamond Blackfan Anemia.

To explore the basis of this reduction, we first evaluated the report of Hoffman and his co-workers who suggested
that CHA is due to the generation of cytotoxic lymphocytes
that attack erythroid precursors in this condition (11).
Table 1 shows that we were unable to detect any evidence
of cytotoxic lymphocytes in this disorder. The growth of
normal bone marrow CFU-E was not inhibited by the lymphocytes of CHA patients, and Table 2 shows that even extra-
ordinary culture conditions in which CHA lymphocytes were
present at a ratio of 20:1 of normal bone marrow cells we
did not depress normal marrow CFU-E formation. Hence, we
have been unable to confirm the impression of Hoffman and
co-workers. In a separate study Freedman and Saunders

Patient Study	CFU-E colonies per 10^5 Normal BM Cells Plated			
	Normal BM	$\dfrac{\text{Normal BM}}{\text{Patient PB}} = \dfrac{9}{1}$	$\dfrac{\text{Normal BM}}{\text{Patient PB}} = \dfrac{2}{1}$	$\dfrac{\text{Normal BM}}{\text{Patient PB}} = \dfrac{1}{1}$
3	185 ± 43	222 ± 36	184 ± 21	235 ± 18
4	1154 ± 124	1172 ± 103	ND	ND
5	800 ± 64	813 ± 97	970 ± 114	810 ± 72
6	520 ± 27	693 ± 53	804 ± 103	578 ± 87

Table 1: The effects of 10, 33 and 50% mixtures of Diamond Blackfan peripheral blood nulceated cells (PB) on the growth of CFU-E in cultured normal marrow (BM). The peripheral blood and marrow cells were mixed immediately prior to co-culture. The results are expressed as the mean and standard errors of the number of CFU-E colonies per 10^5 normal marrow cells plated.

Patient Study	CFU-E Colonies per 10^5 Normal BM or Diamond Blackfan BM Cells Plated			
	Normal PB / Normal BM	Diamond Blackfan PB / Normal BM	Diamond Blackfan PB / Diamond Blackfan BM	Normal PB / Diamond Blackfan BM
4	1530 $\pm$ 123	1081 $\pm$ 90	184 $\pm$ 34	92 $\pm$ 36
5	100 $\pm$ 153	110 $\pm$ 87	18 $\pm$ 4	17 $\pm$ 19
6	543 $\pm$ 68	485 $\pm$ 28	15 $\pm$ 13	49 $\pm$ 33

Table 2: Effects of peripheral blood cells (PB) on the growth of normal and Diamond Blackfan bone marrow (BM) CFU-E. The ratio of peripheral blood to bone marrow was 20:1 and the blood and marrow cells were pre-incubated in a pellet for 2-4 hours prior to co-culture. See text for details of these experiments. The results are expressed as the mean and standard errors of the number of CFU-E colonies per 10^5 marrow cells plated.

have also been unable to detect such lymphocytotoxicity
(12). However, such studies are complex, and there may well
be some cases in which lymphocytotoxicity is present. The
frequency of the finding is presently unknown, but it is
probably unusual.

The bone marrow morphology of CHA patients is most
unusual in that although very few erythroid precursors may
be present, there is, in many cases, an increased absolute
number of proerythroblasts in the marrow. This suggests
that the CHA erythroid precursors that are formed from a
putative CFU-S, albeit reduced in number or function, do
produce some proerythroblasts; but these become frozen in
their development and cannot proceed to the reticulocyte
stage. They die as proerythroblasts in the marrow. To
evaluate such a fundamental disturbance of the erythroid
precursors in CHA, the bone marrows of two patients in
relapse were incubated with varying concentrations of
erythropoietin and the number of CFU-E was determined. The
results are shown in Figure 3. It is clear that a ten fold
increase in the amount of erythropoietin was required for
CFU-E formation in relapsed CHA marrow as compared to
normal marrow. One patient was treated with corticosteroids
and sustained a remission. An increase in the sensitivity
of bone marrow CFU-E to erythropoietin was noted. We,
therefore, suggest that CHA may be due to a diminished response of the CHA erythroid precursor cells to erythropoietin. Steroid therapy may somehow increase the sensitivity of the erythroid precursors to erythropoietin and,
hence, allow erythropoiesis to proceed. Whether the
erythropoietic abnormality in CHA is due to a congenital
dysfunction of the erythropoietin receptor must be explored.

The finding that peripheral blood BFU-E are markedly
decreased in CHA permits us to examine the subset of mononuclear cells that contain these precursors. This could
provide further data on the abnormality in CHA. To
accomplish this, normal peripheral blood cells and CHA
peripheral cells were separated into null, T and B fractions
by immunoaffinity chromatography according to the methods
of Chess and Schlossman (13). Table 3 shows that BFU-E
formation is evident in unfractionated and Ig- cells but not
in separated B or T cells. Some BFU-E are observed in null
cell cultures, but the predominant growth that occurs in
null cells are relatively large numbers of small CFU-E-like

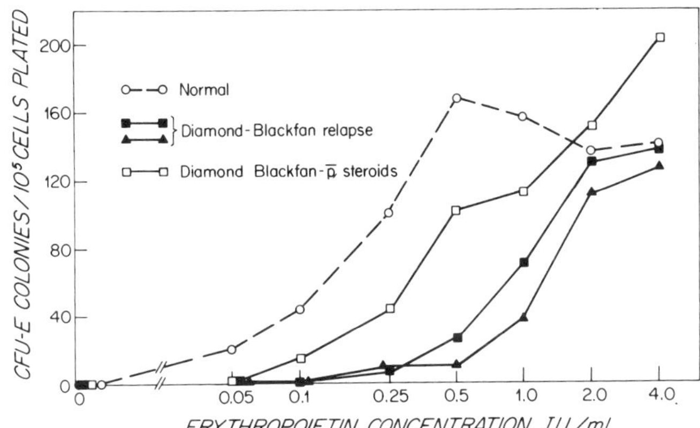

Figure 3: Growth of marrow CFU-E as a function of
erythropoietin concentration in the culture medium. The
normal marrow cells (△··△) were deliberately diluted in
isologous peripheral blood nucleated cells in order to
reduce the maximum CFU-E number to those observed in two
relapsed patients with CHA (●---●, ■---■). This dilution
of normal marrow does not affect the shape of the dose
response curve (data not shown). After steroid induced
remission, the erythropoietin dose response curve on one of
the patients was repeated (○---○). Standard errors range
from 5-15 percent of the means.

colonies that lack the proliferative thrust of BFU-E. This
is shown in Figure 4. However, when T cells are added to
null cells, large numbers of typical BFU-E colonies are
formed. Such results are shown in Figure 5, in which increasing numbers of T cells are added to a constant number
of null cells, and the number of large BFU-E colonies formed
in the culture are scored. When B cells are added, no such
effect is observed. These studies show that the normal
erythroid stem cell, BFU-E, which circulates in peripheral
blood, is found in the null cell fraction, but T cells are
required to stimulate the proliferation and differentiation
of this cell in response to erythropoietin. It is possible
that T cells achieve this function by the production of a
factor which may render the erythropoietin receptor on the
surface of the BFU-E more sensitive to the action of
erythropoietic hormone.

Study Number	Cell Type								
	Unfractionated	Ig–		B		T		Null	
	Numbers of cells plated per ml of clot								
	3×10^6	10^6	5×10^6	10^6	5×10^6	10^6	5×10^6	10^6	5×10^6
	BFU-E colonies per 10^5 cells plated								
1	21	2	15	0	0	0	1	7	20
2	9	0	8	0	0	0	0	0	1
3	7	3	7	0	0	0	0	0	1
4	23	ND*	14	0	0	0	0	8	1
5	16	ND	3	0	0	0	0	15	23

Table 3: BFU-E colony formation in unfractionated and fractionated peripheral blood mononuclear cells from five normal individuals. The cells were plated at the indicated concentrations per ml of clot. The number of BFU-E of a size considered 3+ to 4+ as defined in the legend to Figure 1 are included in the score. The standard errors were less than 10% of the mean in all cases.

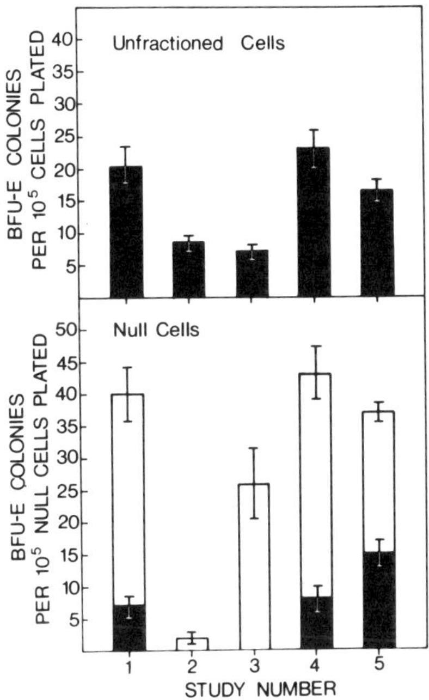

Figure 4:   Total BFU-E and 3-4+ BFU-E colonies in cultures
of (top) unfractionated mononuclear cells and (bottom) null
cell fractions derived from the same samples. The height
of each bar represents the total number of BFU-E colonies
regardless of size. The solid bars represent the proportion
of 3-4+ BFU-E colonies. The data are expressed as the
number of observed colonies per 10^5 cells plated.

That normal T cells produce a differentiating factor
during their proliferative response to mitogens has been
shown by the work of Geha and Merler et al (14) who have
demonstrated that a conditioned medium in which T cells
have divided induces the proliferation and differentiation
of B cells in culture. To determine whether dividing T
cells may, in fact, produce an erythropoietic factor, we
examined the effects of a medium in which normal dividing
T cells responded to tetanus toxoid. The medium was
identical to that described by Geha and Merler. The
medium was mixed in plasma clot culture with normal null
cells at 20% v/v, and a marked stimulation of erythropoiesis

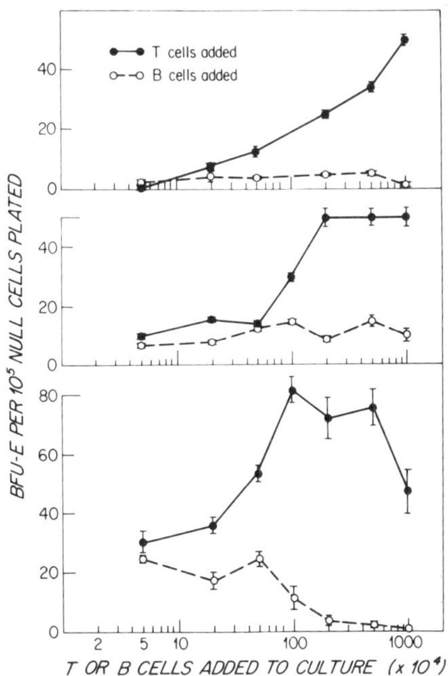

Figure 5: Three examples of the effects of varying numbers of isogeneic T (●) and B (0) cells on the formation of BFU-E colonies. The T or B cells were added to 10^6 null cells per ml of plasma clot in the presence of 2 I.U. of erythropoietin at the cell concentrations shown in the abscissa. The ordinate represents the total number of BFU-E colonies of all sizes observed after 14 days of culture of the cell mixtures. In addition to the numerical increase in BFU-E colonies observed when T cells were added to null cells, there was also an increase in the average size of individual colonies.

occurred as shown in Figure 6. The nature of this erythropoietic factor is yet to be determined, and its interaction with null cells to produce a response to erythropoietin must also be determined.

To examine CHA and the deficiency of erythropoiesis in peripheral blood which characterizes this disorder, we separated null, T and B cells from three patients and mixed the separated null cells with either autologous T cells or

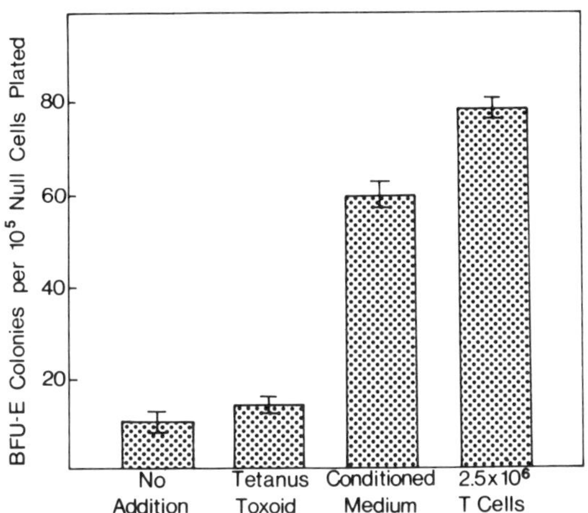

Figure 6: Influence of T cells conditioned medium and intact T cells on 3-4+ BFU-E colony growth in null cells. The null cells were incubated at 10^6 cells per ml of clot in the presence of 2 I.U. erythropoietin. The different additives were tetanus toxoid, at a final concentration of 4 ug per ml of clot, T cell conditioned medium, prepared as described in the text, at 20% v/v or 2.5 x 10^6 T **cells** per ml of clot. The mixtures were cultured for 14 days and the 3-4+ BFU-E colonies were enumerated.

with normal T cells. Conversely, normal null cells were mixed with CHA T cells. CHA T cells were perfectly capable of inducing BFU-E formation in normal null cells, but the CHA null cell could not respond to normal or CHA T cells. Hence, the defect in the Diamond Blackfan anemia appears to reside in the erythroid precursor cells found in the null cell fraction. The CHA T cell is perfectly capable of secreting an erythropoietic factor which induces proliferation in null cells when such cells are exposed to erythropoietin.

Finally, these culture methods permit an analysis of the synthesis of the various hemoglobins within the newly formed colonies. Previous reports on hemoglobin synthesis by the cultured human erythroid precursor cells, BFU-E and CFU-E, have suggested that levels of fetal hemoglobin (HbF) synthesis are elevated by increasing doses of the hormone erythropoiesin (Epo) (7,15). We have investigated the relationship between erythropoietin and the synthesis of fetal hemoglobin in cultured human marrow and blood erythroid cells by performance of radiochromatographic separation of ^{3}H leucine labelled α, β and γ chains. Such measurements of globin chain synthesis were made on cultures of human erythroid precursor cells from both bone marrow and peripheral blood over a range of Epo doses. Even when Epo concentration was varied over a 20 fold range, no significant difference in the γ to β synthetic ratio was observed. Gamma chain production was present only in colonies of peripheral blood BFU-E and not in marrow CFU-E or BFU-E.

These preliminary studies suggest that the peripheral blood BFU-E is a precursor that is programmed to produce fetal hemoglobin and, hence, may represent the precursor to the F-cells observed in the blood of patients with pregnancy or in certain hematologic disorders.

SUMMARY
Two forms of erythroid precursor cells exist in human bone marrow, the BFU-E and CFU-E. The BFU-E are probably precursors to CFU-E. Only BFU-E are found in peripheral blood. Both precursors are markedly deficient as functioning units in CHA, and no lymphocytotoxic basis for this deficiency has been discovered. Very large concentrations of erythropoietin are required to induce any differentiation of CHA erythroid precursor cells. This unresponsiveness is apparently shared by the early differentiated forms, the proerythroblasts. These become frozen in an early stage of development and may, therefore, be present in increasing numbers in the marrow. We believe that corticosteroid therapy may render the erythropoietic precursor cells of CHA patients more responsive to erythropoietin. In further studies we have shown that the erythropoietic precursor cell of peripheral blood (BFU-E) resides in the null cell fraction. Normal T cells are necessary to induce the proliferation and differentiation of such erythropoietic null cells, and this T cell dependence can be replaced by a soluble factor derived from dividing T cells. Utilizing this T cell dependent null cell culture system model, it is possible to study other forms of refractory anemia to determine whether they are characterized by a deficiency in the number or function of null cells or in a helper function derived from T cells.

The pattern of synthesis of hemoglobin subunits in these plasma clots indicates that γ chain synthesis occurs in peripheral blood BFU-E but not in bone marrow BFU-E or CFU-E. The ratio of γ to β chain synthesis in blood BFU-E is independent of the concentration of erythropoietin in the medium.

ACKNOWLEDGEMENT

The authors have performed this work in collaboration with several co-workers who include Dr. Bryan H. Clarke, Dr. David E. Housman, Dr. Blanche P. Alter, Dr. Leonard Chess, Ms. Jacqueline Breard, Dr. Ezio Merler and Dr. Bernard Forget.

REFERENCES

1. Stephenson, J.R., Axelrad, A.A., McLeod, D.L. and Shreeve, M.M.: PNAS 68 (7):1542, 1971.

2. Axelrad, A.A., McLeod, D.L., Shreeve, M.M. and Heath, D.S.: In Robinson, WA (ed). Proceedings of the Second International Workshop on Hematopoiesis in Culture, Airlie, VA 1974. NY Grune & Stratton (In Press).

3. Tepperman, A.D., Curtis, J.E. and MCCulloch, E.A.: Blood 44:659-669, 1974.

4. Clarke, B.J. and Housman, D.: PNAS 74:1105-1109, 1977.

5. Ogawa, M., Grush, O.C., O'Dell, R.F. and Sexton, J.: Exp. Hem. (Suppl)4:41, 1976 (abstract).

6. Gregory, C.J. and Eaves, A.C.: Blood 49:855-864, 1977.

7. Papayannopoulou, Th., Brice, M. and Stamatoyannopoulos, G.: PNAS 73:2033-2037, 1976.

8. Nathan, D.G., Clarke, B.J., Hillman, D.G., Alter, B.P., and Housman, D.E.: J. Clin. Invest. (In Press).

9. McLeod, D.L., Shreeve, M.M. and Axelrad, A.A.: Blood 44:517-534, 1974.

10. Freedman, M.H., Amato, D. and Saunders, E.F. J. Clin. Invest. 57:673, 1976.

11. Hoffman, R., Zanjani, E.D., Vila, J., Zalusky, R., Lutton, J.D. and Wasserman, L.R.: Science 193:899-900, 1976.

12. Freedman, M.H., and Saunders, E.F.: Clin. Res. 25(3):339, 1977 (abstract).

13. Chess, L. and Schlossman, S.F.: Manual of Clinical Immunology, p. 77-80, 1976. N.R. Rose and H. Friedman (ed). Am. Soc. Microbiol., Washington, D.C.

14. Geha, R.S. and Merler, E.: Cellular Immunology 10: 86-104, 1974.

15. Papayannopoulou, Th., Brice, M. and Stamatoyannopoulos, G.: PNAS 74(7):2923-2927, 1977.

DISCUSSION

<u>Dr. Lehman</u>:   I wasn't quite clear in which way does Dr.
George Stammatoyanopoulis differ from you?

<u>Dr. Nathan</u>:   George believes that there is increased fetal
hemoglobin synthesis in marrow erythroid cultures and that
the increase is related to the concentration of epo in the
culture. We do not see significant fetal synthesis in
marrow. We do in blood, but the ratio of γ/β is not a function of the epo concentration.

<u>Dr. Krivit</u>:   Could you grow your cells in a high amount of
glucose, and thus form A_{1c}? Does glucose do anything to
your BFU's or CFU's? Is there any possibility of a difference between you and Dr. Stammatoyanopoulis in Seattle on
conditioning of the media with glucose?

<u>Dr. Nathan</u>: Everybody uses essentially a modification of
the Toronto group's system. NCTC 109 is used as a source of
glucose. We are not prepared to do the HbA_{1c} on this material.

<u>Dr. Ogawa</u>: In the comparison of the marrow and the peripher-
al blood BFU-E, did you remove adherent cell population?
Drs. Aye and Gregory have clearly shown that the colony
stimulating factor alters erythropoietin dose response and
I would imagine the endogenous production of colony stimulating factor differs between blood and bone marrow.

<u>Dr. Nathan</u>: We do not ordinarily add stimulating factor, ex-
cept in so far as marrow and blood cells may make it.
We have used various colony stimulating factors in an attempt to replace T-cell conditioned medium as an erythroid
stimulant. Such colony stimulating factors do not do so.
And furthermore, this T-cell conditioned medium does not
support granulocyte growth. It does not substitute for the
various colony stimulating factors used by those who grow
granulocytes. I'm quite confident that what's coming out
of the T-cell is not classical colony stimulating factor,
in terms of its effects on granulocytes. I don't know what
it is. It is a factor that has been well described by immu-
nologists and is called lymphocyte mitogenic factor or LMF.
It in fact induces the proliferation of B-cells.

The Red Cell, pages 61—62
© **1978 Alan R. Liss, Inc., New York, New York**

<u>Dr. Ogawa</u>: We have compared mouse peripheral blood with bone marrow BFU-E and found that the peripheral blood BFU-E represents only intermediate stages. We examined the number of CFU-E contained in individual bursts.We found that while some of the marrow BFU-E are very immature and are located close to bone marrow stem cells, peripheral BFU-E is mostly restricted to intermediate stages.

<u>Dr. Nathan</u>: It is probably a different population.

POLYMORPHISM IN THE NUMBER OF HEMOGLOBIN α-CHAIN LOCI AND
MECHANISMS GOVERNING THE BALANCE OF CHAIN SYNTHESIS

D. L. Rucknagel, R. M. Baine, S. M. Hanash, and
W. P. Winter
Departments of Human Genetics and Internal
Medicine, University of Michigan Medical School,
Ann Arbor, Michigan 48109

Only a few years ago the genetics of hemoglobin appeared
rather simple and somewhat final. We have known for years,
for instance, that the $\underline{Hb}_\gamma$ and $\underline{Hb}_\beta$ loci were linked, and
these are not closely linked to the $\underline{Hb}_\alpha$ genes. The system
became considerably more complex, however, when Huismann and
Schroeder and colleagues (Schroeder, et al., 1968; Huismann,
et al., 1972) showed that there are at least two $\underline{Hb}_\gamma$ loci,
now known to be closely linked to the $\delta\beta$-complex (Huismann,
Schroeder, and Kendall, 1972).

The complexity of the α-chain structural loci has
evolved perhaps more slowly. It started with a phenomenon
that numerous observers had noted; namely, that heterozygotes
for $\underline{Hb}_\alpha$ mutants possess only 15-20 per cent of abnormal hemoglobin, whereas, among $\underline{Hb}_\beta$ variants the abnormal component
comprises 30-40 per cent of the total hemoglobin (Nute, 1974).
Lehmann and Carrell (1968) proposed that this difference is
due to the presence of two $\underline{Hb}_\alpha$ loci in humans; abnormal α-
chains are therefore diluted with the product of three normal
structural genes. Several individuals have now been reported
to have two different α-chain mutants but also possess Hb A
to confirm that hypothesis (Hollan, et al., 1972; Brimhall,
et al., 1974; DeJong, Khan, and Bermini, 1975). In addition,
homozygotes for Hb Constant Spring (Lie-Injo, et al., 1974)
and Hb Hasheron (Tatsis and Alter, 1976) possess considerable amounts of Hb A.

But not everyone has two $\underline{Hb}_\alpha$ loci. The first evidence
for that was the report of Melanesian homozygotes for Hb J_α
Tongariki who had no Hb A (Abramson, et al., 1970). Since

The Red Cell, pages 63—73
© **1978 Alan R. Liss, Inc., New York, New York**

then two homozygotes for Hb G_α Philadelphia have also been
found who had no Hb A (Shine, 1977; Milner and Huismann,
1976). None of these persons have Hb G-α-thalassemia, in
part because they lack Hb H and other stigmata of thalassemia
intermedia (Rieder, Woodbury and Rucknagel, 1976). This is
a progress report on our efforts to employ heterozygotes for
Hb G-Philadelphia to shed light on the organization of the
$\underline{Hb}_\alpha$ loci.

This mutant, $\alpha 68$ Asn $\rightarrow$ Lys, occurs in approximately 1
in 5,000 American Negroes. We have recognized several
years ago an apparent bimodality in the proportion of this
variant, initially with modes at 30 and 40 per cent Hb G
(Rucknagel and Winter, 1974; Dublin, Cates and Rucknagel,
1974; Rucknagel and Rising, 1975). This started us on a
search for further cases. With the help of friends we have
now studied 70 heterozygotes and the distribution is clearly
trimodal with modes at 20, 30 and 40 per cent Hb G (Baine,
et al., 1976; Baine, et al., 1977). The number of persons
observed in those three non-overlapping modes are 14, 42
and 14, respectively. Proper statistical treatment excludes
a unimodal distribution as an alternative explanation.

Initially, drawing upon the Melanesian experience, we
proposed a gene dosage model to account for this distribu-
tion (Fig. 1), whereby heterozygotes have one $\underline{Hb}_\alpha{}^G$ allele
and 3, 2 or 1 structural gene for α^A chains. Another explanation, however, is that the phenotypes comprising 30 and 40
per cent of Hb G are combinations of one and two α-thalas-
semia genes with the gene for Hb G.

To differentiate these two possibilities we have
examined the hematology accompanying these three phenotypes.
and find that the hematologic data are consistent with the
thalassemia model. The regression of MCV on the percentage
of Hb G is highly significant, $(r = -.77, p < 10^{-4})$, as is
that of MCH, the correlation coefficient being $-.84$,
$p < 10^{-4}$. We have also studied globin synthesis in 32
heterozygotes in the three phenotypic classes (Baine, et al.,
1976; Baine, et al., 1977). In 30 individuals, synthesis
is balanced, including six with 40 per cent Hb G (Table 1);
the differences in the $(\alpha^G + \alpha^A)/\beta$ ratio are not significant.

Two Models for Hb G_α-Philadelphia

Gene Dosage   α-Thalassemia

20% Hb G

$\underline{\alpha^G} \ldots \underline{\alpha^A}$ $\underline{\alpha^G} \ldots \underline{\alpha^A}$

$\underline{\alpha^A} \ldots \underline{\alpha^A}$ $\underline{\alpha^A} \ldots \underline{\alpha^A}$

30% Hb G

$\underline{\alpha^G}$ $\underline{\alpha^G} \ldots$ th

$\underline{\alpha^A} \ldots \underline{\alpha^A}$ $\underline{\alpha^A} \ldots \underline{\alpha^A}$

or   or

$\underline{\alpha^G} \ldots \underline{\alpha^A}$ $\underline{\alpha^G} \ldots \underline{\alpha^A}$

$\underline{\alpha^A}$ $\underline{\alpha^A} \ldots$ th

40% Hb G

$\underline{\alpha^G}$ $\underline{\alpha^G} \ldots \underline{\alpha^A}$

$\underline{\alpha^A}$ th ... th

or   or

$\underline{\alpha^G} \ldots \underline{\alpha^A}$ $\underline{\alpha^G} \ldots$ th

$\underline{\alpha^G} \ldots \underline{\alpha^A}$ $\underline{\alpha^A} \ldots$ th

100% Hb G

$\underline{\alpha^G}$ $\underline{\alpha^G} \ldots$ th

$\underline{\alpha^G}$ th ... th
                                              (Includes Hb H)

<u>Figure 1.</u> Two models to account for the observed trimodality in the proportion of Hb G_α-Philadelphia. Each line represents a chromosome with one or two α-chain structural loci. The so-called α_1-thalassemia gene is now believed to be a deletion of both <u>Hb$_\alpha$</u> structural genes thought to be closely linked. The α_2-thalassemia gene is believed to be due to deletion of one of the two linked <u>Hb$_\alpha$</u> structural genes.

Table 1.

Globin Chain Synthesis in Heterozygotes
For Hb G_α-Philadelphia.

	Phenotype		
	20%	30%	40%
Number	10	15	5
$\alpha^A + \alpha^G/\beta$ (Total Counts)	1.03 ± 0.075*	0.99 ± 0.06	1.0 ± 0.068
$\alpha^A + \alpha^G/\beta$ (Specific Activity)	1.00 ± 0.059	0.98 ± 0.059	1.01 ± 0.091

*$\pm$ 1 s.d.

In only two persons has the α/β ratio been approximately 0.7.
One had obvious iron deficiency. In another with 44 per
cent Hb G the α/β ratio was also 0.7. The family study
showed the nature of the problem. But first it should be
noted that if the gene dosage model is correct a parent
with 40% Hb G could have children with 30 or 40 per cent
Hb G if the parent not having Hb G is a heterozygote for the
two chromosomes in question but no children should have 20
per cent (Fig. 2A). By the same token, one would not
expect a parent with 20 per cent Hb G to have a child with
40 per cent (Fig. 2B). Now, with respect to the heterozygote
with unbalanced synthesis, the mother of this family has
22% Hb G; two of her children have 30 and 44 per cent Hb G
(Fig. 2C). The mother's Hb G gene is clearly on a double
locus chromosome; for her α/β ratio is 1. The α/β ratio
of 0.7 in the child with 44 per cent Hb G, therefore,
suggests that the child's father also has an α_1 thalassemia
chromosome. The fact that the other child has 30 per cent
Hb G indicates that the father also has a single locus
chromosome. Unfortunately, he is not available for study.
The low α/β ratio found in this family also excludes
technical factors as the cause for the high frequency of
balanced synthesis among our subjects. Others have found
similar results. Tatsis (1976) has observed balanced
synthesis in 7 persons with 30% Hb G and one with 40 per

A.

$$\frac{\dfrac{G}{}}{A} \quad 40\%\,G \qquad x \qquad \frac{\dfrac{A}{} \cdots \underline{}}{A \qquad A}$$

$$\downarrow$$

$$+$$

$$\frac{\dfrac{G}{} \cdots \underline{}}{A \qquad A} \quad 30\%\ G \qquad\qquad \frac{\dfrac{G}{}}{A} \quad 40\%\ G$$

B.

$$\frac{\dfrac{G \cdots A}{ \cdots }}{A \qquad A} \quad 20\%\ G \qquad x \qquad \frac{\dfrac{A}{} \cdots \underline{}}{A \qquad A}$$

$$\downarrow$$

$$+$$

$$\frac{\dfrac{G \cdots A}{ \cdots }}{A \qquad A} \quad 20\%\ G \qquad\qquad \frac{\dfrac{G \cdots A}{}}{A} \quad 30\%\ G$$

C.

$$\frac{\dfrac{G \cdots A}{ \cdots }}{A \qquad A} \qquad x \qquad \frac{A}{\mathrm{th} \cdots \mathrm{th}}$$

22% G
$\alpha/\beta = 0.95$

$$\downarrow$$

$$+$$

$$\frac{\dfrac{G \cdots A}{}}{A} \qquad\qquad \frac{G \cdots A}{\mathrm{th} \cdots \mathrm{th}}$$

29.3% G   41.5% G
$\alpha/\beta = 0.95$ $\alpha/\beta = 0.70$

Figure 2. Family configurations of Hb G_α genotypes used to test the gene-dosage hypothesis. A) Theoretical family in which one parent has 40 per cent Hb G, the other Hb A only but is heterozygous for the single and double $\underline{Hb_\alpha}$ locus chromosomes. B) The parent with Hb G has 20 per cent of the abnormal component; the offspring should have only 20 or 30 per cent Hb G. 'C) Actual family in which a mother with 22 per cent Hb G has a child with 44 per cent Hb G and unbalanced synthesis. The α/β ratios shown are based upon total counts of ^{3}H leucine incorporated into the respective chains. The proposed genotype of the father is shown.

cent. Trabuchet, et al. (1976) have found a similar trimodal
distribution for Hb J Mexico in Algerians, although at
values of 30, 40 and 60 per cent Hb J, and synthesis has been
balanced. They proposed that the two $\underline{Hb}_\alpha$ loci do not contribute chains equally and the $\underline{Hb}_\alpha{}^J$ is an allele of the major
locus. On the other hand, Politis-Tsegos, et al., (1976)
have observed unbalanced synthesis in a person with 30 per
cent Hb G. Milner and Huismann (1976) find α/β ratios within
their rather wide range of normal in 3 cases but in a mother
and 5 children found ratios below their normal range. These
findings suggest that the genes for Hb G and α-thalassemia
may be linked in some cases as French and Lehmann (1971)
proposed several years ago. The reported case of Hb G- Hb H
disease in which a woman with thalassemia intermedia pos-
sessed Hb G and Hb H but no Hb A also suggests that the $\underline{Hb}_\alpha{}^G$
can be linked with α-thalassemia (Rieder, Woodbury, and
Rucknagel, 1976). Thus, the $\underline{Hb}_\alpha{}^G$ mutation is found on three
chromosomes, one on the only $\underline{Hb}_\alpha$ gene, on one with two $\underline{Hb}_\alpha$
loci, and in coupling with the α_2-thalassemia allele. One
cannot be certain whether or not these are three independent
mutations; most likely these are due to crossing-over.

We believe that our data support the gene dosage model
for the trimodality of Hb G. This raises a number of questions, however. Chief of these is why is synthesis
unbalanced in α-thalassemia but balanced in these persons
having 30 and 40% Hb G when both entities--40 per cent Hb G
and α_1-thalassemia heterozygotes (Fig. 1)--have the same
number of translatable α-chain genes? An analogous situation
is provided by $\delta\beta$-thalassemia and hereditary persistence of
fetal hemoglobin, both of which are the result of deletions
of the $\underline{Hb}_\delta$ and $\underline{Hb}_\beta$ loci, but one of which results in balanced
synthesis, the other not. The second question is why does
the single locus chromosome result in microcytosis if
synthesis is balanced? Presumably this is due to the deficiency of hemoglobin synthesis rather than chain imbalance.

Finally is the question of the biological significance
of the single and double locus chromosomes. We believe
that we see the answer to this as a result of a study that
we have done in thalassemia for quite different reasons.
Numerous others have shown that in heterozygotes for β-
thalassemia the globin synthesis is grossly unbalanced in
peripheral reticulocytes but much less so in bone marrow
(Chalevelakis, Clegg, and Weatherall, 1975). One possible
explanation that has been invoked for this is that beta

chain mRNA is unstable in β-thalassemia and when the nucleus
has been extruded in late erythroblasts, mRNA for β-chains,
which has presumably been maintained by relatively rapid
transcription, then decreases in amount relative to that
for α-chains. There is evidence against this explanation,
however (Wood and Stamatoyannopoulos, 1975). Another possibility is that proteolysis allows synthesis to be balanced
in the thalassemic marrow but it diminishes in reticulocytes,
allowing the imbalance to become more evident.

We have tested this hypothesis by the following mixing
experiments (Hanash and Rucknagel, 1977). Reticulocytes of
β or $\delta\beta$-thalassemia heterozygotes were pulse labelled and
α/β ratios slightly less than 2 obtained. An aliquot of
cells was then washed and resuspended in unlabelled amino
acids. Unlabelled autologous or heterologous bone marrow
was then added, the mixture was lysed and then incubated for
two hours at 37°C. The α/β ratio of the mixture was then
measured again and found to have decreased considerably
(Table 2). The same effect was obtained when the reticulocyte lysate was incubated with a lysate of nucleated erythroblasts isolated from the peripheral blood of a patient with
β-thalassemia by Ficol-renograffin density centrifugation.
Buffy coat lysates did not produce the effect nor did adding
ATP to the thalassemic lysate alter the ratio. Gel filtration confirmed the nature of these effects. Sephadex G-100
chromatography was performed on one hour incubates; nearly
half of the radioactivity was in a monomer peak. Co-
chromatography with Hb A showed that these were, indeed,
free α-chains. Incubation with marrow or erythroblast
lysates removed the free α-chains.

These observations, at the very least, show that free
α-chains are susceptible to proteolysis. It is well known
that in many cells proteolysis is proportional to the rate
of protein synthesis. These data suggest that proteolytic
enzymes are also active in erythroblasts, but become less
so in reticulocytes and are inactivated in mature erythrocytes. Although initiation of α-chains appears to proceed
more slowly than that of β-chains, ordinarily the two α-
loci still appear to provide an excess of α-chains required
to balance the chains produced by only one $\underline{Hb}_\beta$ locus.
Presumably not all of these get degraded, however, since
there is normally a small pool of free α-chains remaining.
In any event, the proteolytic enzymes appear to function as
a fine tuning mechanism to eliminate the imbalance which is

Table 2.

α/β Ratios of Labelled Hemolysates Reincubated
in Presence of Bone Marrow Lysates.

Experimental	Number	α/β*
Labelled thalassemic reticulocytes	9	2.00 ± 0.15
Labelled reticulocyte lysate incubated without additive	9	1.82 ± 0.10
Labelled reticylocyte lysate incubated with autologous marrow lysate	3	0.96 ± 0.33
Labelled reticulocyte lysate incubated with heterologous (normal) marrow lysate	4	0.96 ± 0.19
Labelled reticulocyte lysate incubated with normoblast lysate	3	1.08 ± 0.15

*Based upon total counts incorporated into each chain as
^{3}H leucine. $\pm$ 1 standard deviation.

otherwise inimicable to red cells. Production of excess
α-chains with degradation of the excess is a more stable
system, more able to withstand unbalancing stresses, such
as iron deficiency, than presumably a system in which
synthesis is balanced by transcriptional or translational
means alone.

The single α locus chromosome is never-the-less common.
The fact that the 30 per cent phenotype can be due to two
possible genotypes has made simple counting of chromosomes
impossible. Never-the-less, by employing family studies
it is possible to utilize the parent and offspring with
Hb G to deduce the genotype of the parent without Hb G.
In this manner we estimate that the frequency of the single
locus chromosome is 0.5 in the American Negro genome. This
implies that selection plays a role in the maintenance of
this polymorphism in the tropics. The nature of that

selection is unclear. Does the high frequency of the single
locus chromosome indicate that selection favors loss of an
α-chain locus or has selection favored addition of an α-
chain locus to that of primitive man? In other words, which
way is man moving evolutionarily, from one locus to two or
vice versa? The fact that many primates have two $\underline{Hb}_\alpha$ loci
suggest that the single locus chromosome has been selected
for.

   In summary, we believe that there is substantial
evidence to support the notion of thalassemic and non-thalassemic deletions of alpha loci, presumably depending upon
whether regulatory material is included in the deletion.
The multiple loci appear to provide an excess of alpha chains
chains, most of which are then degraded by proteolytic
enzymes which provide a fine tuning mechanism to balance
hemoglobin synthesis. There is much yet to be known about
this system, however, and how it relates to the polymorphism
in the number of α-chain loci, although we are convinced
that they are related.

ACKNOWLEDGEMENTS

This research was supported by U.S.P.H.S. Grant NIH-GM-
15419, 5T32-GM-07123, and HL 16008. The authors are
grateful to Ms. Floretta Reynolds and Ms. Dorothy Sweet
for technical assistance.

REFERENCES

Abramson RK, Rucknagel DL, Shreffler DC, Saave JJ (1970).
  Homozygous Hb J Tongariki: Evidence for only one alpha
  chain structural locus in Melanesians. Science 169:194.
Baine RM, Rucknagel DL, Dublin PA Jr, Adams JG III
  (1976). Trimodality in the proportion of hemoglobin G-
  Philadelphia in heterozygotes: Evidence for heterogeneity
  in the number of human alpha chain loci. Proc Natl Acad
  Sci USA 73:3633.
Baine RM, Winter WP, Rucknagel DL, Schneider RG, Ryder H
  (1977). Thalassemic and non-thalassemic deletions of
  hemoglobin α-chain loci. In manuscript.
Brimhall B, Duerst M, Hollan SR, Stenzel P, Szelenyi J,
  Jones RT (1974). Structural characteristics of hemoglo-
  bins J-Buda [α61(E10) Lys $\rightarrow$ Asn] and G-Pest [α74(EF3)
  Asp $\rightarrow$ Asn]. Biochem Biophys Res Comm 336:344.

Chalevelakis G, Clegg JB, Weatherall DJ (1975). Imbalanced globin chain synthesis in heterozygous β-thalassemic bone marrow. Proc Natl Acad Sci USA 72:3853.

DeJong WW, Khan PM, Bernini LF (1975). Hemoglobin Koya Dora: High frequency of a chain termination mutant. Am J Hum Genet 27:81.

Dublin PA Jr, Cates M, Rucknagel DL (1974). Bimodality of the proportion of Hb G_α-Philadelphia due to heterogeneity in the number of hemoglobin alpha chain loci in man. Proc First National Symp. Sickle Cell Disease, Bethesda, Md. DHEW Publ. No (NIH)75-723. p. 173.

French EA, Lehmann H (1971). Is haemoglobin G-Philadelphia linked to α-thalassemia? Acta Haemat 46:149.

Hanash SM, Rucknagel DL (1977). Proteolytic activity in red cell precursors. In manuscript.

Hollan SR, Szelenyi JG, Brimhall B, Duerst M, Jones RT, Koler RD, Stocklen Z (1972). Multiple alpha chain loci for human haemoglobins: Hb J-Buda and Hb G-Pest. Nature 235:47.

Huisman THJ, Schroeder WA, Bannister WH, Grech JL (1972). Evidence for four nonallelic structural genes for the γ chain of human fetal hemoglobin. Biochem Genet 7:131.

Huisman THJ, Schroeder WA, Kendall AG (1972). Hemoglobin Kenya, the product of nonhomologous crossingover of γ and β genes. Blood 40:947.

Lehmann H, Carrell RW (1968). Differences between α- and β-chain mutants of human haemoglobin and between α- and β-thalassaemia. Possible duplication of the α-chain gene. Brit Med J 4:748.

Lie-Injo LE, Ganesan J, Clegg JB, Weatherall DJ (1974). Homozygous state for Hb Constant Spring (slow-moving Hb X components). Blood 43:251.

Milner PF, Huisman THJ (1976). Studies on the proportion and synthesis of haemoglobin G-Philadelphia in red cells of heterozygotes, a homozygote, and a heterozygote for both haemoglobin G and α-thalassemia. Brit J Haemat 34:207.

Nute PE (1974). Multiple hemoglobin α-chain loci in monkeys, apes, and man. Ann N Y Acad Sci 241:39.

Politis-Tsegos C, Lang A, Stathopoulou R, et al. (1976). Is haemoglobin G_α-Philadelphia linked to α-thalassemia? Hum Genet 31:67.

Rieder RF, Woodbury DH, Rucknagel DL (1976). The interaction of α-thalassemia and haemoglobin G-Philadelphia. Brit J Haemat 32:159.

Rucknagel DL, Rising JA (1975). A heterozygote for $Hb\underline{\beta}^S$, $Hb\underline{\beta}^C$ and $Hb\underline{\alpha}^{G-Philadelphia}$ in a family presenting evidence for heterogeneity of hemoglobin alpha chain loci. Am J Med 59:53.

Rucknagel DL, Winter WP (1974). Duplication of structural genes for hemoglobin α and β chains in man. Ann N Y Acad Sci 241:80.

Schroeder WA, et al. (1968). Evidence for multiple structural genes for the γ chain of human fetal hemoglobin. Proc Natl Acad Sci USA 60:537.

Shine I (1977). Personal communication.

Tatsis B (1976). Balanced globin synthesis in hemoglobin G-Philadelphia heterozygotes. Blood 46:1029.

Tatsis B, Alter AA (1976). Homozygosity for hemoglobin Hasheron (α47 Asp $\rightarrow$ His): New evidence for duplicate globin chain genes in man. Abstracts, 19th Ann Meeting, Amer Soc Hemat, Boston, 1976.

Trabuchet G, Dahmane M, Pagnier J, Labie D, Benabadji M (1976). Hb J-Mexico in Algeria: Arguments for an heterogenous distribution of α genes. FEBS Letters 61:156.

Wood WG, Stamatoyannopoulos G (1975). Globin synthesis in fractionated normoblasts of β-thalassemia heterozygotes. J Clin Invest 55:567.

DISCUSSION

<u>Dr. Lehmann</u>: Thank you very much indeed. This has always
been a difficulty for many people to understand why one
person with a single alpha chain should be normal and the
other person should be thalassemic. This would bring us
nearer to understanding that on occasions this should
cause no thalassemic consequences.

<u>Dr. Labie</u>: We have studied about 120 cases of Hb J Mexico
in 8 families. It was a very good family study. We have
also a trimodal distribution, one of the peaks corresponding to homozygotes which have always between 50 and 60
percent of the hemoglobin present. We have a big peak
having 31 percent of the mutant a very homogenous group,
and then we have about 10 cases having 38 and 39 percent
Hb Mexico. Looking at the hematology and the biosynthesis
the group of 31 percent and the group of 55 percent are
absolutely normal, without any difference with normal
controls. The group with 38 percent are at the lower limit
of the normal level. All of them are offsprings of one
parent with 31 percent Hb J and one parent apparently normal
with only Hb A. So we have studied the normal parent when
it was possible. In all of them the α/β ratio was slightly
unbalanced, too. So we think we have evidence now of an
α-thal 2 gene in trans to the J gene. At least in the
Algerian population there are always two genes. Another
approach has been begun this year, not by us but by a
group in Lyons in cooperation with Dr. Williamson of London.
Estimation by hybridization of the number of the genes in
all kinds of these patients: Normal controls, patients
with 55 percent, 31 percent and 38 percent of Hb J. They
found the same level of hybridization in all of them.
Whether a significant difference between three and four
genes can be assessed is not clear.

<u>Dr. Winter</u>: I feel a little bit strange addressing a
comment to this paper since I am a co-author on it. Dr.
Rucknagel had made reference to the Hemoglobin G as being
1 in 5,000. In the work that we are currently doing at
Howard, in 3,000 patients we have now identified six A/G
Philadelphia individuals which is substantially higher
than one would expect for a frequency of 1 in 5,000. We
don't propose that the G-Philadelphia occurs at the same
level as hemoglobin S and that we have been overlooking

The Red Cell, pages 75—78

that much all these years. We do suggest there is a
possibility that depending on how individuals are examined
for heterozygosity for hemoglobin S, that a certain number
of A/G individuals which might be of interest in work of
this sort are being overlooked. So we would just like to
suggest that in looking at all those AS's that many of the
laboratories represented here see, there may be some AG's
and the frequency could be higher and might be of interest
in getting further data on the percentage distribution of
G-Philadelphia.

<u>Dr. Nathan</u>: I am very interested in your studies of hetero-
zygous beta thalassemic peripheral blood and bone marrow
incubations. As I understand it you have actually taken
a lysate of marrow and have been able to change the ratios
in intact cells?

<u>Dr. Rucknagel</u>: No. The peripheral cells and the marrow
cells were mixed, then the two lysed together.

<u>Dr. Nathan</u>: So proteolytic enzymes were free to attack the
newly formed chains. Cividalli has looked at this problem
by examining the rate of degradation of excess alpha chains
in bone marrow and peripheral blood cells in homozygous
thalassemics. As yet, he has not been able to see a difference in the degradation rate of excess alpha chains in
the peripheral blood cells and in the marrow cell. This is
done by pulse labeling and watching the disappearance of the
excess chains, using the same separation technology that you
have used.

<u>Dr. Lehmann</u>: May I now show a slide of my own? There are
known a number of homozygotes for alpha chain abnormal
hemoglobins. The very first one was discovered by our
speaker and there is still a discussion whether the homozygotes for hemoglobin J Tongariki showed thalassemic features
or not. If you take the "two alpha gene" theory seriously,
you would expect that nearly all alpha chain variants would
be present at a 25% ratio in heterozygotes and that homozygotes would show the abnormal alpha chain hemoglobin and
also Hemoglobin A. The homozygotes for Hemoglobin J Tongariki showed Hemoglobin J Tongariki only. Is the absence
of Hemoglobin A explained by the linkage of that hemoglobin
to alpha thalassemia? For hemoglobin G-Philadelphia there
is no doubt that it is very often associated with thalassemia. J-alpha Capetown is a high oxygen affinity hemoglobin.

Dr. M. C. Botha found a child age 5 years which is a homozygote for Hemoglobin J-alpha Capetown and shows no Hemoglobin A. Both parents are heterozygotes, and first cousins.
I am presenting the fingerprint of the child's hemolysate
which shows the typical features of J-alpha Capetown.
$\alpha\Delta$t viii and $\alpha\Delta$t$_p$ viii-ix are missing, and a new peptide
can be seen. The table shows the hematological values of
the family. In the absence of iron deficiency the blood
picture is distinctly hypochromic with low MCH. Up to
now people with this hemoglobin were also iron deficient
and thus did not reach their potential hemoglobin level.
This is a Dutch family living about 500 miles from Capetown.
The two parents are first cousins, and in addition to the
affected child there are two other siblings which were
heterozygous for J-alpha Capetown.

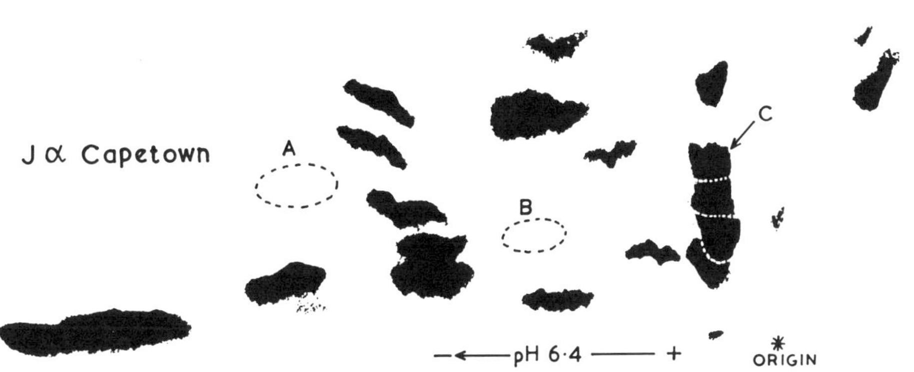

	g/ 100ml	% PCV	% MCHC	$\times 10^6/\text{mm}^3$ RBC	$\times 10^3/\text{mm}^3$ WBC	MCV	MCH	µg/dL Serum Iron	µg/dL TIBC	% Sat.
Pieter Jonker (father)	17.4	55	31.5	7.40	9.8	74	23.5	171	473	36
Marta Jonker (mother)	14.2	48	30	5.72	13.4	84	25	46	385	12
Amy Jonker (age 5 years)	16.2	54	30	7.20	7.7	75	22.5	97	307	31
Daniel Jonker (age 3 years)	13.2	43	31	5.59	13.0	77	24	157	---	--
Edwin Jonker (age 18 mos)	11.9	41	30	5.20	14.8	79	23	---	---	--

HEMOGLOBINOPATHIES

Chairman: E. Russell

HEMOGLOBIN COVENTRY, A $\beta\delta$ CHAIN ?

H. LEHMANN

DEPARTMENT OF CLINICAL BIOCHEMISTRY
UNIVERSITY OF CAMBRIDGE
ADDENBROOKE'S HOSPITAL,CAMBRIDGE.

For the last three years we have been interested in a
child which seemed to possess three different β-chains in
addition to the δ-chain of Hb A_2 and the γ-chain of Hb F.
This child is a patient of Dr. N.K. Shinton of Warwickshire
Hospital, Coventry and has been investigated there and in
the Cambridge University Department of Clinical Biochemistry,
by several of my colleagues who have now left Cambridge,
namely Dr.R. Casey, now in Norwich and Dr.A. Lang now in
Glasgow. Others were Miss P.A.M. Kynoch, who still is a
member of this Department and Drs. G. Nozari and R. Stathopoulou, who are postgraduate research students from Iran
and Greece respectively.

The child, a girl aged seven was admitted to hospital
in Coventry in 1975 with lobar pneumonia. An enlarged spleen
and liver were noticed, but the infection readily responded
to treatment with Cloxacillin and Ampicillin. At the time of
admission, the white blood cell count was considerably raised
$19.9 \times 10^9/l$ and showed all the signs of an acute infection.
The hemoglobin amounted to 8.5 g/dl and the MCV was 88 fl
and the MCH was 29 pg. There were $368 \times 10^9/l$ reticulocytes
counted; whether or not some of them were in fact red cells
containing inclusion bodies was difficult to say later, but
after the child had recovered, about a year later, the hematological values were very similar except that the white cell
count was now normal, and that the reticulocyte count amounted
to only $147 \times 10^9/l$. In the films the red cells showed
polychromasia and occasional schistocytosis. On careful
investigation, a number of cells showed very fine stippling,
which was difficult to reproduce in a photograph and for

The Red Cell, pages 81—89

practical purposes one would have to say that no Heinz bodies
were visible. The bone marrow was normoblastic and showed an
occasional Howell-Jolly body in the red cells. Though it was
difficult to demonstrate inclusion bodies, the hemolysate
showed all the features of an unstable hemoglobin, both by
the 50^{0}/1 hr heat test, and the 37^{0}/15 min. isopropanol
instability test (Carrell, R.W. & Kay, R.C., (1972) and
Dacie, J.V., Grimes, A.J., Meisler, A., Steingold, L.,
Hemsted, E.H., Beaven, G.H. & White, J.C., (1964). This was
supported by the fact that on electrophoresis a faint band
was seen behind the Hemoglobin A_2 where free α-chains would
migrate, a feature which is associated with β-chain unstable
hemoglobin. Similarly, as often seen with these hemoglobins,
the Hemoglobin A_2 level was raised above normal to 4.1% (our
normal range: 2,5-3.6). The fetal hemoglobin also was above
our normal range of up to 0.8% and amounted to 1.4%.

There was no evidence of abnormal hemoglobins in the
parents nor were there abnormal lability tests in the blood
of the parents and the three siblings of the child. The
peripheral blood and the bone marrow of both parents was
considered normal.

Globin from the hemolysate of the child was fractionated
on a CM-23 cellulose 8 M urea column (Clegg, J.B., Naughton, M.A.
& Weatherall, D.J. (1966). The non-α eluted in the same volumes
as normal non-α chains. The same was seen when the globin
prepared from an isopropanol precipitate was treated in this
manner. However, the globin from the precipitate showed a
preponderance of β-chains suggesting the presence of unstable
β-chains, which had preferentially precipitated. The fingerprint of the tryptic peptides of the aminoethylated β-chain
from the precipitate showed several abnormalities (Fig.1.)
Three histidine containing peptides corresponding to βTpIX
(β67-82) βTpVIII-IX (β66-82) and βTpXIV (β133-144) were
duplicated by a companion peptide with similar electrophoretic
but different chromatographic mobility. When the two peptides
corresponding to βTpIX were examined, it was seen that the
lower less hydrophobic peptide had in position β67 an Ala
instead of a Val as shown by amino acid analysis and dansyl-
Edman degradation. The amino acid analysis of the two peptides
in the region of βTpXIV showed that the hydrophobic peptide
had the same composition as β^{A}TpXIV except that the leucine
residue normally found in position β141 could not be demonstrated. (Table 1). Dansyl-Edman degradation of this peptide
confirmed that the amino acid sequence was identical to

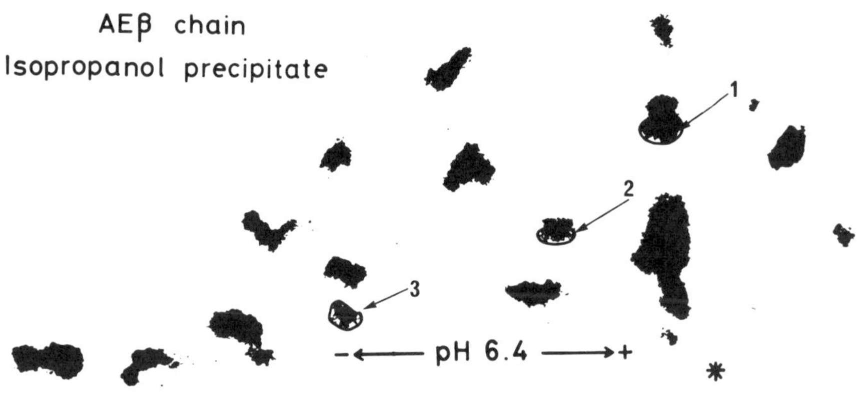

Fig. 1. Fingerprints of tryptic peptides from aminoethylated
β-chains prepared from a 1 min isopropanol precipitate.
* = origin. Peptide 1 is β Sydney TpIX (67-82); 2 is
β Sydney TpVIII-IX (66-82); 3 is β Coventry TpXIV (133-140
and 142-144). In the precipitate which contains no Hb A the
abnormal peptides are enriched but their normal equivalents
are all present. This indicates that the two amino acid
substitutions occur on two different β-chains.

βTpXIV up to residue 142, but that 141 leucine was deleted
(Table 2). Digestion of the two different βXIV peptides
with pepsin yielded a peptide present only in the digest of
the more hydrophilic βTpXIV consisting of 1 Asp (electrophoretic mobility indicated that this was derived from an
Asn), 2 Ala, 1 His, and one Lys.

All the other peptides were in their amino acid
composition identical to the tryptic peptides of normal
β-chain controls. There were thus present two β-chain
abnormalities: β67(E11)Val-Ala, which is the abnormality of
Hemoglobin Sydney (Carrell, R. W., Lehmann, H., Lorkin, P.A.,
Raik, E. & Hunter, E. (1967), and β141(H19) deleted. The
latter abnormality has not been described before and has
been designated "Coventry".

There was no way of determining the proportion of the
different hemoglobins by chromatography, electrophoresis or

TABLE 1.
Amino acid compositions of the abnormal peptides βTpIX
(β67–82) and βTpXIV (β133–143). For details see text.

| | Peptide | | | |
Amino acid	β Sydney TpIX	β[A]TpIX	β Coventry TpXIV	β[A]TpXIV
Asp	3.0	2.9	1.0	1.1
Ser	1.1	0.8	–	1.1
Gly	2.1	2.0	1.0	1.1
Ala	2.9	2.1	3.9	4.0
Val	0.1	0.9	2.8	2.9
Leu	3.9	3.9	–	1.0
Phe	1.0	1.1	–	–
His	0.9	0.9	0.9	1.0
Lys	1.0	1.0	1.0	1.0

TABLE 2.

	67	68	69	70	71	72	73	74	75	76	77	78	79	80	81	82
β[A]TpIX	VAL	Leu	Gly	Ala	Phe	Ser	Asp	Gly	Leu	Ala	His	Leu	Asp	AsN	Leu	Lys
β TpIX Patient	ALA	Leu	Gly	Ala	Phe	Ser	Asp	Gly	Leu	Ala	His	Leu	Asp	AsN	Leu	Lys

	133	134	135	136	137	138	139	140	141	142	143	144
β[A]TpXIV	Val	Val	Ala	Gly	Val	Ala	AsN	Ala	LEU	Ala	His	Lys
β TpXIV Patient	Val	Val	Ala	Gly	Val	Ala	AsN	Ala	–	Ala	His	Lys

even iso-electric focussing, because all behaved as Hb A.

It was therefore attempted to quantitate the abnormal β-chain peptides on two-dimensional chromatograms of the tryptic and other peptides. βTpXIV of Hb Coventry divided by the sum of normal βTpXIV + βTpXIV of β Coventry would equal the percentage of Hb Coventry. Similarly, βTpIX of Hb Sydney divided by the sum of normal βTpIX and the βTpIX of Hb Sydney would equal the percentage of Hb Sydney. In the case of Hb Sydney one would have to take into account also the contribution from the corresponding βVIII-IX peptides. When aminoethylated β-chains from the propositus were "fingerprinted", the Sydney peptide was estimated to be 39% of the sum of the normal and the Sydney peptides. The Coventry peptide appeared as a faint histidine staining peptide calculated to amount to 5-10% of the total of the sum of normal and abnormal βTpXIV present. These results indicated that the Sydney and Coventry abnormalities were not on the same chain. Furthermore, they indicate that in addition to the two abnormal chains amounting to 50% of the total β-chains, Hemoglobin A had to be present. All the other peptides present had the same composition as the normal β-chain peptides. To test this finding, whole hemolysate was submitted to denaturation at 50°C for 2 h. The supernatant was then repeatedly frozen and thawed. Fingerprints of the β-chains isolated from the supernatant showed only the tryptic peptides associated with normal β^A globin; βTpIX Sydney and βTpXIV Coventry were absent.

Fingerprints of globin prepared from whole hemolysates from the propositus parents' gave no indication of the presence of tryptic peptides associated with either of the two abnormal β-chains of their daughter.

To establish whether traces of Hemoglobin Coventry were present in either parents, the following procedure was adopted. We established that with 1 min only incubation in the isopropanol test, no Hemoglobin A precipitated with the unstable components (Fig. 2), though of course only a good deal of the abnormal hemoglobin will still be in solution. If the test is prolonged some Hemoglobin A begins to co-precipitate with Hemoglobin Sydney.

Labelled hemolysates (^{3}H-histidine) were prepared from each of the two parents. These hemolysates were then diluted with unlabelled hemolysate from the red cells of the propositus. The latter provided unlabelled carrier hemoglobin in the subsequent preparation of 1 min isopropanol precipi-

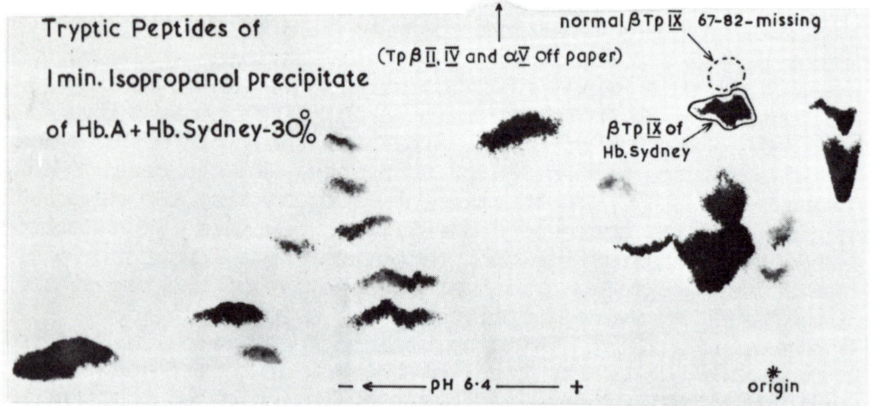

Fig. 2. Fingerprint of a 1 min isopropanol precipitate of
the hemoglobin of a heterozygote for Hemoglobins A and
Sydney. Peptide β^A TpIX is missing. To make certain that it
was not present, chromatography time was prolonged and some
peptides were run "off" the paper.

tates. The β-chains isolated from these precipitates were
then fingerprinted. No significant radioactivity could be
detected in the peptides derived from the mother (normal
βTpIX and βVIII-IX) but in the case of the father a small
but significant incorporation of ^{3}H-histidine was detected
in the peptide associated with Hemoglobin Coventry, i.e.
normal βTpIX and abnormal βTpXIV. We concluded from this
that the propositus' father has the gene coding for the
β-chain of Hemoglobin Coventry. This experiment also
provided additional proof for the non-precipitation of
Hemoglobin A even in the presence of Hemoglobin Sydney in
the 1 min isopropanol test. If it had precipitated β^A TpXIV
should have been labelled above background.

We finally succeeded to demonstrate the physical
presence of Hemoglobin Coventry in the father. Heating
tubes containing 5% hemoglobin of the fathers hemolysate in
0.0125 M phosphate buffer, pH 7 for 75 mins produced a
precipitate which on chain separation yielded a β-chain which
on fingerprinting showed the two histidine containing peptides
in the position of β^A TpXIV and the Coventry βTpXIV. We now
intend to screen the siblings of the propositus by this
method for evidence of this trace hemoglobin.

The propositus unequivocably carries two distinct
genetic aberrations affecting her non-α globin-chain genes.
There is a point mutation changing the codon for β67 valine
to one for alanine and secondly, there is a deletion of
leucine at position β141. These abnormalities are not on
the same globin chain gene for the following reasons: 1 min.
isopropanol precipitates contain no Hb A, yet β-chains
isolated from this precipitate yield on tryptic digestion,
both normal and abnormal βTpIX and normal and abnormal
βTpXIV. Thus normal βTpIX and abnormal βTpXIV must be part
of one β-globin chain and abnormal βTpXIV must be part of
another. Thus the propositus is a heterozygote for two
unstable hemoglobins, Hb Sydney (β67) (E11) Val-Ala) and
Hb Coventry (β141) (H19) Leu deleted).

There remains the enigma of three β-chain genes in one
individual. The β Coventry-chain could have been acquired
recently as a result of duplication of the $β^A$-chain gene,
but considering the following properties of the β Coventry-
chain, it is more likely that, although structurally a
β-chain, it might be genetically, a βδ-fusion chain.

The β Coventry-chain has the same amino acid sequence
as the $β^A$-chain except for the deletion of residue 141
leucine.

The β- and δ-chains differ in sequence by a minimum of
10 out of 146 residues (for refs. see Casey and Lehmann,1976).
If the point of crossing-over follows the last sequence
difference (the codon specifying residue δ126 Met), the
fused βδ gene product is indistinguishable chemically from
$β^A$-chains. This would be the mode of producing a βδ Coventry-
chain. The deletion of residue 141 leucine can also be
explained on the basis of a single crossing-over between
the δ- and β-chain genes (Fig.3).

We discovered Hemoglobin Coventry because of its
accidental coprecipitation with Hemoglobin Sydney. We were
able only to demonstrate in the propositus' father by unusual
non-routine methods, one wonders whether this and similar
hemoglobins are not much more frequent than we realise at
present.

1. β CHAIN

140 141 142 143 144 145 146
ALA LEU ALA HIS LYS TYR HIS TERMINATION CODON
GCC.CUG.GCC.CAC.AAG.UAU.CAC.UAA.GC.............

δ CHAIN

GCC.CUG.GCC.CAC.AAG.UAU.CAC.UAA.......MISALIGNMENT
OF THREE BASES CORRESPONDING TO
141 LEU followed by crossing over

2. βδ COVENTRY
    CHAIN

GCC.GCC.CAC.AAG.UAU.CAC.UAA.....
ALA ALA HIS LYS TYR HIS TERMINATION CODON
140 141 142 143 144 145

Fig. 3. Formation of the βδ Coventry chains by unequal crossing over. The genetic event is illustrated using the nucleotide sequence of the mRNA transcribed from the respective DNA sequences of the known β chain mRNA. The coding is taken from Baralle (1977).

References

Baralle FC (1977). Complete nucleotide sequence of the 5' non-coding region of human α- and β-globin mRNA. Cell (in press, Nov).

Carrell RW, Kay RC (1972). A simple method for the detection of unstable haemoglobins. Brit J Haematol 23:615.

Carrell RW, Lehmann H, Lorkin PA, Raik E, Hunter E (1967). Haemoglobin Sydney β67(E11)valine-alanine: an emerging pattern of unstable haemoglobins. Nature 215:626.

Casey R, Lehmann H (1976). Residues 124 and 125 (H2 and H3) of the human haemoglobin δ-chain. Acta Haematol 56:84.

Clegg JB, Naughton MA, Weatherall DJ (1966). Abnormal human haemoglobins: separation and characterisation of the α and β chains by chromatography and the determination of two new variants Hb Chesapeake and Hb J (Bangkok). J Mol Biol 19:91.

Dacie JV, Grimes AJ, Meisler A, Steingold L, Hemsted EH, Beaven GH, White JC (1964). Hereditary Heinz-body anaemia. A report of studies of five patients with mild anaemia. Brit J Haematol 10:388.

Dacie JV, Lewis SM (1975). Practical Haematology, 5th ed. Churchill, Livingstone, London.

Drysdale JW, Righetti P, Bunn HF (1971). Separation of human and animal hemoglobins by isoelectric focussing in polyacrylamide gel. Biochem Biophys Acta 229:42.

Huisman THJ, Dozy AM (1965). Studies on the heterogeneity of hemoglobin IX. The use of tris(hydroxymethyl)-aminomethane-HCl buffers in the anion exchange chromatography of hemoglobins. J Chromatogr 19:160.

Lehmann H, Huntsman RG (1974). Man's haemoglobins including the haemoglobinopathies and their investigation, 2nd ed. North-Holland, Amsterdam.

DISCUSSION

Dr. Rucknagel: How is it that hemoglobin Myada is not synthesized, yet it has beta chain initiation on the N-terminal
end?

Dr. Lehman: I don't think initiation by itself is so important, and consider that the whole mRNA is involved. If it
were a question of initiation only, one would expect, for
example, that hemoglobin which has the initiation sequence
of δ would be found in just as small amounts as hemoglobin
A_2. But the amount of Hemoglobin Lepore ($\delta\beta$) is about 4 to
10 times more than Hemoglobin A_2 in bone marrow, and in the
circulation amounts to 15%. Hemoglobin Myada is similarly
not formed in reticulocytes but it is formed in the bone
marrow only, although it is similar in sequence to that of
the β -chain. It is a question of the whole of the mRNA
which determines its stability.

Dr. Rosa: Have you an idea on the percentage of the Hemoglobin Coventry in the father?

Dr. Lehman: It must be less than 5%.

Dr. Rosa: But don't you think you would be able to have
very precise information on the percentage of this hemoglobin by studying carefully the very impressive oxygen affinity dissociation curve? Don't you think that by calculation you can, with this experimental data, obtain the precise level of Hemoglobin Coventry?

Dr. Lehman: This might be, I have to confess that this
oxygen affinity was made by the usual classical method by
incubating tonometers with given oxygen concentrations, not
by the machine of Itano. The machine of Itano is in our
department, but it needs a Japanese to run it!

The Red Cell, page 91
© 1978 Alan R. Liss, Inc., New York, New York

THE INTERACTION OF ALPHA THALASSAEMIA WITH SS DISEASE

Annabelle SEWELL, Doreen MILLARD, Graham SERJEANT

Medical Research Council Laboratories, Univ. of

West Indies, Kingston 7, Jamaica.

A group of patients with haematological features intermediate between those of homozygous sickle cell (SS) disease
and the non-Hb A producing type of sickle cell-beta thalassaemia (S beta^0 thalassaemia) has been causing a diagnostic
problem in the Jamaican sickle cell clinic.   Low red cell
indices and elevated Hb A$_2$ levels supported the diagnosis of
sickle cell-beta^0 thalassaemia yet family studies, which
demonstrated the sickle cell gene in both parents, indicated
a diagnosis of homozygous sickle cell disease.   There is
now evidence that this group represents a separate subpopulation resulting from the interaction of SS disease with
alpha thalassaemia.   Some features of this group will be
described in relation to the differential diagnosis of SS
and S beta^0 thalassaemia.

SS disease and S beta^0 thalassaemia have similar
electrophoretic patterns containing only haemoglobins S, F,
and A$_2$, and their differentiation, in the routine laboratory,
depends on family studies, red cell indices, and Hb A$_2$ levels.
The presence of the sickle cell gene as the only abnormality
in both parents or of the beta thalassaemia gene as the only
abnormality in one parent provides unequivocal genetic
evidence for the diagnoses of SS disease and S beta^0 thalassaemia respectively.   However parents may be unavailable
for study and the prevalence of impaternity (18% in the
Jamaican Sickle Cell Cohort Study) may confuse interpretation of data.

In the absence of such evidence, differentiation of
the two conditions depends on red cell indices (MCV, MCH)

The Red Cell, pages 93–102

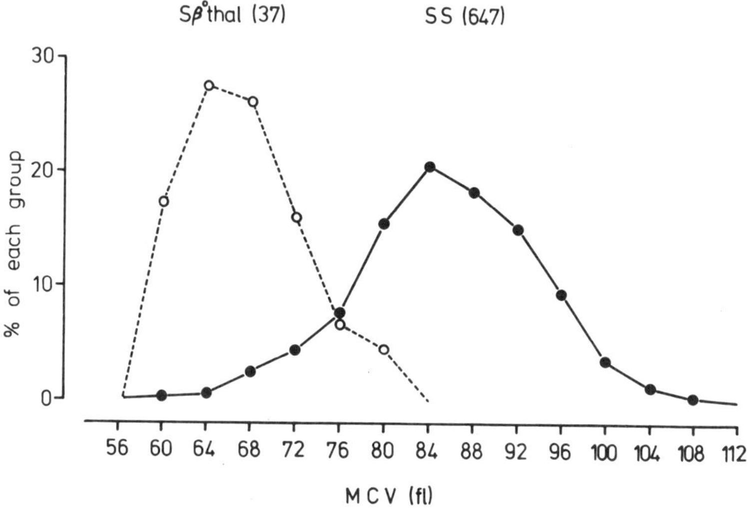

Fig.1.   Distribution of MCV values in SS disease (black
circles) and S beta° thal. (open circles).
Bracketed figures refer to number in each group.
See text for diagnostic criteria for genotypes.

and Hb A_2 levels.   Since these may be influenced by iron
deficiency and other haematological complications, and may
not have reached stable levels in young children, only
steady state observations in non-iron deficient patients
over the age of 4 years are presented in the subsequent
analyses.   For comparison of the two genotypes, SS disease
was defined by a Hb A_2 level below 3.5% or by the presence
of the sickle cell gene in both parents if the Hb A_2 level
exceeded 3.5%, and the data in S beta° thalassaemia was
confined to those cases in which one parent had the beta
thalassaemia trait.   Using these diagnostic criteria,
comparison of MCV in SS disease and S beta° thalassaemia
(Fig.1) indicated considerable overlap of values in the two
conditions even though the means of the two distributions
were significantly different (mean ± S.D; SS disease 80.2 ±
8.1 fl, S beta° thal. 68.7 ± 5.1 fl, p < 0.01).   A similar
though less marked overlap occurred with the MCH (Fig.2)
(mean ± S.D.; SS disease 28.4 ± 3.3 pg, S beta° thal.

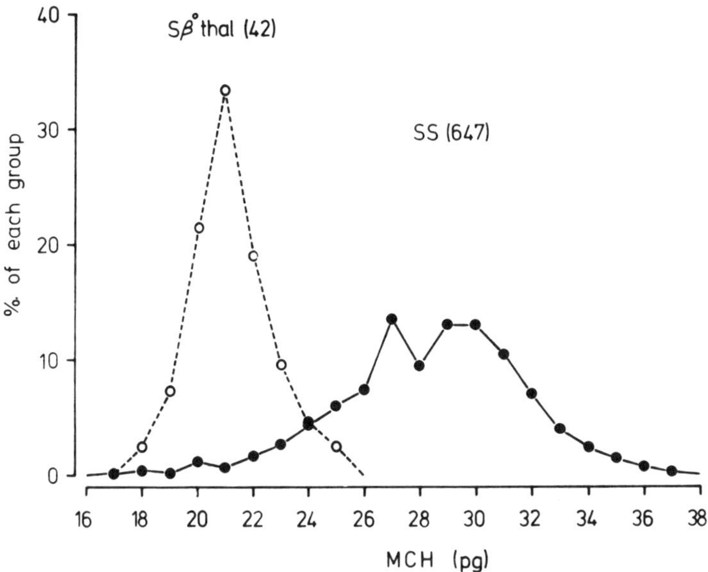

Fig.2.   Distribution of MCH values in SS disease (black circles) and S beta^o thal. (open circles).

21.2 ± 1.5 pg; $p < 0.01$).   The distribution of Hb A_2 levels (Fig.3) indicated better separation of the two conditions (mean $\pm$ S.D.; SS disease $2.80 \pm 0.49\%$, S-beta^o thal. $4.80 \pm 0.52\%$; $p < 0.01$) but some overlap in values still existed.

Further examination of the data indicated that the same patients with SS disease accounted for the overlap between the two genotypes in all three parameters.   With the prevalence of impaternity, it was considered possible that these cases represented sickle cell-beta^o thalassaemia in which the "social father" by chance possessed the sickle cell gene whereas the "biological father" had contributed the beta^o thalassaemia gene.   However, the homogeneity of red cell characteristics and of Hb A_2 levels in this group, their distribution intermediate in level between SS disease and S-beta^o thalassaemia, and the haematological findings in the parents have suggested that these patients represent a separate and distinct group.

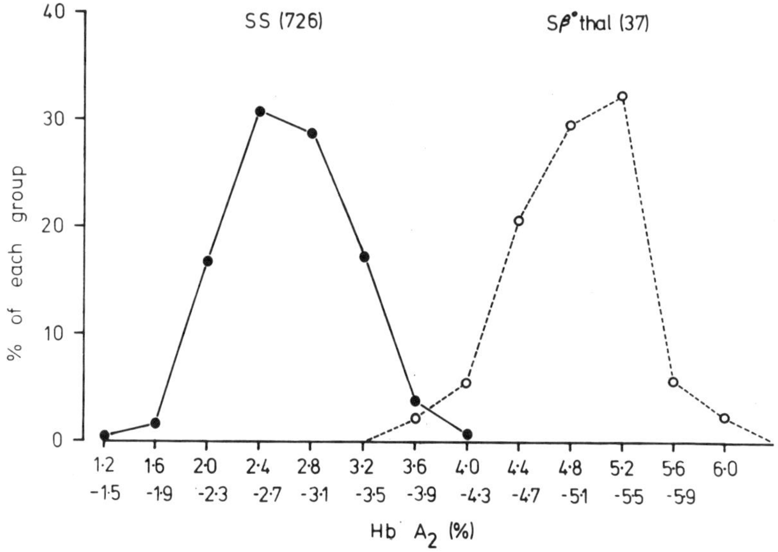

Fig.3.   Distribution of Hb A$_2$ levels in SS disease (black circles) and S beta$^\circ$ thal. (open circles).

Preliminary studies of globin chain synthesis were conducted in a group of these patients to establish evidence for the diagnosis of alpha thalassaemia in SS disease.   Data in all non-iron deficient subjects with SS disease, over 4 years of age, in whom multiple steady state estimates of MCV were available, were ranked in order of MCV and 20 subjects with the lowest values (MCV 65-72 fl) (microcytic group) were matched by age and sex with 20 subjects in whom the MCV exceeded 85 fl (control group).   Some haematological data and globin chain ratios in these groups are presented in Table 1 and Fig.4.

In 18/20 control patients, alpha/non-alpha chain ratios (CPM) varied between 0.88-1.10 similar to the generally accepted normal range.   One control had a low ratio (0.82) and another control had a high ratio (1.30).   These were confirmed on repeated incubations and although they fell outside the normal range, there was no logical reason for

Pt.Age/Sex #	MICROCYTIC GROUP								CONTROL GROUP							
	Hb A$_2$	Hb F	Hb	Retics	MCV	MCH	Fe satn.	alpha/non-alpha ratio	Hb A$_2$	Hb F	Hb	Retics	MCV	MCH	Fe satn.	alpha/non-alpha ratio
	(%)	(%)	(g/dl)	(%)	(fl)	(pg)	(%)		(%)	(%)	(g/dl)	(%)	(fl)	(pg)	(%)	
1 6 F	4.2	3.5	8.6	8	65	20	29	0.74	3.1	5.1	7.3	20	93	30	21	0.82
2 19 F	4.1	1.0	9.0	6	67	20	21	0.75	1.9	11.0	8.8	9	96	32	30	0.96
3 13 F	3.8	8.4	9.7	7	68	22	30	0.86	2.5	8.4	7.4	7	94	32	21	0.99
4 16 M	3.9	3.9	7.4	7	69	22	23	0.94	2.8	9.3	9.4	9	95	32	23	1.02
5 26 M	3.4	1.8	10.9	7	69	21	23	0.78	3.1	4.8	7.4	12	88	30	35	0.94
6 4 M	2.3	10.5	9.3	7	70	22	40	0.84	2.4	5.1	6.0	23	87	26	25	0.88
7 7 M	4.1	3.0	7.5	9	70	21	21	0.71	3.0	.5.5	6.8	17	85	27	21	1.03
8 10 M	3.9	5.4	8.0	9	70	22	24	0.78	2.5	6.7	7.6	9	85	29	21	1.10
9 11 F	3.4	5.7	6.7	10	70	21	29	0.83	3.2	1.7	7.5	8	85	28	20	0.98
10 15 M	3.7	1.5	8.3	6	70	21	33	0.77	2.6	8.6	8.1	11	89	30	23	1.30
11 43 M	3.4	7.6	10.2	7	70	22	32	0.78	2.3	2.7	10.1	13	89	30	35	0.93
12 7 F	4.0	3.6	10.8	5	71	22	26	0.62	2.8	6.5	7.3	12	89	29	28	1.08
13 18 M	3.9	5.9	8.7	7	71	23	30	0.78	2.7	7.5	9.0	17	87	31	22	0.97
14 22 F	4.1	4.3	7.8	6	71	22	22	0.76	2.3	4.6	7.2	16	96	32	30	1.09
15 11 F	4.1	1.6	8.3	13	72	22	27	0.74	3.3	3.5	7.6	21	99	33	37	0.99
16 15 M	3.7	0.8	6.5	8	72	22	24	0.80	3.7	3.6	8.4	12	85	27	22	0.96
17 26 M	3.1	2.1	9.9	6	72	23	22	0.69	2.8	3.9	7.5	18	98	32	36	0.88
18 37 M	3.6	0.6	9.2	9	72	22	27	0.83	3.2	13.6	11.4	6	86	29	26	0.90
19 39 M	4.0	3.4	10.5	7	72	23	36	0.77	3.0	5.1	6.3	8	88	29	43	0.98
20 48 M	4.0	2.1	11.0	3	72	22	22	0.81	3.0	2.6	8.5	9	88	28	23	0.92
Mean±SD	3.74 ±0.45	3.84 ±2.71	8.92 ±1.37	7.35 ±2.06	70.15 ± 1.87	21.75 ±0.85	27.05 ±5.31	0.78 ±0.07	2.81 ±0.42	5.99 ±3.01	7.98 ±1.29	12.85 ± 5.05	90.10 ±4.68	29.80 ±1.99	27.10 ±6.80	0.99 ±0.10

TABLE 1   Some haematological indices and alpha/non-alpha globin chain ratios in microcytic and control groups (see text for further explanation)

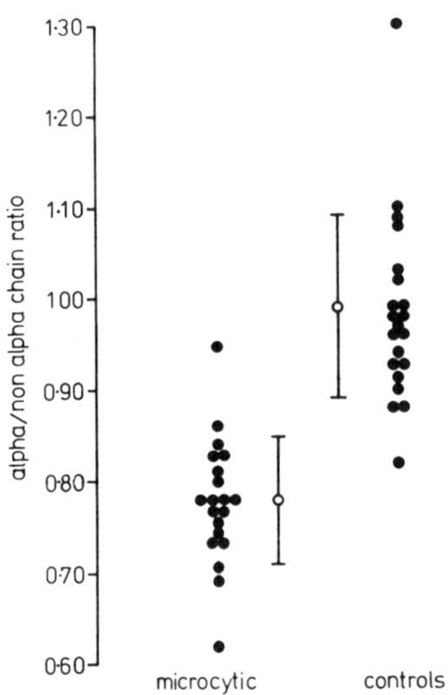

Fig.4.　　Distribution of alpha/non-alpha globin chain ratios
based on CPM in microcytic and control groups.
Mean ± S.D. depicted by circle and vertical line.

excluding them from the control group.　In the microcytic
group, alpha/non-alpha chain ratios varied from 0.62–0.94
(mean 0.78), the ratio in one patient falling in the low
normal range and in 19/20 patients, ratios were compatible
with alpha thalassaemia.

Since the interaction of alpha thalassaemia with the
sickle cell trait lowers the level of Hb S (Steinberg et al
1975), additional evidence for the diagnosis of alpha thalassaemia could be obtained from Hb S levels in the AS
parents (Table 2).　In the microcytic group, Hb S levels
were below 31% in one parent of 10/14 patients in whom
estimates in both parents were available and below 27% in 6
of these, compared to two parents with a Hb S level below
31% in the control group (one of which was associated with
evidence of iron deficiency).　Hb S levels were above 31%
in all remaining parents in the microcytic and control groups
including both parents of 3 patients in the microcytic group.

| | MICROCYTIC GROUP | | | | | | CONTROL GROUP | | | | | |
| | Mother | | | Father | | | Mother | | | Father | | |
	MCV	Fe satn.	Hb S	MCV	Fe satn.	Hb S	MCV	Fe satn.	Hb S	MCV	Fe satn.	Hb S
1	79	25	35.4	66	29	25.0	84	26	38.1	96	17	35.2
2	76	29	31.8	74	21	29.5	98	22	34.9	N.A		
3	78	18	31.8	79	34	24.1	72	11	27.9	N.A		
4	83	11	34.7	N.A			85	21	31.2	N.A		
5	79	13	33.3	N.T			81	14	31.6	95	42	40.2
6	79	25	35.4	66	29	25.0	97	39	38.4	91	35	31.0
7	81	22	34.3	82	35	32.1	88	23	35.3	85	20	36.4
8		SS		72	28	26.1	87	28	38.1	N.T		
9	81	20	31.0	81	35	31.1	86	12	36.0	N.A		
10	N.A			N.A			92	28	37.0	97	49	33.6
11	83	23	35.7	N.A			N.T			N.A		
12	84	21	32.5	88	46	34.0	67	–	34.2	N.T		
13	80	26	29.4	75	42	24.5	86	32	31.6	88	19	35.7
14	71	23	29.3	87	29	30.7	N.T			N.T		
15	77	18	30.1	78	30	30.4	88	35	36.5	N.T		
16	71	14	31.6	88	11	30.8	81	30	32.6	N.T		
17	N.A			N.A			77	27	29.4	100	38	36.4
18	84	35	32.5	89	35	34.0	88	20	36.8	80	21	34.0
19	–	–	25.1	–	–	30.7	N.A			N.T		
20	N.A			N.A			N.A			N.A		

TABLE 2. Mean cell volume (pg), iron saturation (%) and
Hb S levels (%) in AS parents of microcytic and
control groups. Normal Hb S distribution,
mean$\pm$S.D.= 33.9 $\pm$3.7%; n= 493.
N.A. not available (dead, emigrated, unknown,
incompatible genotype).
N.T. not tested.

Low red cell indices were also more common among parents of
the microcytic group, MCV levels $<$80 fl occurring in 15/28
(54%) compared to 3/24 (13%) of the control parents.

The evidence therefore from both globin chain ratios
and parental studies suggests that alpha thalassaemia may
account for some of this subpopulation of patients with SS
disease.   Whereas the interaction of the alpha thalassaemia
gene would explain the thalassaemic red cell characteristics
it would not be expected to cause elevated Hb A_2 levels.
Kim et al (1977) in their report of 4 cases of SS alpha
thalassaemia, also noted that elevated Hb A_2 levels may occur.
It is clearly important to ascertain whether this represents
an absolute or only proportional increase in Hb A_2 especially
in view of the inverse relationship that exists between Hb
A_2 level and the MCV or MCH (Fig.5).   From this it can be

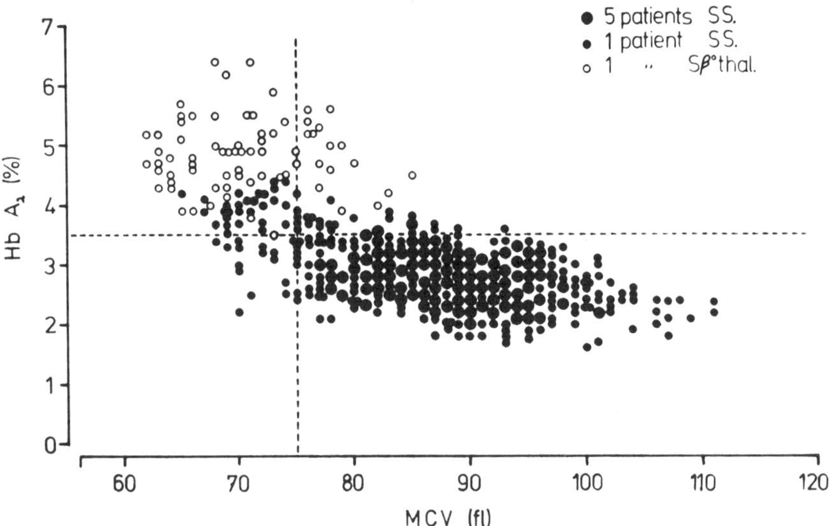

Fig.5.   Relationship between MCV and Hb A_2 levels in SS
disease (solid circles) and S-beta^o thal. (open
circles).   Interrupted lines indicate generally
accepted lower level of MCV and upper level of
Hb A_2.   Subpopulation with presumed SS alpha thal.
lies in upper left quadrant.

seen that there is a steadily rising Hb A_2 level with falling MCV in patients with SS disease and that the population with proposed SS alpha thalassaemia form one end of this continuum. A similar relationship between Hb A_2 and MCH has been reported in the beta thalassaemia trait (Weatherall and Clegg 1972) and although the mechanism is unknown, it serves to maintain an approximately equal amount of Hb A_2 in each cell regardless of size. In the present study, absolute Hb A_2 levels were similar in the microcytic and control groups (0.82 pg and 0.80 pg respectively).

The haematological characteristics of this subpopulation merge with those of SS disease without evidence of alpha thalassaemia and any definition on the basis of haematology is essentially arbitrary. Using the criteria of MCV $<$ 75 fl and Hb A_2 $>$ 3.5% defines a group of 33 (4.9%) of the 690 patients in Fig.5. These criteria almost certainly underestimate the prevalence of alpha thalassaemia in SS disease since family studies and globin chain ratios compatible with SS alpha thalassaemia have been observed in several patients with MCV values between 75–80 fl. This prevalence, however, compares with estimates for alpha thalassaemia of 4–6% in the Jamaican population, obtained on the basis of Hb Barts at birth.

Many questions remain unanswered in relation to SS alpha thalassaemia. The clinical and haematological characteristics of this group must await confident identification of the SS alpha thalassaemia subpopulation, and comparison with cases of SS disease without alpha thalassaemia must be performed in carefully matched and preferably large samples, since without this, the highly variable natural history of SS disease may allow incorrect conclusions. However it is of interest that comparison of the microcytic and control groups in the present study revealed significantly higher haemoglobin levels and lower reticulocyte counts in the SS alpha thalassaemia group. Once identified, the SS alpha thalassaemia subpopulation may be a useful model in which to investigate the effect of the lowered MCV and MCH on the clinical and haematological features of SS disease. It is tempting to postulate that the AS parents with Hb S levels below 26% represent a severe alpha thalassaemia gene and that those with Hb S levels between 29–31% represent a mild alpha thalassaemia but such speculation must await clarification of the alpha thalassaemia syndromes among Negro populations.

<u>SUMMARY</u>

A group of patients with SS disease with red cell indices and Hb A_2 levels intermediate between those of SS disease and sickle cell-beta^o thalassaemia has been described. Globin chain synthesis in 20 of these subjects selected on the basis of low MCV values gave alpha/non-alpha chain ratios in the alpha thalassaemia range (0.62-0.94) compared to 20 age sex matched controls. The AS parents of these subjects with low MCV showed a greater prevalence of low Hb S concentrations (a feature of the interaction of alpha thalassaemia with the sickle cell trait) compared to controls.

These data suggest that this group may represent a subpopulation of SS disease resulting from the interaction with alpha thalassaemia.

<u>REFERENCES</u>

Kim HC, Weierbach RG, Friedman S, Schwartz E (1977) Detection of sickle alpha- or beta^o- thalassemia by studies of globin biosynthesis. Blood 49: 785.

Steinberg MH, Adams JG, Dreiling BJ (1975) Alpha thalassaemia in adults with sickle-cell trait. Brit J Haematol 30: 31.

Weatherall DJ, Clegg JB (1972) "The Thalassaemia Syndromes". (Ed.2) Oxford: Blackwells, p 114.

DISCUSSION

<u>Dr. Castro</u>: Dr. Serjeant, did you find increased hemoglobin F level in your patients with SS α thalassemia?

<u>Dr. Serjeant</u>: In the microcytic and control groups presented, the Hb F was actually lower in both with presumed SS α thalassemia but I don't think we can believe that because of the way in which the cases were selected. However, in general, patients with presumed SS α thalassemia have tended to have low Hb F levels.

<u>Dr. Castro</u>: This is very interesting. Do you believe that the sickle cell anemia patients from Saudi Arabia who have high F levels, in whom there appears to be high frequency of alpha thalassemia by Bart's hemoglobin measurements in cold blood could also have alpha thalassemia?

<u>Dr. Serjeant</u>: It is impossible to predict. There are several unusual genes in that population. Alpha thalassemia assessed by the prevalence of Hb Barts in cord blood samples, appear to affect nearly 50% of the population. I don't know much about the genetics of the high F gene in that population but have assumed that the two genes were independently inherited.

<u>Dr. Nathan</u>: Very interesting data. I take it that you believe that the elevated A_2 levels in the patients with the thalassemia gene probably reflects some increased turnover of the beta chains in excess of the delta chain. Is that how you explain that? Usually in alpha thalassemia we see a lower A_2 when it's related to hemoglobin A

<u>Dr. Friedman</u>: When you're answering that, you might just add to the list of things that might decrease the severity of sickling in alpha thalassemia syndrome the unbalanced synthesis itself, that is, the accumulation of dimers, which in fact may interfere with the sickling process. It may not be the MCH that's the determinant of mildness but rather the mixture in the cell.

<u>Dr. Serjeant</u>: I came here for guidance. I was sure I would find the answers. I know nothing about this relationship between MCV and hemoglobin A_2. It has been described by David Weatherall between MCH and hemoglobin A_2 in the beta thalassemia traits. I don't know whether it is a generally recognized phenomenon that there is an inverse relationship between the two and if so whether it occurs in normal people

The Red Cell, pages 103–107

and what the mechanism of control is. All that I can say
is that we were surprised because these people had propor-
tionately elevated hemoglobin A_2 levels. When we looked at
absolute levels, they appear to be normal but they are not
decreased.

Dr. Shlomo Friedman: We have only four patients with Hb SS
α thalassemia, one of which has an elevated Hb A_2 level.
I wanted to ask, is there a possibility to explain the elevated Hb A_2 level by suggesting that there is a combination
at least in some of your patients of alpha and beta thalassemia? And the reason why I'm suggesting this is several
reasons. First of all, it's a good alternative. The other
thing is that you have 400 patients in Jamaica. You've
shown us that 20 patients, around 5% of your patients, have
alpha thalassemia, in combination with Hb SS disease.

Dr. Serjeant: No. For these studies, we took the bottom 20
out of an MCV distribution based on 680 patients. Thalassemic red cell characteristics as defined by an MCV less than
75 fl. or a Hb A_2 above 3.5% occurred in 33 (4.9%) of the
population.

Dr. Friedman: OK. In other words, your present group of
patients represents less SS alpha thalassemia than you
really have in the population. You studied less than you
really....

Dr. Serjeant: No, no, you can't possibly say that. I said
already that our arbitrary definition with a cut-off point
of 75 fl has excluded people who are already known to have
chain ratios compatible with alpha thalassemia so this figure of 4.9% (33 out of 680) has certainly underestimated
the prevalence of SS alpha thal.

Dr. Friedman: Exactly. I agree. This is an underestima-
tion which means that when you have all patients with Hb SS
α thalassemia you'll have a larger group of patients, and
then some of these with elevated Hb A_2 may represent a combination of alpha-beta thalassemia. Another reason is you
have shown us that it's very easy to differentiate between
SS β^0 thalassemia and SS disease, but we know that the
genetics are not reliable which is usually the case. You
have to base the diagnosis of sickle β^0 thalassemia on
globin synthesis studies. That's the only way you're going
to differentiate between Hb SS disease and Hb S β^0 thalassemia.

And since not enough globin studies are published in patients with sickle β^0 thalassemia some may show a balanced ratio of beta to alpha chains in sickle beta 0 thalassemia, making the differentiation between Hb SS disease and sickle β^0 thalassemia impossible, in all cases.

Dr. Serjeant: I'm sorry, just give me the question again.

Dr. Friedman: Could high A_2 be explained by a combined $HbS\alpha\beta^0$ thalassemia in some of your patients?

Dr. Serjeant: I don't know, I have absolutely no evidence for or against that, I can't say at the moment.

Dr. Lessin: Related to factors that mitigate the severity of disease in the sickle syndromes, it was suggested in a red cell rheology conference a couple of years ago that if sickle cell patients had larger capillaries they would have less severe disease. Here nature has done the converse, they've given the patient smaller cells so that rheologically this would favor easier negotiation of the microcirculation. Have you had an opportunity to look at any of your patients rheologically by filtration studies or other kinds of measurements?

Dr. Serjeant: No, being entirely in vitro techniques this would be something that would be much better done elsewhere I think. We're certainly not equipped to do this. But is it not known, would you not expect, for theoretical reasons, cells in the with low MCVs and MCHs to demonstrate lower rheological properties I mean to move more readily....

Dr. Lessin: You certainly would, in fact, when you compare hereditary spherocytosis, for example, to SS and you do flow versus pressure profiles in a filtration system HS looks very similar to hemoglobin SS cells. However, because the cells are small, one would postulate that vaso-occlusion in the oxygenated state would be unlikely in capillaries but splenic pore blockade likely. The sickle patients with small MCV and MCH would simulate this condition.

Dr. Rucknagel: Well, we've measured synthesis on about 50 or 60 cases of sickle cell anemia, looking at the alpha thalassemia issue and whether that can be protective. We found first of all that we get generally lower alpha/beta ratios in people with sickle cell anemia than we do with

normals and we don't think that all of those have alpha thalassemia. There is something systematic in sickle cell anemics
that lower the alpha/beta ratios and I don't know what it is.
Secondly, in some obvious cases where there's some mild disease and we expected to find lower alpha/beta ratios we did
not. We only have, I believe, one child where we're sure
there's concomitant alpha thalassemia and that individual has
a low A_2. I don't understand why you have high A_2. I rather
suspect that it's technical, but I don't see what it can be.
We have 15 patients from age 40 to 70 with homozygous S and
again, they're all balanced, so we don't think that alpha thalassemia is protective in terms of accounting for the patients
with longer life spans. We do see some sickle β^0 thals with
low ratios and high A_2, what we would expect, although most
black people who have sickle beta thal have $\beta+$.

<u>Dr. Serjeant</u>: I must jump to the protection of my laboratory
here. I would be very reluctant to stand up in front of a
meeting like this if I did not believe there was **very** solid
evidence for elevation fo hemoglobin A_2 in these patients.
These are people who've had repeated estimations. We know
exactly what our normal distributions are and our staff very
competently do about 60 estimations of hemoglobin A_2 every
week, so I don't say that it is likely to be artifactual. I
believe that they are proportionally elevated and this has
been confirmed in some independent laboratories. I'd be
delighted to send some to you, Don.

<u>Dr. Lehmann</u>: It is not really a question of "elevated hemo-
globin A_2". The hemoglobin A_2 per cell is normal, but the
hemoglobin S defaults. It is partially precipitated in the
membranes: both $\alpha_2\beta_2 S$ **and** β^S, and this causes a relative
disproportion.

<u>Dr. Serjeant</u>: I don't know what the answer is. I can only
repeat our two observations. HbA_2 appears to be elevated
when expressed as a proportion but in absolute terms, it
is similar to that in the control group.

<u>Dr. Lubin</u>: I'd just like to mention that in a recent study
in <u>Blood</u> Stamtoyannapoulos and coworkers have shown that
about four or five per cent of black patients seem to have
alpha thalassemia, so one would expect that the sickle cell
patients might have approximately the same incidence. This
would correlate with your data.

Dr. Serjeant: This is the whole point of the operation. If it does   influence the disease for better or for worse the coincidence of the two abnormalities might increase or decrease with advancing age and that's something we just don't know enough about to answer, but it's obviously an important question.

Dr. Brewer: Graham, I agree to tell you what the significance of your finding that the A_2 stays constant per cell is, if you will tell us what the A_2 is there for in the first place.

Dr. Serjeant: Thank you, you strike a hard bargain.

ANTISICKLING EFFECT OF CYSTAMINE AND ITS ACTION ON
THE BIOSYNTHESIS OF HEMOGLOBIN.

Yves BEUZARD, Jean ROSA, Paulo MACHADO,
Waffa HASSAN, Isabelle MAX-AUDIT, Marie-
Claude GAREL.
INSERM. U.91. Hôpital Henri Mondor.
94010 CRETEIL   FRANCE

Cystamine a thiol reagent ($NH_2-CH_2-CH_2-S-S-CH_2-CH_2-NH_2$) has been previously shown to bind to the cystein β93 of hemoglobin (Smithies 1965). The S ethylamine hemoglobin derivative migrated as a single electrophoretic band distinct from that of the unreacted Hb. This property provided a simple means of quantitation of the cystamine reacted fraction (Hassan et al. 1976). The EA-Hb exhibited

Abbreviations : Hb S sickle cell hemoglobin ; S cells, cells containing more than 94% of Hb S ; SA cells, cells containing Hb S and Hb A ; SC cells, cells containing Hb S and Hb C ; MCHC, mean corpuscular hemoglobin concentration ; MCV, mean corpuscular volume ; EA-Hb, S-ethylamine derivative of Hb ; 2,3-DPG, 2,3-diphophoglycerate ; O.D.C., oxygen dissociation curve ; P_{50}, partial pressure of oxygen at which Hb is half saturated with oxygen ; IHP, inositol hexaphosphate ; MGC, minimum gelling concentration ; bis-tris, 2,2-bis (hydroxymethyl) - 2,2',3" - nitroethanol ; RBC, red blood cells ; GSH reduced glutathione ; GSSG, oxidized glutathione ; CSH, cysteamine ; CSSC, cystamine ; NADP, oxidized nicotidamide dinucleotide ; NADPH, reduced nicotidamide dinucleotide ; G6PD, glucose-6-phosphate deshydrogenase ; NCTC, National Cancer Tissue culture medium ; DEAE, diethylaminoethyl ; G6P, glucose-6-phosphate.

The Red Cell, pages 109—126

a high oxygen affinity and a reduced Bohr effect
(Taylor et al. 1966) in view of these properties it
was reasonable to suspect that cystamine could
exert an antisickling effect.

Cystamine is a disulfide comparable to oxidized glutathione. The latter compound is known to
inhibit protein synthesis initiation (Kosower
et al, 1972). Red blood cells rich in reticulocytes were therefore incubated in a complex tissue
culture medium, NCTC 109, widely used for the culture of RBC precursors.

The cystamine binding to hemoglobin was stable for several days in cells incubated in saline
buffers, or in lysate kept at 4°C. However the
percentage of EA-Hb decreased with the duration of
the incubation of the cells in NCTC 109 medium.
This reversion of the binding was found to be the
result of the reduction of the EA-Hb linkage.

This paper describes first the effect of
cystamine on sickling and on the functional properties of A and S cells, second the metabolic
pathway involved to reduce cystamine and the EA-Hb
linkage and third the inhibitory effect of cystamine on protein synthesis in intact cells and in a
reticulocyte cell free system.

METHODS

Incubation of RBCs with cystamine was performed with cells washed thrice with the solutions
used for the incubation i.e., NCTC 109 medium,
0.15 M sodium phosphate or 0.15 M Tris HCl all at
pH 7.45. Incremented amounts of cystamine dichlo-
ride stock solution (1 M) were then added to the
red cell suspensions which had been adjusted to
the final hematocrit value of 5% for the functional studies or 30%. Incubations were performed at
37°C for various periods. The mean corpuscular Hb
concentration (MCHC) was determined from hemoglobin
and hematocrit measurements. Intracellular pH was
determined on packed frozen and thawed cells, at
37°C, with the use of a Radiometer pH meter fitted
with a microelectrode unit (type E 5021a). Erythro-

cyte 2,3-DPG-diphosphoglycerate (2,3-DPG) level was
determined according to Rose and Leibowitz (1970).
Hemolysates were prepared without organic solvent.
Hemoglobin electrophoresis was performed on cellulose acetate strips at pH 8.6 (Garel et al. 1976) ;
the proportions of the various fractions was determined by densitometry.

The cystamine-reacted Hb was purified by chromatography on a DEAE-Sephadex A_{50} (Machado et al.
1977). For the sickling experiments, aliquots (0.1
ml) of washed and packed cells were suspended in
10 ml of 0.15 M phosphate buffer at pH 7.45. The
suspensions were subsequently deoxygenated by eva-
cuation in a 250 ml tonometer at partial oxygen
pressures of 0, 10, 20, 30, 40 or 50 mmHg for 10
min. and incubated at 37°C for a further 10 minutes.
Deoxygenated cells were then anaerobically transferred into a deoxygenated-phosphate-buffered glutaraldehyde solution (5% v/v) for fixation. The percentage of sickle cells was determined by phase contrast microscopy. We have designated sickle cells,
the deformed cells.

Reversible hemolysis to decrease the mean
corpuscular hemoglobin concentration was performed
according May and Huehns (1975).

Oxygen dissociation curves (O.D.C.) were determined on red blood cells and on Hb solutions at
37°C by the spectrophotometric method of Benesch
et al. (1965) as modified by Bellingham and Huehns
(1968) using a Unicam SP 800.

Gelation experiments were performed according
to the method described by Singer and Singer (1953)
as modified by Bookchin and Nagel (1971).

The reduction of S-ethylamine Hb, cystamine
and other compounds by glutathione reductase was
studied according to Beutler (1971).

Cystamine and S-ethylamine Hb are disulfides
which can be reduced or can interchange with other
disulfides. The reaction between cystamine or S-
ethylamine Hb and glutathione was investigated in

order to determine the process involved in their reduction. Characterization of the products of the reaction was performed by electrophoresis on thin layer plates of silica gel (Mauran et al. 1974).

Studies on protein synthesis in intact reticulocytes were performed in the presence or in the absence of hemin (Lingrel and Borsook, 1963). The reticulocyte cell free system was as described by Hunt et al. (1972).

RESULTS

The presence of about 55% of EA-Hb in the cells resulted in a 32% decrease in the P_{50} values of both A and S cells at pH 7.45. The 2,3-DPG levels and pH values, in controls and cystamine-treated cells, were identical. The increase in oxygen affinity of cystamine-treated cells could not therefore be explained by variations in 2,3-DPG concentrations nor in intracellular pH. The oxygen affinity of the S-ethylamine Hb S (or A) solution was considerably greater than that of unreacted Hbs without modification of the cooperativity. The Bohr effect over the pH range 7.15-7.45 was reduced to -0.36 as compared to -0.50 for unreacted Hb S. These results are similar to those obtained by Taylor et al. (1966) on solutions of EA-Hb. A lower interaction with 2,3 DPG for EA-Hb S (or A) was also found. The average effect of different concentrations of 2,3-DPG on the shift towards the right of the O.D.C. of EA-Hb S is 30% less than its effect on that of unreacted Hb S.

Cystamine 1 mM induced a slight increase of the mean corpuscular volume (5%) and the decrease of the hemoglobin concentration. The sickling of cystamine treated cells at a partial oxygen pressure of 10 mmHg was reduced (Fig. 1a). High concentrations of cystamine did not affect the irreversibly sickle cells (ISC) as their number in each sample (3%-12%) remained unchanged. The inhibition of sickling by cystamine inducing 55% of EA-Hb was markedly enhanced when the oxygen pressure was raised from 0 to 20 mmHg as shown in Fig. 1b. This was expected from the high oxygen affinity of cystamine-reacted Hbs. The same data are shown in Fig. 1c, in which the abcissa represents the mean oxygen saturation of S cells from 3 patients. It clearly appears that the proportion of sickle cells is higher at a given oxygen saturation in the un-treated samples than in the cystamine-reacted cells. These results indicate that a part of the antisi-ckling effect of cystamine is independent of its influence on oxygen affinity.

The results of gelation studies are summa-rized in Table I. The values for the minimal gel-ling concentration (MGC) of deoxy Hb S (23.9 g/dl) and for a deoxygenated mixture of 60% Hb A and 40% Hb S (31.5 g/dl) are similar to those previously reported. The minimum concentration of Hb required for gelation of solutions containing S ethylamine Hb S was higher than that for solutions containing unreacted Hb S (Table I). In contrast cystamine-reacted Hb A behaved similarly upon gelation to unreacted Hb A.

The rate of formation and of disappearance of the EA-Hb were studied with erythrocytes of normal adults at 30% hematocrit value, incubated in the presence of cystamine in isotonic solutions of Tris, sodium phosphate or NCTC 109 medium, all at pH 7.45 (Fig. 2). Incubation of RBCs in saline buffers induced a rapid combination of Hb and cys-tamine reaching a plateau of 50% of EA-Hb. Incu-bation of cells in the NCTC 109 medium also showed a rapid binding with a maximum at 10 minutes, but this was followed by a progressive diminution in the EA-Hb level. These experiments indicated that the NCTC 109 medium contained at least one compound necessary to split the disulfide linkage in EA-Hb. The NCTC 109 medium contained several compounds which could be involved in S-ethylamine Hb reduc-tion such as : glutathione, NADP, FAD, cysteine, cystine, riboflavin and glucose. These compounds were therefore added in isolation or in association to fresh red cell lysates containing S-ethylamine Hb. The results indicated that riboflavin, glucose, FAD, or NADP added separately did not decrease the percentage of EA-Hb formed. However addition of both glucose and NADP promoted disappearance of the

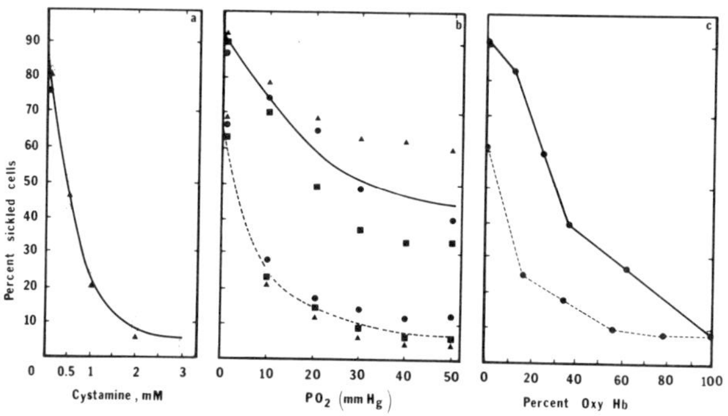

FIG. 1 (a) Effect of increasing concentrations of
cystamine on sickling of S erythrocytes at a PO_2
of 10 mmHg. (b) Influence of oxygen pressure on
sickling of control erythrocytes (solid line) and
erythrocytes treated with 1 mM cystamine (dashed
line). Sickling experiments were done in 0.15 M
phosphate buffer, pH 7.45 at 37°. Different symbols represent results obtained with cells from
different patients. (c) Sickling is related to the
hemoglobin oxygen saturation (same data as shown
in b).

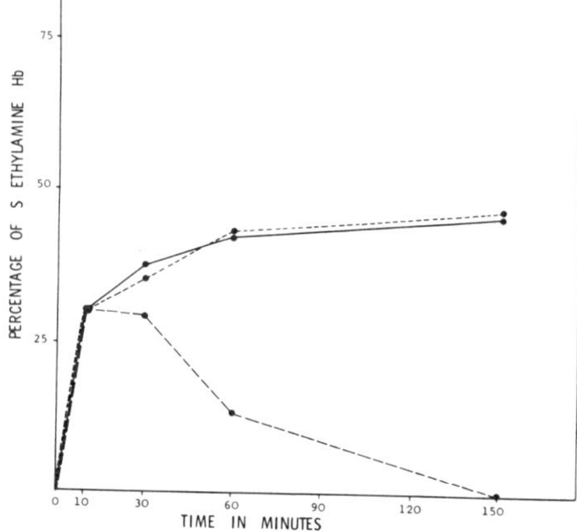

FIG. 2. Kinetics of formation and disappearance
of EA-Hb in cells incubated various media.
Tris ———— Phosphate —————— NCTC 109 — — —

Table I. Effect of cystamine on minimum gelling concentration in g/dl of Hb S and mixtures of Hbs A and S.

% Hb S ($\alpha_2^A \beta_2^S$)	% EA–Hb S ($\alpha_2^A \beta_2$ S–cyst	% Hb A ($\alpha_2^A \beta_2$ A–cyst	% EA–Hb A ($\alpha_2^A \beta_2$ A–cyst	MGC° mean value (g/dl)	Range
100	—	—	—	23.9	23.2–24.0
10	90	—	—	26.6	25.0–28.8
40	—	60	—	31.5	30.4–32.4
40	—	—	60	31.2	30.4–32.0
—	40	60	—	32.7	32.4–33.2
—	40	—	60	32.8	32.4–33.6

° Minimum gelling concentration.

EA-Hb, without any precipitation of Hb, indicating
that the S-ethylamine Hb linkage was cleaved.
Other associations were ineffective. Glucose gives
rise to glucose-6-phosphate. Glucose-6-phosphate
and NADP are both substrates of glucose-6-phosphate
deshydrogenase which reduces NADP. These results
indicated that reduction of the EA-Hb disulfide
bridge probably involved NADPH or a NADPH dependent
reaction. These results were confirmed by the study
performed on G6PD deficient cells obtained from
black males (Fig. 3). G6PD deficient cells exhibited a greater initial binding of cystamine to their
Hb than normal cells. The reduction of their EA-Hb
was impaired. The kinetic differences from those
displayed by the control cells could be explained
by the rapid exhaustion of NADPH in the G6PD-defi-
cient cells. NADPH regeneration would be necessary
to prevent further reaction of Hb with cystamine.

Reduced glutathione when added in isolation
to the lysate induced a rapid disappearance of
EA-Hb.

The structural analogy between oxidized
glutathione and cystamine and the reduction of
GSSG by an NADPH-dependent enzyme prompted us to
investigate the relationship between glutathione
metabolism and the reduction of the EA-Hb or of
the reduction of the cystamine-disulfide bridges.
Purified EA-Hb as well as cystamine were tested as
substrates of glutathione reductase. As shown in
Fig. 4 a EA-Hb was not reduced by NADPH alone or
by glutathione reductase in the presence of NADPH.
In contrast the consumption of NADPH in the presence of EA-Hb and GSH is important. The initial
slope was probably due to the reduction of a small
amount of GSSG contaminating the GSH preparation
and of a compound formed during the preincubation
period. The second part of the curve indicated
that the NADPH consumption persisted but at a
slower rate than during the initial period.

Cystamine was also tested as a putative
substrate of glutathione reductase. This reagent
(1 mM) did not induce NADPH consumption in the
presence of glutathione reductase (Fig. 4b).

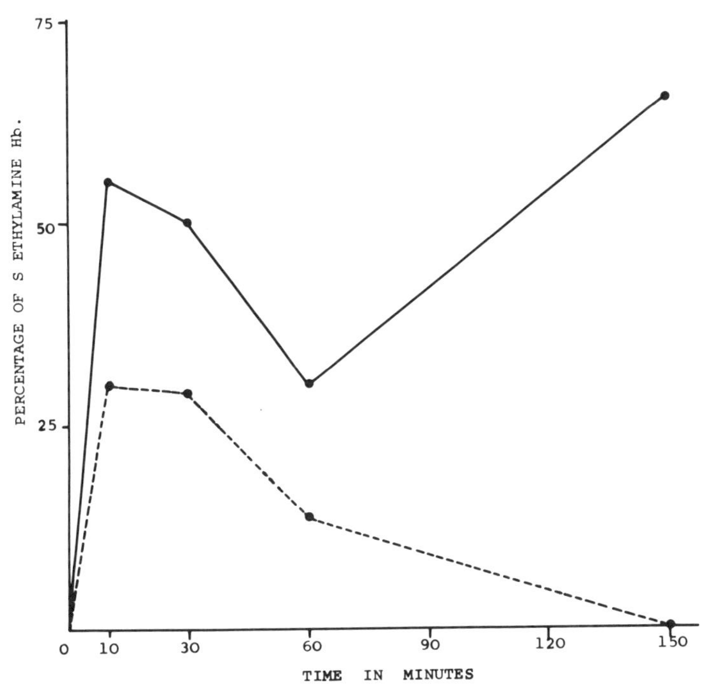

FIG.3. Formation and disappearance of EA-Hb in G6PD deficient RBC ⸻ and normal cells ------- incubated in NCTC 109 medium with cystamine (5 mM). RBCs were at a 30 % hematocrit value.

Addition of GSH promoted the consumption of NADPH ;
the shape of the curve resembling that obtained
by the glutathione reductase reaction in the presence of both EA-Hb and GSH (Fig. 4a). These experiments indicated that EA-Hb and cystamine were
not substrates of glutathione reductase but in the
presence of GSH led to a compound reducible by
glutathione reductase. To determine the nature of
this compound, cystamine or EA-Hb were mixed and
incubated at 37°C for 10 minutes at pH 7.8 with
reduced or oxidized glutathione. The mixtures were
fractionated by electrophoresis on thin layer
plates. Three distinct fractions were obtained
with the glutathione-cystamine incubated mixture :
glutathione, cystamine or cysteamine and a new
compound which was not present in the cystamine nor
in the glutathione preparations but which migrated
between them. This compound incubated with GSH gave
rise to cystamine (or cysteamine) ; these results
indicated that cystamine formed a mixed disulfide
with glutathione by the reaction : GSH + CSSC →
CSSG. The purified complex reacted with GSH in the
following manner : CSSG + GSH → CSH + GSSG. The
glutathione cystamine disulfide was confirmed by
the amino acid analysis of the new compound. The
mixed disulfide CSSG used in the glutathione reductase reaction exhibited the peculiar behaviour
indicated in Fig. 4b. Thus CSSG (0.25 mM) was very
slowly reduced. At a concentration of 1 mM, the
rate of reduction of CSSG increased with time.
Subsequent addition of GSH to the mixed disulfide
(0.25 mM) dramatically increased the speed of the
reaction. These results suggested that CSSG might
be a poor substrate of glutathione reductase.
However, the small amount of GSH formed reacted
with CSSG and released GSSG which was then reduced.
Such reduction progressively increased the amount
of GSH able to react with CSSG. When incubated
with GSH purified EA-Hb restored some cystamine
glutathione complex as shown by the electrophoresis and the amino acid analysis.

    The protein synthesis study indicated that
cystamine inhibits hemoglobin synthesis in intact
cells and in a reticulocyte cell free system. This

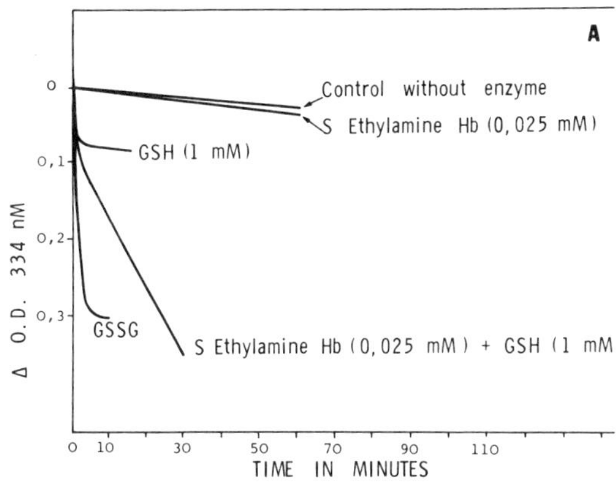

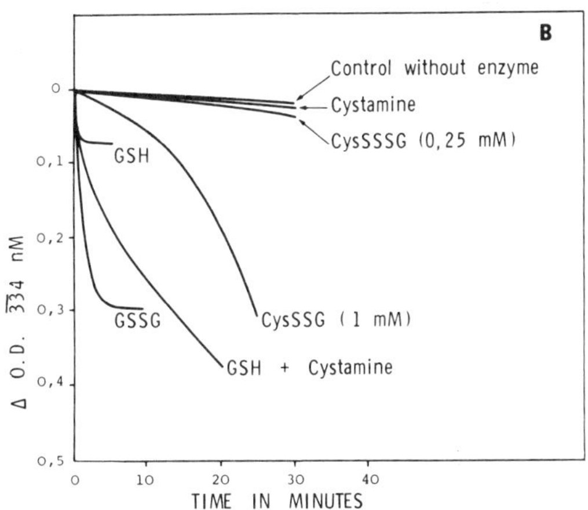

FIG.4. The glutathione reductase reaction in the presence of several compounds as substrates is expressed as the variation in the optical density at 334 nM due to the oxidation of NADPH.

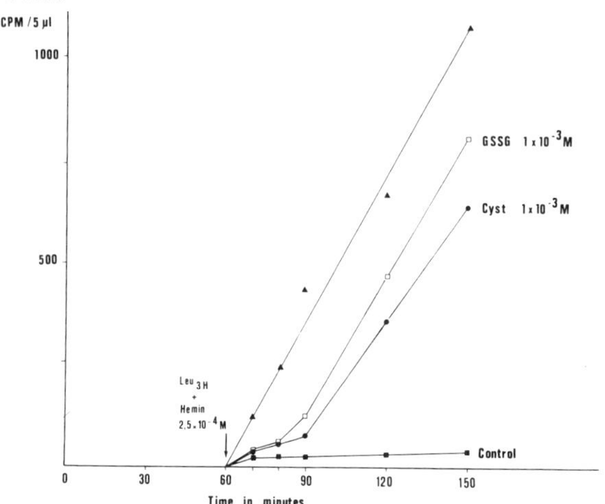

FIG. 5. Effect of cystamine and GSSG on protein synthesis in intact rabbit reticulocytes. The cells were preincubated for one hour before addition of the radioactive leucine.

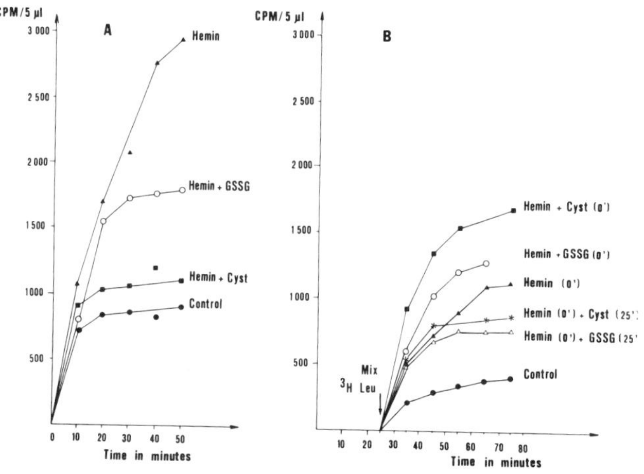

FIG. 6. Effect of cystamine 5 x 10⁻⁵ M and GSSG 5 x 10⁻⁵ M added at zero time on protein synthesis in a rabbit reticulocyte lysate in the presence of hemin 2,5 x 10⁻⁵ M at 33° C.(A) Protein synthesis begin at zero time. (B) Protein synthesis began after a delay of 25 minutes. Cystamine and GSSG are added either at zero time or at 25 minutes.

inhibitory effect is reversible since the reduction of cystamine allows the protein synthesis to
resume (Fig. 5 and Fig. 6).

DISCUSSION

The studies presented in this report provide
evidence that cystamine, a thiol reagent, is a
strong inhibitor of sickling. This agent appears
to modifiy three interrelated processes which underlie the sickling of S erythrocytes : the Hb concentration within the S cells, their oxygen affinity and the gelation of Hb S. Part of our results
were confirmed by Antonini et al. (1977) who found
in addition a similar effect of L. cystine dime-
thylester.

The modifications in the oxygen affinity of
cystamine-reacted cells have to be compared to
those observed with bis (N-maleimido methyl) ether,
an antisickling agent which cross-linked the cysteine β93 to the histidine β97 (Zak et al. 1975).
This substance increased the oxygen affinity but
abolished the cooperativity of oxygen binding in
the S cells. This results contrasts with the normal cooperativity of the cystamine-treated Hb.
Such a discrepancy indicates that these two SH
reagents may play a different role in the inhibition of sickling.

P.OH mercuribenzoate which reacts also with
β93 Cys, raised the O_2 affinity for Hb but did not
alter the MGC of Hb S or of a mixture of S and A
Hb (Nagel and Bookchin, 1975). The modifications
of MGC produced by cystamine suggest alterations
in some bonds which form the polymer or gel. Moreover since the mixtures of Hb S and cystamine-reacted Hb A have the same MGC as mixtures of Hb S
and unreacted Hb A, it seems that Hb S itself must
be altered. This supports a mechanism of conformational change which results from the stabilization
of the quaternary oxy state and is suggested by
the decreased interaction of cystamine-reacted Hb
with 2,3-DPG and by the attenuated spectral changes which occurred in the presence of excess IHP
(Hassan et al. 1976). This hypothesis is consis-

tent with the conclusions of Bookchin and Nagel (1973) in studies of the MGC of half liganded Hb S.

The present results provide also evidence that the binding of cystamine to Hb is a reversible process. EA-Hb is reduced in the presence of GSH and cannot be directly by glutathione reductase. Furthermore we have shown that S-ethylamine Hb as well as cystamine may react with GSH to form a CSSG mixed disulfide and that the isolated hybrid was slowly reduced by glutathione reductase. This reaction was however more rapid in the presence of GSH. EA-Hb contained two molecules of S-ethylamine, each bound to a β93 residue (Garel et al. 1974).

The sequence of reactions involved in the reduction of EA-Hb can be summarized as follows :

$$EA\text{-}Hb + 2\ GSH \rightarrow Hb\ SH + 2\ CSSG$$
$$2\ CSSG + 2\ GSH \rightarrow 2\ GSSG + 2\ CSH$$
$$2\ GSSG + 2\ NADPH + 2\ H^+ \rightarrow 4\ GSH + 2\ NADP$$

The lack of reduction of EA-Hb in cells incubated without glucose can be easily explained. In such cells, glucose-6-phosphate is rapidly exhausted and the reduction of NADP by the hexose monophosphate pathway is halted. Consequently, the GSH and NADPH involved in the reduction of S-ethylamine Hb are rapidly consumed. The observation that G6PD-deficient cells are unable to reduce S-ethylamine Hb as well as normal cells emphasized the role of NADPH. The mixed disulfide CSSG which was formed when GSH or GSSG was added to cystamine, was slowly reduced by glutathione reductase. This result may be explained in one of three ways : firstly, CSSG is a substrate of glutathione reductase and is directly reduced at a low rate. Secondly, small amounts of GSH may contaminate the CSSG fraction and induce a thiol disulfide interchange. The glutathione concentration would then be the limiting factor in the reaction ; thirdly, the mixed disulfide CSSG could participate in a

slow disulfide interchange thus producing both
GSSG and cystamine. GSSG could then be reduced
and could itself induce a thiol disulfide interchange with CSSG. The rate of the reaction,
initially slow, would increase with the formation
of GSH. The rate of NADPH consumption would then
depend on the initial concentration of the CSSG
hybrid and would increase with time. This is
consistent with the results described. The binding of cystamine to haemoglobin is reversible
only in the presence of GSH. This result differs
from that obtained with the haemoglobin glutathione disulfide which is a substrate of glutathione reductase (Srivastava and Beutler, 1970).
EA-Hb does not seem to be a substrate of this
enzyme under the conditions employed but is reduced via thiol disulfide interchanges and
reduction of GSSG as shown in the present study.

The inhibition of protein synthesis by
cystamine is difficult to interpret. The inhibition of protein synthesis could be either an
indirect effect of cystamine in increasing the
GSSG concentration or a direct effect of cystamine
very similar to the inhibition induced by GSSG.
Upon reduction both cystamine and GSSG are reduced.

Preliminary studies of the action of cystamine on erythrocyte enzyme activities revealed no
major modification. However extensive studies are
required to determine the extent of the cellular
alterations induced by cystamine.

SUMMARY

The studies presented in this report provide
evidence that cystamine as a thiol reagent is a
strong inhibitor of sickling which affects three
interrelated processes which underlie the sickling
of S erythrocytes : the Hb concentration within the
cells, their oxygen affinity and the gelation of
Hb S. Cystamine crosses the red cell membrane and
reacts with hemoglobin within the cells. Cystamine
did not affect the intracellular pH nor the 2,3-
DPG level.

The reduction of intracellular S-ethylamine
Hb was impaired in the absence of glucose or in
cells deficient in glucose-6-phosphate dehydrogenase (G6PD). In both cases the NADPH regenerating system was decreased ; the presence of both
glucose and NADP was required for the reduction of
S-ethylamine Hb in the haemolysate.

The mechanism of reduction of S-ethylamine
Hb A seem to involve the following steps : reduced
glutathione (GSH) reacts with ethylamine-Hb or
cystamine to form a mixed disulfide, CSSG. This
compound reacts with GSH to form oxidized glutathione (CSSG) ; GSH can be recovered from GSSG by
treatment with glutathione reductase, a NADPH dependent enzyme. Neither S-ethylamine Hb nor cystamine were substrates of glutathione reductase.

The inhibition of protein synthesis by cystamine in reticulocyte is similar to the effect of
oxidized glutathione. It is a reversible process
when the disulfide is completly reduced.

AKNOWLEDGMENT.

We thank Mrs. CACHELEUX for excellent technical assistance and INSERM for financial support.

REFERENCES.

Antonini, E., Ioppolo, C., Giardina, B., Brunori,
    M. 1977. Chemical modifications of SH groups
    of intraerythrocytic hemoglobin. Biochem.
    Biophys. Res. Comm. 74:1647.
Bellingham, A.S., Huehns, E.R. 1968. Compensation
    in haemolytic anaemias caused by abnormal hae-
    moglobin. Nature, 218:924.
Benesch, R., Macduff, G., Benesch, R.E. 1965.
    Determination of oxygen equilibria with a ver-
    satile new tonometer. Analytical Biochemistry
    11:81.

Beutler, E. 1971. Red cell metabolism p. 64
    GRUNE   STRATTON, New York.
Bookchin, R.M., Nagel, R.L. 1971. Ligand-induced
    conformational dependence of hemoglobin in
    sickling interactions. J. Mol. Biol. 60:263.
Bookchin, R.M., Nagel, R.L. 1973. Conformation re-
    quirements for the polymerization of hemoglo-
    bin S : studies of mixed liganted hybrids. J.
    Mol. Biol. 76:233.
Garel, M.C., Cohen-Solal, M., Blouquit, Y., Rosa,
    J. 1974. A method for isolation of abnormal
    haemoglobins with high oxygen affinity due to
    a frozen quarternary R structure : application
    to Hb Creteil. $\alpha_2^A \beta_2$ (F5) 89 Asn. FEBS Letters
    43:93.
Hassan, W., Beuzard, Y., Rosa, J. 1976. Inhibition
    of erythrocyte sickling by cystamine a thiol
    reagent. Proc. Nat. Acad. Sci. 73:3288
Hunt, T.   , Vanderhoff, G.A., London, I.M. 1972.
    Control of globin synthesis : the role of heme.
    J. Mol. Biol. 66:471.
Kosower, N.S., Vanderhoff, G.A., Kosower, E.M.
    1972. Glutathione VIII. The effects of gluta-
    thione disulfide on initiation of protein syn-
    thesis. Biochim. Biophys. Acta, 272:263.
Lingrel, J.B., Borsook, M. 1963. A comparison of
    aminoacid incorporation into the hemoglobin
    and ribosomes of marrow erythroids cells and
    circulating reticulocytes of severely anemic
    rabbits. Biochemistry 2:309.
Machado, P., Beuzard, Y., Audit, I., Rosa, J.
    Submitted. Reduction of S ethylamine in human
    red blood cells.
May, A., Huehns, E.R. 1975. The concentration de-
    pendence of the oxygen affinity of haemoglo-
    bin S. Brit. J. Haemat. 30: 317.
Nagel, R.L., Bookchin, R.M. 1975. Mechanisms of
    hemoglobin S gelation structural restrictions
    to supramolecular models of the polymerization
    of Hb S. In LEVERE, R.D. ed. "Sickle cell ane-
    mia and other hemoglobinopathies". New York
    Academic Press.
Rose, Z.D., Liebowitz, J.,1970. Direct determina-
    tion of 2-3 diphosphoglycerate. Analyt. Bio-
    chem. 35:177.

Singer, K., Singer, L. 1953. Studies on abnormal
    hemoglobins : VIII the gelling phenomenon of
    sickle cell hemoglobin : its biological and
    diagnostic significance. Blood, 8:1008.
Smithies, O. 1965. Disulfide bond cleavage and
    formation in proteins. Science, 150:1595.
Srivastava, S.K., Beutler, E. 1970. The enzymatic
    cleavage of glutathione haemoglobin prepara-
    tions by glutathione reductase. Biochem. J.
    119:353.
Taylor, J.F., Antonini, E., Brunori, M., Wyman, J.
    1966. Studies on human hemoglobin treated with
    various sulfhydril reagents. J. Biol. Chem.
    241:241.
Zak, S.J., Geller, G.R., Finkel, B., Tukey, D.P.,
    Mc Cormack, M.K., Krivit, W. 1975. Bis (N -
    Maleimidomethyl) ether : an antisickling rea-
    gent. Proc. Nat. Acad. Sci. (USA) 72:4153.

DISCUSSION

<u>Dr. London</u>: I find these studies of great interest and I'd
like to comment particularly on the last portion with regard
to the inhibition of protein synthesis by cystamine. We've
been studying the mechanism by which oxidized glutathione
is inhibitory. As many of you know this inhibition can be
overcome by the addition of the specific initiation factor,
EIF-2. This inhibition of protein synthesis by oxidized
glutathione is very similar to that which one observes with
double stranded RNA and with that which has been most studied,
namely the deficiency of hemin. In these three conditions
one can observe the activation of a specific cyclic-AMP-
independent protein kinase which phosphorylates the 38,000
dalton subunit of the initiation factor, EIF-2. It is not
clear at present whether the protein kinase activities induced
under these three inhibitory conditions are the same or different entities. Now, in the light of the impressive similarity between the results of cystamine and glutathione, it would
be interesting to see whether cystamine treatment also leads
to the activation of protein kinase activity. In addition,
I think one has to distinguish between the effects of glucose
and NADP in the reduction of the cystamine-hemoglobin-bond
and the effect of glucose in overcoming the inhibition of
protein synthesis. Dr. Vivian Ernst in our laboratory has
shown that the addition of glucose-6-P alone in the absence
of added NADP overcomes the inhibition of protein synthesis
induced by GSSG or by heme-deficiency. In the case of GSSG-
induced inhibition, glucose-6-P appears to be acting in two
ways. Initially glucose-6-P appears to overcome inhibition
by reducing GSSG to GSH. However, glucose-6-P also restores
synthesis, when added after the onset of inhibition, by a
mechanism which is independent of NADPH production. Moreover, in heme-deficiency the effect of glucose-6-P in overcoming inhibition appears to be unrelated to the ability to
generate NADPH.

<u>Dr. Winterbourn</u>: Have you been able to tell whether the effect
of cystamine on protein synthesis is direct or is due to its
oxidizing the GSH that would be present to GSSG?

<u>Dr. Beuzard</u>: Yes, your point is right. It is impossible in
this experiment to know if there is only the formation of
oxidized glutathione or if cystamine is acting itself on
protein synthesis initiation.

The Red Cell, pages 127—129

<u>Dr. Winterbourn</u>: It may be possible to block the GSH, say
with iodoacetamide, and distinguish between the two possibilities.

<u>Dr. Smith</u>: I would like to take this opportunity to give the
conference an update on another sulfhydryl reagent which
possesses antisickling potency, bis-maleimidomethyl ether (BME).
It is a bifunctional (2 reactive sites per molecule) maleimide compound which reacts with free sulfhydryl groups in an
irreversible fashion with high specificity. The drug easily
enters the red cell adn does have significant non-hemoglobin
sulfhydryl binding reacting with the fastest liganding sulfhydryl groups first i.e. glutathione. Like cystamine it increases the oxygen affinity of reacted red cells and hemolysates.

It will decrease the sickled and intermediate forms by one-
half in thoroughly deoxygenated samples after 25% of the
red cell sulfhydryl groups **have** been bound. This effect is
not appreciably augmented by increasing the sulfhydryl
ligation. The most interesting observation we have made
is that about one half of its "antisickling effect" resides
in the production of an <u>eccentrocyte</u> cell i.e. a disco-
stomatocytic cell in which the hemoglobin is unevenly distributed to one side of the cell leaving a large slip of hemoglobin sparse membrane. It looks like a half-sickle cell with
asynchrony of hemoglobin and membrane. This is specific for
BME-deoxygenated sickel red cells and is not observed with
AA red cells or monofunctional sulfhydryl blockade reagents.
Upon reoxygenation the cells assume their usual discoid form.
The percentage of these cells is more or less constant after
25% of the sulfhydryl groups have been liganded. Our preliminary experiments do not suggest an easy explanation for this
cell. Permeability measurements (MCHC, K+) and membrane
pliability measurements (filterability and micropipette)
performed on a 50% liganded cell are not unusual. We have
verified the irreversibility of the chemical bond within the
red cell and assured ourselves of adequate deoxygenation of
the sample by spectral assessment. We do not see significant
changes in minimum gelling concentration at this dosage of
the drug. Our current working assumption is that BME alters
the usual sickle red cell hemoglobin-membrane relationship
or affects some later stage in hemoglobin polymer organization. My question to the group is whether anyone has observed
this type of cell in various manipulations of sickle red cells
or in AA red cells. We would like to obtain some sort of a

lead into more specific arenas of future investigation.

Dr. Brewer: I have one question of Dr. Beuzard. Do you think that the antisickling effects that you're seeing are primarily oxygen-affinity related?

Dr. Beuzard: It's probably a combination of different mechanisms. Maybe the more important is the effect of the oxygen affinity but cystamine has also a direct effect on polymerization in the absence of oxygen and it has also an effect on the Bohr effect and the 2,3-DPG effect, and all are concurring to inhibit the sickling. The last effect I did not speak about is a slight swelling of the cell and a decrease of 1% on the Hb concentration of the cell which also diminishes the sickling process.

POST-TRANSLATIONAL CONTROL OF HUMAN HEMOGLOBIN SYNTHESIS;
THE NUMBER OF α CHAIN GENES AND THE SYNTHESIS OF HB S.

A. Felice, E. C. Abraham, A. Miller, N. Cope,
M. Gravely, and T.H.J. Huisman
Departments of Cell and Molecular Biology, and
Medicine, and Comprehensive Sickle Cell Center,
Medical College of Georgia, and Veterans Admin-
istration Hospital, Augusta, Ga. 30901.

INTRODUCTION

Numerous studies have shown that the synthesis of hemoglobin α chains in man is under the control of two structural
genes per chromosome (for references see Milner and Huisman,
1976). However, some persons may have four α genes (the
αα/αα arrangement), others three (-α/αα) and others two
(-α/-α). A person with the -α/-α genic arrangement has hematological features resembling those of the thalassemia-1
heterozygote of East Asian populations (with the --/αα genic
arrangement). The basic difference between these two α-thal-
assemic conditions will readily explain the rarity of Hb H
disease (with the --/-α arrangement) and the absence of
hydrops fetalis (with the --/-- arrangement) in a population,
such as the black population of the USA, in which the incidence of the --/αα type of α-thalassemia is extremely low
but that of the -α/-α type is perhaps 2 to 3% (Huisman, 1977).
Alpha-chain deficiency due to the -α/-α genic arrangement
results in the presence of about 5% Hb Bart's (γ_4) at birth
and an unbalanced *in vitro* chain synthesis which is evident
throughout adult life (Altay *et al*, 1977). The milder form
of deficiency (the -α/αα genic arrangement) results in the
presence of much smaller quantities of Hb Bart's at birth
(1-2%) and a nearly balanced *in vitro* chain synthesis; Extension of these data to children with a Hb S or Hb C heterozygosity who, at birth, had 5% Hb Bart's showed low percentages of the β chain variant (< 30%), decreased MCV and MCH
values, and an unbalanced *in vitro* chain synthesis (Huisman,
1977). Thus, it appears that a decrease in active number of
α chain genes affects the level of (certain) β chain variants

The Red Cell, pages 131—153

in heterozygotes. This was even more clearly demonstrated through studies of a large number of families with a heterozygosity for Hb S, Hb C and Hb Leslie ($\alpha_2\beta_2$ ^{131}Gln$\rightarrow$0 (Lutcher *et al*, 1976)) in which a trimodality for these variants was observed (Huisman, 1977). Variation in α gene dosage apparently affects the percentages of these β chain variants in heterozygotes mainly through a post-translational control mechanism because an overt preference of α^A chains for β^A chains over β^{Leslie} and β^S chains was observed when the relative affinities of these β chains for α chains were measured in appropriate mixtures of isolated chains (Abraham and Huisman, in press).

This communication describes the results of quantitative analyses in heterozygotes within families, and in persons who are heterozygous for an α chain variant and are either heterozygous or homozygous for Hb S. Data from *in vitro* recombination experiments involving various isolated abnormal α chains and normal β chains suggest that post-translational control is also a factor in determining the level of certain α chain variants in heterozygotes. *In vitro* chain synthesis and degradation kinetics were studied in the reticulocytes from four patients with sickle cell anemia, two with the assumed $\alpha\alpha/\alpha\alpha$; β^S/β^S genic arrangement, one with the $-\alpha^G/-\alpha$; β^S/β^S, and one with the $-\alpha/-\alpha$; β^S/β^S genic arrangement. The results of these analyses indicate that post-translational control is an important phase in protein synthesis in the reticulocyte; a reduced α gene dose (as in the $-\alpha/-\alpha$; β^S/β^S genic arrangement) results in excess β^S chains which are readily hydrolyzed by (ill-defined) proteolytic mechanisms, and in a decreased cellular content of Hb S which is potentially of benefit in sickle cell anemia.

MATERIALS AND METHODS

Patients

Numerous members of several black families, all but the caucasian families with either the Hb St. Luke's (α_2 ^{95}Pro$\rightarrow$Arg β_2 (Bannister *et al*, 1972)) or the Hb Rampa (α_2 ^{95}Pro$\rightarrow$Serβ_2 (de Jong *et al*, 1971)) variant residing in the state of Georgia, participated in this study. Some were heterozygous for Hb G-Georgia (α_2 ^{95}Pro$\rightarrow$Leuβ_2 (Huisman *et al*, 1970)), Hb G-Lloyd ($\alpha_2^x\beta_2$), Hb G-Montgomery (α_2 ^{48}Leu$\rightarrow$Argβ_2 (Brimhall *et al*, 1975)), Hb G-Philadelphia (α_2 ^{68}Asn$\to$Lysβ_2 (Baglioni *et al*, 1961)), or Hb S, or had a heterozygosity for both Hb S and one of these α chain variants. Identification of the variant in each family was made with standard procedures which are reviewed in Huisman and Jonxis, 1977; the radio-immunoassay recently developed in this laboratory by Garver *et al* (1977) greatly aided the identification of Hb G-Philadelphia. The identity of Hb G-Lloyd is still uncertain but the abnormality likely involves an Asp$\to$Asn substitution in αT-9. Four SS patients were also included; three were regular visitors to the out-patient facilities of the Center, and one young girl who is also heterozygous for Hb G-Philadelphia was attending the Pediatric out-patient clinic. Informed consent was obtained. Usually 5 to 20 ml of blood was collected in a vacutainer with EDTA as anticoagulant.

Hematological Methods and Hemoglobin Analysis

Blood counts and red cell indices were obtained with a Coulter Counter Model S. Hemoglobin electrophoresis was performed on starch gel (Efremov *et al*, 1969) and Hb F was determined by alkali denaturation (Betke *et al*, 1959). Hemoglobins were quantified by elution from DEAE-cellulose columns (Abraham *et al*, 1976). This method gives excellent separations; for instance, it allows the quantitation of eight different hemoglobins in a blood sample of a patient with the Hb S-G-Georgia condition (Fig. 1, top panel). Similar results were obtained for persons with the Hb S-G-Philadelphia condition except that the Hbs A$_2$ and SG ($=\alpha_2{}^G\beta_2{}^S$) did not separate (Fig. 1, bottom panel). Accurate and reproducible data were obtained when the blood sample was analyzed within a few days after collection, stored at 4°C, while the red cell lysate was immediately dialyzed for 24 hrs at 4°C against the first developer.

Recombination of Isolated α and β Chains

The α and β chains (with heme attached) of the six α chain variants (see above) and Hb S have been isolated as PMB derivatives by CM-cellulose or DEAE-cellulose chromatography, and the relative affinities of the β^A and β^S chains for normal and variant α chains determined through quantitation by chromatography of the hemoglobins that were formed when mixtures of the different chains were prepared. The method has been described in detail before (Abraham and Huisman, in press).

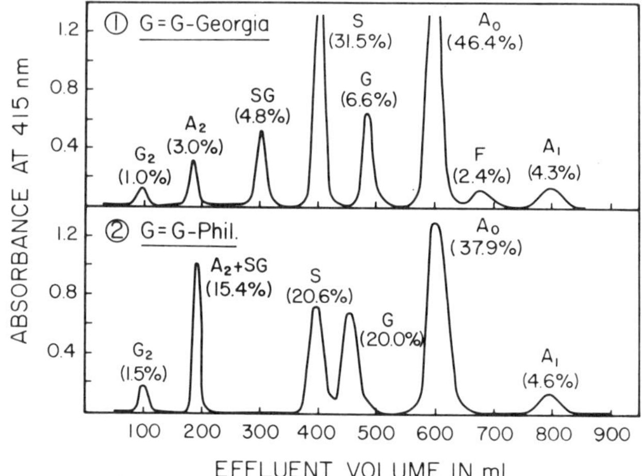

Fig. 1   Separations of hemoglobins in red cell hemolysates
from patients with the S-G-Georgia or the S-G-Philadelphia
condition by DEAE-cellulose chromatography. For details,
see Abraham *et al*, 1976.

Globin Chain Synthesis Analyses

These analyses were limited to blood samples of the four
SS patients. The red cells (with over 10% reticulocytes)
were washed three times in cold reticulocyte saline and incubated with a medium supporting protein synthesis as previously
described (Huisman and Jonxis, 1977). One tenth ml ^{14}C-leu-
cine solution (50 μCi/4 mg/ml) per one ml of cells was added
after 5 minutes of pre-incubation. Aliquots were collected
at various times as indicated later. One larger aliquot of
cells was taken at 20 minutes, washed three times with cold
reticulocyte saline for about 30 minutes, and re-incubated
under the same condition except that 0.1 ml of ^{12}C-leucine
(4 mg/ml) was added per one ml of cells. Again aliquots
were collected at various times as discussed later. All
aliquots were washed three times with cold reticulocyte
saline at 4°C, lysed by addition of an equal volume of distilled water, and whole cell globin was prepared with ice-
cold acid acetone (Anson and Mirsky, 1930). This material
(about 30 mg) was analyzed by chromatography on 0.9 x 8 cm
columns with 8 M urea-phosphate developers (150 ml Developer
A = 8 M urea, 0.005 M sodium phosphate, 0.05 M β-mercapto-

ethanol, pH 6.5, and 150 ml Developer B = same solution but
0.04 M in sodium phosphate). Flow rate was 18 ml/hour. OD
readings were made at 280 nm, and radioactivity counting was
done as described before (Huisman and Jonxis, 1977). The results were expressed as the total radioactivity incorporated
into the chains, the specific activity per unit of OD at
280 nm of the individual chains, and as ratios between these
values. Counting errors were less than 10% for all samples.

RESULTS AND DISCUSSION

A. Quantities of Some α Chain Variants in Heterozygotes

The open symbols in Fig. 2 represent the relative quantity of one of six different Hb G-like α chain variants in
each of 77 heterozygotes, and Table 1 summarizes the hematological and hemoglobin composition data. The 14 persons with
Hb G-Georgia were members of two families; all but one had a
Hb G level varying between 12 and 15.5% with normal hemato-

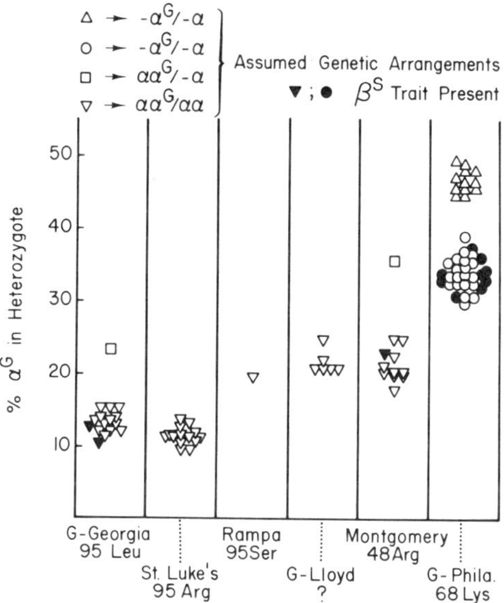

Fig. 2   The percentages of various α chains in heterozygotes.

logy suggesting the presence of four active α genes of which
one is mutated (the $\alpha\alpha^G/\alpha\alpha$ arrangement). One person, the
original Hb G-Georgia heterozygote described before (Huisman
et al, 1970), had consistently higher values over many years
of study; the value of 23.5% given in Table 1 was from a most
recent blood sample. This person always had a slight microcytosis without an overt iron deficiency. It seems probable
that he has only three active α genes (one mutated) and that
the $\alpha\alpha^G/-\alpha$ arrangement fits the available data.

The two additional variants with a substitution at position $\alpha95$ also occur in low quantities in heterozygotes. Hematological data, not listed in Table 1, support the possible
presence of four active α genes in the Hb St. Luke's heterozygotes (the $\alpha\alpha^G/\alpha\alpha$ arrangement) but the number of α chain
genes in the Hb Rampa heterozygote is uncertain.

TABLE 1

Hematological and hemoglobin composition data on persons
heterozygous for one of four α chain variants (average values
only).

Condition	n	Hb g%	PCV l/l	RBC $10^{12}/l$	MCV fl	MCH pg	G_2 %	A_2 %	G %	Total G %
AG-Georgia	13	13.1	.396	4.83	82	26.7	0.8	1.9	13.0	13.8
AG-Georgia	1	14.6	.440	5.55	79	25.9	1.1	1.9	22.4	23.5
AG-Lloyd	6	14.3	.422	4.83	88	29.5	0.3	1.8	21.4	21.7
AG-Montg.	10	13.0	.380	4.44	85	28.3	0.7	2.1	20.3	21.0
AG-Montg.	1	12.7	.389	4.58	83	26.3	0.9	2.0	34.7	35.6
AG-Phil.	19	13.0	.388	4.65	82	26.7	0.9	1.6	33.0	33.9
AG-Phil.	12	12.6	.399	5.64	74	22.0	1.0	1.2	46.0	47.0

The six Hb G-Lloyd heterozygotes (of one family) and ten
of the Hb G-Montgomery heterozygotes (of four families) had
slightly more than 20% of the variant, and a completely normal
hematology. Thus, these persons likely have four active α
genes with one being mutated. One Hb G-Montgomery heterozygote had nearly 36% Hb G; genetic evidence, to be presented
later in Fig. 6, suggests the presence of three active α
genes in this person (the $\alpha\alpha^G/-\alpha$ arrangement).

Data on the 31 Hb G-Philadelphia heterozygotes belonging
to 15 families suggested a bimodal distribution with average
values of 34% and 47%, respectively (Fig. 2 and Table 1). In
none of these the % Hb G was less than 30%. Some of these
families have been discussed before (Milner and Huisman, 1976),
and the $-\alpha^G/\alpha\alpha$ and $-\alpha^G/-\alpha$ genic arrangements have been proposed for the two groups, respectively. The hematological
data given in Table 1 indicated an appreciable decrease in
both the MCV and MCH values of the heterozygotes with the 47%
Hb G-Philadelphia; these values were comparable to those presented earlier.

The assessment of the genetic α chain gene arrangement
in these heterozygotes is based on the relative amounts of
the variant, the hematological observations, and on data from
family studies (*f.i.* one Hb G-Philadelphia heterozygote with
35% G has a Hb G homozygote who does not make Hb A (Milner and
Huisman, 1976) The data of Fig. 2 indicate not only differences in quantities of α chain variants within families but
also between persons with presumably the same number of active
α genes but with different types of α chain variants (the same
has been observed for many other α chain variants, Huisman
and Jonxis, 1977; Rucknagel and Winter, 1974). Two groups
can be recognized; in one (heterozygotes for Hbs G-Georgia,
St. Luke's, and perhaps Rampa with the $\alpha\alpha^X/\alpha\alpha$ arrangement)
the average percentage of Hb G is about 13% while in the
second (heterozygotes for Hbs G-Lloyd, G-Montgomery, and
likely also G-Philadelphia (Baine *et al*, 1976) with the
$\alpha\alpha^G/\alpha\alpha$ arrangement) the average percentage of Hb G is 21 to
22%. These differences may in part be explained by an instability of certain variants (for ref. see Huisman and Jonxis,
1977; Bunn *et al*, 1977)); however, the Hbs G-Georgia, St.
Luke's and Rampa are not heat labile and their occurrence is
not associated with a Heinz Body type of hemolytic anemia. Another contributing factor to be considered is the possibility
that the nature of the substitution in the α chain affects
the rate of dimer ($\alpha^X\beta$) or tetramer ($\alpha_2^X\beta_2$) formation. Data
from *in vitro* recombination experiments involving β^A and α^A
chains and α^X chains, presented in Fig. 3, indicate that indeed considerable differences do exist in the quantities of
hemoglobin variant recovered from these mixtures. The first
experiment was designed to maintain a constant ratio between
α^A and α^X chains but to vary the ratio between β and total
α chains. The % Hb G present in mixtures involving either
one of the three variants G-Lloyd, G-Montgomery or G-Philadelphia was independent of the β/α ratio and averaged about

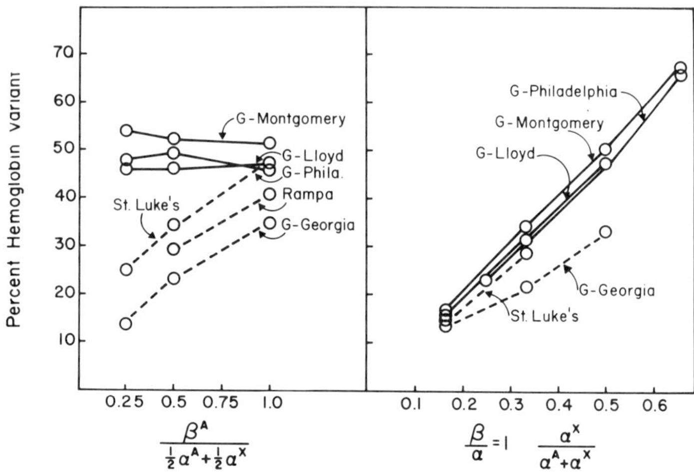

$$\frac{\beta^A}{\frac{1}{2}\alpha^A + \frac{1}{2}\alpha^X} \qquad\qquad \frac{\beta}{\alpha} = 1 \qquad \frac{\alpha^X}{\alpha^A + \alpha^X}$$

Fig. 3   The relative amounts of the α chain variants present in mixtures prepared by combining free α chains with free β chains in ratios as indicated. The percentages are based on the amount of hemoglobin isolated from each DEAE-cellulose column.

the expected 50%. However, when α chains of the Hbs G-Georgia, St. Luke's or Rampa were mixed with α^A and β^A chains, the formation of the variant was greatly dependent upon the β/α ratio and only some 15–25% of Hb G was present in mixtures in which the ratio between β^A chains and a mixture of equal amounts of α^A and α^X chains was 4 to 1 (Fig. 3). These data suggest that in conditions of relative α chain deficiency the formation of Hb A is favored over that of the G-Georgia, St. Luke's or Rampa variants. The results obtained for similar mixtures but with a constant β/α ratio and a variable ratio of α^A and α^X chains are shown in the right panel of Fig. 3. The expected percentages were obtained for mixtures involving either G-Lloyd, G-Montgomery or G-Philadelphia but the limited number of experiments with G-Georgia (and perhaps with St. Luke's) again suggests a decreased formation of the variant. These results indicate that for certain α chain variants with rather critical substitutions such as those involving prolyl residue in position 95 the formation of

dimers and/or tetramers is impaired and that the formation
of Hb A is favored over that of the variant.

B. Quantities of Some α Chain Variants and of Hb S in Persons
    with a Heterozygosity for Both (designated as ASAG).

This study involved 10 persons with the ASAG-Philadelphia
condition (from five families; two families had one case each,
two had two cases each, and one had four ASAG members (see
also Fig. 7)), two with the ASAG-Georgia condition (one in
each of the two families), and one with the ASAG-Montgomery
condition (see also Fig. 6). Hematological data and hemoglobin composition data are given in Table 2. All persons with
ASAG-Philadelphia had slightly decreased MCV and MCH values.
The % total Hb G (=G+G_2) averaged 35.6% (range 33.8-37.5);
these values are comparable to those of Hb G-Philadelphia
heterozygotes of the "35% G" category with the $-\alpha^G/\alpha\alpha$ genic
arrangement (Fig. 2). Similar values have been obtained by
others (Huisman and Jonxis, 1977; Rucknagel and Winter, 1974;
Baine *et al*, 1976; Rucknagel and Rising, 1975; McCurdy *et al*,
1975; Charache *et al*, 1977, *a.o.*).

Results from previous analyses involving Hb S heterozygotes which were described before (Huisman, 1977) and referred
to earlier in this paper, have indicated that persons with
a more limited number of active α genes have lesser amounts
of Hb S and lower MCV and MCH values. These and additional
data are again illustrated in Fig. 4; the study involved 34
AS persons with the assumed αα/αα genic arrangement, 28 with
the -α/αα arrangement and 8 with the -α/-α genic arrangement.
Distinct differences were apparent between the -α/-α; β^A/β^S
and αα/αα; β^A/β^S categories and between the -α/-α; β^A/β^S
and -α/αα; β^A/β^S categories but the differences between the
-α/αα; β^A/β^S amd αα/αα; β^A/β^S categories were considerably
less striking, except for that between the percentages of
Hb S. As expected, the percent Hb S in the persons with
ASAG-Philadelphia who presumably have the $-\alpha^G/\alpha\alpha$; β^A/β^S genic
arrangement varied between 30.7 and 37.5 (average 34.1%,
Table 2) and was the same as that in Hb S heterozygotes without the G-Philadelphia variant but the presumed -α/αα genic
arrangement. *In vitro* recombination experiments involving
mixtures of α^A, β^A, and β^S chains, to be published elsewhere
(Abraham and Huisman, in press) have suggested a decreased
formation of Hb S in conditions of a relative α chain

TABLE 2

Hematological and hemoglobin composition data on persons who are heterozygous
for Hb S and for either Hb G-Philadelphia, Hb G-Georgia or Hb G-Montgomery.

Case	Sex Age	Hb g/dl	PCV l/l	RBC $10^{12}/l$	MCV fl	MCH pg	MCHC %	G_2 %	A_2+SG[a] %	S %	G %	Total G %	Total S %
Subjects with Hb S and Hb G-Philadelphia													
L.Z.	F-7	12.6	.377	4.96	75	24.0	32.7	0.8	14.5	19.5	22.0	35.3	32.0
K.C.	F-11	13.0	.388	4.89	78	25.2	32.7	0.9	14.5	21.6	20.2	33.8	34.1
H.K.	F-30	10.7	.314	3.92	78	25.8	33.2	1.1	16.9	19.2	21.5	37.5	34.1
J.K.	M-8	11.6	.342	4.42	76	24.9	33.2	1.1	16.8	20.6	20.7	36.6	35.4
C.H.	F-39	14.0	.400	5.42	72	24.5	34.4	0.8	16.8	22.7	20.7	36.3	37.5
C.C.	F-24	14.4	.438	5.35	80	25.5	32.1	0.9	15.1	20.3	20.2	34.2	33.4
M.C.	M-6	13.6	.405	5.34	74	24.1	32.9	1.0	15.5	20.0	19.7	34.2	33.5
J.H.	M-2	–	.265	–	–	–	–	1.2	14.0	18.7	24.0	37.2	30.7
W.R.	M-12	15.6	.416	5.29	77	28.0	36.8	1.4	15.4	20.6	20.0	34.8	34.0
G.R.	M-14	14.9	.435	5.75	74	24.5	33.4	1.5	16.4	21.6	20.5	36.4	36.0
(average)		(13.4)	(.378)	(5.04)	(76)	(25.2)	(33.5)	(1.1)	(15.6)	(20.5)	(21.0)	(35.6)	(34.1)
Subjects with Hb S and Hb G-Georgia													
J.L.	M-11	11.9	.347	4.72	73	24.8	34.5	0.8	2.9±3.9	31.4	5.6	10.3	35.3
J.N.	M-5	11.1	.316	4.35	72	25.1	35.3	1.0	3.0±4.8	31.5	6.6	12.4	36.3
(average)		(11.5)	(.332)	(4.54)	(73)	(25.0)	(34.9)	(0.9)	(3.0±4.4)	(31.5)	(6.1)	(11.4)	(35.9)
Subject with Hb S and Hb G-Montgomery													
L.W.	F-13	13.3	.392	4.53	85	27.9	33.3	0.4	10.6	30.2	14.6	23.6	38.8

a. Samples from persons with the ASAG-Philadelphia condition or with the ASAG-Montgomery
condition are assumed to contain 2.0% Hb A_2.

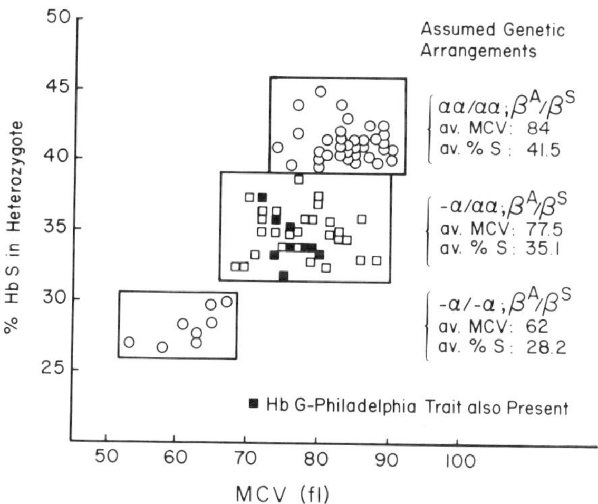

Fig. 4 The relationship between the MCV values and the percentages of Hb S in heterozygotes. For details, see text.

deficiency. The data presented in Fig. 5 indicate among others that less than 35% Hb S (instead of the expected 50%) was present in a mixture with α^A, β^A and β^S being present in a ratio of 1:1:1. (Even more striking decreases were observed when the β^S chain was replaced by the β chain of the Hb Leslie variant, but were absent when mixtures of α^A, β^A and β^N chains were analyzed). Thus, it appears that a relative α chain deficiency due to a limited number of α chain structural genes may influence the level of Hb S in heterozygotes through this mechanism to the extent that less than 30% is present in persons with the $-\alpha/-\alpha$; β^A/β^S genic arrangement and slightly more than 40% in persons with the $\alpha\alpha/\alpha\alpha$; β^A/β^S genic arrangement. The simultaneous presence of Hb G-Philadelphia apparently does not affect the level of Hb S in heterozygotes.

Similar observations have been made in the two children with ASAG-Georgia (Table 2). Both had slightly decreased MCV and MCH values but Hb G percentages as expected for persons with the $\alpha\alpha^G/\alpha\alpha$ genic arrangement. The percentages of Hb S (= sum of % SG and % S) were surprisingly low because values above 40% have consistently been found in persons with

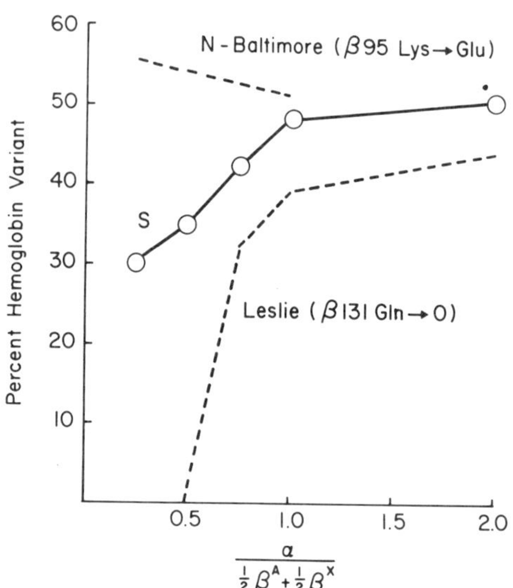

Fig. 5 The relative amounts of Hb S present in mixtures prepared by combining free α chains with a mixture of equal amounts of free β^A and β^S chains in ratios as indicated (from Abraham and Huisman, in press).

the $\alpha\alpha/\alpha\alpha$; β^A/β^S genic arrangement (Fig. 4). The low values of about 36% cannot easily be explained without additional data from *in vitro* recombination experiments which have not been carried out.

Fig. 6 presents the pedigree of the family of a 13 year old girl with the ASAG–Montgomery condition, while hematological and hemoglobin composition data are summarized in Table 3. Two siblings of the proposita (a 1 year old half-sister, S.M., and F.W., a 9 year old brother) had a Hb G heterozygosity with 23 to 25% Hb G suggesting an $\alpha\alpha^G/\alpha\alpha$ genic arrangement (the low MCV value of 68 fl in S.M. is inconsistent but might be due to a nutritional deficiency). The mother, P.M., with near normal hematological values had a surprisingly high level (35.6%) of Hb G and, consequently, had only three active α structural genes (the $\alpha\alpha^G/-\alpha$ genic arrangement). The proposita apparently inherited an $\alpha\alpha^G$ cistron from her mother and an $\alpha\alpha$ cistron from her father (who is deceased) because both the % Hb G (23%) and the %

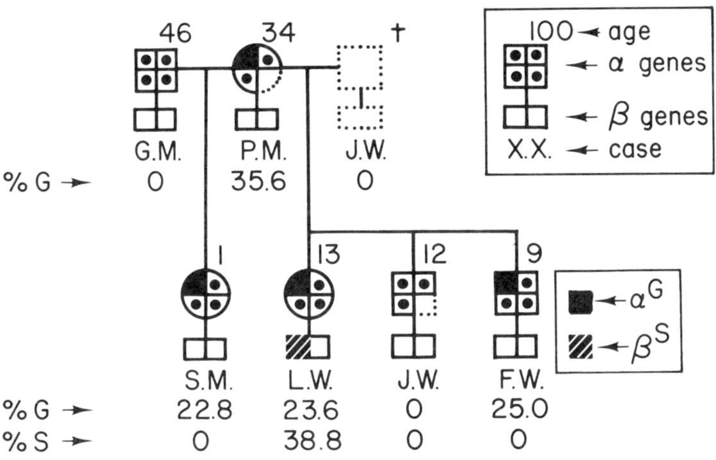

Fig. 6   Pedigree of family M. with Hb S and Hb G—Montgomery.

Hb S (39%) as well as the hematological values were consis-
tent with the $\alpha\alpha^G/\alpha\alpha$; β/β^S genic arrangement. If these genetic considerations are correct her brother, J.W., who has no
Hb variant(s), obligatorily has the $\alpha\alpha/-\alpha$ genic arrangement.

TABLE 3

Hematological and hemoglobin composition data on
members of Fam. M. with Hb G—Montgomery

Case[a]	Condition	Hb g%	PCV l/l	RBC $10^{12}/l$	MCV fl	G_2 %	A_2(+SG) %	G %	S %
G.M.	AA	16.2	.479	5.51	85	0	2.6	0	0
P.M.	AG	12.7	.389	4.58	83	0.9	1.9	34.7	0
S.M.	AG	11.5	.369	5.33	68	0.3	1.4	22.5	0
L.W.	ASAG[b]	13.3	.392	4.53	85	0.4	10.6[c]	14.6	30.2
J.W.	AA	13.2	.397	4.87	80	0	2.7	0	0
F.W.	AG	11.6	.348	3.97	86	0.4	1.7	24.6	0

a) See pedigree of Fig. 6; *b*) Indicates heterozygosity for
Hb G(=Montgomery) and for Hb S; *c*) Assumed to contain 2% Hb A_2.

C. Quantity of Hb G-Philadelphia in a Patient with a Hetero-
    zygosity for Hb G and a Homozygosity for Hb S (designated
    as SSAG, the A indicating the presence of one or more
    normal α chain structural gene(s)).

Patient D.C.H., a six year old female, was diagnosed at
an early age as having Hb G-Philadelphia and a homozygosity
for Hb S. This child is clinically well without the well-
known symptoms often inherent to the presence of a SS condition. Hematological evaluations were made on numerous occasions, and the data listed in Table 4 are from a sample collected in 1977. A significant finding was the persistantly
low MCV value and the low MCH value. The percentage of Hb SG
($=\alpha_2{}^G\beta_2{}^S$ including Hb A_2) was high, namely 47.2% which placed
this patient in the "45% Hb G" category. Fortunately, exten-
sive family studies were possible (Fig. 7). The patient's
brother (J.H.), cousin (M.C.), mother (C.H.), and aunt (C.C.)
had the ASAG-Philadelphia condition (hematological data can
be found in Table 2); the levels of Hb G (averaged at 35.5%)
and Hb S (averaged at 34%) suggested that all four had the
$-\alpha^G/\alpha\alpha$; β/β^S genic arrangement. The father of the patient
had a Hb S heterozygosity with an intermediate value for Hb S
which likely placed him in the category of Hb S traits with
three active α genes (the $-\alpha/\alpha\alpha$; β/β^S genic arrangement).
These observations together with the hematological data and
the percentage of Hb SG strongly suggest that this girl has
only two active α chain structural loci of which one is mutated, thus the $-\alpha^G/-\alpha$; β^S/β^S genic arrangement.

The condition of this patient is in sharp contrast to
that of a 15 year old black girl, described by Charache *et
al* (1977); the latter patient also had the SSAG condition but
suffered from a rather severe disease with many complications
and hospital admissions. Hematological values, reported in
Table 1 of the quoted reference were: Hb 6.6 g/dl; PCV
0.187 l/l; RBC 1.97 x $10^{12}/l$; MCV 94 fl; MCH 33.4 pg; MCHC
35.2% while the proportion of electrophoretically separable
hemoglobin components showed a Hb SG(+ Hb A_2) level of 32.9%
and a Hb G_2 level of 1.7% (Table 2 of same reference). Un-
doubtedly, the $-\alpha^G/\alpha\alpha$; β^S/β^S genic arrangement fits the published data. The difference in clinical expression of these
two closely related conditions is most striking but rather
difficult to explain without further investigations.

TABLE 4

Hematological data of four patients with Sickle Cell Anemia.

	D.C.H.*	S.B.	B.H.	E.E.
Sex and age	F-6	F-23	F-21	F-17
Electrophoresis	S+SG	SS	SS	SS
Hb A_2 (%)	–	3.3	2.6	3.1
Hb F_{AD} (%)	7.2	5.6	1.9	5.1
Hb (g/dl)	9.9	11.5	7.6	9.1
PCV (l/l)	0.296	0.329	0.201	0.248
RBC ($10^{12}/l$)	4.33	4.70	2.46	2.49
MCV (fl)	67	68	88	97
MCH (pg)	21.7	23.3	30.4	34.8
MCHC (%)	32.8	34.3	34.4	35.9
% Hb S in father	33*	35	42	46
% Hb S in mother	37*	34	44	42
Assumed genic arrangement	$-\alpha^G/-\alpha;$ β^S/β^S	$-\alpha/-\alpha;$ β^S/β^S	$\alpha\alpha/\alpha\alpha;$ β^S/β^S	$\alpha\alpha/\alpha\alpha;$ β^S/β^S

*   See Figure 7.

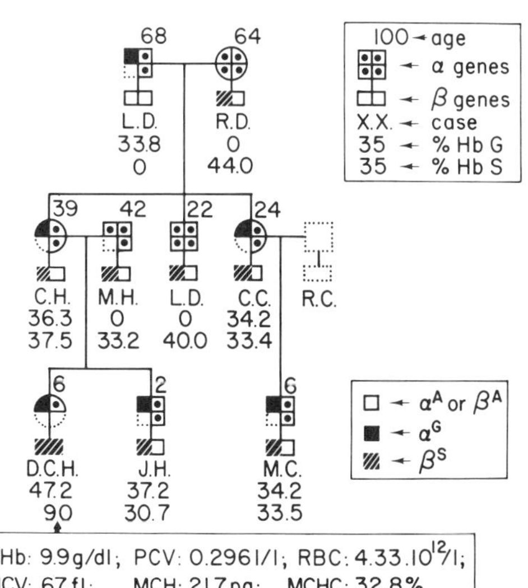

Fig. 7   Pedigree of family H. with Hb S and Hb G-Philadelphia.

D. Synthesis Analyses in Sickle Cell Anemia Patients with
   Different Number of Active α Chain Structural Genes.

These studies were made in four patients (Table 4) of
whom patient D.C.H. was discussed above. The other three
were females belonging to large families which have recently
been studied in great detail (P. F. Milner *et al*, in preparation). Results of these family studies, the hematological
data, and the quantitative data in the parents of the patients
(some of this information is included in Table 4) had led to
the conclusion that one girl (S.B.) has the $-\alpha/-\alpha$; β^S/β^S
genic arrangement while the other two (E.E. and B.H.) have
four active α chain gene loci (the $\alpha\alpha/\alpha\alpha$; β^S/β^S genic arrangement). The latter two patients had normal MCV and MCH values
and a rather severe course of the disease while S.B. had low
MCV and MCH values comparable to those of D.C.H. (see above)
and a relatively mild clinical course.

The ratios between the total radioactivities incorporated
into the β^S chains and into the α^A chains (E.E., B.H. and S.B.)
or the $\alpha^A + \alpha^G$ chains (D.C.H.) are shown in Fig. 8. The subjects fell into two groups with ratios below and above unity,
respectively. The two patients with the assumed $\alpha\alpha/\alpha\alpha$; β^S/β^S
genic arrangement (E.E. and B.H.) had ratios which at early
incubation times were comparable to those observed in β-thal-
assemia heterozygotes. The apparent imbalance (average value
at 5 to 20 minutes: 0.65) improved slightly with continuous
incubation with ^{14}C-leucine (average value at 120 and 180
minutes: 0.80). The two patients with only one-half the full
complement of active α genes (S.B. and D.C.H.) initially had
ratios of 1.8 at 5 minutes, which fell to about 1 after more
than 120 minutes of incubation. The specific activity ratios
fell in similar patterns, except that the ratios for patients
E.E. and B.H. (with the $\alpha\alpha/\alpha\alpha$; β^S/β^S genic arrangement) were
about 1.0 throughout the entire incubation period (Fig. 8).

The specific activities of the β^S and α^A chains in E.E.
and B.H. increased at comparable rates but the specific activities of the α^A chains in S.B. and of the $\alpha^A + \alpha^G$ chains in
D.C.H. were at all incubation times less than those of the
β^S chains (Fig. 9). The lower specific activity of α chains
in S.B. and D.C.H. supports the assumed genic arrangement in
these patients which were previously assigned on the basis
of hematology, hemoglobin composition analyses, and family
studies. Thus, it appears that β^S chains were synthesized

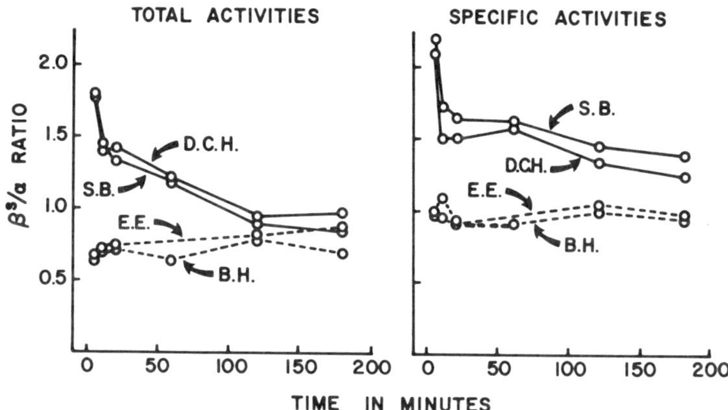

Fig. 8   The ratios of radioactivities of β^S and α chains during *in vitro* incubation of reticulocytes with ^{14}C-leucine. The four patients are identified in Table 4.

in excess of α chains because of a reduced number of active α genes, and that uncombined β^S chains were degraded during the post-translational metabolism of chains without giving rise to severe hematological stigmata of thalassemia except for microcytosis and hypochromia.

The specific activities of the chains observed during re-incubation with ^{12}C-leucine of previously labelled reticulocytes are given in Fig. 10. These experiments were designed to study the fate of previously labelled chains because this type of study will identify chains that are preferentially degraded after their synthesis on ribosomes. The data of Fig. 10 shows that the activity of the β^S chains in the two patients with the $\alpha\alpha/\alpha\alpha$; β^S/β^S genic arrangement (E.E. and B.H.) was largely constant, but that there was a slight loss of α chain activity. These observations are consistent with the slight increase in the *in vitro* synthesis ratio observed during continuous incubation with ^{14}C-leucine (Fig. 8). On the other hand, there was a fall in the specific activity of the β^S chains in D.C.H. and to a lesser extent in S.B., both having a reduced *in vitro* α chain synthesis (see above) while the specific activity of the α chains did not change.

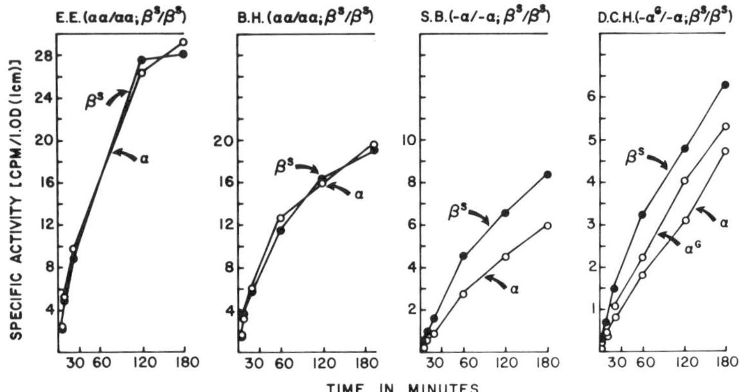

Fig. 9   The specific activities of the β^S, α^A and α^G chains during *in vitro* incubation of reticulocytes with ^{14}C-leucine.   The patients are identified in Table 4.

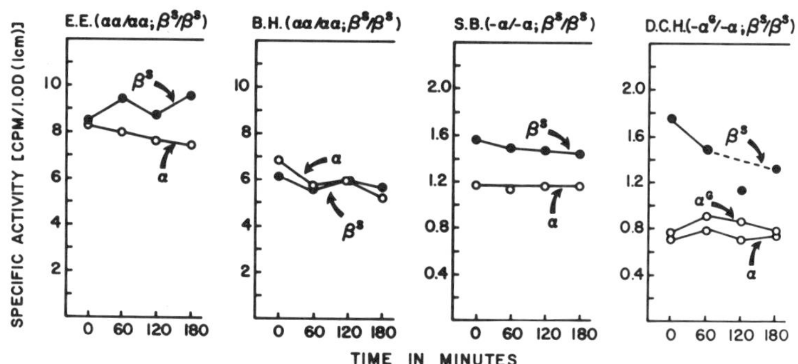

Fig. 10   The specific activities of the β^S, α^A and α^G chains during *in vitro* incubation with ^{12}C-leucine of previously labelled reticulocytes.   The patients are identified in Table 4.

All data are consistent with the hypothesis that S.B. and D.C.H. have a reduced complement of active α genes. The synthesis studies, the finding of Hb G–Philadelphia in the high mode (D.C.H.), and the degree of microcytosis and hypochromia in both patients suggest the presence of only two active α genes; hence, the $-\alpha/-\alpha$; β^S/β^S genic arrangement. The data also indicate that β^S chains which are synthesized in excess of the available α chains are preferentially degraded; thus, after continuous incubation with ^{14}C-leucine a nearly balanced synthesis is observed despite an initial discrepancy.

CONCLUSIONS

Considerable insight has been gained into the polymorphism of α chain loci, the genetics of α thalassemia in black Americans and oriental populations and the interaction between β chain variants and α chain deficiencies (α-thalassemia) in heterozygotes. Thus, variation in the number of active α chain genes on a pair of chromosomes in human erythroid precursors can adequately explain the hematological heterogeneity of α thalassemia and the finding of several α chain variants in different modes of concentration, with or without hematological abnormality. The expression of a single α chain gene depends very much on the presence or absence of a functioning α chain gene *in cis*, and on the homologous chromosome bearing none, one, or two active α chain genes.

The finding that the α chain variants St. Luke's, Rampa, and G-Georgia in heterozygotes with completely normal hematology and, hence, with the $\alpha\alpha^G/\alpha\alpha$ assumed genic arrangement occur in relatively low concentrations may be indirectly due to the structural abnormality that is present. These hemoglobins have in common a substitution of a prolyl residue in position α95 which is part of the critical $\alpha^1-\beta^2$ contact, and which presumably plays an important role in the stabilization of tetramers. Probably the reduced binding of these abnormal α chains with β chains is caused by a diminished ability of the $\alpha^X\beta$ dimers to form tetramers resulting in a reduction of the relative concentration of these variants from the 20-25% expected, to the 10-13% observed. Somewhat similar observations have been made for some β chain variants in heterozygotes, such as Hb S, Hb C, and Hb Leslie which in *in vitro* recombination experiments were found to have a reduced affinity

for α chains. Thus, the nature of the amino acid substitution
can have a profound effect on the ultimate quantity of the
abnormal hemoglobin that is produced. Some determinants of
primary or higher order structure upon which depends the
relative affinity of α and non-α chains for each other apparently need to be retained by the molecular conformation of
the hemoglobin chains.

The concept of one gene one peptide has in the past been
quantitatively understood to mean that the relative concentration of the products of a polymorphic system reflects the
number of respective structural genes. This may not always
be the case because post-transcriptional or post-translational
control, or both, may have relevant effects on the quantities
of abnormal hemoglobins that are produced. Hemoglobin variants which are found in lower than expected concentration,
and chains synthesized in excess because of a thalassemia
determinant may be somehow degraded after synthesis on ribosomes. This mechanism is believed to be responsible for the
observed trimodality in the relative concentration of some β
chain variants in heterozygotes with four, three, or two
active α chain genes. The study of subjects who are heterozygous for Hb G–Philadelphia and Hb S is of considerably interest in this respect because these persons have features
which are consistent with the $-\alpha^G/\alpha\alpha$ genic arrangement and a
relative concentration of Hb S in the intermediate mode of
concentration. A somewhat higher concentration of Hb S is
present in the subject with the Hb G–Montgomery–Hb S condition
supporting hematological features consistent with the $\alpha\alpha^G/\alpha\alpha$
genic arrangement.

In vitro synthesis and degradation studies of the present investigation concerned four Hb S homozygotes of whom
two have been assigned the $\alpha\alpha/\alpha\alpha$; β^S/β^S genic arrangement,
while the third presumably has the $-\alpha^G/-\alpha$; β^S/β^S and the
fourth the $-\alpha/-\alpha$; β^S/β^S genic arrangement. Although all four
have nearly balanced *in vitro* synthesis ratios after prolonged
incubation with ^{14}C–leucine, important differences are observed in the pattern of synthesis kinetics. The data clearly
show that the ratios at early incubation times more accurately
reflect the different genetic status. This finding has important practical and theoretical significances. First, the
finding of a balanced or nearly balanced *in vitro* synthesis
ratio after 120 minutes incubation in Hb S homozygotes does
not necessarily exclude the diagnosis of an α chain deficiency. Secondly, it appears that in these patients too, post-

translational degradation of excess β^S chains plays an important part in determining the ultimate amount of Hb S that is
formed. Whereas the two subjects with four active α chain
genes have an [MCH-β^S] of 14.9 and 16.5 pg/cell, respectively,
those with two active α chain genes have an [MCH-β^S] of only
10.1 and 11.0 pg/cell, respectively. A reduced number of
active α chain genes (or α thalassemia) has a beneficial effect on the hematological and clinical expression of sickle
cell anemia because the post-translational control of hemoglobin synthesis is modified in such a way that the proteolytic degradation of free β^S chains is promoted and the production of Hb S is decreased.

ACKNOWLEDGEMENT

The authors thank Cordell Bragg, Mrs. M. Stallings, and
Mrs. S. M. Mayson for capable technical assistance. This
research was in part supported by U. S. Public Health Service Research Grants HLB-05168 and HLB-15158.

REFERENCES

1. Abraham EC, Huisman THJ (in press). Differences in
     affinity of variant β chains for α chains: A possible
     explanation for the variation in the percentages of β
     chain variants in heterozygotes. HEMOGLOBIN
2. Abraham EC, Reese A, Stallings M, Huisman THJ (1976).
     Separation of human hemoglobins by DEAE-cellulose
     chromatography using glycine-KCN-NaCl developers.
     HEMOGLOBIN 1:27.
3. Altay C, Ringelhann B, James L, Gravely M and Huisman THJ
     (1977). Hemoglobin α chain deficiency in black children
     with variable quantities of hemoglobin Bart's at birth.
     Ped Res 11:147.
4. Anson ML, Mirsky AE (1930). Protein coagulation and its
     reversal. The preparation of insoluble globin
     and heme. J Gen Physiol 13:469.
5. Baglioni C, Ingram VM (1961). Abnormal human haemoglo-
     bins. V. Chemical investigation of haemoglobins A, G,
     C, X from one indifidual. Biochim Biophys Acta 48:253.
6. Baine RM, Rucknagel DL, Dublin PA Jr., Adams JG III (1976).
     Trimodality in the proportion of hemoglobin G-Philadel-
     phia in heterozygotes: Evidence for heterogeneity in
     the number of human α chain loci. Proc. Natl. Acad.

Sci USA 73(10):3633.

7. Bannister WH, Grech JL, Plese CF, Smith LL, Barton BP, Wilson JB, Reynolds CA, Huisman THJ (1972). Hemoglobin St. Luke's or α_2 ^{95}Arg(G2)β_2. Europ J Biochem 29:301.

8. Betke K, Marti HR, Schlicht I (1959). Estimation of small percentages of foetal haemoglobin. Nature 184:1877.

9. Brimhall B, Jones RT, Schneider RG, Hosty TS, Tomlin G, and Atkins R (1975). Hemoglobin Alabama [β 39 (C5) Gln→Lys] and hemoglobin Montgomery [α 48 (CD6) Leu→Arg]. Biochimica Biophys Acta 379:28.

10. Bunn HF, Forget BG, and Ranney HM (1977). "Human Hemoglobins." Philadelphia:Saunders.

11. Charache S, Zinkham WH, Dickerman JD, Brimhall B, Dover GJ (1977). Hemoglobin SS, SS/G$_{Philadelphia}$ and SO$_{Arab}$ Diseases. Am J Med 62:439.

12. DeJong WWW, Bernini LF, Meera Khan P (1971). Haemoglobin Rampa: α ^{95}Pro→Ser. Biochim Biophys Acta 236:197.

13. Efremov GD, Huisman THJ, Smith LL, Wilson JB, Kitchens JL, Wrightstone RN, Adams HR (1969). Hemoglobin Richmond, a human hemoglobin which forms hybrids with other hemoglobins. J Biol Chem 244:6105.

14. Garver FA, Baker MM, Jones CS, Gravely M, Altay G, Huisman THJ (1977). Radioimmunoassay for abnormal hemoglobins. Science 196:1334.

15. Huisman THJ (1977). Trimodality in the percentages of β chain variants in heterozygotes: The effect of the number of active Hb α structural loci. HEMOGLOBIN 1:349.

16. Huisman THJ, Adams HR, Wilson JB, Efremov GD, Reynolds CA, Wrightstone RN (1970). Hb G Georgia or α_2 ^{95}Leu(G2)β_2. Biochim Biophys Acta 200:576.

17. Huisman THJ, Jonxis JHP (1977). "The Hemoglobinopathies, Techniques for Identification." New York:Marcel Dekker, Inc.

18. Lutcher CL, Wilson JB, Gravely ME, Stevens PD, Chen CJ, Lindeman JG, Wong SC, Miller A, Gottlieb M, Huisman THJ (1976). Hb Leslie, an unstable hemoglobin due to deletion of glutaminyl residue β131 (H9) occurring in association with β^0-thalassemia, Hb C and Hb S. Blood 47:99.

19. McCurdy PR, Sherman AS, Kamuzora H, Lehmann H (1975). Globin synthesis in subjects doubly heterozygous for hemoglobin G-Philadelphia and hemoglobin S or C. J Lab Clin Med 85:891.

20. Milner PF, Huisman THJ (1976). Studies on the proportion
    and synthesis of haemoglobin G Philadelphia in red cells
    of heterozygotes, a homozygote, and a heterozygote for
    both haemoglobin G and α thalassaemia. Brit J Haemat
    34:207.
21. Rucknagel DL, Rising JA (1975). A heterozygote for
    Hb-β^S, Hb- β^C and Hb-α^G Philadelphia in a family pre-
    senting evidence for heterogeneity of hemoglobin alpha
    chain loci. Am J Med 59:53.
22. Rucknagel DL, Winter WP (1974). Duplication of structural
    genes for hemoglobin α and β chains in man. Annals
    N Y Acad Sci 241:80.

DISCUSSION

<u>Dr. Carrell</u>: I would first like to make a comment and then ask a question. The comment partly reflects on the earlier talk by Dr. Rucknagel. This morning we found several cases of hemoglobin G Philadelphia with a percentage of about 20 per cent in a family from an island next door to the island of Tangariki and undoubtedly of the same genetic stock as the Tangariki people. This is evidence that in the Melanesian, the situation is the same as one suspects in the Negro.. There may be, within the one small population, some individuals with four alpha chain genes as this family with 20 per cent G Philadelphia obviously has, and again some instances of people with just the 2 genes as in the homozygous instances of hemoglobin Tangariki. I want to congratulate Professor Huisman on the quality of his quantitative evidence and to stress how important this is. It's very easy, particularly with earlier DEAE sephadex techniques, to include with your abnormal hemoglobin or with the hemoglobin A, the modified hemoglobins from the preceding peak. That is Hb S_1 will contaminate HbA_0 and Hb A_1 will contaminate Hb J. I would imagine the same problem arises with the glycine buffer separation technique?

<u>Dr. Huisman</u>: Before the analysis is made, one of the first things to do is to collect the blood and store it on ice, and make your hemolysate as soon as possible, and dialyze overnight to remove the glutathione. If you do this, and analyze the sample within 24 hours, then the excess production of fast components, both of the normal and of the abnormal type, is minimized. After that you find small quantities of what I call C1, S1, or Leslie L. Usually you can separate these by this new technique and incorporate them into the calculation of the total quantity of the variant.

<u>Dr. Rucknagel</u>: Well, there are some obvious differences, one being the frequency of the 20% phenotype. I thought that you and Paul published in that British Journal of Hematology paper that you had seen 20%?

<u>Dr. Huisman</u>: I guess I have to go back and read that over again. It was an earlier version, but the family that was listed in this slide was of hemoglobin Lloyd. On subsequent structural analysis, it turned out not to be G-Philadelphia.

The Red Cell, pages 155—157

Dr. Rucknagel: Oh, so you didn't have the structure then. Well, we do have the structure on all of ours and we believe that they all are G-Philadelphia. Among your 100 cases there is undoubtedly a large amount of family data. How many independent genes would that reduce to if you correct for ascertainment?

Dr. Huisman: I would assume about 30-40 families. If these families are related or not, we would never know in that area.

Dr. Rucknagel: Well, I didn't say so far because of the short amount of time, but in addition to estimating the double, the 2 A's and the 2 alpha A's and the single alpha A we estimated the alpha A, alpha G chromosome and the single alpha G. There are only 16 independent chromosomes that I can estimate and the ratio is 10:6. I believe it's the 10 double to 6 single with the G on one or the other. So you have a small sample here and I will confess that we had looked at nearly 50 G-Philadelphia before we saw our first 20%.

Dr. Huisman: Maybe I should continue looking for this.

Dr. Rucknagel: You obviously are going to have to continue. The evidence of course is the difference in the alpha/beta ratios and I don't have a good explanation for that either.

Dr. Huisman: Before the chromatographic analysis of the samples have you removed your membranes first? It is important that the stroma is not removed; you may be losing some chains stroma-bound. So the technique is critical.

Dr. Rucknagel: That may be a technical difference between us. We've looked at that in the past and haven't really seen a difference. Have you seen a significant effect?

Dr. Huisman: We have really convinced ourselves that it will make a difference.

Dr. Black: Given that you have two alpha genes on each of two chromosomes, it would seem that the possibility of some sort of misalignment and crossing over is much greater, in which case one of the products would contain a single alpha gene, the other product would contain 3 alpha genes. Have you considered the possibility of more than two alpha genes on one chromosome?

Dr. Huisman: We are very good at that. We have considered four γchain genes on one chromosome. Now we are inclined to drop one of these and add another one instead. It becomes very much speculation.

Dr. Tatsis: Dr. Rucknagel mentioned earlier that I reported about a year ago a set of patients with G-Philadelphia and I found them to have balanced globin chain synthesis. The fact is after I reported it, Dr. Milner mentioned to me that he had several patients with imbalanced globin chain synthesis and also Dr. Lehmann sent me some reprints of his cases. So, I went back and I repeated the synthetic studies and I found that there is statistically significant difference between the normal controls and the G-Philadelphia patients. The Hb G-Philadelphia carriers, as a group, have imbalanced globin chain synthesis with a defect in the αchain production.

Dr. Huisman: Did you separate the stroma?

Dr. Tatsis: Yes, I did. In other words, I don't separate the stroma for the preparation of globin. What perhaps is another technical problem is the fact that during the warm season, beta chains may elute from the column in the void volume so you lose some counts from the beta chain and so you may have balanced synthesis. With respect to the 20% G-Philadelphias, maybe they are an independent mutation of G-Philadelphia. I don't know how many cases there are.

Dr. Rucknagel: There are several from all over the U.S.

Dr. Tatsis: This doesn't exclude independent mutation, if there was a family which then spread all over the U.S. What you expect actually, if you accept Dr. Stamatoyannopoulos' data, is that you should have about 5% of the total G-Philadelphia carriers to have 45% Hb G-Philadelphia, because these are the people that have one αchain gene or an αthal gene in combination with the G-Philadelphia gene.

Dr. Friedman: I would like to add our small experience to that of Professor Huisman. We have studied about 10 or 12 patients in 2 families with alpha G-Philadelphia. They all have balanced globin synthesis and we haven't seen any with 20% alpha G.

KINETICS OF SICKLING OF INTACT ERYTHROCYTES

Hiroshi Mizukami and Betsy Adams

Division of Regulatory Biology and Biophysics,
Department of Biology, Wayne State University,
Detroit, Michigan 48202   USA

INTRODUCTION

It is well known that erythrocytes obtained from anemic
homozygous sickle cell patients undergo sickling upon deoxygenation, and desickling upon oxygenation. However, information is scarce as to the degree of deoxygenation necessary
for the cells to sickle, the degree of reoxygenation necessary for desickling, the rates of sickling and desickling,
and even the reversibility of the oxygen dissociation equilibrium curves of these cells (S-rbc) (Cameron et al., 1975).
In order to answer these questions, we have developed two
instruments, i.e., the rapid oxygen association-dissociation
equilibrium curve analyzer (ROADEA), and the monolayer kinetic
analyzer (MKA). In the former instrument we obtain the oxygen association-dissociation equilibrium curves of the same
small quantity of erythrocytes under both deoxygenating and
reoxygenating conditions. In the latter we obtain the rate
of light intensity loss and gain, which are related to the
sickling and desickling processes of S-rbc.

INSTRUMENTATION FOR EQUILIBRIUM STUDIES

Various methods exist for the continuous determination
of either oxygen association or oxygen dissociation equili-
brim of rbc (Longmuir and Chow, 1970; Duvelleroy et al.,
1970; Rossi-Bernardi et al., 1975; Kiesow et al., 1974).
However, none of these methods allows the determination of
both using the same sample. The instrument described herein
uses less than a drop of blood to obtain continuous curves

The Red Cell, pages 159–174

for both oxygenation and deoxygenation equilibria starting
from any desired level of oxygen saturation. Less than 5 min
is required for each direction of equilibrium determination
(Mizukami et al., 1977).

A simplified diagrammatic sketch of this instrument is
shown in Fig. 1. Whole blood is suspended as a thin liquid
film on EMI micromesh in the thermostated chamber (Fig. 2).

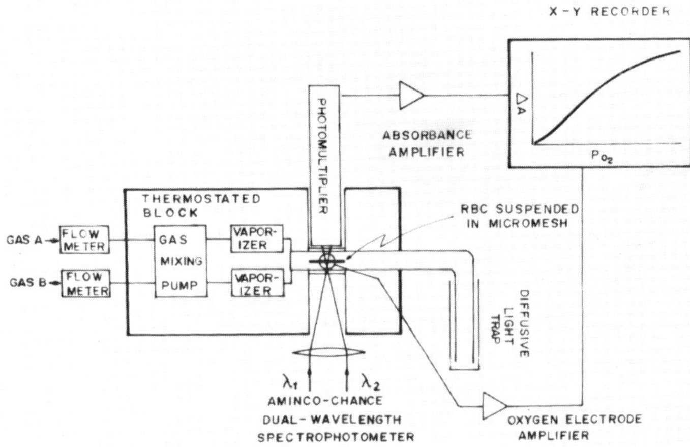

Figure 1. A simplified diagrammatic sketch of the instrument.

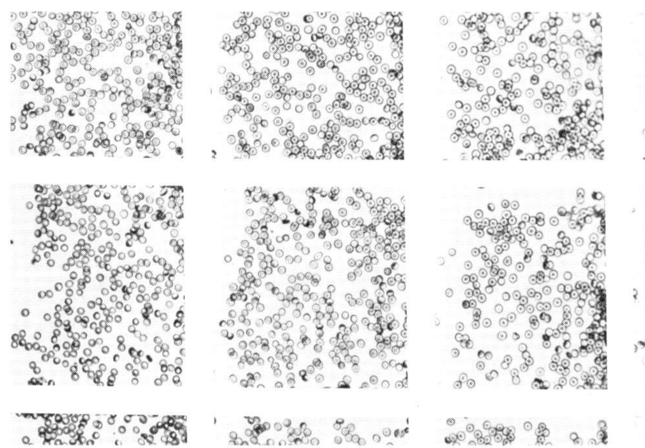

Figure 2. Microscopic photograph of red blood cells suspended
in EMI micromesh No. 100.

The suspended rbc within this reenforced thin film quickly
establish gaseous equilibrium with the surrounding gas. Two
types of gases, A and B, are mixed, saturated with water vapor,
and then pumped at a near-constant net flow rate from the left
of the thermostated chamber. The mixing ratio of the gases
changes continually. However, the rate of change of mixing
is maintained so that rbc suspended in the thin liquid film
are always in equilibrium with the gas, and the rate does not
exceed the response time of the Clark-type electrode. The
electrode, mounted close to the rbc suspension, monitors the
partial pressure of oxygen. The depolarizing current from
the electrode is amplified and fed into the X axis of an
X-Y recorder. Two independent wavelengths, λ_1 and λ_2, are
obtained from an Aminco-Chance dual wavelength spectrophotometer. Normally, λ_1 is set at 431 nm (the Soret band of deoxygenated rbc), and λ_2 is set at 396.5 nm (the isosbestic point).
Spectral changes observed with the end-on photomultiplier
are amplified and fed to the Y axis of the recorder.

EQUILIBRIUM EXPERIMENTS WITH NORMAL AND S-RBC

Blood samples were collected from healthy subjects into
heparinized Vacutainer tubes and were used immediately. All
experiments were carried out at $28 \pm 0.5^{\circ}C$.

One drop of the sample was placed on the micromesh, and
excess blood was removed. The mesh was placed into the reaction chamber which was preflushed with a gas mixture composed
of 5% CO_2, 25% O_2, and 70% N_2 (henceforth referred to as
5% CO_2-O_2 gas). By activating the gas mixing pump, a mixture
composed of 5% CO_2 and 95% N_2 (henceforth referred to as
5% CO_2-N_2 gas) was gradually introduced while the pumping
rate of 5% CO_2-O_2 was reduced. In general, complete exchange
of the two gases was accomplished within approximately 5 min.
The net flow of the gas mixtures was maintained at ca. 200 ml
per min throughout the experiment. After completion of the
gas exchange, i.e., deoxygenation, the process was reversed
by reintroducing 5% CO_2-O_2 gas. Several more experiments were
carried out with the same sample and P_{50} values obtained.

The Bohr effect was tested by performing experiments in
gas mixtures containing 2.5, 5.0 and 10.0% CO_2.

Typical oxygen-rbc equilibrium curves obtained during
the process of deoxygenation (the arrow going from right to

left) and that of reoxygenation (the arrow going from left
to right) are shown in Fig. 3. The X-axis of the recorder was
calibrated with gases containing 25% and 0% O_2, and was converted to read P_{O_2} in mmHg after correcting for vapor pressure

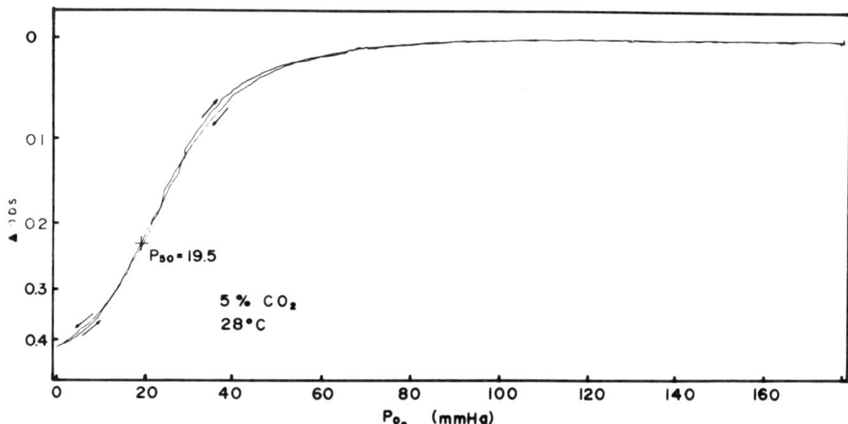

Figure 3. Oxygen association-dissociation equilibrium curves
of whole blood at 28°C in 5.0% CO_2. The direction
of the arrows indicate the change of partial pressure of oxygen.

at that temperature and atmospheric pressure. The Y axis of
the recorder monitored oxygen saturation of rbc's, assuming
the rbc's were fully saturated in gas containing 25% O_2 and
deoxygenated in gas containing 0% O_2. As can be seen in Fig.
3, the equilibrium curves obtained during the process of
deoxygenation and reoxygenation are nearly identical, con-
firming that equilibrium was maintained at all times. The
half-saturation point, P_{50}, thus obtained, is 19.5 mm Hg, and
is close to that tabulated elsewhere (Altman and Dittmer,
1971) at this temperature and CO_2 content.

Figure 4 shows the saturation curves obtained during the
process of deoxygenation using a gas mixture containing 2.5,
5.0 and 10.0% CO_2. The fact that all three curves do not have
identical total absorbance change is primarily due to the differences in the populations of rbc's seen by the photomultiplier. The average P_{50} for gas mixtures containing 2.5, 5.0
and 10.0% CO_2 are 16.8, 19.3 and 24.5 mmHg, respectively.

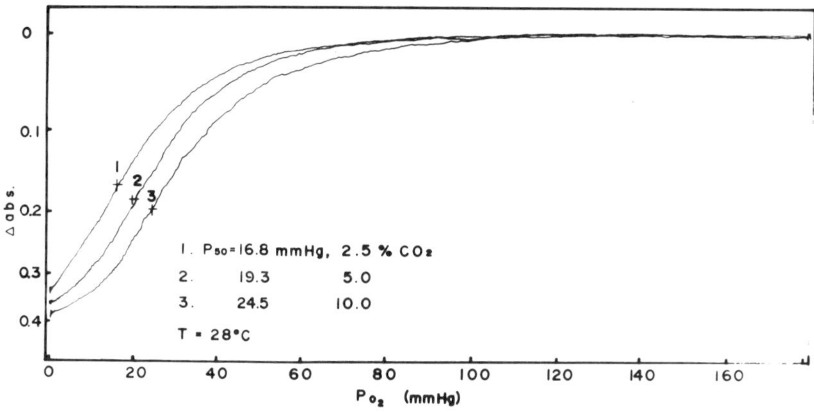

Figure 4. The oxygen dissociation equilibrium curves of whole blood in 2.5, 5.0 and 10.0% CO_2 and at 28°C.

After correcting for temperature and P_{CO_2}, the values obtained are similar to those reported by Altman and Dittmer (1971).

S-rbc were obtained from a homozygous sickle cell anemia patient (HbS 87.0% and HbF 10.5%), and the sample was used within 4 hr after collection of the blood in heparinized Vacutainers. Homozygous sickle cell blood from two other individuals was also tested. However, due to the variability of hemoglobin composition in each individual blood sample, no quantitative comparison among the subjects will be attempted at this time. The tracing of the curve in the direction of either deoxygenation or reoxygenation took approximately 10 min. Although not shown, temporary maintenance at any particular partial pressure of oxygen did not show any significant change in absorbance, indicating that the S-rbc and the environmental gases were in equilibrium.

Typical oxygen association-dissociation equilibrium curves for S-rbc are shown in Fig. 5. The curves obtained during deoxygenation are shown in continuous lines, and those obtained during reoxygenation are shown in broken lines. The heavy lines represent experiments in 10.0% CO_2 and the thin lines represent those in 5% CO_2. As can be seen in each CO_2 system, the curve obtained at the time of reoxygenation is shifted to the right of those obtained during deoxygenation,

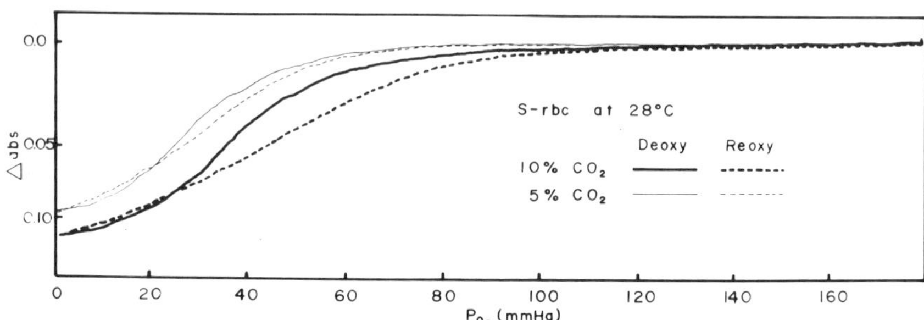

Figure 5.   The oxygen association-dissociation equilibrium of sickle cells at 28°C. The curves obtained during deoxygenation are shown in continuous lines, and those obtained during reoxygenation are shown in broken lines. The heavy lines represent experiments in 10.0% CO_2 and thin lines are for 5.0% CO_2.

thereby displaying hysteresis-like phenomena. Similar experimental results were obtained for the two other homozygous patients.

After replotting the Fig. 5 results as Hill plots, the P_{50} and Hill constant, n (at P_{50}), of each curve are obtained. The results are summarized in Table 1.

TABLE 1

Oxygen Affinity (P_{50}) and Hill's Constant (n) of
Homozygous Sickle Cells Determined at 28°C (Avg. of 3 Runs)

CO_2 (%)	P_{50} (mnHg)		n (at P_{50})	
	Deoxy	Reoxy	Deoxy	Reoxy
5.0	28.2	31.3	3.0	2.7
10.0	31.8	43.7	3.25	2.5

The P_{50} of blood depends upon 2,3-diphosphoglycerate, pH, P_{CO_2}, temperature, and the content of hemoglobin variants. Accordingly, P_{50} values reported here are not necessarily representative of S-rbc. In addition to the hysteresis-like phenomena described, it can be seen that the Hill constants at P_{50} for both CO_2 systems are less at the time of reoxygenation than are those of deoxygenation. The change in the constant was greater for the 10.0% CO_2 system. As has been observed by others (Seakins <u>et al.</u>, 1973; Jayalaskshmi and Seakins, 1976), the Hill constant at P_{50} is relatively small for the equilibrium curve at the time of reoxygenation, but increases considerably as the degree of oxygen saturation increases. This apparent increase in cooperativity in the higher region of oxygenation may be related to the depolymerization of HbS.

KINETIC STUDIES WITH S-RBC

The instrument in use is similar to what has been described earlier, and the reaction chamber is shown in Fig. 6.

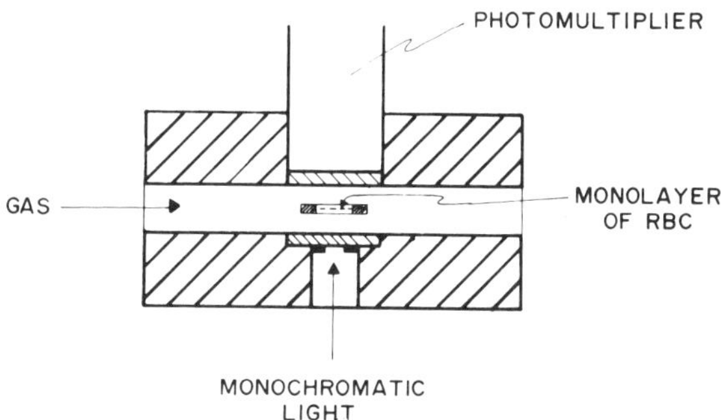

Figure 6.　Schematic representation of the main components of the instrument.

In this procedure, the purging vaporized gases are quickly changed with a solenoid valve from a gas containing oxygen

(25% O_2, 5% CO_2, and 70% N_2) to another without (5% CO_2 and 95% N_2), and _vise_ _versa_. The proper single wavelength is selected with a Bausch and Lomb high intensity grating mono- chromator and the spectral changes are recorded on a storage oscilloscope.

Blood samples obtained were spun, the red blood cells diluted with Krebs- Henseleit buffer (pH 7.4) by a factor of 6, and the plasma concentration adjusted to 2-3%. All experi- ments were performed at $25^{\circ}C \pm 0.5^{\circ}C$.

Three wavelengths (440, 542 and 522 nm) were selected to observe the spectral change. 522 nm is the isosbestic point for oxygenated and deoxygenated red blood cells (Kiesow _et al._, 1972). The flow rates of both purging gases were kept con- stant at 435 ml/min. The estimated lag period for the gas to reach the rbc at this flow rate was 0.25 sec.

Samples from four different subjects were examined and similar results were obtained. Fig. 7 represents oscillo- scope traces at 440 nm. The trace going downward is deoxy- genation and that going upward is reoxygenation. The hori- zontal sweep is 0.2 sec/div. Fig. 8 shows similar oscillo- scope tracings at 542 nm. Fig. 8a is deoxygenation at a sweep of 0.5 sec/div, and Fig. 8b is reoxygenation at 0.2 sec/div. Fig. 9 shows similar traces at 522 nm. Fig. 9a is deoxygenation at a sweep of 0.5 sec/div, and Fig. 9b is re- oxygenation at 0.2 sec/div.

Since the absorbance change at 440 nm arises from the spectral change of the soret band, the electronic gain has been reduced by a factor of approximately five, as compared with other wavelengths observed. Hence, at this wavelength most of the absorbance change arises from the ligand inter- action under the present experimental conditions. It can be seen, however, that the t_{50} (the time required for 50% absor- bance change) for deoxygenation is 0.56 sec. This is much greater than that obtained by other methods, such as stopped flow analysis (Rotman _et al._, 1974; Harrington _et al._, 1977), and is thus not true representation of ligand kinetic inter- pretation. However, the spectrophotometric change observed here is still an indication of the degree of oxygenation of S-rbc suspended in the liquid.

The spectral changes at 542 nm (Fig. 8) indicate there are at least two types of reactions involved for each direc-

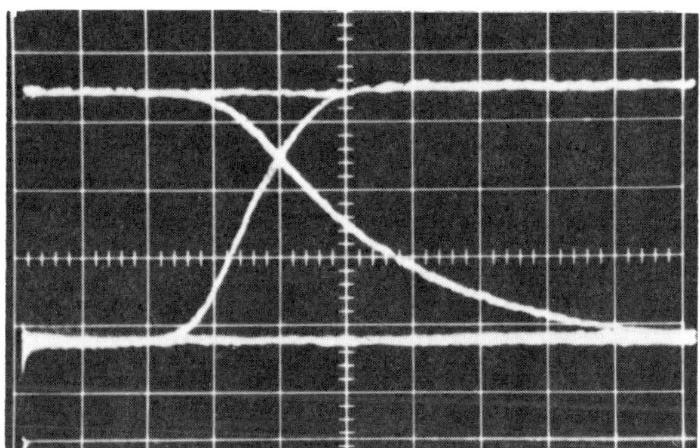

Figure 7.   Oscilloscope traces at 440 nm of deoxygenation
(downward curve) and reoxygenation (upward curve)
of S-rbc diluted 1/6 with Krebs-Henseleit buffer,
pH 7.4, and temperature $25^{O}C$. The gas over the
thin film of rbc was exchanged from one composed
of 20% O_2, 5% CO_2 and 70% N_2 to one containing
5% CO_2 and 95% N_2 for deoxygenation, and _vice_
versa for reoxygenation. The flow rate of the
gases for all reactions was 435 ml/min. Vertical
input represents the change in absorbance. The
straight horizontal trace is the dark current.
Each horizontal division corresponds to 0.2 sec.

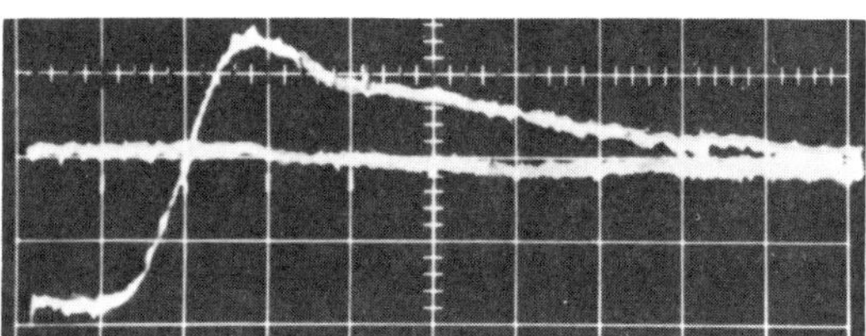

Figure 8a.   Oscilloscope trace of deoxygenation of S-rbc at
542 nm, with horizontal sweep of 0.5 sec/div.

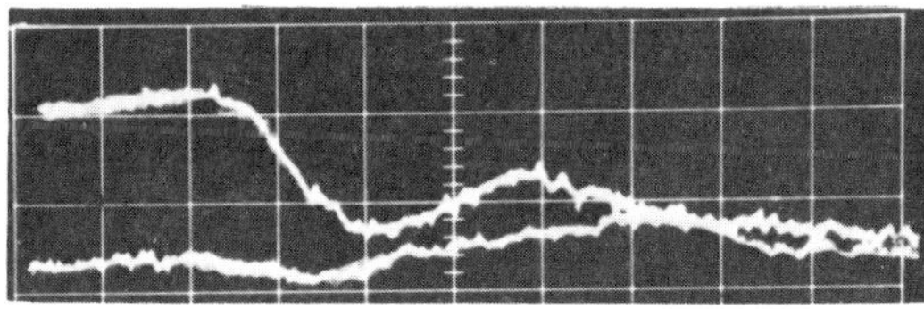

Figure 8b.   Oscilloscope trace of reoxygenation of S-rbc at
542 nm, with horizontal sweep of 0.2 sec/div.

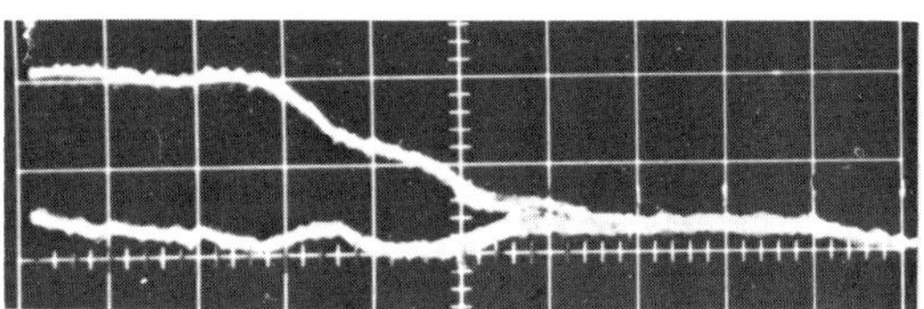

Figure 9a. Oscilloscope trace of deoxygenation of S-rbc at
522 nm (the isosbestic point), with horizontal
sweep of 0.5 sec/div.

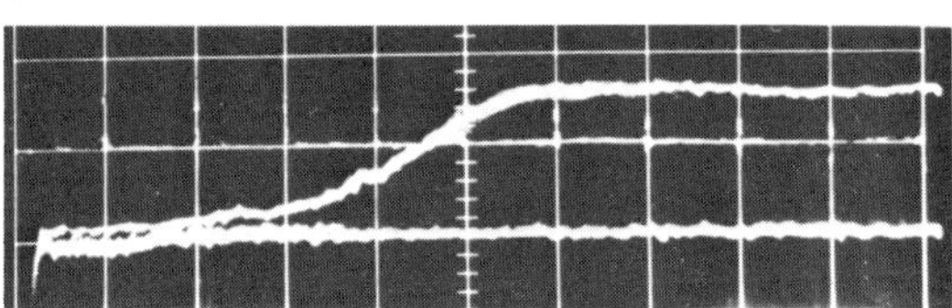

Figure 9b. Oscilloscope trace of reoxygenation of S-rbc at
522 nm, with horizontal sweep of 0.2 sec/div.

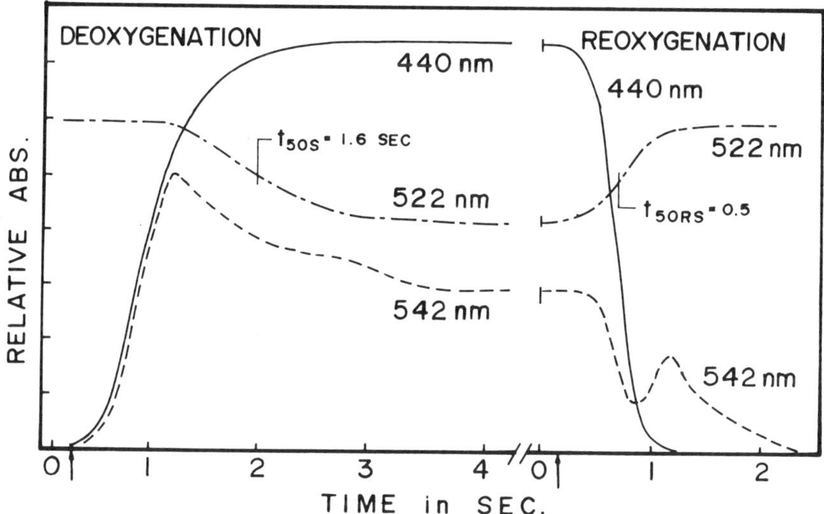

Figure 10. Normalized summary of Figs. 7, 8 and 9. The direction of change of absorbance at 440 nm has been reversed so that it can be compared with the results at 542 and 522 nm. The abscissa is time in seconds, and the ordinate is relative absorbance. The lag time (time required for the complete exchange of gases) is indicated by arrows along the abscissa. The t_{50S} for deoxygenation is 1.6 ± 0.2 sec, and the t_{50RS} for reoxygenation is 0.5 ± 0.04 sec at 522 nm. Each is indicated on its respective curve.

tion of reaction. Upon deoxygenating, there is a rapid
spectral change which corresponds to that observed at 440 nm,
followed by a slow reverse spectral change. When the sample
is reoxygenated, there is again rapid ligand interaction
which is almost immediately interrupted by a reverse spectral
change, followed finally by a slow spectral change in the
same direction as that of the ligand reaction. These observations suggest that the ligand interaction is followed by a
light-scattering interaction. The light loss by scattering
after deoxygenation is almost entirely recovered by reoxygenating.

The change of light-scattering alone can be measured if
the wavelength is set at 522 nm, the isosbestic point of
ligand interaction. Fig. 9 clearly demonstrates this change
of absorbance arising from only the light-scattering. The
apparent lag periods are longer during both deoxygenation and
reoxygenation reactions, indicating no absorbance change takes
place during the ligand interaction. Subsequent absorbance
changes correspond closely to the reverse absorbance changes
observed in Fig. 8 at 542 nm for each reaction.

The results shown in Figs. 7, 8 and 9 are normalized and
summarized in Fig. 10. The direction of the change of absorbance at 440 nm has been reversed so that it can be compared
with the results at the other two wavelengths. As is expected, the rates of deoxygenation observed at 440 nm and 542 nm
are nearly identical, but the scattering light loss at 542 nm
takes place before complete deoxygenation of the sample.
This scattering change coincides with that observed at 522 nm.
The t_{50S} (time required to complete 50% scattering change) is
1.6 $\pm$ 0.2 sec for the four samples observed.

Comparison of the rate of reoxygenation observed at 440
and 542 nm is difficult, since the scattering change also
takes place shortly after the initiation of reoxygenation –
the results at 542 nm being a complex of these two phenomena.
For reoxygenation, the t_{50RS} (time taken to recover 50% loss
of light scattering determined at 522 nm is 0.5 $\pm$ 0.04 sec
for the four samples examined.

Further studies of the effect of cell age and MCHC on
the rates of light-scattering change for both deoxygenation
and reoxygenation process is now being studied.

DISCUSSION

It has been observed that the oxygen dissociation equilibrium curve of dilute HbS in solution resembles that of normal
hemoglobin (HbA) in solution (Allen and Wyman, 1954; Bunn and
Briehl, 1970). The oxygen dissociation equilibrium curve of
S-rbc, on the other hand, is shifted to the right of that
of normal rbc (Bromberg and Jensen, 1967). The cause of this
hysteresis-like behavior, among others, was suggested to be
the difference in the physical state of oxy- and deoxy-erythro-
cytes - the degree of the hysteresis being dependent on how
the polymers were formed (Mizukami et al., 1977 ; Winslow,
1976). For example, if sickling is caused by a rapid deoxygenation process, the polymers formed are less ordered, or
inhomogeneous. In order to demonstrate this assumption, S-rbc
which had previously been quickly deoxygenated by insertion
of the sample into the deoxygenation chamber, were reoxygenated in the usual manner. Curve 1 in Fig. 11 was obtained.
Immediately after completion of reoxygenation, curve 2 was
obtained by slowly deoxygenating the same sample in the usual
manner. Curve 3 was obtained by reoxygenating the sample a
second time. Curves 1 and 2 are similar in that they are
both sigmoidal and have approximately the same oxygen affinity, whereas only curve 3 shows an apparent reduction in the
sigmoidal shape and a decrease in oxygen affinity.

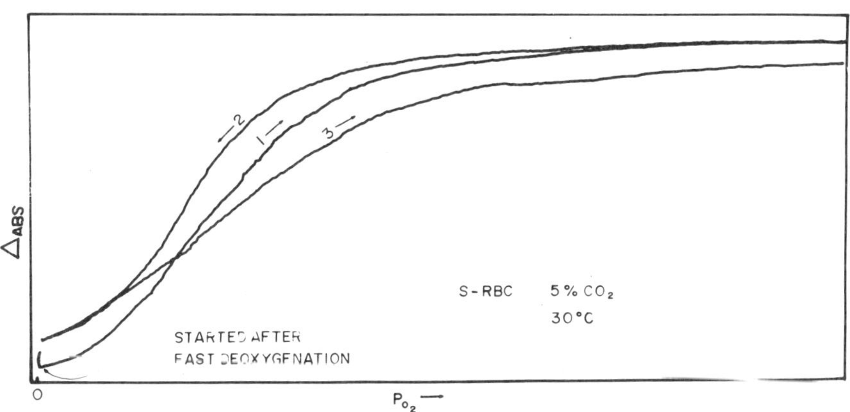

Figure 11. For description see text.

The rate of scattering light intensity change reported herein is similar to that of Zarkowsky and Hochmuth (1975) for sickling - their t_{50S} being about 1.5 sec ; and that of Messer _et al_., (1976) for desickling - their t_{50RS} being less than 0.5 sec. However, the exact cause of the scattering change of light could arise from the optical change due to aggregation of hemoglobin molecules, the structural change of cells, or both. No such extent of light-scattering change has been observed for normal red blood cells, and light microscopic analysis using videotape has shown that after complete deoxygenation of the sample on micromesh, a large percentage of sickle cells (>90%) become sickled. Reoxygenation of the same sample results in a large percentage (>90%) of the sickled cells recovering their normal shape, inducing little, if any, irreversibly sickled cells.

Both the equilibrium and kinetic studies indicate that the sickling process proceeds prior to complete deoxygenation and that desickling is being initiated prior to complete oxygenation. The changes observed here are statistical averages of whole blood and any effect of cell age remains to be studied. However, preliminary microscopic observation suggests that the cell age has a considerable effect on both equilibrium and kinetic results. As the change in intracellular constituents is age dependent, this is to be expected.

SUMMARY

Two instruments which measure the interaction of intact erythrocytes with oxygen are described. One determines the oxygen association-dissociation equilibrium curve of less than one drop of blood in the directions of both deoxygenation and reoxygenation in less than 10 minutes. The other determines the rate of sickling and desickling of sickle erythrocytes. Using these two instruments for the analysis of erythrocytes obtained from homozygous sickle cell anemia patients, it has been shown that: (a) The oxygen association-dissociation equilibrium curve determined at the time of reoxygenation is shifted to the right of that of deoxygenation (hysteresis), and the degree of hysteresis is dependent on how sickle erythrocytes are being deoxygenated to form hemoglobin polymers; (b) The time required to cause 50% light-scattering loss (t_{50S}) by sudden deoxygenation at 25°C is 1.6 ± 0.2 sec for the four samples tested, and that the light-scattering gain (t_{50RS}) by sudden reoxygenation is 0.5 ± 0.04 sec. Visual observation suggests that these light-scattering changes are directly related to the sickling and desickling of erythrocytes; _(c)_ The sickling takes place under partial deoxygenation, and desickling is initiated prior to complete reoxygenation of the erythrocytes.

ACKNOWLEDGMENTS

The authors are investigators of the Comprehensive Sickle Cell Center of Wayne State University, and acknowledge the technical assistance rendered by David Bartinicki, A. Gerald Beaudoin and William Casey.

REFERENCES

Allen DW, Wyman J Jr (1954). Equilibre de l'hemoglobine de dreponocytose avec l'oxygene. Rev hemat 9:155.
Altman PL and Dittmer DS (eds) (1971). "Blood and Other Body Fluids." Bethesda: Fed Amer Soc Exp Biol.
Bromberg PA, Jensen WN (1967). Blood oxygen dissociation curves in sickle cell disease. J Lab Clin Med 70:480.
Bunn HF, Briehl RWJ (1970). The interaction of 2,3-diphosphoglycerate with various human hemoglobins. J Clin Invest 49:1088.
Cameron BF, Zucker R (1975). Oxygen binding to human erythrocyte cell populations. Am NY Acad Sci 244:60
Duvelleroy MA, Buckles RG, Rosenkaimer S, Tung C, Laver MB (1970). An oxyhemoglobin dissociation analyser. J Appl Physiol 28:227.
Harrington JP, Elbaum D, Bookchin RM, Wittenberg JB, Nagel RL (1977). Ligand kinetics of hemoglobin S containing erythrocytes. Proc Natl Acad Sci 74:203.
Jayalakshmi M, Seakins M (1976). The concentration dependence of the hemc heme interaction of hemoglobin S. Biochem Med 15:115.
Kiesow LA, Bless JW, Nelson DP, Shelton JB (1972). A new method for the rapid determination of oxygen dissociation curves in small blood samples by spectrophotometric titration. Clin Chim Acta 41:123
Kiesow LA, Shelton JB, Bless JW (1974). The determination of O_2-dissociation curves in hemoglobin solutions with a

liquid fluorocarbon O_2 transport system. Anal Biochem 58:14.

Longmuir IS, Chow J (1970). Rapid method for determining effects of agents on oxyhemoglobin dissociation curves. J Appl Physiol 28:343.

Messer MJ, Hahn JA, Bradley TB (1976). The kinetics of sickling and unsickling of red cells under physiologic conditions: rheologic and ultrastructural correlations. In "Proceedings of the Symposium on Molecular and Cellular Aspects of Sickle Cell Disease," Bethesda:HEW, p225.

Milner PF (1974). Oxygen transport in sickle cell anemia. Arch Intern Med 133:565.

Mizukami H, Beaudoin AG, Bartnicki DE, Adams B. (1977) Hysteresis-like behavior of oxygen association-dissociation equilibrium curves of sickle cells determined by a new method. Proc Soc Exp Biol Med 154:304.

Rossi-Bernardi L, Luzzana M, Samaja M, Davi M, DaRiva-Ricci D, Minoli J, Seaton B, Berger RL (1975). Continuous determination of the oxygen dissociation curve for whole blood. Clin Chem 21:1747.

Rotman HH, Klocke RA, Andersson KK, D'Alecy L, Forster RE (1974). Kinetics of oxygenation and deoxygenation of erythrocytes containing hemoglobin S. Resp Physiol 21:9.

Seakins M, Gibbs WN, Milner PF, Bertles JF (1973). Erythrocyte hg-s concentration. An important factor in the low oxygen affinity of blood in sickle cell anemia. J Clin Invest 52:422.

Winslow RM (1976) Blood oxygen equilibrium studies in sickle cell anemia. In "Proceedings of the Symposium on Molecular and Cellular Aspects of Sickle Cell Disease," Bethesda: HEW, p235.

Zarkowsky HS, Hochmuth RM (1975). Sickling times of individual erythrocytes at zero P_{O_2}. J Clin Invest 56:1023.

DISCUSSION

Dr. Morse: How does the sickling and desickling time compare to the length of time that the cells are actually in the capillaries?

Dr. Mizukami: This is really a very difficult question to answer. We know that the red blood cell has pulsating motion and it stops and goes in the capillaries. However, it seems to be agreeable to people these days in that it takes one second or less in tissue capillaries and probably much less in the alveolar capillaries.

Dr. Brewer: I'm a little confused by the relationship of the first data, which I believe you have called hysteresis, in which the reoxygenation curve does not trace back over the same curve, and the fact that the recovery of the sickle cell by light scattering is so rapid. On the basis of the hysteresis effect would you not expect desickling to take longer? If you did slow deoxygenation would the desickling be slower?

Dr. Mizukami: I think this is a very good point. Under the kinetic condition what I can do is a very fast exchange of gases, that is similar to what has been shown in the last slide. So, I expect to see in the deoxygenated state and under kinetic conditions, very poor aggregates. It makes sense that deaggregation is much faster than what I expected in the perfect aggregates. So if I have done this experiment as you have suggested, that is to do a very slow deoxygenation, then do the pulsating change in the gas, I would expect to see much longer T50 for deaggregation.

The Red Cell, page 175

THE DETERMINANTS OF SICKLE ERYTHROCYTE SURVIVAL IN SICKLE
CELL PATIENTS AND AN ANIMAL MODEL OF SICKLE CELL DISEASE

Eric B. Schoomaker[*], and George G. Brewer

Department of Human Genetics, University of Michi-
gan, Ann Arbor.
[*]Present address: Department of Medicine, Duke
University, Durham.

INTRODUCTION

Very few correlations have been observed among characteristics of the sickle red blood cell (RBC) and the clinical
state of the sickle cell anemic (SCA) patient. This extends
even as far as hematologic variables which correlate with RBC
destruction, as measured by erythrocyte ^{51}Cr survival. One
important relationship is that between the proportion of
irreversibly sickled cells (ISC) and the hemolytic rate. It
has been proposed that the rate of overall RBC destruction is
determined to a considerable extent by the ISC count (Serjeant
et al., 1969). This may be the tip of a unifying concept in
SCA clinical pathology, for the ISC count covaries with the
level of fetal hemoglobin (HbF) on the one hand (Serjeant,
1970; Bertles and Milner, 1968), and at least two measures of
organ damage--the development if ischemic fibrosis of the
spleen (Serjeant, 1970) and the degree of vascular injury to
the conjunctiva (Serjeant et al., 1972)--on the other.

One method of investigation which may shed some light on
the determinants of SCA RBC survival is the Castro animal
model of sickle cell disease (Castro et al., 1973). This
technique permits the controlled study of the survival of
human SCA erythrocytes in a mammalian circulation. Laboratory
rats, whose immune and erythrophagocytic functions have been
blocked by prior chemotherapy, are transfused with labeled
human RBC and erythrocyte survival is determined. Thus far,
work with this model has been directed toward the study of
two, newly discovered, sub-populations of sickle cells which
are categorized according to their survival in extreme

The Red Cell, pages 177–193

hypoxia (Castro et al., 1974; Castro et al., 1976). Additionally, we have used the model to study the anti-sickling properties of elemental zinc (Schoomaker et al., 1976) and have proposed its use as an in vivo test for anti-sickling agents.

However, no one has demonstrated that the determinants of RBC survival in the animal model are the same as and of equal magnitude as those in the human patient. This is an important relationship to prove if data obtained from the model are assumed to reflect the behavior of cells in the human. We have undertaken to answer the questions: 1) what are the factors which influence sickle RBC survival in the animal? and 2) how do these compare with the determinants of erythrocyte loss in the donor patients?

MATERIALS AND METHODS

Subjects

Blood used for these studies was obtained with informed, written consent from 15 adult SCA patients and 4 non-SCA, non-anemic healthy adults. At the time of sampling all patients were in a stable, non-crisis state and had not been transfused for at least three months prior to the study. Blood was drawn into heparinized containers and used promptly. The ^{51}Cr RBC survivals in the animals and patients, and the remainder of the hematologic variables described below were determined simultaneously or within a span of time which approximated simultaneous measurements.

Erythrocyte survival

A modification of the method of Castro and his coworkers (1973), which has been fully described elsewhere (Schoomaker et al., 1976), was employed to measure ^{51}Cr RBC survival in the animals. Briefly, this technique permits the long-term survival of ^{51}Cr-labeled human RBC transfused into donor rats by prior blockade of the reticuloendothelial system (RES) with ethyl palmitate and depletion of the complement system with cobra venom factor. Both are administered by intravenous injections eight and two hours, respectively, before transfusion. Following a fifteen minute mixing period, base line ^{51}Cr activity of the animals' blood is determined with a

micro-sample and a conventional RBC survival curve is constructed through serial sampling over the next eight to twenty-four
hours.

From knowledge of the size of transfusion, the size of
the animal and the ^{51}Cr activity in the blood after the fifteen minute equilibration period, recovery of the transfused
SCA RBC in the circulation of rats is computed. Experience
has taught us (Schoomaker et al., 1976) that the slope of the
survival curve, λ_S, called the sequestration rate constant, is
a more accurate measure of the rate of sequestration of the
transfused cells than the conventional half life. Accordingly,
λ_S has been used for data analyses in these studies. It should
be noted that λ_S and the more traditional half-time of survival
($t\frac{1}{2}$) are inversely related: when λ_S is large, $t\frac{1}{2}$ is small and
vice versa. The mean RBC survival in the patients was deter-
mined by standard labeling techniques. To avoid confusion with
λ_S, this measure is called the ^{51}Cr RBC survival.

Hematologic variables

Counts of ISC were made from air-dried blood smears using
a modification of the Hellerstein et al., (1974) criteria for
defining an ISC. Erythrocyte survival studies of high and
low ISC blood were performed using blood which had been enriched or depleted of ISC by ultracentrifugation (Bertles and
Milner, 1968).

Hemoglobin fractionation was performed by conventional
techniques in which HbA$_2$ was eluted and measured spectropho-
mometrically at 415 nm after electrophoresis on cellulose
acetate and HbF levels were determined by the one minute alkali denaturation method (Singer et al., 1951). The per cent
of total hemoglobin remaining after HbF and HbA$_2$ were removed
was designated HbS.

The partial pressure of oxygen (pO$_2$) at which 50% of the
Hb is deoxygenated (p50) was calculated by measuring the per
cent saturation, pH, and pO$_2$ as the blood was slowly desatura-
ted in a tonometer. The Hb oxygen saturations were corrected
to pH 7.4 and a curve drawn in the usual fashion.

ABO and RhD blood types were determined by conventional
techniques. The hemoglobin, hematocrit (Hct), mean cell
hemoglobin concentration (MCHC) and mean cell volume (MCV)

were all determined using a Coulter particle counter.

RESULTS

Erythrocytes from SCA patients were found to have significantly shorter survival in the animals relative to normal
controls. The λ_S for the SCA RBC were significantly greater
than the λ_S of normal RBC by the Student's t-test. This is
graphically depicted in Figure 1.

Erythrocyte survival in the animal model was determined
for eight SCA patients on more than one occasion over a
period ranging from one day to one year. Overall, 103 λ_S
measurements were made. A nested, one-way analysis of variance was performed to determine the degree and statistical
significance of differences 1) among replicate λ_S measurements
made on different animals for a given experiment, 2) among
different mean λ_S measurements for a given patient, and
3) among different patients. A highly significant difference
was found only among patients. The degree of experimental
variability exhibited by different animals during a single
experiment and by different estimates of λ_S for a single
patient was not statistically significant. This patient-
specificity of SCA RBC survival is shown in Figure 2.

Trivial explanations for the abbreviated survival of
sickle RBC in the animals and for the patient-specificity of
λ_S based upon major blood group antigens or cell size differences were not found . No pattern of control or sickle RBC
survival in the animal as a function of the major blood groups,
A, B, O or RhD, was observed. Similarly, MCV did not correlate with λ_S. As a further demonstration of the independence
of donor cell size, recipient (animal) cell size, and λ_S,
guinea pigs were transfused with SCA RBC in several experiments.
No influence upon λ_S was observed when guinea pigs were used.
The MCV of guinea pigs $(77\mu^3)$(Altman and Dittmer, 1961) is
intermediate between the rat $(61\mu^3)$ and human $(94\mu^3)$. If
physical characteristics of the donor cells and capillary
beds of the recipient animal based upon size were major determinants of λ_S, variation in λ_S would have been introduced by
use of the guinea pig.

The correlation coefficients between λ_S and the hematologic variables of the donor RBC are given in Table I.

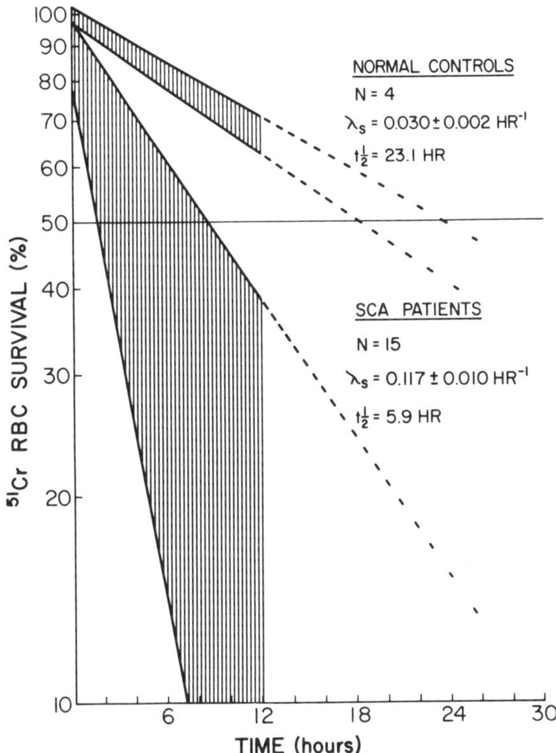

Figure 1. Composite illustration of the RBC ^{51}Cr survival in pre-treated rats for erythrocytes from SCA patients (lower range) and HbAA controls (upper range). The curves were drawn to include the range of observed extrapolated zero time values and λ_S for both groups. The shaded areas describe the period during which samples are taken; the broken lines are extrapolated beyond the observation period. In actuality, the animals begin to recover from the CVF and EP after 12-14 hours and the λ_S change markedly.

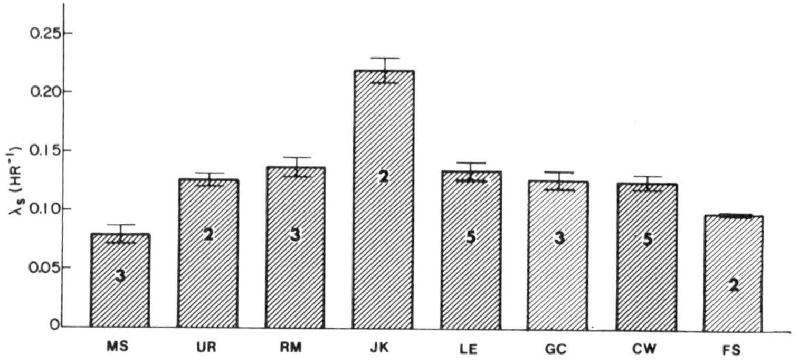

Figure 2. Bar graph demonstrating the patient-specificity of sickle RBC survival in the animal model (λ_S). Shown are the mean $\lambda_S \pm 1$ S.E.M. for a number of experiments conducted on different days for each patient. The number of experiments is shown on the bars. Each experiment employed 3 - 7 animals.

Table 1

	λ_S	^{51}Cr RBC Survival	%HbA$_2$	%HbF	%HbS	ISC	p50
λ_S	1						
^{51}Cr RBC Survival	NS	1					
%HBA$_2$	NS	NS	1				
%HbF	NS	0.860 (p=0.01)	NS	1			
%HbS	NS	-0.872 (p=0.01)	NS	-0.996 (p=0.01)	1		
ISC	NS	-0.692 (p=0.05)	NS	-0.733 (p=0.05)	0.760 (p=0.05)	1	
p50	0.918 (p=0.01	NS	NS	NS	NS	NS	1

Product-moment correlation coefficients (r) for pairs of variables measured on 15 SCA patients. Values for r are given in each cell. The probability levels are in parentheses.

The rate of SCA RBC sequestration in the animals (λ_s) did not correlate with the hemolytic rate of similar cells in the donor patient (51 RBC survival). Of all of the variables measured in these cells, only the regression of λ_s on p50 was statistically significant (Figure 3).

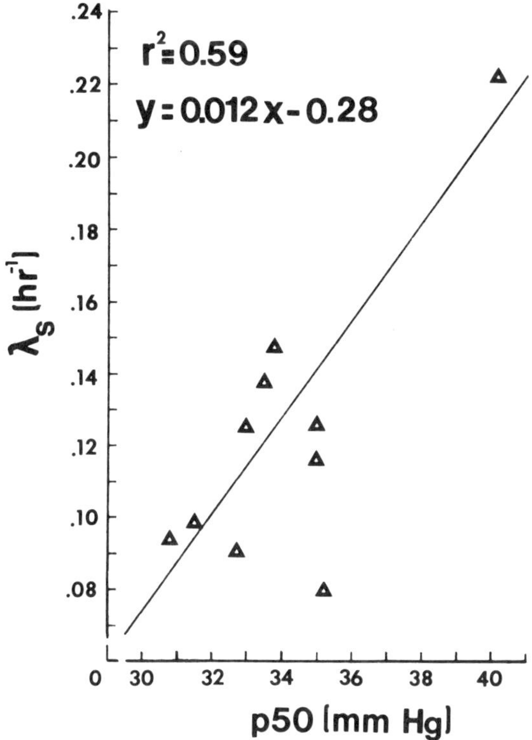

Figure 3. Regression of sequestration rate constant (λ_s) for sickle RBC survival in the animal model on p50. The regression equation and coefficient of determination (r^2) are also given.

The recovery of transfused SCA cells in the animals after the first 15 minute equilibration period was quite variable across patients, ranging from 36.6% to 92.4%. In contrast, recovery of cells from three normal controls was very close to 100%. The per cent base line recovery was observed to covary closely with the relative number of ISC in the transfused blood (Figure 4).

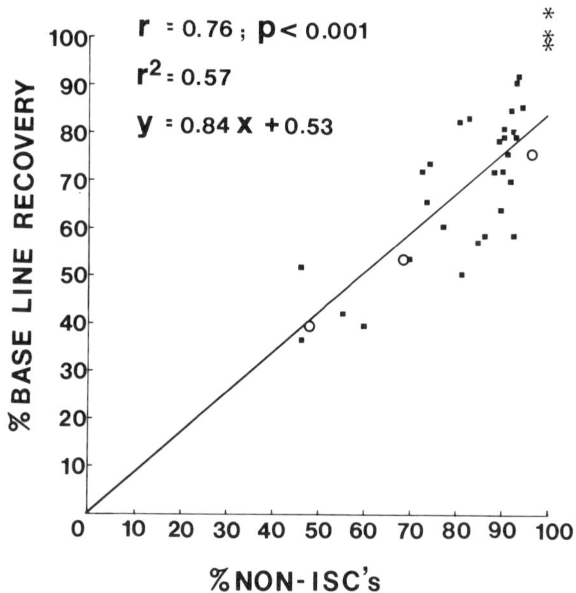

Figure 4. Scatter plot of per cent recovery of transfused RBC after the 15 minute equilibration period (% base line recovery) and drawn for values derived from experiments with SCA patients (■). Stars (*) represent values for three normal (AA) controls. The open circles (O) describe the relationship between base line recovery and non-ISC for the ISC fractionation experiment.

Ultracentrifugation of SCA blood from a single donor resulted in an ISC-rich (51.9% ISC) and an ISC-poor (3.8% ISC) fraction (Figure 5). When these two fractions and a mixture of the two (30.1% ISC) were labeled with ^{51}Cr and transfused into rats in the usual fashion, the recovery of cells was directly proportional to the per cent non-ISC (Figure 6) as observed across patients (Figure 3).

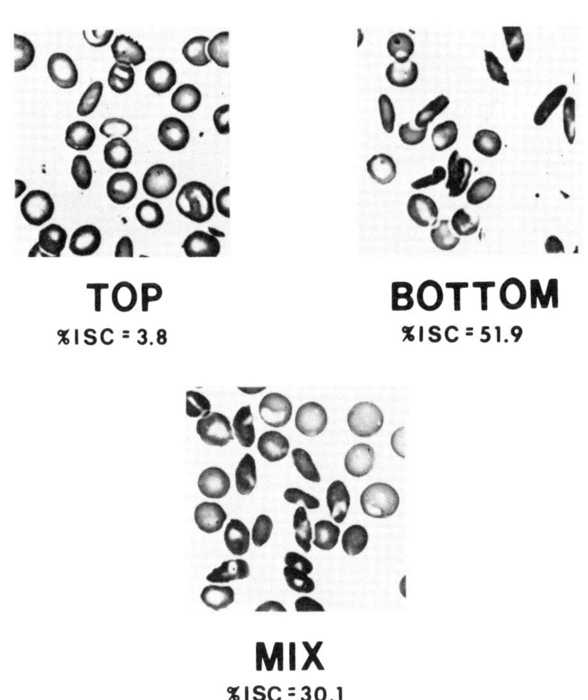

Figure 5. Photomicographs of air-dried blood smears, stained with Wright's stain, made from the top, ISC= 3.8% and bottom, ISC= 51.9% fraction of ultracentrifuged whole blood from a single SCA patient (Hct= 0.75; 54,000 x G for 60 minutes at 4° C) and a mixture of top and bottom, ISC= 30.1%. All cells with more than one sharp projection, holly forms and cells with one dimension greater than twice the lesser dimension are classified as ISC.

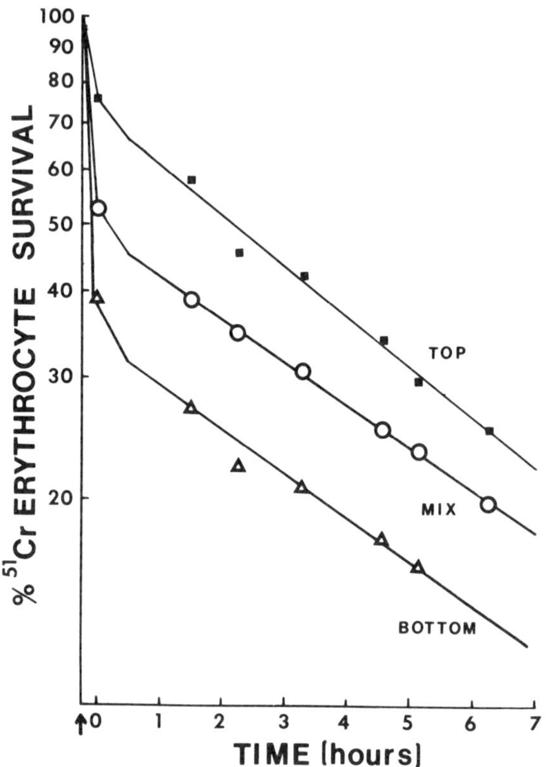

Figure 6. RBC ^{51}RBC survival curve for three fractions of ultracentrifuged whole blood from a single SCA patient. The transfusions were performed at the arrow; zero time values are the per cent recovery of cells at the base line. Shown are the survival curves for the top fraction ($\blacksquare$; λ_s=0.167± 0.111(±1.S.E.M.); 3.8% ISC) bottom fraction ($\triangle$; λ_s=0.151± 0.039; 51.9% ISC) and mixture of top and bottom ($\bigcirc$; λ_s=0.143 ± 0.008; 30.1% ISC). The points represent the mean values of three animals used in each group.

Erythrocyte survival in the patients was found to covary
closely with the %HbS, %HbF and %ISC (Table 1). However,
large correlations were found among %HbS, %HbF and %ISC as
well. (The large inverse correlation between %HbS and %HbF
is not surprising given the arithmetic relationship between
them.) The observed correlations between ^{51}Cr RBC survival
and each of the variables may result from mutual covariation
with a common variable. For example, the observed correlation between erythrocyte survival and %ISC may be the result
of mutual correlation of each with %HbS, and not through any
independent relationship between the two. A multivariate
analysis was undertaken to assess the contribution to overall
[51]Cr RBC survival of each variable alone. Multiple regression
of erythrocyte survival on %HbS and %ISC was performed. The
level of HbS rather than HbF was selected because of its
larger coefficient of correlation with erythrocyte survival.

Multiple regression yields a statistically significant
partial regression coefficient of ^{51}Cr RBC survival on %HbS
(-0.75, p=0.05). However, the level of ISC has an insignificant independent partial regression with patient erythrocyte
survival once the influence of %HbS is removed. Thus, the
main reason for the large negative correlation between %ISC
and ^{51}Cr RBC survival (r=-0.708) is 1) the correlation between
%ISC and %HbS and 2) the significant regression of ^{51}Cr RBC
survival on %HbS.

DISCUSSION

The Castro animal model of SCA may be viewed as a living
mammalian circulatory filter of human sickle erythrocytes
which is devoid of idiosyncracies of the patients' circulatory
systems. These idiosyncracies, e.g. variations in splenic
function, splenic and pulmonary arterio-venous shunts, may
play a major role in the hematologic severity of the disease
(erythrocyte survival). From this perspective, the model may
serve to distinguish determinants of overall RBC survival
which are inherent in the erythrocyte, from vascular components which are patient specific and unpredictable.

This work confirms the earlier observations of the
Castro group that sickle erythrocyte survival is abbreviated
relative to the survival of non-SCA RBC and that the reduction is of a magnitude similar to that observed in ^{51}Cr RBC
survival (Figure 1). A new finding (Schoomaker et al., 1976)

is that RBC survival in the animal is quite patient-specific (Figure 2). Thus, factors which are intrinsic to the RBC and specific for the donor patient determine λ_S. A compartmentalization of the overall variance in λ_S reveals that the greatest source of variance is that due to differences between patients.

Despite the patient-specificity of λ_S, erythrocyte survival in the animal does not correlate significantly with ^{51}Cr RBC survival. This answers one question about the utility of the animal model: it cannot substitute for isotopic or other measures of erythrocyte survival in the patient. How can the apparent inconsistency of two separate patient-specific yet uncorrelated degrees of RBC filterability in the mammalian circulation--λ_S in the rat and ^{51}Cr RBC survival in the human--be explained?

The first and most readily discarded explanation lies in physical and immunologic characteristics of the cell. The mean corpuscular volume of a rat erythrocyte is two-thirds that of the SCA patients under study-- $61\mu^3$ versus $94\mu^3$. While no good measurements of "mean capillary radius" have been performed in rats, it is not unreasonable to assume that vascular size is matched with erythrocyte volume (Krogh, 1959). Ultimate survival of heterologous sickle cells in the rat may then be closely linked to their ability to negotiate tight passages in the recipient's circulation, which may, in turn, be a function of the MCV of the donor cells. Two experimental observations refute this hypothesis. The first and most direct is that λ_S does not correlate with MCV. The second and more indirect observation is the result of RBC survival studies in the guinea pig. The MCV of the guinea pig is intermediate between the rat and human--$77\mu^3$. According to the above reasoning, λ_S in the guinea pig should be less than in the rat, i.e. RBC survival should be prolonged. In fact, sickle erthrocyte survival is not different in these two species.

Can the differences in λ_S across SCA patients and the failure of λ_S and ^{51}Cr RBC survival to correlate be explained by immunologic differences in the cells? Despite the depletion of C3-C9 and RES paralysis, antibody attachment to certain blood group antigens may hasten or prevent RBC trapping. Evidence against this is found in the absence of any pattern of sickle RBC survival in the animal as a function of the major blood groups, A, B, O or RhD.

The failure of SCA erythrocyte survival in the animal model and in the patient to correlate lies in different determinants of survival for these cells in the two systems. Through measurements of a number of characteristics of the sickle RBC which may play an important role in survival we have shown that λ_S and ^{51}RBC survival are largely determined by two different variables. Sickle erythrocyte survival in the animal appears largely determined by Hb oxygen affinity while RBC survival in the donor patients is a function of the concentration of HbS in the RBC.

Serjeant and his coworkers (1969) undertook a similar investigation of the determinants of ^{51}Cr RBC survival. Although a multivariate approach was not used, they observed an inverse correlation between %ISC and ^{51}Cr RBC survival of -0.68 (versus r=-0.692 in the present work). Consequently, they proposed a major determining role for %ISC on ^{51}Cr RBC survival. The underlying relationships between %HbS and RBC survival and between %HbS and %ISC were not observed by these investigators. Thus, the role of %HbS in SCA RBC survival evident in the present work was not described.

Although quantitative electrophoresis of HbA_2 and HbF was performed by these investigators, %HbS was not calculated, nor were correlations between the levels of Hb types and ^{51}Cr RBC survival or ISC examined. Using their published data, correlations among the key variables were computed and are shown, along with the results of the present study, in Table 2. Other than the ISC-^{51}Cr RBC survival correlation, no significant correlations were observed in their data. Besides our work, this is in conflict with two other studies of HbF and ISC. Bertles and Milner (1968), in their study of the distribution of HbF in ISC and non-ISC, found a significant inverse correlation between %HbF and %ISC (r=-0.65; p<0.01). The same is true of Seakins and his coworkers (r=-0.734; p<0.01)(1973). While Serjeant and his coworkers do not report the method used for HbF quantitation, Bertles and Milner used a one-minute alkali denaturation method identical to the one used here. Minor changes in this method may significantly alter the measurement of HbF and subsequent computation of HbS; Serjeant's mean %HbF is less than the mean %HbF in Bertles and Milner's group and the Seakin's group and the present study. Alternatively, the SCA patients studied by Serjeant may have had other, more fundamental differences from our patients.

TABLE 2

	Serjeant et al. (1969) (N=22)	Schoomaker and Brewer (1977) (N=10)
CRS	7.4 ± 0.5 days	8.1 ± 1.1 days
ISC	16.1 ± 1.7 %	26.4 ± 3.8 %
HbA_2	2.75 ± 0.12%	2.89 ± 0.11%
HbF	4.08 ± 0.68%	5.63 ± 1.18%
HbS	93.16 ± 0.64%	91.48 ± 1.11%
$r_{crs-isc}$	-0.655 (p<0.01)	-0.708 (p<0.05)
$r_{crs-HbS}$	-0.212 (NS)	-0.872 (p<0.01)
$r_{crs-HbF}$	0.100 (NS)	0.860 (p<0.01)
$r_{isc-HbS}$	0.324 (NS)	0.760 (p<0.05)
$r_{isc-HbF}$	-0.264 (NS)	-0.733 (p<0.05)

Comparison of ^{51}Cr RBC survival (CRS), %ISC, Hb quantitation
and correlation coefficients between pairs of these variables,
between the present study and work by Serjeant et al., (1968).
Values for the five variables are the mean±1 S.E.M. Significance levels for each r are given in parentheses.

Although multiple regression analysis reveals an insignificant independent role for ISC in ^{51}Cr RBC survival,
it is reasonable that ISC should contribute to overall
sickle erythrocyte survival. They are part of the labeled
sample measured by the test and previous studies have
shown (Bertles and Milner, 1968) that they are a short-lived
cell form. Our results must be interpreted as showing that
the formation of ISC is but one reflection of the general
tendency of a sickle patient's erythrocytes to sustain terminal injury and to undergo hemolysis or to be trapped in the
RES. This overall propensity for injury is a result of the
mean concentration of HbS in the patient's RBC. The generation of ISC, while serving in the patient as one means of
hastening erythrocyte loss, is not the key determinant in
overall RBC survival.

In marked contrast to erythrocyte survival in the patient,
sickle RBC survival in pretreated animals does not correlate
significantly with %ISC or %HbS. The lack of a correlation
with the level of ISC in the transfused cells is explained
by the almost immediate removal of these cells from the cir-

culation. Direct proof of this was not accomplished, but
the indirect evidence is overwhelming. First, there is a
significant positive regression of recovery of cells after
the 15 minute equilibration period on %non-ISC in the transfused cells across patients (Figure 4). This is not a nonspecific immunologic effect; normal RBC will give 100%
recovery. This regression does not rule out the possibility
that factors other than the level of ISC, but closely correlated with it, differ across patients and determine the recovery of transfused cells. The fact that transfused cells
with differing levels of ISC from a single patient retain
the same relationship between recovery and %non-ISC (Figure
6) eliminates this alternate explanation.

The large coefficient of determination of λ_S by p50
($r^2=0.59$) is evidence that the major determinant sickle RBC
survival in the animals is Hb oxygen affinity. This may be
interpreted to mean that the presence of HbS is enough to
hasten sequestration of sickle RBC relative to normal cells
and that the factor which adjusts the rate at which this
loss occurs is the Hb oxygen affinity. Even pretreated, the
rat is a better filter of SCA erythrocytes than the donor
patient. Witness the almost immediate trapping of ISC in
the animals. Small variations in the mix of HbF and HbS
must be overshadowed by the p50.

SUMMARY

The Castro animal model of SCA is an _in vivo_ filter of
sickle erythrocytes which measures a small number of factors
intrinsic to the RBC. The factors determining RBC survival
in the animal and the patient, while patient-specific, are
fundamentally different. Sickle erythrocyte survival in
the patient is largely a function of the mean HbS concentration. Individual cells may be destroyed following their
transformation into ISC but this step is a marker of the
overall survival of RBC and does not make an independent
contribution to it. In contrast to the situation in the
patient, the major determinant of sickle RBC survival in
the animal is Hb oxygen affinity as measured by the p50.
Irreversibly sickled cells are rapidly removed from circulation in the animals, further emphasizing the abbreviated survivability of these cells in circulation. The model should
prove most useful in studies of the influence of HbS oxygen
affinity upon sickle RBC survival in the mammalian circula-

tion, or in screening for therapeutic agents which affect
this parameter.

ACKNOWLEDGEMENTS

We wish to acknowledge the valuable assistance of
Dr. Donald Rucknagel in performing the hemoglobin fractionation, Dr. Henry Gershowitz in performing the blood typing
and Ms. Lucia F. Brewer in performing the counts of ISC.

This work was supported by a generous grant from the
Allen H. Meyers Foundation, by NIH research grant No. HL 16008
from the Sickle Cell Disease Branch, National Heart and
Lung Institute, DHEW; NIH contract No. NO1-HB-2-2918-B; and
NIH training grant 5T01-GM-0071.

BIBLIOGRAPHY

Bertles, J.F. and Milner, P.F. (1968). Irreversibly sickled
  erythrocytes: a consequence of the heterogeneous distribution of hemoglobin types in sickle cell anemia. J Clin
  Invest 47: 1731-1742.

Castro, O., Orlin, J., Rosen, M. and Finch, S.C. (1973).
  Survival of sickle cell erythrocytes in heterologous
  species: response to variations in oxygen tension.
  Proc Nat Acad Sci USA 70: 2356-2359.

Castro, O., Finch, S.C., and Osbaldiston, G. (1974). Sickle
  cell resistance to in vivo hypoxia. Nature 251: 620-621.

Castro, O., Osbaldiston, G.W., Aponte, L., Roth, R., Orlin, J.,
  and Finch, S.C. (1976) Oxygen-dependent circulation of
  sickle erythrocytes. J Lab Clin Med 88: 732-744.

Hellerstein, S. and Bunthrarungroj, T. (1974). Erythrocyte
  composition is sickle-cell anemia. J Lab Clin Med 83:
  611-624

Krogh, A (1959). "The Anatomy and Physiology of Capillaries."
  New York: Hafner Publishing Co., p. 30.

Schoomaker, E.B., Brewer, G.J. and Oelshlegel, Jr., F.J. (1976).
  Zinc in the treatment of homozygous sickle cell anemia:
  studies in an animal model. Am J Hematol 1: 45-57.

Seakins, M., Gibbs, W., Milner, P.F. and Bertles, J.F. (1973).
Erthrocyte Hb-S concentration: an important factor in
the low oxygen affinity of blood in sickle cell anemia.
J Clin Invest 52: 422-432.

Serjeant, G.R , Serjeant, B.E. and Milner, P.F. (1969). The
irreversibly sickled cell; a determinant of haemolysis
in sickle cell anaemia. Brit J Haematol 17: 527-533.

Serjeant, G.R. (1970). Irreversibly sickled cells and
splenomegally in sickle-cell anemia. Brit J. Haematol 19:
635-641.

Serjeant, G.R., Serjeant, B.E. and Condon, P.F. (1972). The
conjunctival sign in sickle cell anemia. J Am Med Assoc
219: 1428-1431.

Singer, K., Chernoff, A.I., and Singer, L. (1951). Studies
on abnormal hemoglobins II Their identification by means
of the method of fractional denaturation. Blood 6: 429-435.

DISCUSSION

<u>Dr. Castro</u>: Credit for the development of the model belongs
to Dr. Stuart C. Finch of Yale University. We became involved
with it primarily by applying it to the study of sickle cell
anemia. Our own experience with the survival of the irreversibly sickled cells in the model clearly support your conclusions: We injected blood of SCA patients into the animals and
then followed their survival directly by counting irreversibly
sickled cells. We found, as you did, that approximately one
half of the transfused irreversibly sickled cells were no longer
present in the rats' blood 15 minutes after transfusion. Furthermore, during the first hour or so after the transfusion experiment the half-life of the irreversibly sickled cells was
about 1/2 of that of the whole sickle cell population. Thereafter, however, the survival curve of the irreversibly sickled
cells was identical to that of the non-irreversibly sickled
RBCs suggesting to us that some irreversibly sickled cells may
have adapted to the stress of a sturdier circulation that is
not even all that physiological. Perhaps some of these irreversibly sickled cells accumulate in the blood of patients
precisely because they somehow have acquired properties that
allow them to circulate despite their shape, low level of
fetal hemoglobin and other anomalies. Incidentally, the RBCs
from patients with Hb SC disease and Hb Sβ^+ thalassemia show
very short survival in the rat although there are no ISCs
in these patients. This confirms that the rat model measures
mainly reversible sickling.

<u>Dr. Schoomaker</u>: Thank you for your comments. These studies
on the abbreviated survival of ISCs are very important; at
the membrane workshop yesterday interest was expressed in
using the animal model to examine the kinetics of ISC survival. This fraction is further separable if you do even more
extensive ultracentrifugation or separation experiments.
Maybe what you are observing and which I was not equipped to
study is that there is differential survivability of that
fraction which I've shown you up here as a single fraction,
if it is broken down even further by more extensive separation procedures. The presentations yesterday demonstrated
that the most dense fraction by one hour ultracentrifugation
without a gradient medium is actually made up of several
easily separable fractions if gradient media are used.

<u>Dr. Kurantsin-Mills</u>: The cells flow through capillaries and

The Red Cell, pages 195—196

yet there seem to be no concern about that. I wonder whether
you have attempted transfusing ISCs or sickle cells into normal
people. I ask this question because we all have the experience
that some patients don't have any major problems. There are
some walking in Africa who don't even know they have the disease. And so I wonder if one transfused sickled cells into
normal people what type of survivability of ^{51}Cr-tagged cells
would you see? Alternatively if you transfused cells from
clinically severe patients in steady state into patients who
are clinically mild and vice versa, what will be the survivability of these cells? Such an experiment will attempt to
find out whether or not the micro vessels of these patients
have unique characteristics that make the two patient types,
clinically severe and clinically mild, different? Have you
tried or have you talked about such an experiment?

Dr. Schoomaker: We have not attempted such an experiment.
I recall that many years ago, Doctor Singer did a limited
experiment in which sickle cells were labelled and transfused
into normal controls. This served as early proof that there
is differential hemoglobin S and F concentration in a population of sickle cells. However, I take exception with your
first comment that we are not concerned with the intact living
circulation. I think that's what prompted the development of
the animal model. It's an attempt to find a well controlled,
intact, mammalian circulation that removed a lot of the difficulty that we had in studying filterability or viscosity of
sickled cells at the bench.

Dr. Cameron: You gave a t 1/2 for these survivals. Was this
calculated from the slope, that is the half-life for survival
of those cells after the ISCs have been removed?

Dr. Schoomaker: That's right.

Dr. Cameron: Your correlation of the animal model to the
cell sample is with P-50. Have you modified the P-50 of the
cells, for example, by using stored cells in which DPG is
reduced and P-50 shifted. to see if survival still correlates?

Dr. Schoomaker: No, I have not.

ERYTHROCYTE METABOLISM, GENERAL

Chairman: D. Paglia

ERYTHROCYTE CYTOCHROME b_5: STRUCTURE, ROLE IN METHEMOGLOBIN
REDUCTION, AND SOLUBILIZATION FROM ENDOPLASMIC RETICULUM

Donald E. Hultquist, Shelley R. Slaughter,
Richard H. Douglas, Lucy Jean Sannes, and
G. Gary Sahagian
Department of Biological Chemistry
The University of Michigan
Ann Arbor, Michigan 48109

DETECTION OF ERYTHROCYTE CYTOCHROME b_5

Several years ago we detected in erythrocytes a soluble
hemeprotein with spectral properties indistinguishable from
microsomal cytochrome b_5 of other cells (Hultquist et al.,
1969). We first isolated this cytochrome from human
erythrocytes (Passon et al., 1972; Hultquist et al., 1974),
then from rabbit erythrocytes and reticulocytes, from bovine
erythrocytes (Hultquist and Douglas, 1974; Hultquist et al.,
1975), and most recently from mouse erythrocytes (Slaughter
and Hultquist, 1977).

The liver microsomal cytochrome b_5 and the erythrocyte
cytochrome b_5 are indistinguishable in terms of the visible
spectra of the isolatable ferric form (absorbance maximum
at 413 nm) and the dithionite-reduced form (absorbance
maxima at 423, 527, and 556 nm, with a shoulder at 560 nm).
The erythrocyte and liver proteins are also indistinguishable in terms of EPR spectra, ability to be reduced by
dithionite, lack of reactivity with sulfite and carbon monoxide, a protoheme IX prosthetic group, ability to serve as
the substrate for microsomal cytochrome b_5 reductase, and
reaction of the ferrous form with oxygen and methemoglobin.

In most cells cytochrome b_5 is a hydrophobic protein
which is embedded in the endoplasmic reticulum membrane.
This cytochrome b_5 functions as a part of the microsomal
electron transfer system which desaturates fatty acids
(Oshino and Omura, 1973). In contrast, erythrocyte cytochrome b_5 is a water-soluble protein present in the cytoplasm.

The Red Cell, pages 199—211

Its molecular weight is smaller than the microsomal b_5 of other cells. It is obviously not a microsomal protein since erythrocytes are devoid of endoplasmic reticulum.

ROLE OF CYTOCHROME b_5 IN METHEMOGLOBIN REDUCTION

In the erythrocyte the function of soluble cytochrome b_5 is to reduce methemoglobin. The methemoglobin reduction system is the soluble enzyme system of erythrocytes that uses the electrons of NADH to reduce methemoglobin back to the physiologically active ferrous form which is capable of binding oxygen. These reactions of hemoglobin may be summarized as follows:

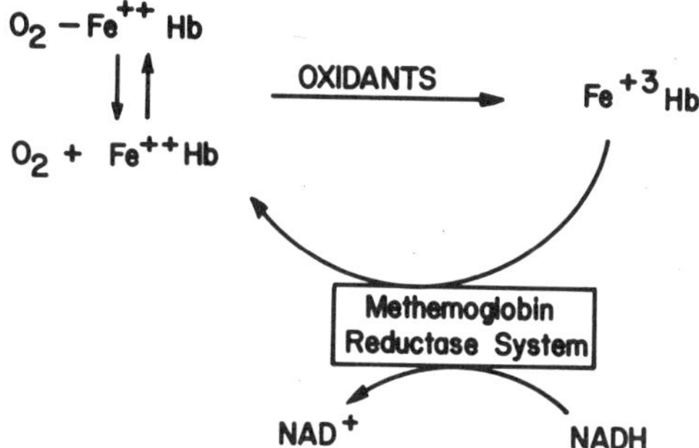

An NADH-dependent methemoglobin reductase (Scott and McGraw, 1962; Sugita et al., 1971; Kuma and Inomata, 1972) is essential for this reduction. It was previously believed that the reductase catalyzed the direct transfer of electrons between NADH and methemoglobin.

Using purified proteins, however, we showed that human erythrocyte cytochrome b_5 markedly stimulated the reductase-catalyzed reduction of methemoglobin (Hultquist and Passon, 1971). The reductase-catalyzed transfer of electrons from NADH to methemoglobin is very slow in the absence of cytochrome b_5 but quite rapid in the presence of concentrations of b_5 comparable to those present in the erythrocyte. The absence of NADH, reductase, or methemoglobin from this system resulted in no reduction. There is a linear relationship between rate of the reaction and amount of cytochrome b_5 added as the b_5 concentration varies from 0 to 0.8 micromolar.

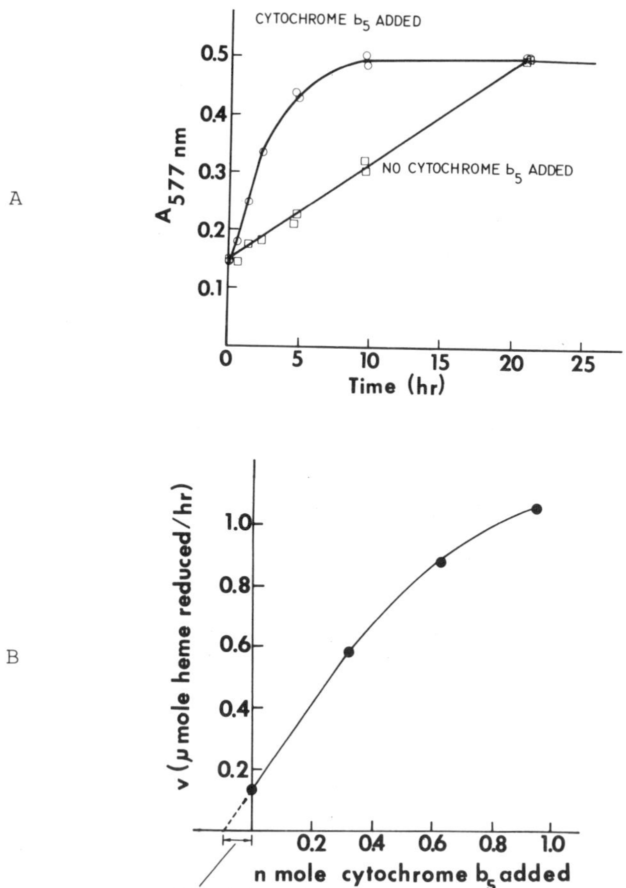

Figure 1. Stimulation by cytochrome b_5 of methemoglobin reduction catalyzed by crude hemolysate. Nitrite-treated cells were hemolyzed with 3 volumes of water. See text for details. To 1.0 ml of the resulting hemolysate were added 4.8 μmoles of NADH and (where indicated) purified cytochrome b_5 from human erythrocytes. The final volume was 1.2 ml. The reaction was allowed to proceed at 37°C. (A) Production of oxyhemoglobin with time as measured by the increase in absorbance at 577 nm. □———□, in the absence of added cytochrome b_5; 0———0, in the presence of 0.32 nmole of added cytochrome b_5. (B) Velocity of methemoglobin reduction versus amount of added cytochrome b_5.

A similar stimulation of reduction by cytochrome b_5 is seen when the reaction is carried out in crude hemolysate. Hypotonic lysates were obtained from outdated human erythrocytes which had been treated with sodium nitrite to oxidize hemoglobin to methemoglobin and then had been washed repeatedly to remove the excess nitrite. Figure 1A shows that the rate of absorbance change in the presence of added cytochrome b_5 is considerably greater than the rate where the only b_5 present is that which was present in the hemolysate. Figure 1B shows the relationship between rate of reduction and the amount of cytochrome b_5 added to the hemolysate. Extrapolation of this curve back to a rate of zero suggests that cytochrome b_5 is present in the outdated human erythrocyte at a concentration of approximately 0.37 micromolar. This is in agreement with the amount of cytochrome b_5 (0.20 to 0.33 nmole/ml) which can be isolated in crude form from outdated erythrocytes. The approximation of b_5 from the above curve is based on the assumptions that the relationship between rate and concentration is linear at low b_5 concentrations and that the rate would be zero in the absence of cytochrome b_5.

We believe that the rate of methemoglobin reduction is dependent on cytochrome b_5 concentration not only in the crude hemolysate and in the system reconstituted from purified proteins but also within the intact erythrocyte. From kinetic studies with hemolysates and with the reconstituted system we have concluded that methemoglobin is reduced by the ferrous form of cytochrome b_5. The reduction of b_5 is in turn catalyzed by the reductase. Thus, the reduction of methemoglobin occurs by the transfer of electrons in the sequence:

NADH $\longrightarrow$ Cytochrome b_5 $\longrightarrow$ Cytochrome b_5 $\longrightarrow$ Methemoglobin
                reductase

The NADH-dependent reductase essential for the reduction of methemoglobin has long been known as "NADH methemoglobin reductase". We have shown that the enzymatic properties of this water-soluble, cytoplasmic reductase (Passon and Hultquist, 1972) are very similar to those of microsomal cytochrome b_5 reductase from liver and other cells (Strittmatter and Velick, 1957). The erythrocyte soluble reductase and microsomal cytochrome b_5 reductase both contain FAD prosthetic groups and show the same substrate specificity, pattern of inhibition, and pH dependency.

On the basis of these similarities we have changed the
name of the enzyme from "methemoglobin reductase" to "erythrocyte soluble cytochrome b$_5$ reductase".

IDENTIFICATION OF ERYTHROCYTE CYTOCHROME b$_5$ AS A SEGMENT OF
MICROSOMAL CYTOCHROME b$_5$

The similarities between the enzymatic properties of
erythrocyte and liver microsomal cytochrome b$_5$ reductases
and the strikingly similar physical properties of erythrocyte and liver microsomal cytochrome b$_5$ led us to compare
in greater depth these liver and erythrocyte proteins. We
therefore undertook a structural comparison of these forms
of cytochrome b$_5$. First we compared human liver microsomal
and human erythrocyte cytochrome b$_5$, and then bovine liver
and bovine erythrocyte cytochrome b$_5$. The same picture
emerges from the comparison of the human proteins as from
the comparison of the bovine proteins. We have collected
more data with the bovine system, however, and it is these
data which will be presented in this paper.

Multiple forms of bovine erythrocyte cytochrome b$_5$ have
been purified by successive chromatography on DEAE-cellulose,
Bio-Gel P-60, and DEAE-Sephadex (Hultquist and Douglas, 1974;
Hultquist et al., 1975). The structure of only one of the
forms of bovine erythrocyte cytochrome b$_5$ (form I) will be
discussed here. This form was separated from the other
forms and purified to homogeneity by repeated chromatography
on DEAE-Sephadex.

The structure of bovine liver microsomal cytochrome b$_5$,
deduced from the work of laboratories of Strittmatter and
Ozols, is shown in Figure 2. The protein is a single peptide
chain with 145 amino acid residues and one heme. The N-
terminus is non-reactive with dansyl chloride. The two-
thirds of the molecule beginning at the N-terminus is hydrophilic whereas the one-third of the molecule at the C-terminus
is very hydrophobic. It is this hydrophobic part of the
molecule that is embedded in the membrane of the endoplasmic
reticulum (Ito and Sato, 1968; Ozols, 1974). Trypsin
degrades this molecule to the hemepeptide containing residues
7 through 88 (Strittmatter and Ozols, 1966).

```
                              7                 10
(Glx,Glx,Ala)-Ser-Ser-Lys-Ala-Val-Lys-Tyr-Tyr-Thr-Leu-Glu-
                   20
Gln-Ile-Glu-Lys-His-Asn-Asn-Ser-Lys-Ser-Thr-Trp-Leu-Ile-
    30                                          40
Leu-His-Tyr-Lys-Val-Tyr-Asp-Leu-Thr-Lys-Phe-Leu-Glu-Glu-
                        50
His-Pro-Gly-Gly-Glu-Glu-Val-Leu-Arg-Glu-Gln-Ala-Gly-Gly-
              60                                    70
Asp-Ala-Thr-Glu-Asp-Phe-Glu-Asp-Val-Gly-His-Ser-Thr-Asp-
                           80
Ala-Arg-Glu-Leu-Ser-Lys-Thr-Phe-Ile-Ile-Gly-Glu-Leu-His-
              88        90                 95        97
Pro-Asp-Asp-Arg-Ser-Lys-Ile-Thr-Lys-Pro-Ser-Glu-Ser-Ile-
    100                                      110
Ile-Thr-Thr-Ile-Asx-X-Asx-Pro-Ser-Ser-Val-Leu-Thr-Asx-Trp-
                      120
Leu-Ile-Pro-Ala-Ile-Ile-Leu-Asx-Ala-Ser-His-Leu-Tyr-(Phe,
       130                                  140
Cys)-Met-Trp-Gln-Pro-Ser-Val-Ala-Leu-Ile-Tyr-Ala-Leu-Phe-
          145
Thr-Ser-Glu-Asx
```

Figure 2. The amino acid sequence of bovine liver microsomal cytochrome b_5. Data taken from the structures most
recently reported by Corcoran and Strittmatter (1977),
Ozols <u>et al</u>. (1976), and Ozols (1975).

Bovine erythrocyte cytochrome b_5 form I has a molecular
weight of approximately 12,000 daltons. Trypsin degrades
this hemeprotein to a hemepeptide of approximately 10,000
daltons. This hemepeptide co-migrates on disc gel electrophoresis with the tryptic hemepeptide derived from bovine
liver microsomal cytochrome b_5 (Hultquist <u>et al</u>., 1975),
suggesting that liver and erythrocyte b_5 have a hemepeptide
in common. The tryptic hemepeptide derived from the
erythrocyte cytochrome b_5 was purified to homogeneity and
shown to have the same amino acid composition as the liver
tryptic hemepeptide. Like the liver tryptic hemepeptide,
alanine is the N-terminal residue (Hultquist <u>et al</u>., 1976).

Chemical analysis of the intact bovine erythrocyte
cytochrome b_5 suggested that this protein corresponds to
a segment of the larger liver microsomal cytochrome b_5.
The amino acid composition of the erythrocyte hemeprotein
was shown to agree very well with the composition of
residues 1 through 97 of the liver protein. End group

analysis supported this hypothesis. Like residue #1 of
the liver protein, the N-terminus of the erythrocyte protein
is non-reactive with dansyl chloride. Moreover, like residue
#97 of the liver protein, the C-terminal residue of the
erythrocyte protein is serine.

Analysis of the tryptic peptides derived from apo-
cytochrome b$_5$ has provided further evidence for the proposed
structure. Removal of the heme was necessary in order to
expose all of the arginine and lysine residues of cytochrome
b$_5$ to trypsin. The resulting peptides have been mapped and
the amino acid compositions of the isolated peptides have
been determined. These results provide strong evidence that
the erythrocyte cytochrome b$_5$ does indeed correspond to
residues 1 through 97 of the microsomal protein. The
erythrocyte protein has the structure of microsomal cytochrome b$_5$ minus the hydrophobic one-third of the molecule
that is embedded in the endoplasmic reticulum membrane. It
has the structure of the hydrophilic two-thirds of the liver
protein. This readily explains why the erythrocyte protein
is water-soluble whereas the liver protein is water-insoluble.

DETECTION OF MICROSOMAL CYTOCHROME b$_5$ IN ERYTHROLEUKEMIA
CELLS

What is the significance of the finding that a water-
soluble protein that functions in erythrocytes to reduce
methemoglobin is a piece of a water-insoluble, membrane-bound
protein which in other cells functions to desaturate fatty
acids? We should remember that the immature red cell is a
cell with a full complement of subcellular organelles,
including endoplasmic reticulum. At some early point in the
maturation, the endoplasmic reticulum disappears by some
unknown process. We have postulated (Passon and Hultquist,
1972) that the soluble cytochrome b$_5$ and soluble cytochrome
b$_5$ reductase of erythrocytes are derived from the endoplasmic
reticulum of immature erythroid cells by proteolytic degradation during the process of cell maturation. To make such an
idea believable we need to show that particulate cytochrome
b$_5$ and cytochrome b$_5$ reductase are present in immature
erythroid cells and that there is a protease which solubilizes these microsomal proteins.

We chose the mouse Friend virus-infected erythroleukemia
cell as the cell from which to attempt to isolate microsomes.

The erythroleukemia cell is a model for a very immature
erythroid cell since its maturation has been arrested at an
early stage of development (Friend et al., 1971). A small
amount of endoplasmic reticulum can be seen in electron
micrographs of erythroleukemia cells (see Figure 3).

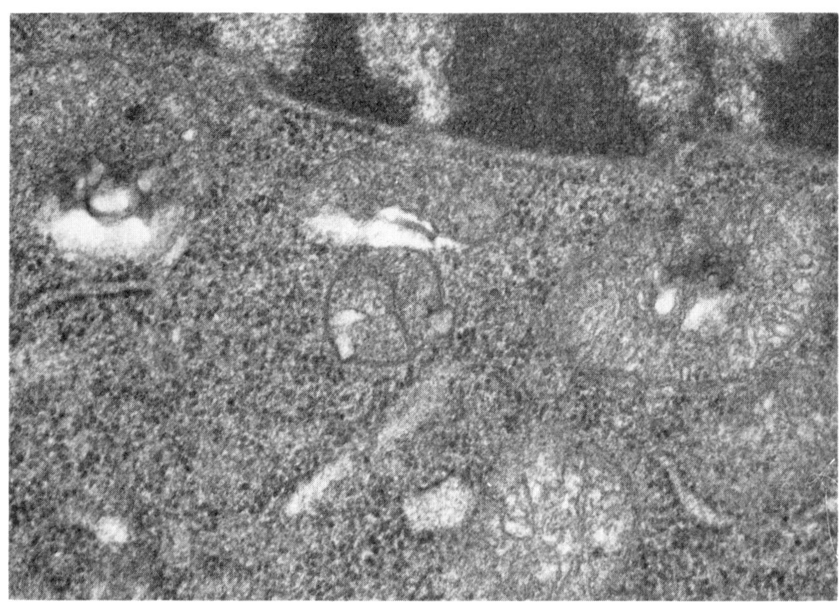

Figure 3. Electron micrograph of a murine Friend virus-
infected erythroleukemia cell showing part of the nucleus,
numerous mitochondria, and a small amount of endoplasmic
reticulum. X 60,000. The cells were collected by centrifugation, fixed with glutaraldehyde, post-fixed in osmium
tetroxide, embedded in Epon, post-stained with uranyl
magnesium acetate and lead citrate, and examined with an
AEI Corinth 275 electron microscope.

The erythroleukemia cells were grown in culture,
harvested, washed, and frozen. The isolation of microsomes
was achieved from the thawed cells by homogenization and
centrifugation of the homogenate at 105,000 x $\underline{g}$. The
resulting pellet was shown to contain microsomes as evidenced by the presence of the microsomal markers cytochrome
b_5, cytochrome b_5 reductase, and cytochrome P-450. The
cytochrome b_5 and cytochrome P-450 were identified and
quantitated by difference spectrophotometry; cytochrome b_5

reductase was identified and quantitated by its NADH-cyto-
chrome c reductase activity. The amounts of these proteins
detected in erythroleukemia cells are summarized in Table 1.
To our knowledge, this is the first isolation of microsomes
from an erythroid cell.

Table 1
Microsomal Redox Proteins of Mouse Erythroleukemia Cells

Protein/10^9 cells	Erythroleukemia cells	Erythrocytes	Hepato-cytes*
Microsomal protein (mg)	8.6	None	118
Microsomal cytochrome b$_5$ (nmole)	0.12	None	71
Cytoplasmic cytochrome b$_5$ (nmole)	None	0.05	–
Microsomal cytochrome P-450 (nmole)	0.22	None	123
NADH-cytochrome c reductase (μmole cytochrome c reduced/min)	0.80	–	–

*Based on the work of Dr. Kostas Vatsis.

Whereas the erythroleukemia cells contained microsomal
cytochrome b$_5$, no soluble cytochrome b$_5$ was detected in the
cytoplasmic fraction of these cells. Conversely, cytoplasmic but no microsomal b$_5$ was detected in mouse erythrocytes. The amounts of microsomal redox proteins in the
erythroleukemia cells are small relative to the liver cell
(see Table 1). This is in agreement with the small amount
of total protein in the microsomal pellet and the small
amount of endoplasmic reticulum observed upon electron
microscopic observation of the cells. However, the amount
of particulate cytochrome b$_5$ in the immature cell is greater
than the amount of soluble cytochrome b$_5$ in the erythrocyte.
These values are compatible with the hypothesis that
particulate cytochrome b$_5$ of immature erythroid cells is
the source of the soluble b$_5$ of erythrocytes.

CONVERSION OF MICROSOMAL CYTOCHROME b_5 TO SOLUBLE CYTOCHROME b_5 BY LYSOSOMAL PROTEASE

If particulate cytochrome b_5 is solubilized during erythroid maturation, what is the solubilizing agent? One reasonable possibility for the solubilizing agent would be a cathepsin provided by the lysosomes of the immature erythroid cell. We have used liver lysosomes as a model for erythroid lysosomes. Bovine liver lysosomes were incubated with bovine liver microsomes under conditions that lyse the lysosomes. Several forms of soluble cytochrome b_5 were obtained by this procedure and among them were forms which co-migrated on disc gel electrophoresis with the forms of cytochrome b_5 isolated from bovine erythrocytes.

Recently we have isolated a protease fraction from bovine liver lysosomes which solubilizes microsomes to give predominantly forms of cytochrome b_5 which co-electrophorese with the forms of erythrocyte cytochrome b_5. It appears that the protease fraction is especially effective in cleaving the bond between residues 97 and 98 of the liver microsomal cytochrome. We are further purifying the protease and are performing peptide mapping on the derived hemepeptides.

Figure 4 depicts what we believe is happening to the cytochrome b_5 during erythroid maturation. At an early point in the maturation of the red cell a cathepsin of the lysosome is believed to attack the endoplasmic reticulum, cleaving the cytochrome b_5 and cytochrome b_5 reductase at the points where these proteins emerge from the membrane. Such action by the protease might occur within the lysosome or upon release of the protease from the lysosomes as depicted in the figure. The hydrophobic parts of the mole- cules would be expected to remain with the membranes and be discarded; the hydrophilic portions of cytochrome b_5 and cytochrome b_5 reductase become the components of the methemoglobin reduction system. The conversion of the particulate redox system to a soluble system should serve as a very useful probe for studying erythroid maturation. Studies of the protease may likewise be of great value in understanding the maturation of both normal and abnormal erythroid cells.

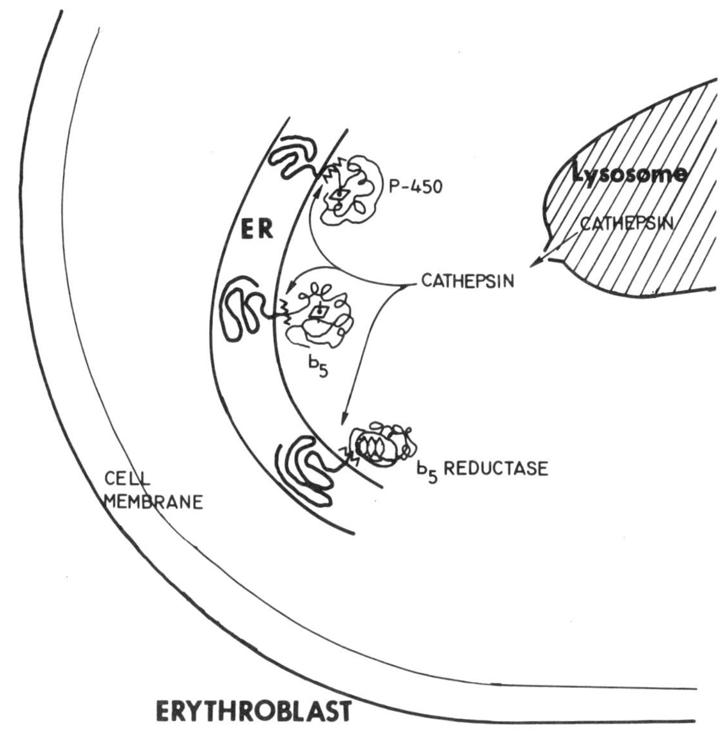

Figure 4. Hypothetical scheme for the solubilization of endoplasmic reticulum redox proteins during erythroid maturation.

ACKNOWLEDGEMENTS

We wish to acknowledge the work, insight, and dedication of Dr. Dan Reed, Dr. Philip Passon, and Dr. Richard Dean who, as former investigators in this laboratory, initiated and carried out many of the early studies. We also wish to acknowledge the collaboration of the laboratory of Dr. Raymond Ruddon in growing and harvesting the erythroleukemia cells, the laboratory of Dr. Charles Williams in mapping and analyzing the tryptic peptides, and the laboratory of Dr. Robert Gray in performing the electron microscopic studies.

This work was supported by U.S. Public Health Service
Research Grant AM-09250, U.S. Public Health Service Training
Grant GM-00187, American Cancer Society Institution Grants,
an Institutional Equal Opportunity Award, and a Faculty
Research Grant from the University of Michigan.

REFERENCES

Corcoran D, Strittmatter, P (1977). Amino acid sequence of
  the nonpolar segment of calf liver cytochrome b_5. Fed
  Proc 36:897.
Friend C, Scher W, Holland JG, Sato T (1971). Hemoglobin
  synthesis in murine virus-induced leukemic cells in vitro:
  stimulation of erythroid differentiation by dimethyl
  sulfoxide. Proc Nat Acad Sci USA 68:378.
Hultquist DE, Dean RT, Douglas RH (1974). Homogeneous
  cytochrome b_5 from human erythrocytes. Biochem Biophys
  Res Commun 60:28.
Hultquist DE, Douglas RH (1974). Cytochrome b_5 from human
  and bovine erythrocytes. 168th Meet Am Chem Soc BIOL-103.
Hultquist DE, Douglas RH, Dean RT (1975). The methemoglobin
  reduction system of erythrocytes. In Brewer GJ (ed):
  "Proceedings of the Third International Conference on Red
  Cell Metabolism and Function," New York: Alan R. Liss,
  p 297.
Hultquist DE, Douglas RH, Slaughter SR (1976). Evidence
  that the two forms of cytochrome b_5 from bovine erythrocytes are identical to segments of microsomal cytochrome
  b_5. Fed Proc 35:1424.
Hultquist DE, Passon PG (1971). Catalysis of methemoglobin
  reduction by erythrocyte cytochrome b_5 and cytochrome b_5
  reductase. Nature New Biol 229:252.
Hultquist DE, Reed DW, Passon, PG (1969). Isolation,
  characterization, and enzymatic reduction of cytochrome B
  (556) from human erythrocytes. Fed Proc 28:862.
Ito A, Sato R (1968). Purification by means of detergents
  and properties of cytochrome b_5 from liver microsomes.
  J Biol Chem 243:4922.
Kuma F, Inomata H (1972). Studies on methemoglobin reductase.
  II. The purification and molecular properties of reduced
  nicotinamide adenine dinucleotide-dependent methemoglobin
  reductase. J Biol Chem 247:556.
Oshino N, Omura T (1973). Immunological evidence for the
  participation of cytochrome b_5 in microsomal stearyl-
  CoA desaturation reaction. Arch Biochem Biophys 157:395.

Ozols J (1974). Cytochrome b$_5$ from microsomal membranes of equine, bovine, and porcine livers. Isolation and properties of preparations containing the membranous segment. Biochem 13:426.

Ozols J (1975). Structural studies on microsomal proteins: isolation and the primary structure of the membranous segment of cytochrome b$_5$. In Laursen RA (ed): "Solid-Phase Methods in Protein Sequence Analysis. Proceedings of the First International Conference," Rockford, Illinois: Pierce Chemical Company.

Ozols J, Gerard C, Nobrega FG (1976). Proteolytic cleavage of horse liver cytochrome b$_5$. J Biol Chem 251:6767.

Passon PG, Hultquist DE (1972). Soluble cytochrome b$_5$ reductase from human erythrocytes. Biochim Biophys Acta 275:62.

Passon PG, Reed DW, Hultquist DE (1972). Soluble cytochrome b$_5$ from human erythrocytes. Biochim Biophys Acta 275:51.

Scott EM, McGraw JC (1962). Purification and properties of diphosphopyridine nucleotide diaphorase of human erythrocytes. J Biol Chem 237:249.

Slaughter SR, Hultquist DE (1977). Demonstration of microsomal cytochrome b$_5$, cytochrome b$_5$ reductase, and cytochrome P-450 in Friend erythroleukemia (FL) cells. Fed Proc 36:928.

Strittmatter P, Ozols J (1966). The restricted tryptic cleavage of cytochrome b$_5$. J Biol Chem 241:4787.

Strittmatter P, Velick SF (1957). The purification and properties of microsomal cytochrome reductase. J Biol Chem 228:785.

Sugita Y, Nomura S, Yoneyama Y (1971). Purification of reduced pyridine nucleotide dehydrogenase from human erythrocytes and methemoglobin reduction by the enzyme. J Biol Chem 246:6072.

DISCUSSION

<u>Dr. Goldstein</u>: Do you know the pH optimum of the protease?
Is it acid as one would expect for lysomal hydrolases?

<u>Dr. Hultquist</u>: We have not determined the pH optimum. The
only thing we did was to take fractions off a gel filtration
column and looked for the protease that would cleave microsomes to give us the right product. Obviously we must now
characterize the enzyme.

<u>Dr. Brewer</u>: In congenital methemoglobinemia, I take it that
the defective protein is usually the reductase, is that right?

<u>Dr. Hultquist</u>: Yes, in several hundred patients, that is the
case. Either the reductase is absent or there is an abnormal
form of the reductase.

<u>Dr. Brewer</u>: If I understand what you are saying, the cytochrome
b-5 is shared by the liver cell and the red cell. The liver
cell has it attached to the endoplasmic reticulum with the
tail still on it. Do these cell types also share the cytochrome b-5 reductase and if they do what happens to the liver
in congenital methemoglobinemia?

<u>Dr. Hultquist</u>: There are two cases of congenital methemoglo-
binemia in which apparently the reductase is normal. One is
in Rochester; one is in Israel. I would very much like to
know in those two cases if the cytochrome b-5 itself is deficient. I think that there is another possibility- erythrocytes in which the reductase is deficient may also be deficient in b5; this could result from a defect in the protease
or in the mode of solubilizing both of the proteins. In fact,
one kinetic study which we have done, with cells from a family
with congenital methemoglobinemia, indicates that this may
indeed be the case. The kinetics just don't make sense unless
both the reductase and the b5 are missing.

<u>Dr. Carrell</u>: The question I was going to ask was partly put
by Dr. Brewer. Is there a practical measurement technique
in terms of the blood volume that could be obtained from a
patient for cytochrome b-5 in human red cells?

<u>Dr. Hultquist</u>: If there had been a good method we would have
immediately looked at these patients in which we think the

The Red Cell, pages 213—216

cytochrome b5 might be deficient. We have worked out an
assay but it is really not very good. In the slide which
shows reduction by a crude hemolysate, you may have noticed
that we extrapolated back to the X-axis to calculate how much
b-5 was present in the hemolysate. We got a value of 0.39 micromolar. The answer to your question is "no." We need an immunological assay.

Dr. Carrell: The second point, I wonder if you could comment
on because I think it will be of particular interest to people
whose prime interest is in the area of hemoglobin. This is
the question of the finding I understand by some Japanese
that the reduction occurs more efficiently in hemoglobin that
is combined with IHP, that is when methemoglobin is put into
the T-conformation.

Dr. Hultquist: The slide which showed the course of methemoglobin reduction by hemolysate showed that there was no
change in the rate of reduction all the way up to the point
where the reduction was essentially complete. This indicates
that in hemolysates methemoglobin reduction is independent
of methemoglobin concentration. So it is not a bimolecular
reaction between cytochrome b-5 and methemoglobin, in which
methemoglobin concentration is determining the rate of the
reaction. We would like to think that perhaps there is a
complex formed and we will try to get at this with stop-flow
experiments. If we could indeed get a complex, this would
be terribly exciting in that the structure of b-5 has been
determined by x-ray crystallography; the structure of methemoglobin has been determined. Hopefully, we could form a
complex between the two. Structural analysis of that complex
would be terribly exciting.

Dr. Rucknagel: As an exciting example of how a gene product
seems to be packaged in two different ways in delivery to
two different tissues, do you think that the microsomal b-5
would work in the red cells if it still had that tail on?
The second question is do you have any evidence on the specificity of the peptides that are released from that protease?
Could it be that that tail is simply uncoiled since it is so
hydrophobic, and is more accessible? Do you have any notions
about the specificity?

Dr. Hultquist: In terms of specificity of the protease remember that we are isolating microsomes and there is a question
of whether microsomes look to the protease anything like

endoplasmic reticulum of the cell. I don't know how natural
the situation is. I think the protease cleaves where it does
because that is an available point which is not buried in the
hydrophobic segment. The structure of the hydrophobic portion
is very tight. Scott Matthews has shown by x-ray diffraction
that it's a very tight molecule. There aren't many bonds
available for cleavage. So, it's probably a combination of
specificity and bond availability.

I think it's interesting that in previous studies incubation of
pancreatic, "lipase" with liver microsomes gave two soluble
hemepeptides, corresponding to residues,1 through 97 and 1
through 95. Apparently, pancreatic "lipase" contains pancreatic proteases. I think that erythrocyte cytochrome b-5
results from cleavage at these same points. I didn't mention
that we have isolated a second form of erythrocyte b-5 that
could possibly result from cleavage at 95 instead of 97. So
the cleavage we are postulating has been observed before.
But, to answer your question, I think that a combination of
a tightly coiled molecule and protection within the ER, explains why the bond between residues 97 and 98 is one of the
few places where cleavage can occur.

Dr. Rucknagel: Would the microsomal system work in red cells?

Dr. Hultquist: In one experiment we took microsomes and tried
to make them reduce methemoglobin.   Reduction did not occur. But there may be a problem of transport into the microsomes, which may be very different from the E.R.

Dr. Mansouri: In answer to Dr. Carrell's question regarding
conformational change and reduction, I just wanted to mention
about what I did in this reduction reaction. I was interested in studying the reduction of methemoglobin in terms
of conformational change, and I found that reduction of the
methemoglobin in the absence of oxygen is somehow, about
thirty per cent faster than the reduction of hemoglobin in
the presence of oxygen or in the presence of carbon monoxide. Also, as you mentioned, there is not doubt that IHP
increases the rate of the reduction reaction, but that's as
far as I have gone.

Dr. Hultquist: It's interesting that carbon monoxide and oxygen will affect a reaction of methemoglobin. Oxygen and
carbon monoxide are affecting the rate of reduction?

<u>Dr. Mansouri</u>: The question was that, of course, methemoglobin
has conformation under the oxy or deoxy condition. But as
it is reduced to hemoglobin, in the absence of oxygen or
carbon monoxide, it assumes T conformation whereas in the
presence of one of the above ligands, it does not undergo
much of a conformational change.

UNSTABLE ENZYMES IN ERYTHROCYTES OF A FAMILY WITH THE
HUTCHINSON-GILFORD PROGERIA SYNDROME

Samuel Goldstein and Elena J. Moerman

Depts. Medicine & Biochemistry
McMaster Univerity Medical Centre
Hamilton, Ontario, Canada L8S 4J9

INTRODUCTION

Hutchinson-Gilford progeria syndrome is a rare and
obscure disorder of infancy with catastrophic consequences
(DeBusk, 1972; Goldstein, 1978). Following the onset of
severe growth stunting, as a rule in the first year of life,
several phenotypic characteristics of accelerated aging
appear with death ensuing in the teens, most often the result
of advanced coronary or cerebrovascular disease. We have
recently demonstrated that circulating erythrocytes of a
child with progeria contain an increased heat-labile fraction
of two genetically distinct enzymes, glucose-6-phosphate
dehydrogenase (G6PD) and 6-phosphogluconate dehydrogenase
(6PGD) (Goldstein & Moerman, 1978). Additionally, both
parents have values intermediate to those of their daughter
and controls consistent with genetic transmission of an
autosomal recessive trait. Studies in tissue culture of this
family and other unrelated progeric subjects have demonstrated similar enzyme instability as well as diverse
abnormalities of non-enzymatic proteins (Goldstein &
Moerman, 1976; Goldstein, 1978). In the present report,
we review and extend the previous data on G6PD and 6PGD
in peripheral erythrocytes, and present additional results
on a third enzyme, hypoxanthine-guanine phosphoribosyl-
transferase (HGPRT). We also provide a detailed analysis
of G6PD heat-lability in red cells fractionated according
to circulating age.

The Red Cell, pages 217—228

<u>METHODS</u>

<u>Subjects</u>

The progeria family was of Caucasian origin (Table 1).
Both parents were clinically normal and denied a history of
consanguinity or any progeria-like disorder. The female
proband was the product of a single uncomplicated pregnancy.
A second pregnancy ended in spontaneous first trimester
abortion. Progeria was first diagnosed at age 2 following
clinical presentation with severe growth failure to the
extent that the child was and still remains below 3 percentile
for height and weight. Studies reported here were initiated
when the patient was 3 years of age and conducted over an
interval of 30 months.

TABLE 1. SUBJECTS IN ERYTHROCYTE STUDY

PROGERIA FAMILY

Subject		Age (Years)
B.S.	Proband	5
A.S.	Mother	31
R.S.	Father	43

CONTROLS

Normal

M.B.		9
D.E.		25
E.M.		34
S.G.		38
A.S.		65

Abnormal

T.Dù	FUO	8
T.Da	Hodgkin's	9
G.R.	Myelofibrosis	78

Controls

Normal controls were healthy and denied any history of
metabolic disease or family history of disorders associated
with shortening of the lifespan (Table 1). Abnormal controls
were included because chronic illness could have influenced
erythrocyte turnover and enzyme instability.

Laboratory Studies

Non-fasting blood was obtained by venipuncture without
anticoagulants. The procedure of Murphy (1973) was used
in slightly modified form (Goldstein & Moerman, 1978). In
brief, blood was defibrinated at room temperature by gentle
rotary shaking in a glass beaker containing glass beads. The
supernatant blood was decanted and centrifuged at 200g to
remove the buffy coat followed by careful mixing and
recentrifugation. This procedure was repeated 3 times, at
which time leukocytes were found to comprise less than .01%
of the erythrocyte count. Erythrocytes were then suspended
in homologous serum and adjusted to a hematocrit of 85%. An
aliquot of the whole erythrocyte population (WEP) was removed
and held on ice. The remainder was centrifuged in a fixed
angle rotor in a Sorvall centrifuge for 1 hour at 30°C.
Efficacy of fractionation was confirmed by ^{59}Fe kinetic
studies on two of the abnormal control subjects, as well as
enzyme activities and reticulocyte counts (Marks et al,
1958; Fornaini et al, 1969; Turner et al, 1974; Goldstein
& Moerman, 1978). Young cells in the top fraction or 6
equal fractions in total were recovered by careful manual
removal using a pasteur pipet. The WEP and each fraction
were then hemolysed, the hemolysate was cleared by
ultracentrifugation and assayed for G6PD and 6PGD heat-
lability exactly as described (Goldstein & Moerman, 1978).
HGPRT was assayed as for cultured fibroblasts (Goldstein &
Moerman, 1975) except that the heating temperature was 73°C.
The fraction of heat-labile enzyme and half-life of the
stable component were derived by linear regression analysis
of values falling on the linear portion of the curves as
described below.

Results

Routine blood tests including hemoglobin, hematocrit,

reticulocyte fractions, white blood count and differential,
were normal in the proband and both parents. Starch and
polyacrylamide gel electrophoresis for G6PD revealed normal
(type B) patterns. Similarly, electrophoretic banding
patterns for 6PGD were normal. Electrophoresis of HGPRT
was not carried out.

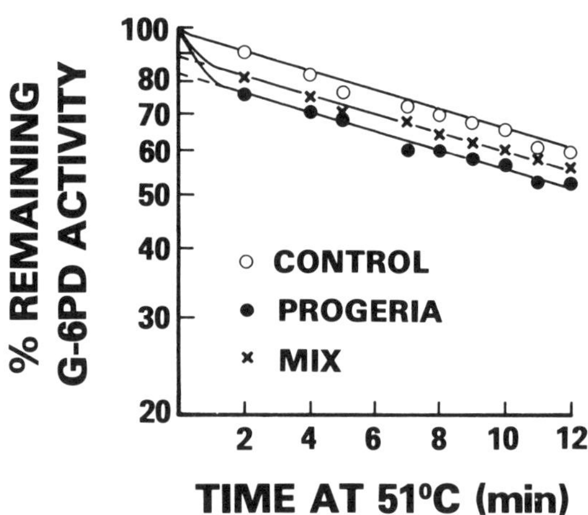

Figure 1. Heat-lability of glucose-6 phosphate dehydrogenase
in hemolysates of whole erythocyte populations. Shown here
is a representative experiment on samples from a 9 year old
normal control, the proband and an equal part mixture of
these two samples. See text for details.

Increased heat-lability of G6PD in progeric erythrocytes
is shown in Figure 1. A two phase phenomenon was always
apparent for all 3 enzymes in the proband and both parents:
an initial component showing rapid loss of activity followed
by a second larger component of linear exponential decay.
The half-life and the heat-labile fraction were calculated
from the slope-intercept values, respectively, derived from
linear regression analysis. Values obtained in this manner
agreed closely with the manual method of drawing a line that
best fit the points, extrapolating the linear portion back
to the ordinate at zero time, and subtracting the intercept
value from 100%. In Figure 1, the heat-labile fraction of
G6PD in WEP of the proband was 18.70±1.67% (mean ± S.D.)
and 2.24±1.48% for the control. The half-life of the stable

component was $18.48^{+}1.08$ min. for the proband and 16.78^{+} 0.73 min. for the control. The intermediate line, an equal part mixture of hemolysates from progeric and control samples, gave a heat-labile fraction of $12.20^{+}1.02\%$, not far from that obtained by averaging progeria and control data (10.4%). Similarly, the half-life of the stable component in this mixing experiment was $19.50^{+}0.71$ mins. These findings strongly suggest that progeric hemolysates did not contain proteolytic or other detrimental factors, or alternately, were not deficient in essential stabilizing factors.

Combined results on the heat-labile fractions of G6PD, 6PGD and HGPRT are shown in Table 2. In WEP, the proband showed the highest heat-labile fraction for all 3 enzymes. This was followed by values in the parents which were inter- mediate to those of the daughter and controls; the single exception was the higher heat-labile fraction of HGPRT in the father. The percent heat-lability for control HGPRT was somewhat higher than for the two dehydrogenases which relates to a dialysis step required to deplete endogenous purines prior to HGPRT assay. A similar phenomenon was observed in cultured skin fibroblasts (Goldstein & Moerman, 1975) but as in fibroblasts, heat-labile fractions in erythrocytes were significantly higher in progeria. Young erythrocytes contained heat-labile fractions that were not statistically different from WEP for all 3 enzymes. But once again, corresponding values were significantly elevated in the progeric child and intermediate in both parents.

Control erythrocytes contained slightly higher G6PD activity than erythrocytes of the proband (Table 3) both in WEP and 6 fractions of WEP. Although in both cases activity dropped progressively on descending the gradient, the percent activity remaining relative to fraction 1 was not significantly different in the proband and control. However, heat-lability experiments on G6PD in these same fractions showed several interesting differences (Table 4). First, the percent heat-lability of G6PD was significantly higher in fraction 1 of progeric erythrocytes compared to the control. Second, this percentage decreased progressively in progeric cells to fraction 5 of the gradient, while in contrast, the initially small percent of heat-labile enzyme in control cells changed very little. Third, in both samples, the stable component of G6PD maintained the same half-life into the older erythrocytes of fractions 5 and 6 where progeric G6PD had a half-life shortened by about 50% compared

TABLE 2. FRACTION OF HEAT-LABILE ENZYMES IN CIRCULATING ERYTHROCYTES *

Enzyme	Cell Type	Controls	Progeria Family					
			Proband	P [+]	Mother	P	Father	P
G6PD	WEP	3.43 ± 0.75 (8)	22.26 ± 4.33 (5)	.001	13.83 ± 3.79 (5)	.001	11.57 ± 1.36 (4)	.001
	young	3.05 ± 0.71 (10)	24.55 ± 2.96 (5)	.001	11.96 ± 5.71 (2)	.005	9.51 ± 3.17 (3)	.005
6PGD	WEP	5.05 ± 1.40 (6)	22.31 ± 8.09 (3)	.005	9.13 ± 2.58 (2)	.1	9.69 ± 1.84 (2)	.05
	young	4.12 ± 1.77 (6)	29.90 (n=1)	−	13.65 ± 3.01 (2)	.02	13.78 ± 1.94 (2)	.01
HGPRT	WEP	11.68 ± 4.41 (5)	21.20 ± 1.84 (2)	.05	19.69 ± 4.04 (3)	.1	28.05 ± 4.76 (3)	.02
	young	7.44 ± 3.88 (5)	23.82 ± 3.33 (2)	.02	19.11 ± 11.27 (2)	.1	13.28 ± 1.27 (2)	.1

* Data are mean percent $\pm$ S.E.M. (number of experiments on separate blood samples)

+ Significance of difference: family member versus controls (P < values shown)

TABLE 3. G6PD activity in WEP and erythrocytes
fractionated according to age
(International units/ml packed cells) *

Cell Type	CONTROL		PROGERIA	
	Enzyme Activity	Relative to Fr. 1 (%)	Enzyme Activity	Relative to Fr. 1 (%)
WEP	2.21	80	2.00	83
Fr. 1	2.78	100	2.41	100
Fr. 2	2.61	94	2.21	92
Fr. 3	2.41	87	2.21	92
Fr. 4	2.14	77	2.00	83
Fr. 5	1.80	65	1.57	65
Fr. 6	1.60	57	1.19	50

* Data obtained from blood samples worked up simultaneously
from a 9 year old normal subject and the proband. Fraction
1 is the top of the gradient descending through fraction 6
at the bottom.

TABLE 4. Percent heat-lability of unstable component and half-life of stable component of G6PD in erythrocyte populations fractionated according to age *

Fraction Number	CONTROL		PROGERIA	
	Heat-Labile Fraction (%)	$t\frac{1}{2}$ (mins)	Heat-Labile Fraction (%)	$t\frac{1}{2}$ (mins)
1	$3.49^{+}_{-}1.49$	$16.15^{+}_{-}0.68$	$21.80^{+}_{-}1.09$	$16.23^{+}_{-}0.57$
2	$3.83^{+}_{-}1.25$	$16.50^{+}_{-}0.59$	$18.80^{+}_{-}1.41$	$15.93^{+}_{-}0.69$
3	$0.08^{+}_{-}2.00$	$16.54^{+}_{-}0.95$	$16.10^{+}_{-}1.25$	$17.80^{+}_{-}0.73$
4	$1.31^{+}_{-}2.22$	$15.68^{+}_{-}0.96$	$14.40^{+}_{-}0.81$	$17.90^{+}_{-}1.20$
5	$2.05^{+}_{-}1.90$	$14.33^{+}_{-}0.68$	$13.30^{+}_{-}2.67$	$8.22^{+}_{-}0.34$
6	$5.71^{+}_{-}3.10$	$13.40^{+}_{-}0.99$	$16.03^{+}_{-}2.62$	$8.31^{+}_{-}0.35$

* Values shown ($^{+}_{-}$ S.D.) were calculated from linear regression analysis as in Methods and Results. All regression coefficients were between r = -0.981 and -0.996. Data derived from samples analyzed in Table 3.

to fraction 1. In contrast, control G6PD was reduced by less than 20% in corresponding fractions consistent with earlier reports on normal subjects under comparable conditions (Fornaini et al, 1969).

DISCUSSION

The current findings extend our earlier observations demonstrating a widespread defect of genetic expression in progeric cells. The presence of an increased fraction of heat-labile G6PD, 6PGD and HGPRT in progeric erythrocytes, as well as qualitatively similar enzyme defects and other alterations in non-enzymatic proteins of cultured skin fibroblasts, indicates that the problem in progeria affects a diversity of gene products and cell types in vivo and in vitro.

Although several enzymes show progressive deterioration in several physical-chemical parameters during erythrocyte aging in the circulation (Marks et al, 1958; Fornaini et al, 1969; Turner et al, 1974), the present observations appear to be distinctive for two major reasons. First, all members of the family had normal blood indices and reticulocyte counts. Second, all three enzyme activities in young cells and WEP were similar in the family and controls (Goldstein & Moerman, 1978). If erythrocytes were merely turning over more slowly in this family, it would be reasonable to expect abnormalities in one or more of these parameters.

The possibility of simultaneous mutations in structural genes for these three enzymes must be considered. Inherited changes in the primary sequence of amino acids are usually associated with increased thermolability of various enzymes, although in such instances the entire population of enzyme molecules is labile rather than a fraction (Goldstein & Moerman, 1978). However, the second phase of decay, which represents the normal majority of enzyme molecules, was not different in WEP and young erythrocytes of each family member versus controls (Goldstein & Moerman, 1978, and see Fig. 1 and Table 4). Thus, the present results taken together with those in cultured fibroblasts indicate that a unique defect exists in progeria cells.

Mutation in a single gene which controls a critical step

of macromolecular turnover is a plausible explanation. If
for example, an enzyme involved in protein synthesis were
defective in progeric cells, this could lead to the production of a mixture of normal and abnormal proteins. The
latter proteins would contain a random array of amino acid
substitutions which might explain our negative electrophoretic
studies: heterogeneously altered proteins would be dispersed
into many positions in the gel and not be detectable on
staining. Still another possibility is a defect in
proteolysis, a process now believed to selectively identify
and degrade abnormal proteins (Goldstein et al, 1976).
However, the coexistence of a linked defect in synthesis and
degradation, i.e. protein turnover, cannot be ruled out
either.

A mechanism leading to diverse post-translational
alterations could also yield an increased fraction of
altered proteins. The shortened half-life of G6PD in the
oldest progeric erythrocytes (Table 4) is consistent with
either a post-translational defect or an abnormality in
protein turnover. But the presence of the highest heat-
labile fraction in young progeric erythrocytes and its
progressive fall with time in the circulation seems best
reconciled with a primary defect in protein synthesis
followed secondarily by increased denaturation and/or
proteolysis.

Evidence also exists for abnormal DNA repair in progeric
fibroblasts (reviewed in Goldstein, 1978). Such a defect
could result in a generalized increase in mutability and
account for the widespread abnormality of genetic expression
in progeric cells. But this has been a controversial area,
and more recent studies suggest that the putative defect in
DNA repair may only be a consequence of abnormal protein
turnover (Goldstein et al, 1976; Goldstein, 1978; Goldstein
et al, in preparation).

More definitively, the presence of increased fractions
of heat-labile enzymes in clinically normal parents of the
progeric child is consistent with autosomal recessive
inheritance. This is of great practical importance with
regard to genetic counselling. In this family, therefore,
the probability that future progeny might be affected is 1
in 4, in contrast to an etiology based on fresh dominant
mutation (Jones et al, 1975) which would carry an extremely
low risk of the order of 1 in 10^6.

Finally, the promise that heat-labile enzymes represent a screening test for progeria must be viewed with caution. Indeed, similar data have now been obtained in Werner's syndrome, both in skin fibroblasts (Holliday et al, 1974; Goldstein & Moerman, 1975) and circulating erythrocytes (Goldstein & Moerman, in preparation). Moreover, progeria itself may be a genetically heterogeneous disorder. In any case, this simple test on blood and cultured cells should be a valuable adjunct to clinical criteria in expediting the diagnosis of progeria and other disorders or premature aging.

ACKNOWLEDGMENT

We thank Dr. A. Bailey of the Toronto Hospital for Sick Children for referring the progeria family, Dr. N. Rudd and Dr. M. Buchwald of the same institution for their generous assistance throughout these studies and Mr. Calvin Harley for help with statistical analysis. Supported by Grant MT-3515 from the Medical Research Council of Canada.

REFERENCES

DeBusk FL (1972). The Hutchinson-Gilford progeria syndrome. J Pediatr 80: 697..

Fornaini G, Leoncini G, Segni P, Calabria GA, Dacha M (1969). Relationship between age and properties of human and rabbit erythrocyte glucose-6-phosphate dehydrogenase. Eur J Biochem 7: 214.

Goldstein S (1978). Human genetic disorders which feature accelerated aging. In Schneider EL (ed): "The Genetics of Aging", New York, Plenum Press (in press).

Goldstein S,,Moerman E (1975). Heat-labile enzymes in skin fibroblasts from subjects with progeria. New Engl J. Med 292: 1305.

Goldstein S, Moerman E (1975). Heat-labile enzymes in Werner's syndrome fibroblasts. Nature 255: 159.

Goldstein S, Moerman EJ (1976). Defective proteins in normal and abnormal human fibroblasts during aging in vitro. Interdiscip Topics Geront 10: 24.

Goldstein S, Moerman EJ (1978). Am J Hum Genet (in press).

Goldstein S, Stotland D, Cordeiro RAJ (1976). Decreased proteolysis and increased amino acid efflux in aging human fibroblasts. Mech Ageing & Develop 5: 221.

Holliday R, Porterfield JS, Gibbs DD (1974). Premature aging and occurrence of altered enzyme in Werner's syndrome fibroblasts. Nature 248: 762.

Jones KL, Smith DW, Harvey MA, Hall BD, Quan L (1975). Older paternal age and fresh gene mutation: data on additional disorders. J Pediatr 86: 84.

Marks PA, Johnson AB, Hirschberg E (1958). Effect of age on the enzyme activity in erythrocytes. Proc Nat Acad Sci 44: 529.

Murphy JR (1973). Influence of temperature and method of centrifugation on the separation of erythrocytes. J Lab Clin Med 82: 334.

Turner BM, Fisher RA, Harris H (1974). The age related loss of activity of four enzymes in the human erythrocyte. Clin Chim Acta 50: 85.

DISCUSSION

Dr. Carrell: The changes that are taking place occur in such a wide range of enzymes that they must surely be post-translational, so this suggests several mechanisms. One attractive one would be a failure to remove the pre-peptides that are now known to be attached to most proteins to allow formation on the endoplasmic reticulum. Failure to remove this hydrophobic portion would increase lability. The other mechanism could be polymerization. Both of these mechanisms would be indicated very simply by molecular weight measurements. Is there any alteration in the molecular weights?

Dr. Goldstein: We would have to purify the enzymes to look carefully at the molecular weight of subunits. Since we're dealing with a rather labile subfraction, we are afraid that it may be "purified out". We have made a number of attempts at purification using conventional chromatographic techniques, with a rather quick disappearance of the labile subfraction. I agree that there is a possibility of a post-translational mechanism, but I am not quite as certain that these are definitely post-translational. That remains to be proven. There could still be a synthetic defect, even a pre-translational defect.

Dr. Rosa: If I have understood, you have made your heat-stability test on whole hemolysate? Yes. Okay. Have you made the same stability test on purified or pre-purified G6PD?

Dr. Goldstein: This is the problem that I have just alluded to. If you begin to purify these enzymes you lose the altered subfraction. So, you really can't go after it by conventional techniques. As you know, when you purify an enzyme from red cells, you end up with yields variously reported say for G6PD, of anywhere from ten to fifty percent. In the fifty to ninety percent that you lose, you are definitely losing the "weaker" species of molecules such as a labile subfraction. That's the major problem in pursuing this.

Dr. Rosa: I would just like to know if you have tried just to strip your hemolysate, and then made your stability test?

Dr. Goldstein: Well, we have dialyzed hemolysates. When we do there is increased heat lability of the overall enzyme.

The Red Cell, pages 229—231

That is the difference in heat labile subfractions between
the progeric samples and controls are preserved. We don't
think it's a small molecule problem although we can't really
rule this out. The mixing experiments are also against that
idea.

Dr. Paglia: Dr. Goldstein, may I ask, have you tried any
stabilizing agents to see if you could prevent the increased
lability? Substrates, cofactors or sulfhydryl reagents, for
example?

Dr. Goldstein: Well, the hemolysates are produced in the
presence of twenty micromolar NADP. We've increased that
to a hundred micromolar and it doesn't make much difference.
β-mercaptoethanol and E-amino caproic acid are also present,
but it doesn't seem to make much difference.

Dr. Winterbourn: Have you observed any effects of oxygen
on the protein stability? I realize that red cells would
not be appropriate to study, but the fibroblasts might
reveal something.

Dr. Goldstein: We have been doing some collaborative work
on superoxide dismutase which relates to the oxygen tension.
We don't have any direct observations on the survival capacity
but we have evidence of inducing the superoxide dismutase in
normal cells with increased oxygen. Preliminary results
suggest that progeria cells may be a little impaired in
responding to oxygen reduction. But we believe this reflects a generalized abnormality of proteins rather than a
primary defect of superoxide dismutase.

Dr. Lessin: I may have missed it. Do these children
clinically have hemolytic anemia and if not, why not?

Dr. Goldstein: There appears to be no hemolytic anemia
because enzyme activities are all pretty normal. Now the
question is, would they have hemolytic anemia if they had
a febrile type of illness, especially when prolonged? I
don't know. We simply don't have enough observations of that
kind. I would think if they did have a febrile illness and
began to inactivate enzymes leading to hemolysis, they could
compensate adequately by just increasing erythropoiesis. So
I don't think it would become clinically apparent.

Unidentified speaker: What about hemoglobin stability?

<u>Dr. Goldstein</u>: In collaboration with Dr. Shu Wong, the
Hemoglobinopathy Lab at S. Joseph's Hospital in Hamilton
has a preliminary result, which means one experiment. There
seems to be increased heat-lability of hemoglobin in the
progeric child compared to one control.

<u>Dr. Labie</u>: I wonder if you have studied your enzymes by
isoelectrofocusing?

<u>Dr. Goldstein</u>: Starch gel, cellagel and polyacrylamide gel
electrophoretic patterns of G6PD and 6PGD are all normal
for progeric samples. Isoelectric focusing experiments are
in progress.

RED CELL ACID PHOSPHATASE: MODULATION OF ACTIVITY BY PURINES

E. Mansfield and G. F. Sensabaugh

Dept. of Genetics and School of Public Health,

University of California, Berkeley

The presence of acid phosphatase activity in red cells
was first demonstrated over 50 years ago (Martland, Hansman,
and Robinson, 1924). It has since been established that the
enzyme responsible for this activity is encoded at a single
genetic locus (Hopkinson, Spencer, and Harris, 1963). It has
also been shown that this red cell acid phosphatase (RCAP) is
genetically distinct from the acid phosphatases found in
lysosomes, being products of different genetic loci; RCAP
is further distinguished from the lysosomal acid phosphatases
by a distinctive set of molecular and catalytic properties
(Abul-Fadl and King, 1949; Sensabaugh, 1975). There is both
biochemical and genetic evidence indicating that this acid
phosphatase is found in the cytoplasm of many tissues (Neil
and Horner, 1963; Swallow, Povey, and Harris, 1973; Sensabaugh, 1975) and thus the designation "red cell" acid
phosphatase is somewhat misleading; nevertheless, we shall
use it in this paper.

Evidence of a specific metabolic role for the RCAP has
been lacking until recently. Based on earlier studies
(Luffman and Harris, 1967; Scott, 1966; Sensabaugh, unpublished) showing that flavin mononucleotide (FMN, riboflavin-
5-phosphate) appears to be significantly better as a
substrate for this enzyme than any of the other natural
phosphate esters tested; we had hypothesized that RCAP might
act in vivo as an FMN phosphatase (Sensabaugh, 1974, 1975).
We have recently developed several new pieces of evidence in
support of this hypothesis (Sensabaugh and Mansfield, in
preparation). In red cells, at least, all the detectable
FMN phosphatase activity co-chromatographs on Sephadex G-100

The Red Cell, pages 233—247

columns with the RCAP activity. The FMN phosphatase activity
in red cells parallels the acid phosphatase activity in pH
profile, and the two activities are also parallel in their
profiles of activation and inhibition by purines, folic acid,
and formaldehyde. The most convincing evidence that RCAP
possesses specificity for FMN is provided by the finding that
RCAP is specifically adsorbed onto affinity columns containing
FMN or riboflavin covalently attached to Sepharose; the FMN
phosphatase activity co-elutes from these columns with RCAP
on a gradient of increasing salt concentration. Moreover,
preliminary experiments with tissues containing other types
of acid and alkaline phosphatases have indicated RCAP is the
only phosphatase adsorbed to these affinity supports. Thus
there is evidence indicating that RCAP possesses a specific
binding site for riboflavin and that this enzyme is the only
specific FMN phosphatase in red cells and other tissues.

The assignment of this metabolic role to RCAP generates
questions relating to the genetic polymorphism of the enzyme
in humans and its possible physiological significance. The
genetic polymorphism of RCAP was first described in 1963 by
Hopkinson, Spencer, and Harris and has been subsequently
studied by many workers. In Caucasian populations, there
are three common alleles (P^a, P^b, and P^c) segregating at an
autosomal locus. The three alleles give rise to six
phenotypes, A, BA, B, CB, CA, and C, which can be distinguished by electrophoresis; of these, the C homozygote type
is rarely seen due to the low frequency of the P^c allele.

Of particular interest from a physiological perspective
is the activity variation associated with the polymorphism
(Spencer, Hopkinson, and Harris, 1964; Eze, et. al., 1974).
The acid phosphatase activity levels in red cells vary
according to RCAP phenotype; the activities of the three
homozygote types, A, B, and C, vary in the ratio 2:3:4,
respectively. The effect is gene dose additive; the
heterozygote types have RCAP activity levels intermediate to
those of the two appropriate homozygote types. The biochemical basis of this activity variation has not been
elucidated; there are small differences in kinetic properties
between the allelic forms of RCAP but these differences are
not sufficient to explain the activity variation (Scott,
1966; Fenton and Richardson, 1971). Whatever the basis of
this activity variation, it seems possible that an effect of
this magnitude might have some physiological consequence.

In this article, we describe a second kind of activity variation associated with the red cell acid phosphatase; this is a genotype dependent activity modulation by purines. That purines might modulate RCAP activity was suggested by the work of DiPietro and Zengerle (1967) who noted that certain purines including adenine, hypoxanthine, and guanine stimulated the activity of a low molecular weight acid phosphatase isolated from human placenta. We have shown that this placental enzyme and RCAP are one and the same, part of the evidence for this identity being that the activity of RCAP from red cells was similarly affected by purines (Sensabaugh, 1975). Additional studies have shown that the extent of activity modulation by these purines is highly genotype dependent. In an effort to gain further insight into the purine modulation effect and its possible physiological significance, we have extended the scope of our analysis to the level of enzyme mechanism; a preliminary account of our findings is presented here.

MATERIALS AND METHODS

Blood was collected from adult donors into tubes containing EDTA as the anticoagulant. Whole blood samples were stored refrigerated until analysis which was usually within 48 hours of collection. Following centrifugation of the whole blood, the plasma and buffy coat were removed from the red cells and the cells were washed three times in cold 0.9% saline. Hemolysates were prepared by the addition of two volumes distilled water to a volume of packed red cells; unlysed cells and debris were removed by centrifugation for 15' at 12,000 RPM at 4°C. Hemolysates were then dialyzed 8 hours against pH 7.4 tris buffered isotonic saline (0.01 M in tris) containing 0.1% Triton X-100 and 7 mM mercapto-ethanol (MSH); Triton X-100 and MSH have been shown to stabilize the enzyme (Tsuoubi and Hudson, 1955).

Red cell acid phosphatase genotypes were determined by starch gel electrophoresis on freshly prepared hemolysates using the phosphate-citric buffer system described by Swallow, et. al. (1973). The RCAP activity was detected on the gels by the hydrolysis of 4-methylumbeliferone phosphate (4 mM in 0.1 M acetate buffer, pH 5.5) to the fluorescent product, 4-methylumbeliferone.

Acid phosphatase activity was determined by a standard procedure reported previously (Sensabaugh, 1975). Generally, 0.1 ml hemolysate was assayed in a total volume of 1.5 ml of sodium acetate (pH 5.5) containing 2 mM p-nitrophenyl phosphate. The reaction was terminated by addition of 1.5 ml 10% trichloroacetic acid (TCA). Precipitated protein was removed by centrifugation and 2.0 ml of the supernatent added to 1.3 ml of 1.0 M NaOH. The p-nitrophenol produced was determined spectrophotometrically at 410 nm using the molar extinction coefficient of 16,200 at the end of the procedure. In experiments involving activity modulation by purines, the purines were added to the reaction mixture to achieve the desired concentration.

RESULTS

Modulation of RCAP Activity by Purines

The effect of a number of purines on RCAP (B genotype) activity is indicated in Table 1. Most of the purines and purine containing compounds that were tested exhibited some effect on RCAP activity, either as activators or inhibitors. The most potent activator among the purines tested is

Table 1

Modulation of Red Cell Acid Phosphatase Activity by Purines.

Purine[1]	Relative Rate[2]	Purine[1]	Relative Rate[2]
hypoxanthine	2.12	xanthine	1.01
allolpurinol	2.05	adenosine	1.01
6-methyladenine	1.51	AMP	.98
6-mercaptopurine	1.50	uric acid	.71
inosine	1.50	6-amino-2-mercapto-	
c-AMP	1.25	purine	.55
theophyllin	1.25	alloxan	.50
adenine	1.20	2,6-diaminopurine	.15
caffeine	1.10		

1. All purines were at 5 mM in the assay mixture except uric acid which was at 2.5 mM.
2. Rates are reported relative to the rate in the absence of purine. All determinations employed partially purified B type RCAP.

hypoxanthine; in the presence of this purine, RCAP activity
is effectively doubled. At the other end of the scale, 2,6-
diaminopurine is a potent inhibitor of RCAP activity, the
enzyme activity in the presence of this purine being about
85% inhibited. These two extremes illustrate the degree to
which RCAP activity can be modulated by purines.

The structural basis of the purine effect is not immediately evident; it is clear that different additions to the
purine nucleus greatly alter the direction and extent of
activity modulation. Additions at the 6 position appear to
be critical: adenine (6-amino purine), 6-methyl adenine
(6-methylamino purine), and hypoxanthine (6-hydroxypurine)
are activators of increasing potency. However, the addition
of a second amino group to adenine at the 2- position yields
the inhibitor, 2,6-diamino purine. The nucleosides, adenosine
and inosine, are less effective as modulators than the purines
they contain; this may be due to the addition to the purine
but may also be due to steric hindrance in the interaction of
nucleoside with enzyme. It is apparent then, that more work
is needed to clarify the relationship between purine structure
and RCAP activity modulation.

Phosphate, a competitive inhibitor of the phosphatase
reaction (Scott, 1966; Fenton and Richardson, 1971), has
been found to influence the purine modulation of RCAP activity
in red cell hemolysates. The effect of phosphate is
illustrated in figure 1; the figure shows RCAP activity in an
extensively dialysed hemolysate in the presence of three
purines, -adenine, 6-methyl adenine, and hypoxanthine- as a
function of added phosphate. In the dialysed hemolysate, the
extent of acid phosphatase activity enhancement by these
purines is maximal. As phosphate is added back, the degree
of activation diminishes until at some critical phosphate
concentration no activation is seen; at yet higher phosphate
concentrations the presence of purines actually appears to
inhibit (Sensabaugh, 1975). The concentration of phosphate
required to neutralize the purine activation varies with the
activator used; 1 mM phosphate is sufficient to counter the
adenine activation effect, 15 mM phosphate is required for
6-methyl adenine, and 25 mM phosphate for hypoxanthine. It
should be noted that the concentration of phosphate required
to neutralize the activation by a purine directly correlates
with the activation potential of that purine.

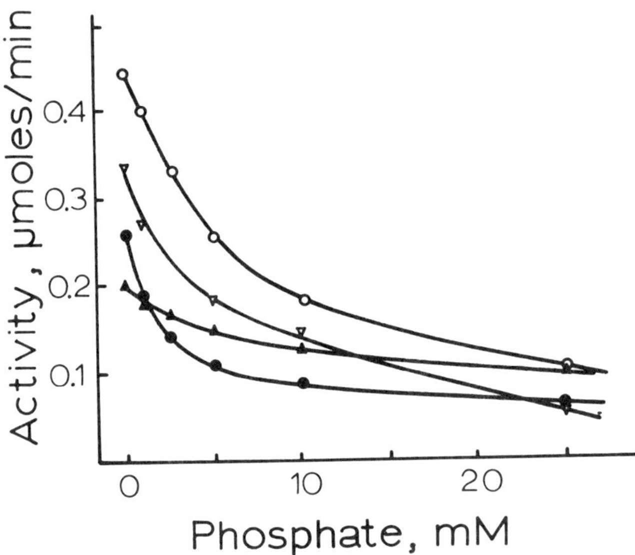

Figure 1. Effect of phosphate concentration on modulation of acid phosphatase activity by purines. RCAP, freed of phosphate ion, was assayed in the presence of added back phosphate at the indicated concentrations. The curves represent activity (μmoles p-nitrophenol released per minute) with no added purine ($\blacktriangle$ — $\blacktriangle$), adenine ($\bullet$ — $\bullet$), 6-methyladenine($\triangledown$ — $\triangledown$), and hypoxanthine (o — o); purines were at 5 mM.

Kinetic analyses have been done in an attempt to gain some insight into the mechanism of the RCAP activity modulation by purines. The results to date have yielded a rather interesting picture. Using RCAP partially purified on an FMN-Sepharose affinity column, double reciprocal plots such as shown in Figure 2 have been obtained; this particular plot is of the hypoxanthine effect. The parallel line plots are characteristic of an uncompetitive activation or inhibition (Mahler and Cordes, 1966). The conventional interpretation of an uncompetitive effect in terms of phosphatase mechanism is that the modulator is binding to the phosphoryl enzyme intermediate; activators facilitate and inhibitors slow down

the breakdown of this intermediate. The purine modulators
are uncompetitive with respect to the substrate (p-nitrophenyl
phosphate) because they interact with the enzyme only after
the enzyme has reacted with the substrate. If the kinetic
analysis is done in the presence of exogenous phosphate, a
more complex result is obtained: the plotted lines are not
parallel but rather intersect in a way that indicates mixed
activation and inhibition effects. This result is not unexpected given the expression of purine modulation in the

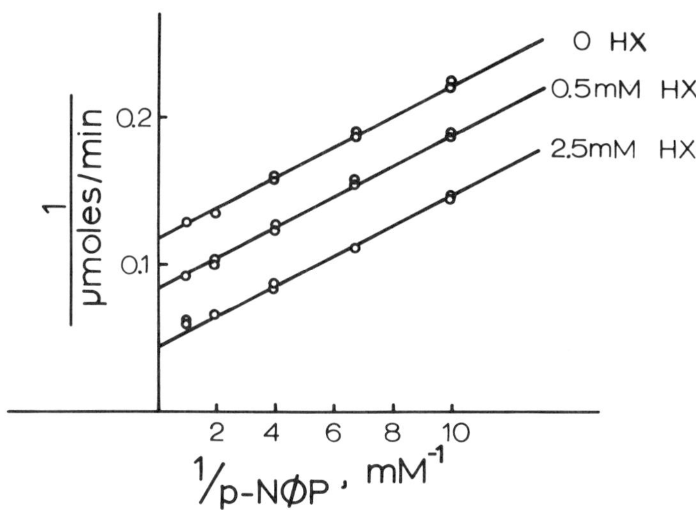

Figure 2. Kinetic analysis of hypoxanthine activation of red
cell acid phosphatase. Assays were done at the indicated
concentrations of hypoxanthine (HX). The source of enzyme was
a partially purified preparation from an FMN-affinity column.
Activity is expressed as umoles p-nitrophenol produced per
minute.

presence of phosphate illustrated in figure 1. Interestingly, when extensively dialysed hemolysate is used as the enzyme source for the kinetic analysis, the same mixed type effects are seen; it is possible that some endogenous phosphate is not removed by dialysis but alternatively it is possible that the hemolysate contains some nondialysable component which modulates RCAP activity.

Genotype Dependent Effects

In the course of studying the purine modulation of acid phosphatase activity, it was apparent that the extent of activity modulation varied with acid phosphatase genotype. (The results reported up to this point have been obtained using enzyme from the common homozygous type, the B type.) To determine the extent of the genotype dependent variation, the modulation of RCAP activity by purines was measured in lysates from a panel of individuals representing each of the common acid phosphatase phenotypes; the genotype dependent activation by adenine is illustrated in figure 3. The differences in the extent of activity modulation by adenine for the different RCAP genotypes are strikingly apparent. The mean values for adenine activation by genotype are summarized in Table 2 as are the values for 6-methyladenine activation, hypoxanthine activation, and uric acid inhibition. A one-way analysis of variance of these data indicates that the genotype differences are highly significant ($p < .005$ in all cases) for each of these purines.

Using the data in Table 2, it is possible to test whether the purine modulation effects are additive with respect to gene dosage. Let us represent the mean activation or inhibition increment for each genotype as $\bar{A}$, $\overline{BA}$, $\bar{B}$, etc. If the modulation effects are additive, then the two following relationships should hold:

(1) $1/2\ \bar{A} + 1/2\ \bar{B} = \overline{BA}$

(2) $\overline{CA} - 1/2\ \bar{A} = \overline{CB} - 1/2\ \bar{B}$

In the case of the adenine activations, the sum, $1/2\ \bar{A} + 1/2\ \bar{B}$, yields a prediction for $\overline{BA}$ of 1.31 which is very close to the observed value of $\overline{BA}$, 1.33. Similarly we find that $\overline{CA} - 1/2\ \bar{A}$ = 1.15 and $\overline{CB} - 1/2\ \bar{B}$ = 1.14. Thus the observed values of adenine activation are consistent with a simple gene dose

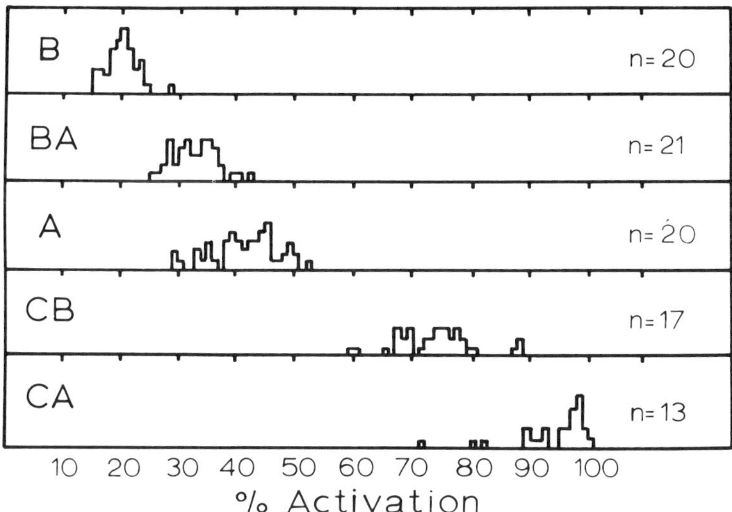

Figure 3. Genotype dependent activation of red cell acid phosphatase by adenine (5 mM). The samples were hemolysates from individuals representing each of the common acid phosphatase phenotypes; the hemolysates were extensively dialysed against pH 7.4, 10 mM tris buffered saline prior to the assay to remove phosphate ion.

additive situation. It is then possible to calculate the degree of adenine activation expected for the type C homozygote; both sides of the equation (2) estimate the C gene contribution and the prediction for the C homozygote is simply twice this, $\underline{i.e.}$, $\overline{C}$ = 2.29. The modulation effect produced by the other three purines also shows gene dose additivity.

An interesting pattern emerges from the evaluation of the genotype dependent activity modulation by purines. Since the modulation effects are additive, the contributions of the three alleles, P^a, P^b, and P^c, can be compared directly. In the case of adenine, 6-methyladenine, and uric acid, the

Table 2

Genotype Dependent Modulation of Red Cell Acid Phosphatase Activity by Purines[1]

Genotype (n)	Adenine	6-Methyladenine	Hypoxanthine	Uric Acid
E (20)	$1.20^{\pm}.06$	$1.51^{\pm}.11$	$2.12^{\pm}.08$	$.71^{\pm}.07$
BA (21)	$1.33^{\pm}.06$	$1.58^{\pm}.06$	$2.10^{\pm}.08$	$.68^{\pm}.05$
A (20)	$1.42^{\pm}.06$	$1.64^{\pm}.07$	$1.99^{\pm}.07$	$.60^{\pm}.07$
C3 (17)	$1.74^{\pm}.09$	$1.95^{\pm}.10$	$1.64^{\pm}.08$	$.65^{\pm}.05$
CA (13)	$1.86^{\pm}.09$	$2.03^{\pm}.09$	$1.58^{\pm}.07$	$.55^{\pm}.09$
C (predicted)[2]	2.29	2.41	1.16	.34

1. The data is given as mean ± standard deviation for activity in the presence of purine relative to activity in the absence of purine. All purines were at 5 mM concentration except uric acid which was at 2.5 mM.
2. Prediction of activity from C homozygote type based on estimate C gene dose as described in text.

extent of activity modulation is ordered $\overline{B} < \overline{BA} < \overline{A} < \overline{CB} < \overline{CA}$; the contribution of the alleles is thus $P^b < P^a < P^c$. In the case of the hypoxanthine, the order of activation is reversed, i.e., $\overline{CA} < \overline{CB} < \overline{A} < \overline{BA} < \overline{B}$; this indicates the allelic contributions are $P^c < P^a < P^b$. In either case, this pattern of activity modulation places the common B and CA genotypes at opposite extremes (with the predicted rare CC phenotype being even more extreme from a type B). This ordering contrasts to the ordering seen with the genotype dependent variation in activity levels which is $P^a < P^b < P^c$; in terms of activity levels in red cells, the $\overline{CA}$ and $\overline{B}$ genotypes approximately equal.

DISCUSSION

It has been recognized for many years that the genetic polymorphism of RCAP is accompanied by quantitative variation in enzyme activity levels (Spencer, Hopkinson, and Harris, 1964). In this report, we outline some features of a second kind of enzyme activity variation associated with this polymorphism, the genotype dependent variation in the modulation of enzyme activity by purines. These two types of variation differ in several respects, the most notable of which is the different ordering of the alloenzymes with respect to the contribution of each to the observed variation. In the quantitative variation of RCAP activity levels, the contribution of the alloenzymes is, in increasing order: $A < B < C$. In contrast, the alloenzyme contribution to the purine modulation effect is ordered either $B < A < C$ or $C < A < B$. This difference in ordering indicates that the two kinds of activity variation represent independent effects.

Genetically determined variation in enzyme behavior is of considerable interest for this variation may have physiological consequences; the hemoglobin variants and glucose-6-phosphate dehydrogenase variants are well known examples. Many of the red cell enzyme polymorphisms have been found to have associated activity variation (Battistuzzi, et. al., 1974); whether physiological significance can be attached to any of these is an open question. Nevertheless, it is a question worth asking for the answers will provide insight into individual variation in physiology and into the mechanisms by which polymorphisms are maintained.

In this vein, we may speculate on the role of RCAP in
the red cell and upon the significance of its genetic variation. We had previously suggested that the in vivo function
of the enzyme was as an FMN phosphatase (Sensabaugh, 1974,
1975). This would put the enzyme into the context of flavin
coenzyme metabolism as indicated below:

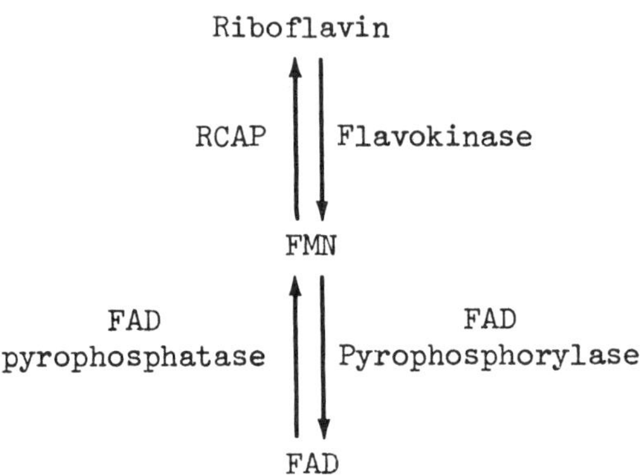

It has been shown that the activity of the enzymes in this
metabolic cycle can be altered by dietary conditions and by
manipulation of hormone levels (for reviews, see Rivlin, 1970,
1975) and that a consequence of this is a change in the levels
of the flavin coenzymes. This in turn may lead to an alteration in the activity levels of flavoenzymes.

In red cells, several flavoenzymes have been shown to
play key roles in the maintenance of cellular integrity
(Beutler, 1969). Notable among these is glutathione reductase,
an FAD dependent enzyme (Icen, 1967). This enzyme acts to
maintain glutathione in a reduced state; impairment or
absence of glutathione reductase activity results in a net
accumulation of oxidized glutathione followed by red cell
lysis (Kosower, et. al., 1971). Buetler (1969) has shown
that red cells are chronically deficient in FAD; in vivo
or in vitro supplementation of riboflavin or FAD increases
the activity of glutathione reductase.

From this point, it can be speculated that RCAP, acting
in its role as FMN phosphatase, may be involved with the
regulation of flavin coenzyme levels. The genetic variation
in RCAP activity would lead to the prediction that flavin
coenzyme levels, and glutathione reductase activity ought to

vary with the RCAP genotype. The modulation of RCAP activity
by purines and by folic acid (Sensabaugh and Golden, in
preparation) similarly leads to predictions that dietary or
hormonal influences might be significant. Although the
modulation effects we have described here require super-
physiological concentrations of purines, the same pattern of
genotype dependent variation might be expressed at physiological levels of as yet unrecognized compounds. In this
regard, Bottini, et. al., (1971, 1973) have provided evidence
that the incidence and severity of hemolytic favism in glucose-
6-phosphate dehydrogenase deficient individuals varies with
RCAP type; the pattern of variation places A and CA type
individuals at greatest risk and B type individuals at least
risk. Similarly, Bottini, et. al., (1976) have recently
reported that hospital admissions for neonatal jaundice and
serum bilirubin levels in neonates show this same pattern,
i.e., CA type infants are at one extreme and B type infants
are at the other. The pattern of variation exhibited by the
purine modulation effect may thus be the key to the interpretation of Bottini's observations. Although these
correlations are highly speculative, they provide a point of
departure by providing testable hypotheses covering the
functions of the acid phosphatase in red cells.

REFERENCES

Abul-Fadl MM, King EJ (1949). Properties of the acid
    phosphatases of erythrocytes and of human prostate gland.
    Biochem J 45:51.
Battistuzzi G, Scozzari R, Santolamazza P, Terrenato L,
    Modiano G (1974). Comparitive activity of red cell
    adenosine deaminase allelic forms. Nature 251:711.
Beutler E (1969). Effect of flavin compounds on glutathione
    reductase activity: in vivo and in vitro studies. J Clin
    Invest 48:1957,
Beutler E (1969). The effect of flavin coenzymes on the
    activity of erythrocyte enzymes. Experimentia 25:804.
Bottini E, Lucarelli P, Agostino R, Palmarino R, Businco L,
    Antognori G (1971). Favism: association with erythrocyte
    acid phosphatase phenotype. Sci 171:409.
Bottini E (1973). Favism: current problems and investigations.
    J Med Genet 10:154.
Bottini E, Scacchi R, Gloria-Bottini F, Mortera J, Palmarino
    R, Carapella-deLuca E, Lapi AS, Noclari D (1976). Neonatal
    jaundice and erythrocyte acid phosphatase phenotype
    (letter). Lancet 1:918.

DiPietro DL, Zengerle FS (1967). Separation and properties of three acid phosphatases from human placenta. J Biol Chem 242:3391.

EZE LC, Tweedee MCK, Buller MF, Wren PJJ, Evans DAP (1974). Quantitative genetics of human red cell acid phosphatase. Ann Hum Genet 37:333.

Fenton MR, Richardson KE (1971). Human erythrocyte acid phosphatase: resolution and characterization of the isozymes from three homozygous phenotypes. Arch Biochem Biophys 142:13.

Hopkinson DA, Spencer N, Harris H (1963). Red cell acid phosphatase variants: a new human polymorphism. Nature 199:969.

Icen A (1967). Glutathione reductase of human erythrocytes. Purification and properties. Scand J Clin Lab Invest Suppl 96:1.

Kosower NS, Marikovsky Y, Wertheim B, Danon D (1971). Glutathione oxidation and biophysical aspects of injury to human erythrocytes. J Lab Clin Med 78:533.

Luffman JE, Harris H (1967). A comparison of some properties of human red cell acid phosphatase in different phenotypes. Ann Hum Genet 30:387.

Mahler HR, Cordes EH (1966). "Biological Chemistry" New York: Harper and Row, p 219.

Martland M, Hansman FS, Robinson R (1924). The phosphoric esterase of blood. Biochem J 18:1152.

Neil MW, Horner MW (1964). Studies on acid hydrolases in adult and foetal tissues. Biochem J 92:217.

Rivlin RS (1970). Riboflavin metabolism. New Eng J Med 283:463.

Rivlin RS (1975). Hormonal regulation of riboflavin metabolism in Rivlin ES (ed): "Riboflavin", New York, Plenum Press, p 393.

Sensabaugh GF (1974). Studies on red cell acid phosphatase. Amer J Hum Genet 26:78a.

Sensabaugh GF (1975). Genetic and non-genetic variation of human acid phosphatases. In Markert CL (ed): "Isozymes I: Molecular Structure," New York: Academic Press, p 367.

Scott EM (1966). Kinetic comparison of genetically different acid phosphatases of human erythrocytes. J Biol Chem 241:3049.

Spencer N, Hopkinson DA, Harris H (1964). Quantitative differences and gene dosage in the human red cell acid phosphatase polymorphism. Nature 201:299.

Swallow DMS, Povey S, Harris H (1973). Activity of the "red cell" acid phosphatase locus in other tissues. Ann Hum Genet 37:31.
Tsuboi KK, Hudson PB (1955). Acid phosphatase. V. Nature of inactivation and stabilization of purified human red cell phosphomonoesterase. Arch Biochem Biophys 55:206.

DISCUSSION

<u>Dr. Brewer</u>: In the G6PD deficient red cell the glutathione
reductase activity should be lower in people with AC type
compared to BB, if the activity has been modulated by FAD
levels, which in turn has been affected by the processes you
have been talking about?

<u>Ms. Mansfield</u>: That is correct, however, the acid phophatase
activity alone cannot explain this effect because the AC and
the BB genotypes have the same activities. However, if it is
due to modulation by adenine, or molecules similar to adenine
where the AC type is more strongly activated then you would
expect and thus this genotype has higher phosphatase activity and therefore lower glutathione reductase activity
which maybe reflected in a reduced red cell stability.

<u>Dr. Brewer</u>: Could one test your hypotheses by measuring the
glutathione reductase activity of the two types?

<u>Ms. Mansfield</u>: This has been done and a published report
indicates a negative correlation between acid phosphatase
activity and glutathione reductase activity. Therefore
the C type individuals show the lowest glutathione reductase activity because they have the highest acid phosphatase
activity. But experiments from this lab did not find any
correlation. I think that it probably should be looked at
again.

<u>Dr. Hultquist</u>: What is the subcellular localization of the
liver and the red cell phosphatase?

<u>Ms. Mansfield</u>: It is cytoplasmic in all tissues.

<u>Dr. Brewer</u>: I must compliment you on a beautiful piece of
work. We have all wondered for a long time what the acid
phosphatase is doing and now we are beginning to get some
place with figuring it out.

<u>Dr. Paglia</u>: I would like to echo Dr. Brewer's compliment!
This is why we at U.C.L.A. consider Berkeley one of the up
and coming institutions.

The Red Cell, page 249
© 1978 Alan R. Liss, Inc., New York, New York

STUDIES ON A LARGE KINDRED WITH HEMOLYTIC ANEMIA AND LOW
ERYTHROCYTE 2,3-DPG*

D.R. Harkness, S. Roth, P. Goldman,
C. Kim and R.E. Isaacks
Veterans Administration Hospital, Department
of Medicine, University of Miami School of
Medicine, Miami, Florida 33125

INTRODUCTION

Eight years ago we had the opportunity to study for a
short period of time a mother and her two children who
suffered from nonspherocytic hemolytic disease. Their
erythrocytes contained approximately one-half the normal
concentration of 2,3-diphosphoglyceric acid (2,3-DPG).
At that time we were unable to define the underlying abnormality in their erythrocytes. Recently we restudied these
patients and examined other members of the kindred.

In this paper we report the results of our efforts to
elucidate the biochemical lesion which causes the shortened
red cell survival and the low erythrocyte 2,3-DPG in this
family

MATERIALS AND METHODS

Dowex-1-chloride and hydroxylapatite were obtained from
BioRad Laboratories and diethylaminoethylcellulose DE52 from
Whatman Biochemicals Ltd. EDTA, Tris, Bis Tris, trietha-
nolamine (TEA) and β-mercaptoethanol were purchased from
Sigma Chemical Company. General Biochemicals was the
supplier of 2-phosphoglycolate (P-glycolate). All cofactors,

*Supported by the Veterans Administration, a grant
(RR 00261) from the General Clinical Research Centers
Program of the Division of Research Resources, NIH,
and by US Public Health Service Grant HL-15999.

The Red Cell, pages 251—269

substrates and reagent enzymes were obtained from Calbiochem
or Sigma. The other chemicals, all of reagent grade, were
products of Fisher Scientific Company. 3-Phosphoglyceric
acid (3-PGA) was freed of 2,3-diphosphoglyceric acid (2,3-DPG)
and P-glycolate of Pi by chromatography on Dowex-1-chloride,
eluting with a linear gradient of HCl (0.005 to 0.080 N).

Oxyhemoglobin dissociation curves were performed in
0.16 M sodium phosphate buffer at pH 7.4, pCO_2 of 40 torr,
and 37°C by a modification of the continuous recording method
of Longmuir and Chow (1970) as described previously (Lian
et al, 1971). When studying hemoglobin solutions 0.05M Bis
Tris was used as buffer. The P_{50} and n values were determined
by computor employing a program developed by Dr. Bruce Cameron
of the Papanicolaou Cancer Research Institute. Organic
phosphates were removed from hemoglobin ("stripped" Hb) by
passage of hemoglobin which had been dialyzed against 0.05M
Tris chloride buffer, pH 7.4, through small columns of DE52
equilibrated with the same buffer. Carboxyhemoglobin (CO-Hb)
was measured in an IL Co-Oximeter. Enzymatic assays were
employed to measure 2,3-DPG (Rose and Liebowitz, 1970a) and
ATP (Lamprecht and Trautschold, 1963).

2,3-$D^{32}PG$ was prepared as previously described (Harkness
et al, 1970) for use as substrate in the assay of 2,3-DPG
phosphatase. 2,3-DPG phosphatase was assayed in the presence
of P-glycolate as activator. Reaction mixtures, 0.5 ml,
containing 100 mM Tris chloride (pH 7.5), 0.02 µM P-glycolate,
0.25-1.0 mM 2,3-$D^{32}PG$ and enzyme were incubated at 37°C for
60 min. The details of the assay have been published previously (Harkness et al, 1970). Activity is expressed as
µmoles/hr/ml rbc.

Diphosphoglycerate mutase (DPGM) was measured in a
Cary 15 recording spectrophotometer at ambient temperature
by the method of Schröter and Kalinowsky (1969). The reaction
mixtures contained in a volume of 1.0 ml: 60 mM TEA buffer
(pH 7.6), 10 mM KPO_4 (pH 7.5), 10 mM fructose-1,6-diphosphate,
4.3 mM 3-PGA (2,3-DPG free), 2.5 mM NAD, aldolase (50 µg,
0.60 units), glyceraldehyde-P dehydrogenase (50 µg, 3.0 units),
and triose-P isomerase (50 µg, 327 units). After equilibrium
is attained, the reduction of 1 µmole NAD represents the
formation of 1 µmole 2,3-DPG.

2-Phosphoglycolate phosphatase was assayed by the method
described by Badwey (1976). Saline-washed erythrocytes were

hemolyzed by an equal volume of distilled water and centrifuged at 15,000 g for 20 min. The supernatant fractions were dialyzed overnight against 5 mM Tris chloride (pH 7.5) containing 1 mM β-mercaptoethanol. One mililiter reaction mixtures containing 50 mM Tris chloride (pH 7.5), 2.5 mM Mg Cl_2, 100 mM KCl, 3.2 mM P glycolate (free of Pi) and 0.2 to 0.4 ml dialyzed hemolysate were incubated at 37°C for 60 min. Reactions were terminated by adding 0.5 ml 6% perchloric acid. Inorganic phosphate was determined on the supernatant fluid and the results expressed as µmoles Pi/hour/gm Hb. Identical reactions with 4 mM α-glycerophosphate produced less than one-tenth the Pi formed with P-glycolate, indicating that the hydrolysis of P-glycolate was not catalyzed primarily by the red cell acid phosphatase.

The efflux of radioactive Na^+ from erythrocytes was measured by a slight modification (Harkness and Grayson, 1969) of the method described by Jacob and Jandl (1964). Lipids were extracted from washed erythrocytes by the method of Rose and Oklander (1965). The phospholipids were separated by thin layer chromatography and quantitated as described by Dodge and Phillips (1967). Cholesterol was determined after Zlatkis et al (1953).

The protein possessing both DPGM and DPG phosphatase activities (2,3-DPG phosphatase-mutase) was partially purified by a procedure described in detail elsewhere (Harkness et al, 1977).

RESULTS

Clinical Evaluation and Initial Studies

In 1969 the 14 year old propositus (III-18), her 16 year old brother (III-17) and their 35 year old mother (II-13) were admitted to the Clinical Research Unit at the University of Miami for investigation of nonspherocytic hemolytic anemia. During the previous 8 years the propositus had experienced intermittent episodes of abdominal pain accompanied by fatigue, jaundice, and passage of dark urine. Her hemoglobin was usually within the lower limits of normal and the reticulocyte count ranged from 3-9%. The brother and mother had experienced similar episodes but the abdominal pain was less severe. Neither had been found to be anemic. A number

Table 1. Initial Evaluation of Propositus and Her
Brother and Mother

	Proband III-18	Brother III-17	Mother II-13	Normal Value
Hemoglobin, gm%	13.7	16.2	14.3	14-18
Reticulocytes, %	5.0	6.7	5.2	0.5-2.0
WBC, (X10^{-3})	9.2	12.5	11.0	5.0-10.0
Platelet count, (X10^{-3})	392	320	479	150-300
Bilirubin, dir/tot, mg%	0.4/1.6	0.4/6.0	0.4/1.7	<0.4/1.0
Serum haptoglobin, mg%	117		119	50-175
RBC survival, T/2 in da	19	13.5	15.5	27-33
Ferrokinetic studies				
Serum Fe, μg%	102	135	105	60-160
Fe binding capacity, μg%	344	253	283	250-350
Clearance, T/2 in min.	60	35	60	60-120
Utilization, % in 6 da*	87	90	92	>80%
Turnover, mg/da	45	96	49	∿25
Autohemolysis				
No addition	2.44	3.47	2.06	<1.0
Glucose, 0.02 M	0.43	0.22	0.44	<0.5
ATP, 0.02 M	0.18	0.02	0.44	<0.5
RBC 2,3-DPG, μmole/ml rbc	3.09	3.19	2.82	4.0-5.0
RBC ATP, μmole/ml rbc	1.11	1.08	0.95	0.8-1.0

  * Values given at 6 days since counts at 10-14 days were
lower due to the shortened erythrocyte survival.

of years earlier an open liver biopsy had been performed on
the brother because of jaundice but the results were never
made available to us. Physical examination of the three
revealed no abnormal findings except that the boy was
clinically jaundiced at the time and his liver was slightly
enlarged. Their spleens were not palpable.

Some of the pertinent initial laboratory data are given
in Table 1. All had normal hemoglobin values and elevated
reticulocyte and platelet counts. The red cell indices
were normal. Red cell morphology was normal except for the
presence of a few (2-3%) small dense crenated cells
(similar to those sometimes seen with deficiencies of
pyruvate kinase, hexokinase and phosphoglucose isomerase)

and rare spherocytes. There was indirect hyperbilirubinemia
and urine urobilinogen was elevated. Serum haptoglobins
were normal and there was no hemosiderinuria. All were blood
group 0 Rh positive; the Coombs tests were negative.

X-rays revealed thickened calvaria with slight "hair-on-end"
pattern. Gallstones were not present. Bone marrow aspirates
revealed marked normoblastic erythroid hyperplasia. Serum
folate and B_{12} values, serum protein electrophoresis, immunoglobulin levels and coagulation studies were normal. Iron
kinetic studies demonstrated rapid clearance and efficient
utilization and the red cell survival was significantly
decreased in all three family-members.

Autohemolysis studies indicated mild hemolysis totally
corrected by glucose or ATP. Osmotic fragility, before and
after incubation, was normal. Hemoglobin electrophoresis on
cellulose acetate, pH 8.6, and citrate agar, pH 6.2, Hb F
quantitated by alkali denaturation, and Hb A_2 assayed by
microcolumn chromatography were all normal. Heinz bodies
were not observed and hemoglobin instability was not detected.
Erythrocyte 2,3-DPG was significantly decreased (40-60% of
normal) and ATP was slightly elevated (appropriate to the
degree of reticulocytosis).

The activities of all of the enzymes of the glycolytic
pathway, the hexosemonophosphate shunt and glutathione
reductase were assayed in the erythrocytes of all three
patients and were found to be the same or slightly greater
than normal controls run simultaneously. 2,3-DPG phosphatase
activity with 20 mM sodium bisulfite as activator was normal.
We were not assaying DPGM in the laboratory at that time.
Erythrocyte reduced glutathione levels were normal.

It seemed evident that all three family members were
afflicted with the same hemolytic process. Because of the
apparent dominant mode of transmission and lack of evidence
of an abnormal hemoglobin, a membrane abnormality was
considered most likely. The membrane phospholipids were
separated and their distribution was nearly normal (Table 2)
as were cholesterol and the ratio of total phospholipids
to cholesterol (Table 3). Red cell ghosts were prepared;
the proteins were solubilized with detergent and subjected
to SDS disc gel electrophoresis. The protein bands were
indistinguishable from normal controls. The rate of loss
of radioactivity from $^{22}Na^+$ loaded red cells was the same

Table 2.   Distribution of Phospholipids of Erythrocytes
(Mole %)

Phospholipid	Propositus III-18	Brother III-17	Mother II-13	Control (n=12)
PE*	32.3	32.4	26.8	28.6 ± 2.0
PS**	13.3	12.4	15.0	15.3 ± 1.9
Lecithin	29.6	30.5	33.1	27.6 ± 3.4
Sphingomyelin	22.1	22.2	22.5	24.3 ± 2.6
Lyso-lecithin	2.4	1.5	1.2	2.5 ± 2.1

* Phosphatidyl ethanolamine; ** Phosphatidyl serine

Table 3.   Cholesterol and Phospholipid Composition of the
Erythrocytes

Subject	Cholesterol µmole/ml rbc	Phospholipid µmole/ml rbc	P:C
III-18 (propositus)	4.16	4.00	0.96
III-17 (brother)	3.67	4.15	1.13
II-13 (mother)	4.63	4.70	1.02
Control (n=12)	4.17 ± 0.31	4.13 ± 0.30	0.99

Table 4.   Erythrocyte Sodium Efflux

Subject	0 time %	60 min %	120 min %	180 min %
III-18 (propositus)	100	67.6	51.0	42.2
III-17 (brother)	100	65.7	49.6	42.0
II-13 (mother)	100	66.7	50.7	43.0
Control	100	69.5	52.3	43.9

as from normal cells (Table 4). It was concluded that an
abnormality of the erythrocyte membrane did not give rise
to the hemolysis.

Shortly after discharge from the Clinical Research Unit
the family left Miami. In 1974 the propositus was diagnosed
elsewhere as having hereditary spherocytosis and underwent
splenectomy with no apparent improvement. In 1976 she was
found to have gallstones and a cholecystectomy was performed.

In the spring of 1977 she developed a urinary tract infection
and returned to the University of Miami Hospital for treatment.
At that time it was possible to perform further studies on
the three persons studied in 1969 and to examine 13 other
members of the family and the father of the propositus.

Recent Studies

The oxygen-binding properties of the erythrocytes were
measured on the three patients studied originally (Table 5).
A left shift, consistent with the low 2,3-DPG, was noted.
The P_{50} of the hemoglobin freed of organic phosphates was
normal as was the response to added 2,3-DPG (Table 6). The
somewhat lower values for the P_{50} and the lower Hill constant
in II-13 are undoubtedly due to the elevated CO-Hb levels
associated with heavy cigarette smoking.

Table 5. Hemoglobin Functional Studies on Intact Erythrocytes

Subject	P_{50}	n	CO-Hb	2,3-DPG
	torr		%	μmole/ml rbc
III-18 propositus	24.4	2.8	3.0	2.94
III-17 brother	23.6	2.6	5.0	2.71
II-13 mother	21.8	2.2	9.6	2.14
Normal	27.0 ± 1.0	2.4-2.9	<2.0	4.0-5.0

Table 6. Functional Studies on Stripped Hemoglobin[*]

Subject	No 2,3-DPG	2,3-DPG added
II-13	16.9	21.2
III-17	18.8	23.0
Normal	18.7	23.4

[*] Data expressed as P_{50} in torr.

Eleven of the thirteen additional members of this kindred
studied are also affected (Fig. 1). In each the 2,3-DPG
levels and the P_{50} of intact erythrocytes were decreased and

Table 7. Enzyme Activities of the Erythrocytes of the Propositus*

Enzyme	Propositus	Control	Normal Mean ± S.D.
Hexokinase	0.18	0.19	0.25 ± 0.05
Glucose-P isomerase	16.2	14.2	12.1 ± 1.53
Phosphofructokinase	4.9	3.1	3.25 ± 0.45
Aldolase	1.2	0.98	0.9 ± 0.1
Triose isomerase	133.0	140.0	156 ± 10
Glyceraldehyde-3-P dehydrogenase	30.5	30.5	31.8 ± 3.7
Phosphoglycerate kinase	41.5	45.2	28.4 ± 1.35
D-phosphoglyceromutase	6.5	7.4	7.1 ± 0.9
Enolase	6.8	6.0	4.0 ± 0.5
Pyruvate kinase (3.0 mM PEP)	7.5	7.8	5.1 ± 1.2
(0.4 mM PEP)	6.0	5.9	3.1 ± 0.7
Lactate dehydrogenase	60.1	51.1	53.1 ± 14.4
Glucose-6-P dehydrogenase	4.5	3.7	2.65 ± 0.5
Phosphogluconate dehydrogenase	2.9	2.4	1.94 ± 0.40
Glutathione reductase	3.0	2.5	2.15 ± 0.3
Glutathione peroxidase	9.7	4.9	6.8 ± 1.2
Adenylate kinase	86.1	74.0	85.8 ± 12.3
Ribose-P pyrophosphokinase	57.0	25.2	30.5 ± 3.8
Adenine P-ribosyltransferase	2.63	3.17	3.4 ± 0.4
Pyrimidine nucleotidase (UMP)	8.6	10.2	9.9 ± 2.5
(CMP)	7.9	9.0	7.4 ± 1.8
Glutamic oxalacetic transaminase	2.55	1.33	-----
Malic dehydrogenase	5.1	4.7	4.7 ± 0.4
Adenosine deaminase	0.33	0.27	-----
Nucleoside phosphorylase	15.6	17.7	-----

* Performed in the laboratory of William N. Valentine; activities are expressed as μmoles/ min/10^{10} cells at 37°.

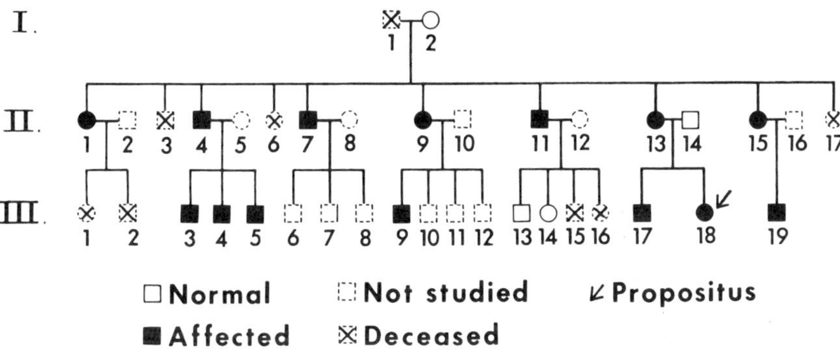

Fig. 1. Kindred with Hemolytic Anemia and Low Erythrocyte 2,3-DPG.

the reticulocytes were increased. Most had thrombocytosis and about half had elevated leukocyte counts. Hemoglobin levels, Hb electrophoresis, Hb F, Hb A_2 and red cell indices were normal in all. The erythrocytes of II-4 and his three sons (III-3, III-4, and III-5) contained somewhat higher levels of 2,3-DPG (3.51 to 3.61 μmoles/ml rbc) than did the other affected individuals (from 2.14 to 3.35 μmoles/ml rbc; average, 2.76 μmoles/ml rbc).

Blood from the propositus and a control were sent to Dr. William N. Valentine's laboratory for repeat enzyme analyses. The activities of the enzymes of glycolysis, including DPGM, and the hexosemonophosphate shunt and several other enzymes were again found to be normal (Table 7). The activity of P-glycolate phosphatase was measured in our own laboratory and found normal in several family members (Table 8), as were repeat assays of 2,3-DPG phosphatase (Table 9).

Table 8. Phosphoglycolate Phosphatase Activity of
                    Erythrocytes

Subject	Activity
	μmole/ml rbc/min
II-1	0.44
II-4	0.47
II-15	0.36
Normals (n=6)	0.33 ± 0.05

Table 9.   2,3-DPG Phosphatase Activity of Erythrocytes[*]

Subject	Activity
	μmole/ml rbc/hr
III-18 (propositus)	1.72
II-13 (mother)	1.64
Normal	1.60
Normal	1.61

* Assayed in presence of 2μM P-glycolate.

Because of the striking similarities between our
patients and some of those described with proven heterozygous
DPGM deficiency (Cartier et al, 1972; Travis et al, 1976)
we felt that a closer look at the 2,3-DPG phosphatase
mutase was indicated. This enzyme was partially purified
from 30 ml erythrocytes from II-13 and 32 ml erythrocytes
of a normal donor. Purification involved removal of the
bulk of hemoglobin by batch adsorption of the enzymes to
DEAE cellulose, elution from the cellulose after it had
been washed free of hemoglobin, acetone precipitation at
-20°C and then column chromatography on hydroxylapatite.
The final step completely separates phosphoglyceromutase
from 2,3-DPG phosphatase-mutase. Purification was monitored
by the phosphatase assay. DPGM and DPG phosphatase assays
on the fractions eluted from the hydroxylapatite column had
identical profiles in both preparations, as expected.
There were no significant differences noted in the purification of the enzyme from the affected (Table 10) and
normal (Table 11) erythrocytes. Note that the activities
in the starting hemolysate are the same.

The kinetic properties of the two enzyme preparations
are presented in Table 12. In the phosphatase assay the
optimal pH, Km for 2,3-DPG, activation by sodium bisulfite
and P-glycolate and inhibition by 3-PGA are comparable.
Because the coupled reaction employed for measuring DPGM
activity is not suitable for meaningful kinetic studies,
we were limited in the properties that could be compared.
The optimal pH for the overall reaction and the concentra
tion of 3-PGA allowing optimal activity were the same for
both enzyme preparations. The ratio between DPGM and 2,3-DPG
phosphatase activities in the peaks eluted from the two

Table 10.   Purification of 2,3-DPG Phosphatase from
            Normal Erythrocytes of II-13*

Step	Total Activity	Total Protein	Specific Activity	Purification	Recovery
	μmole/hr	mg	μmole/hr/mg	fold	%
Hemolysate	36.80	9983	0.004	----	100
DE-52 eluate	34.30	171	0.20	54.5	93
Acetone ppt.	26.53	102	0.26	70.4	72
Hydroxyl-apatite	22.37	12.2	1.83	495	61

* Starting with 32 ml leukocyte-free erythrocytes.

hydroxylapatite columns which contained the highest activities
were identical (Table 12).

A number of studies on the stability of 2,3-DPG were
performed on red cell suspensions. Erythrocytes from III-18
and II-13 suspended at 37°C in isotonic Tris-saline (pH 7.4)
with added glucose had no drop in 2,3-DPG at 2 hr and only a
very slight drop at 4 hr. When 20 mM bisulfite was added the
rate of fall in 2,3-DPG (though starting at lower levels)
paralleled that of normal cells. Cells incubated without
glucose had a slow fall in 2,3-DPG similar to normal cells.

Table 11.   Purification of 2,3-DPG Phosphatase from
            Normal Erythrocytes*

Step	Total Activity	Total Protein	Specific Activity	Purification	Recovery
	μmole/hr	mg	μmole/hr/mg	fold	%
Hemolysate	34.61	10850	0.003	----	100
DE-52 eluate	32.04	216	0.15	46.5	93
Acetone ppt.	24.21	118	0.20	64.1	70
Hydroxyl-apatite	15.99	19.4	0.82	258	46

* Starting with 30 ml leukocyte-free washed erythrocytes.

Table 12. Comparison of Properties of Purified Enzymes

	Normal	Affected
Phosphatase Activity		
pH optimum	7.3	7.5
K_m for 2,3-DPG ($X10^5$)	2.17	2.13
% inhibition by 2 mM 3-PGA	100	86
% activation by 20 mM HSO_3^-	781	934
% activation by 2 µM P-glycolate	1121	1272
DPG Mutase Activity*		
pH optimum	8.5	8.5
optimal 3-PGA concentration (mM)	4.3	4.3
Mutase/phosphatase activity*	0.470	0.472

* Assayed on fraction eluted from hydroxylapatite column
containing maximal activity.

2,3-DPG remained unchanged in both patient and control cells
when incubated in Tris-saline buffer, 5 mM inosine, 5 mM
pyruvate and glucose at pH 7.4 without added Pi. Assays
for ATP and analysis of experiments performed at higher pH
with added Pi (2,3-DPG generation studies) have not yet
been completed. The latter require separation of the
organic phosphates by anion chromatography before quantitation
because of the interference by the Pi in the enzymatic
determination of 2,3-DPG.

DISCUSSION

We have been unable to determine the abnormality underlying the hemolysis and the reasons for the low 2,3-DPG in
this family. Because of the dominant mode of transmission,
initially we pursued in some depth the possibility of a
primary membrane defect. Although the autohemolysis data
were compatible with a membrane problem, the normal osmotic
fragility, the normal amount and distribution of the

phospholipids, the normal cholesterol and especially the normal Na^+ efflux are strong evidence that this is not the case. Furthermore it was difficult to understand how a membrane abnormality could give rise to low cellular 2,3-DPG. The 2,3-DPG level is normal in hereditary spherocytosis (Travis et al, 1976) and was normal in one of the children with hemolytic disease associated with altered phospholipids in the erythrocytes reported by Jaffé et al (1968).

It seemed unlikely that a hemoglobinopathy could explain the low 2,3-DPG. Hemoglobin electrophoresis was normal at two pH's, no unstable hemoglobin was detected, and no Heinz bodies were seen in the erythrocytes of the propositus before or after splenectomy. Since DPGM is inhibited by product, we did consider the possibility of there being an amino acid replacement which prevented binding of 2,3-DPG with secondary reduction of 2,3-DPG synthesis. However, the P_{50} of the stripped hemoglobin of two affected family-members was normal as was the increment increase in P_{50} upon addition of 2,3-DPG. In reviewing the literature describing 14 hemoglobin variants with amino acid substitutions at or near the 2,3-DPG binding sites, the 2,3-DPG levels were reported in only 5 and all were normal. We concluded that a mutant hemoglobin could not explain the findings in this kindred.

At this point it seemed that the most plausible explanation for the hemolysis and the low 2,3-DPG was the presence of an enzyme abnormality. As pointed out above under Results, the findings in this family are strikingly similar to those few patients who have been studied thoroughly and shown to have a partial (heterozygous) deficiency of DPGM, especially those reported by Cartier et al (1972) and Travis et al (1976). For this reason we tried rigorously to rule out the presence of an abnormality of this enzyme. The protein which catalyzes the formation of 2,3-DPG has been demonstrated to also possess the specific 2,3-DPG phosphatase activity (Rosa et al, 1975; Sasaki et al, 1975; Kappel and Hass, 1976). In one patient with proven partial DPGM deficiency, a parallel decrease in 2,3-DPG phosphatase activity was demonstrated (Rosa et al, 1975). Though this need not be so in every instance, it would be most probable.

In our family we found the DPGM and 2,3-DPG phosphatase activities to be normal. However the assay of DPGM activity in hemolysates has not always been satisfactory in our laboratory. In addition, the activity of an enzyme _in vitro_

need not imply its normal function within the intracellular
environment. The DPG mutase-phosphatase from the abnormal
cells behaved identically with the enzyme from normal cells
during purification and the kinetic properties of both
partially purified enzymes were the same in the phosphatase
assays. In the mutase assay the optimal pH and 3-PGA
concentration were the same. Perhaps of most importance,
the ratio of phosphatase to mutase activities of the tubes
eluting from the hydroxylapatite columns containing the
highest activities were precisely the same. To summarize,
we could detect no quantitative or qualitative abnormality
in 2,3-DPG phosphatase-mutase.

Increased activity of 2,3-DPG phosphatase within the
cell would also lower 2,3-DPG. P-glycolate is a potent
stimulator of this enzyme (Rose and Liebowitz, 1970b).
Although there has been controversy about the actual
presence of this compound in human erythrocytes, the recent
demonstration of phosphorylation of glycolate (presumably
by pyruvate kinase) by human erythrocyte suspensions with
subsequent fall in the 2,3-DPG levels (Rose, 1976) and the
demonstration of a specific P-glycolate phosphatase in
human erythrocytes (Badwey, 1976) give credence to a
possible regulatory role of this phosphate ester within
the human red blood cell. The activity of P-glycolate
phosphatase activity in the erythrocytes of three affected
members of this kindred was not found to be diminished.

A large Dutch kindred has been reported in which
numerous individuals had mild hemolytic anemia and whose
erythrocytes contained very low levels of 2,3-DPG (about
30% of normal), a two-fold increase in ATP and elevated
pyruvate kinase activity. The pattern of transmission
was consistent with autosomal dominance. That increased
pyruvate kinase activity can induce high ATP and low 2,3-DPG
was clearly demonstrated by Oelshlegel et al (1975a) in
malaria-infected erythrocytes of monkeys and mice. Not
only were the 2,3-DPG decreased and the ATP and pyruvate
kinase activity increased, but a new isozyme of pyruvate
kinase, presumably contributed by the parasite, was
demonstrated in the infected cells. It has been well-
established that 2,3-DPG concentration is increased in
pyruvate kinase deficiency (Robinson et al, 1961; and many
others) and in PGA kinase deficiency (Valentine et al, 1969;
Hjelm and Wadman, 1970; Cartier et al, 1971; and others).

As is discussed elsewhere in this volume, Badwey and
Westhead (1976) have shown recently that the activity of
pyruvate kinase oscillates and may play a role in increasing
2,3-DPG while the erythrocyte is in the tissues and decreasing
2,3-DPG as the cell passes through the lung. The Dutch
family seemed clearly different from the patients with high
ATP but no hematologic abnormality reported by Brewer (1965).
However subsequent studies have lead to the suggestion that
these persons also have increased pyruvate kinase activity,
perhaps due to an enzyme with an altered Km for phosphoenol
pyruvate (Oelshlegel et al, 1975b). The pyruvate kinase
activity in the erythrocytes of three of our kindred was
found to be normal in several determinations in our
laboratory and in the propositus by Dr. Valentine's laboratory.
Both laboratories tested the activity of the enzyme with
high and low substrate concentrations. Also the ATP levels
in our patients are probably normal, considering the increase
in reticulocytes.

The 2,3-DPG has also been reported to be low in the
erythrocytes of patients with hemolytic anemia due to
hexokinase deficiency (Keitt, 1969; Oski et al, 1971) and
phosphoglucose isomerase deficiency (Miwa et al, 1973).
The activities of these enzymes were found to be normal in
the erythrocytes of several members of our kindred in our
laboratory and in the propositus in Dr. Valentine's
laboratory. In addition all patients with hemolytic anemia
due to these enzyme deficiencies are homozygous recessives.

Finally it should be noted that the affected members
of this kindred have a mild hemolytic process. The marrow
erythroid hyperplasia and the results of the ferrokinetic
studies indicate an appropriate and normal marrow response
to the hemolysis. Judging by the hemoglobin levels, the
hemolysis could be termed "fully compensated". However
one must take into account the moderate decrease in the
P_{50} and therefore physiologically these persons are mildly
anemic.

Whereas the study of this family has been interesting
we have been frustrated by our inability to delineate the
pathogenesis of the hemolysis. However, this family is
not unique in our experience for we find that we are unable
to define the etiology of the hemolysis in at least half
of the families referred to us with hereditary nonspherocytic

hemolytic anemias.

SUMMARY

Fourteen of sixteen members of a large kindred were
found to have mild hemolytic anemia with approximately
half-normal concentrations of 2,3-DPG in their erythrocytes.
Inheritance follows a pattern of autosomal dominance. Red
cell morphology was normal except for the presence of
2-3% crenated cells. Chromium tagged red cell half-survival
time was between 13.5 and 19 days. The hemoglobin values
were in the normal range despite the hemolysis. There was
a left-shift in the oxygen dissociation curve, the magnitude
of which was appropriate for the level of 2,3-DPG.

Autohemolysis was mildly abnormal and corrected by
glucose and ATP. Osmotic fragility, total red cell phospholipids and their distribution, cholesterol, and Na^+ efflux
were normal.

Hemoglobin electrophoresis and Hb A_2 and Hb F levels
were normal. Heinz bodies were not present and no unstable
hemoglobin was detected. Stripped hemoglobin had a normal
P_{50} and its response to 2,3-DPG was normal.

The activities of the red cell enzymes of glycolysis,
the hexosemonophosphate shunt, diphosphoglycerate mutase,
2,3-DPG phosphatase, P-glycerate phosphatase and numerous
others were normal. Because of the striking similarity
between these patients and those reported with heterozygous
diphosphoglycerate mutase deficiency, the 2,3-DPG
phosphatase-mutase was partially purified from abnormal
cells and its properties compared to that of the normal
enzyme. No differences were detected.

The biochemical abnormality underlying the low
erythrocyte 2,3-DPG and the hemolytic process in this
family remains undefined.

Acknowledgements: The authors wish to thank Dr. W.N. Valentine
for measurement of the activities of the erythrocyte enzymes
in the propositus, Dr. B.F. Cameron for providing the
computer program for determination of P_{50} and n values, and
Dr. D. Sheps who determined the carboxyhemoglobin levels.

REFERENCES

Badwey JA (1976). Phosphoglycolate phosphatase in human
    erythrocytes. J Biol Chem 252:2441.
Badwey JA, Westhead EW (1976). Hysteretic response of
    human erythrocyte pyruvate kinase to phosphoenol-
    pyruvate. J Biol Chem 251:5600.
Brewer GJ (1965). A new inherited abnormality of human
    erythrocytes: elevated erythrocytic adenosine
    triphosphate. Biochem Biophys Res Commun 18:430.
Cartier P. Habibi B, Leroux JP, Marchand JC (1971).
    Anemic hémolytique congenitale associe a un déficit
    en phosphoglycerate-kinase dans les globules rouge,
    les polynucleaires et les lymphocytes. Nouv Rev
    Franc Hémat 11:565.
Cartier P, Labie D, Leroux JP, Najman A, Demaugre F (1972).
    Déficit familial en diphosphoglycerate-mutase: étude
    hématologique et biochemique. Nouv Rev Franc Hémat
    12:269.
Dodge JT, Phillips GB (1967). Composition of phospholipids
    and of phospholipid fatty acids and aldehydes in human
    red cells. J Lipid Res 8:667.
Harkness DR, Grayson V (1969). Erythrocyte metabolism in
    the bottlenosed dolphin, Tursiops truncatus. Comp
    Biochem Physiol 28:1289.
Harkness DR, Isaacks RE, Roth S (1977). Purification and
    properties of 2,3-DPG phosphatase-mutase from
    erythrocytes of day-old chicks. Europ J Biochem
    (In press).
Harkness DR, Thompson W, Roth S, Grayson V (1970). The
    2,3-diphosphoglyceric acid phosphatase activity of
    phosphoglyceric acid mutase purified from the human
    erythrocyte. Arch Biochem Biophys 138:208.
Hjelm M, Wadman B (1970). Nonspherocytic haemolytic
    anaemia with phosphoglycerate kinase deficiency.
    Proc VIIIth Internat Cong Haemat, Munich, p 121.
Jacob HS, Jandl JH (1964). Increased cell membrane
    permeability in the pathogenesis of hereditary
    spherocytosis. J Clin Invest 43:1704.
Jaffé ER, Gottfried EL (1968). Hereditary nonspherocytic
    hemolytic disease associated with an altered phospho-
    lipid composition of the erythrocytes. J Clin Invest
    47:1375.
Kappel WK, Hass LF (1976). The isolation and partial
    characterization of diphosphoglycerate mutase from
    human erythrocytes. Biochemistry 15:290.

Kayne FJ (1974). Pyruvate kinase catalyzed phosphorylation
    of glycolate. Biochem Biophys Res Commun 58:8.
Keitt AS (1969). Hemolytic anemia with impaired hexokinase
    activity. J Clin Invest 48:1997.
Lamprecht W, Trautschold I (1963). Adenosine Triphosphate.
    Determination with hexokinase and glucose-6-phosphate
    dehydrogenase. In Bergmeyer H (ed): "Methods of
    Enzymatic Analysis," New York:Academic Press, p 543.
Lian C-Y, Roth S, Harkness DR (1971). The effect of
    alteration of intracellular 2,3-DPG concentration upon
    oxygen binding of intact erythrocytes containing normal
    and mutant hemoglobins. Biochem Biophys Res Commun
    45:151.
Longmuir IS, Chow J (1970). Rapid method for determining
    effect of agents on oxyhemoglobin dissociation curves.
    J Applied Physiol 28:343.
Miwa S, Nakashima K, Oda S, Oda E, Matsumoto N, Ogawa H,
    Fukumoto Y (1973). Glucosephosphate isomerase
    deficiency hereditary hemolytic anemia. Report of
    the first case found in Japanese. Acta Haemat Jap 36:65.
Oelshlegel FJ, Sander BJ, Brewer GJ (1975a). Pyruvate
    kinase in malaria host-parasite interaction. Nature
    255:345.
Oelshlegel FJ, Sander BJ, Brewer GJ (1975b). Role of in vivo
    pyruvate kinase activity: A. Inheritance of elevated
    red cell ATP levels B. Red cell malarial parasite
    interactions. In Brewer GJ (ed): "Erythrocyte Structure
    and Function," New York: Alan R. Liss, p 199.
Oski FA, Marshall BE, Cohen PJ, Sugarman HJ, Miller LD
    (1971). Exercise with anemia. The role of the left-
    shifted or right-shifted oxygen-hemoglobin equilibrium
    curve. Ann Int Med 74:44.
Robinson MA, Loder PB, deGruchy GC (1961). Red cell
    metabolism in nonspherocytic congenital haemolytic
    anaemia. Brit J Haemat 7:327.
Rosa A, Audit I, Rosa J (1975). Evidence for three
    enzymatic activities in one electrophoretic band of
    3-phosphoglycerate mutase from red cells. Biochimie
    57:73.
Rose HG, Oklander M (1965). Improved procedure for the
    extraction of lipids from human erythrocytes. J Lipid
    Res 6:428.
Rose ZB (1976). A procedure for decreasing the level of
    2,3-biophosphoglycerate in red cells in vitro.
    Biochem Biophys Res Commun 73:1101.

Rose ZB, Liebowitz J (1970a). Direct determination of 2,3-diphosphoglycerate. Anal Biochem 35:177.

Rose ZB, Liebowitz J (1970b). 2,3-Diphosphoglycerate phosphatase from human erythrocytes. General properties and activation by anions. J Biol Chem 245:3232.

Sasaki R, Ikura K, Sugimoto E, Chiba H (1975). Purification of biphosphoglyceromutase, 2,3-biphosphoglycerate phosphatase and phosphoglyceromutase from human erythrocytes. Eur J Biochem 50:581.

Schröter W, Kalinowsky W (1969). Erythrocyte 2,3-diphospho-glycerate mutase: an optical test in hemolysates. Clin Chim Acta 25:283.

Travis SF, Martinez J, Garvin J (1976). Study of a kindred with red cell 2,3-diphosphoglyceromutase (DPGM) deficiency and compensated hemolysis. Blood 48:993.

Valentine WN, Hsieh HS, Paglia DE, Anderson HM, Baughan MA, Jaffe′ ER, Garson OM (1969). Hereditary hemolytic anemia associated with phosphoglycerate kinase deficiency in erythrocytes and leukocytes. New Eng J Med 280:528.

Zlatkis A, Zak B, Boyle AJ (1953). A new method for the direct determination of serum cholesterol. J Lab Clin Med 41:486.

Zürcher C, Loos JA, Prins HK (1965). Hereditary high ATP content of human erythrocytes. Proc 10th Congr Int Soc Blood Transf, Stockholm 1964, p 549.

DISCUSSION

Dr. Keitt: In the assessment of the upper glycolytic enzymes did you or Dr. Valentine perform kinetic studies as well as V_{max}?

Dr. Harkness: That is a pertinent question and the answer is no. I am aware of your paper in which you demonstrated kinetic abnormalities (but normal V_{max}) in hexokinase in two relatives with hereditary non-spherocytic hemolytic anemia. In view of the dominant mode of transmission in our family, the likelihood that we are dealing with the type of patients you described seems small.

Dr. Keitt: I agree that it's small. The dominant inheritance leads me to my next comment. George Palek I think some years ago demonstrated low 2,3, DPG levels in hereditary spherocytosis. He was at some difficulty in explaining the mechanism and I don't think it's ever been satisfactorily explained but I do believe that the DPG level rose again to normal after splenectomy. I don't think your patient has hereditary spherocytosis, but I wonder if the same phenomenon might apply here. Did you get a chance to measure DPG in the propositus after splenectomy?

Dr. Harkness: The 2,3-DPG levels in the erythrocytes of the propositus were unchanged following splenectomy.

Dr. Keitt: Do you have any comments on the HS situation?

Dr. Harkness: We have recently studied one family in which five members had hereditary spherocytosis and all had very slight elevations of 2,3-DPG in keeping with mild anemia. Three were splenectomized after which the 2,3-DPG fell very slightly to the normal range. Travis and co-workers from the Cardeza Foundation, who presented a paper on a family with low 2,3-DPG and heterozygous deficiency of DPG mutase at the American Society of Hematology meetings in Boston last December, reported the values for 2,3-DPG in the erythrocytes of a group of patients with hereditary spherocytosis to be normal.

Dr. Shine: I notice you stated that the hemolytic anemia is an autosomal dominant, but as it doesn't segregate in your family doesn't that suggest that it isn't an autosomal

The Red Cell, pages 271—274

dominant and perhaps isn't even genetic?

Dr. Harkness: Although I'm moderator of the next session on red cell genetics, I am not a geneticist and I'm afraid I really cannot answer that ! It did bother me that nearly every member of the family studied possessed the abnormality and I can recall from my college genetics that the probability of getting the results we obtained in the second generation would be something like $(1/2)^7$. Would you care to elaborate on your point that this might not be genetic?

Dr. Shine: Well, one way of restating Mendel's law is "that which does not segregate is not genetic".

Dr. Harkness: I see. Very good!

Dr. Mansouri: I wonder if you measured the 2,3 DPG hemoglobin binding affinity. Because, just adding 2,3-DPG to the patients' hemoglobin which normalized its affinity for oxygen does not prove that its binding affinity for 2,3-DPG is normal.

Dr. Harkness: We did not measure 2,3-DPG binding constants. To rigidly exclude an alteration of the binding site this would have to be done. However, the functional response to added 2,3-DPG is a pretty good screening procedure for examining 2,3-DPG-hemoglobin interaction. This information, plus the knowledge that red cell 2,3-DPG is normal in red cells containing high affinity hemoglobins with mutations of the 2,3-DPG binding site, steered us away from looking further at hemoglobin.

Dr. Mansouri: I agree that the effect is the same but that still is not satisfactory because perhaps a smaller amount of DPG could do the same job to that patient's hemoglobin.

Dr. Harkness: Again, strictly speaking, you are correct. However, let me restate what we found. The P_{50} of the "stripped" hemoglobin was normal and the increment increase in P_{50} with added 2,3-DPG was normal. Therefore I ascribe the whole cell left shift to the low 2,3-DPG and not to an abnormal hemoglobin in addition to the low 2,3-DPG.

Dr. Freedman: Despite the data you have presented, I still think that there might be a silent hemoglobin mutation present. I wonder if it wouldn't be valuable to actually do a sequence analysis of the hemoglobin?

Dr. Harkness: You may be right. Because of the data we have
presented I think it would be hard to convince another laboratory (and since we do not do structural work we'd have to
get someone else to agree to perform the studies) to undertake the task!

Dr. Freedman: I have one other suggestion. Someone mentioned
a hemolytic anemia somewhat similar to your family in which
there was increased calcium flux. Of course the red cell
morphology was much more abnormal than in your patients.
But would it not be worthwhile measuring calcium flux in
your patients?

Dr. Harkness: Yes, I believe it would. Fortunately Dr.
Bruce Cameron is at our medical center and I am certain
that we can prevail upon him to do this for us.

Dr. Fairbanks: As you know from the workshop, Dr. Harkness,
the patients that we're studying have a clinical and metabolic picture that is extraordinarily similar to that you
just reported; but , in addition, they show a selective potassium leak and a modest cellular dehydration. I wonder
if you've noted that in your patients. And, secondly, although we haven't done the work on the enzymes that you've
done, we think we have seen some subtle changes in the membrane proteins. In view of what you've done, I would take
those even more seriously.

Dr. Harkness: Yes, there certainly are many similarities
between this family and the one you are studying. But there
are differences also. Osmotic fragility was normal in our
patients whereas it was quite abnormal in your family. We
looked at Na^+ and K^+ content of the red cells and that was
normal. We reported Na^+ efflux to be normal but did not
look at K^+ leak. You presented a very convincing story and
it is possible that there may be some abnormal enzyme-mem-
brane binding in this family. Perhaps we should look at
this but I hardly know where to begin!

Dr. Rosa: You are surely not dealing with an abnormal hemoglobin variant with high oxygen affinity for the 2,3-DPG
is normal in all of these. I am not certain that you have
totally excluded an abnormality of 2,3-DPG mutase and I think
you should perform electrophoresis and stain for both 2,3-DPG

mutase and 2,3-DPG phosphatase activities. I also think
that phosphorylated intermediates should be measured.

<u>Dr. Harkness</u>: Yes. Dr.Rosa and I discussed this earlier and
he has kindly offered to perform the electrophoretic studies
for us. The only phosphorylated intermediate we quantitated
was fructose diphosphate which we could identify from our
column chromatographs. It was only slightly elevated. Dr.
Valentine's lab did measure others but this was done on acid
extracts mailed across the country at ambient temperatures.
There were no remarkable variations from normal.
    I would like to make note of an error in the manu-
script in Table 7. DPGM activity was not measured in Dr.
Valentine's laboratory and the values given represent activity of PGA mutase. The values were inadvertently reported
as DPGM activity.

HEREDITARY PERSISTENCE OF FETAL ERYTHROCYTE PYRUVATE KINASE
IN THE BASENJI DOG

John A. Black, Marvin B. Rittenberg, Robert J.
Standerfer and James S. Peterson
Department of Biochemistry and Department of
Microbiology and Immunology
University of Oregon Health Sciences Center
Portland, Oregon 97201

Over 200 human cases of hemolytic anemia due to an
erythrocyte deficiency in the glycolytic enzyme, pyruvate
kinase have been described in the literature. From these
reports it is clear that there is a wide range of altered
molecular function and phenotypic expression. Pyruvate
kinase deficiency is not a single entity. The functional
deficiency may be due to a mutation directly affecting the
activity of enzyme present in normal quantities or there
may be a reduced quantity of normal enzyme due to a problem
in protein synthesis.

Figure 1 shows an electrophoretic separation of the
pyruvate kinase isozymes present in normal human tissues.
The L isozyme is the major component in liver. The enzyme
present in human erythrocytes gives two bands designated
R_1 and R_2 in this electrophoretic system. M_1 is the
isozyme present in skeletal and heart muscle. M_2 is the
major isozyme found in kidney and is a minor component in
liver. This is the isozyme which is present in fetal
tissues (Imamura and Tanaka, 1972).

The M_1 and M_2 isozymes are immunologically identical.
They can, however, be distinguished by their electrophoretic
mobility and their kinetic parameters. The M_1 isozyme
has Michaelis Menton kinetics whereas the M_2 isozyme demonstrates some allosteric properties.

The Red Cell, pages 275—290
© 1978 Alan R. Liss, Inc., New York, New York

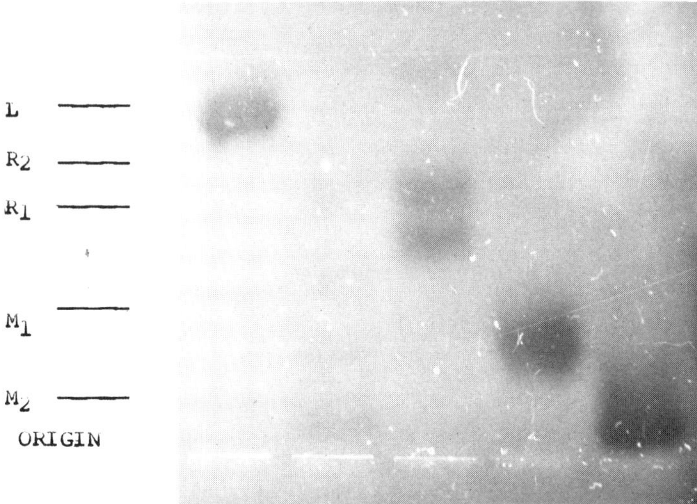

Figure 1.   The electrophoretic separation of the human
            pyruvate kinase isozymes according to Imamura
            and Tanaka (1972).

The R and L isozymes are also immunologically identical. There is no cross reaction of R or L with M_1 or M_2.
The R and L isozymes are kinetically similar both showing
allosteric properties. The genetic relationships between
the isozymes are unknown. Nakashima (1974) has demonstrated conversion of R_1 to R_2 and subsequently L by
repeated freezing and thawing or treatment with a liver
homogenate. Marie, Garreau and Kahn (1977) have recently
shown that this conversion is probably due to proteolytic
modification.

The isozyme pattern in dogs is equivalent to that in
humans with the exception that the red cell isozyme gives
only a single band on electrophoresis. The canine R
isozyme is equivalent to the human isozyme in its kinetic
properties and immunological reaction to anti-human anti-
serum. It gives allosteric kinetics with respect to
phosphoenol pyruvate, is activated by fructose-1,6-diphos-
phate and is inhibited by ATP (Black, Chern, and Rittenberg,
1975). These properties are consistent with a rate controlling function in erythrocyte glycolysis. This rate
controlling function in the erythrocyte is presumably

related to the need to regulate 2,3-diphosphoglycerate
levels since there is no need for separate control of
glycolysis and gluconeogenesis such as occurs in the liver.

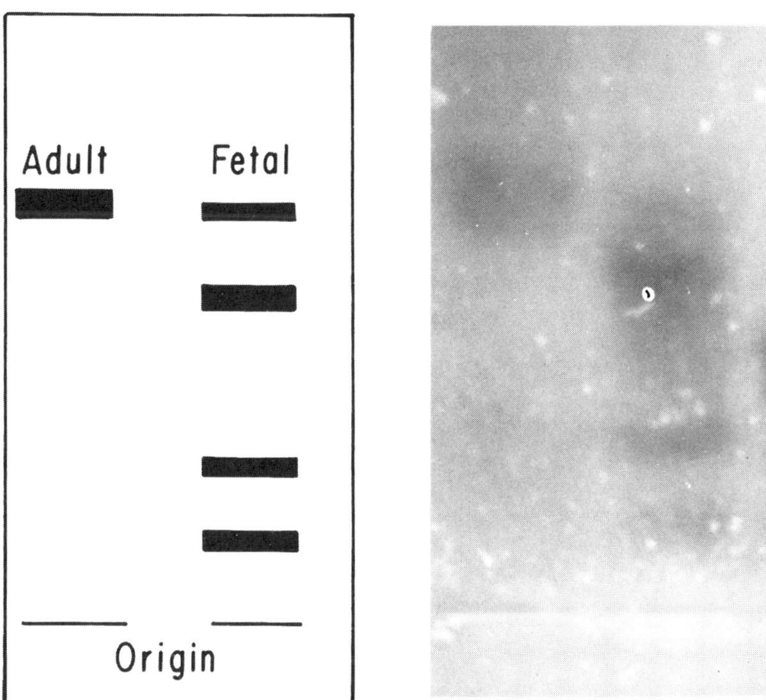

Figure 2.   The electrophoretic pattern of adult canine
            erythrocyte pyruvate kinase and the isozymes in
            late-gestation fetal erythrocytes.

Figure 2 compares the electrophoretic pattern of the
enzyme from red cells of an adult dog and a late-gestation
fetal animal. The slowest migrating band in the fetal
sample corresponds to the M_2 isozyme and the fastest migrating to the adult R isozyme. The identity of the two intermediate bands has not been established. After birth the
isozyme pattern changes with loss of the slower migrating
components and at six months of age is indistinguishable
from the adult pattern.

The results of immunological inactivation of the enzyme
activity in fetal and newborn animals are shown in Figure 3.

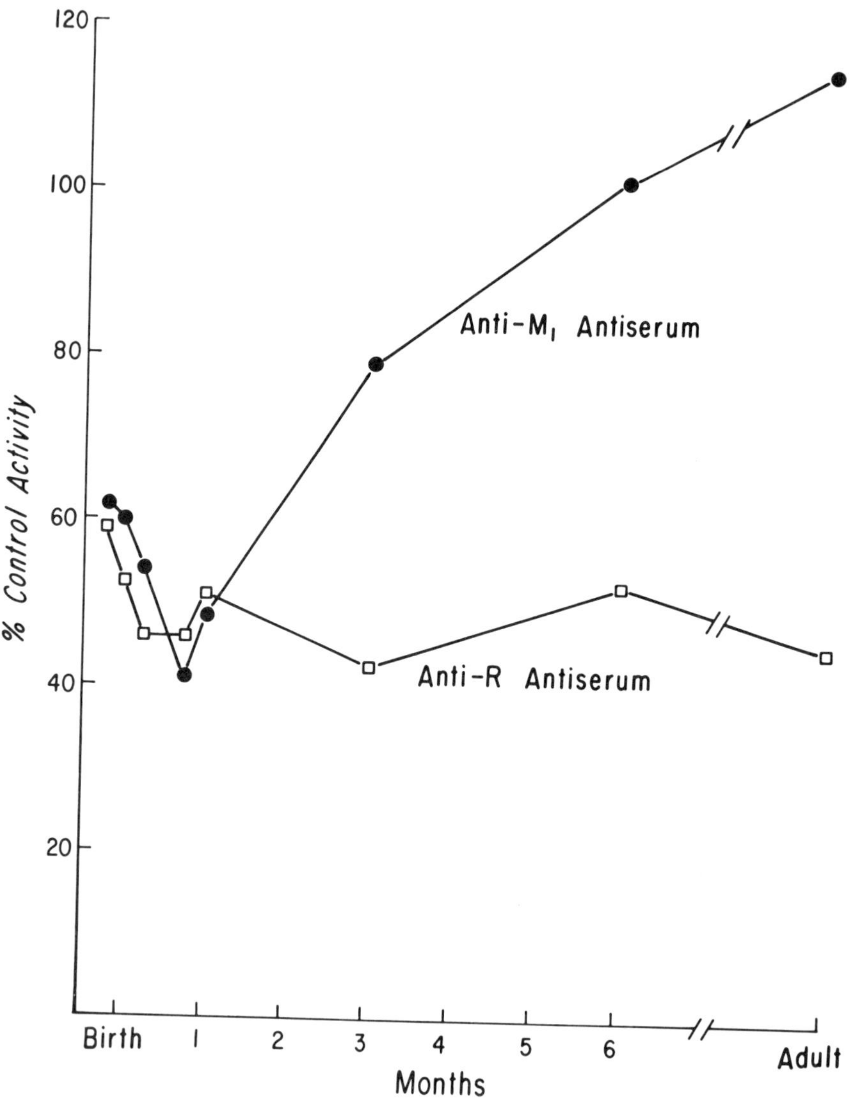

Figure 3. The inactivation of pyruvate kinase from fetal and post-natal canine erythrocytes by anti-human R and anti-human M_1 antisera.

Anti-human R and anti-human M1 antibodies were used in the
inactivation experiments. These inactivate the Canine R
and M2 isozymes respectively. There is no cross-inactivation.
These quantitative results agree with the qualitative electrophoretic results. The full adult pattern is achieved
around six months of age. The developmental shift in pyruvate kinase isozyme pattern is similar to the shift observed
in humans from fetal hemoglobin to adult hemoglobin and must
be related to the altered physiological requirements of the
red canine red cell after birth.

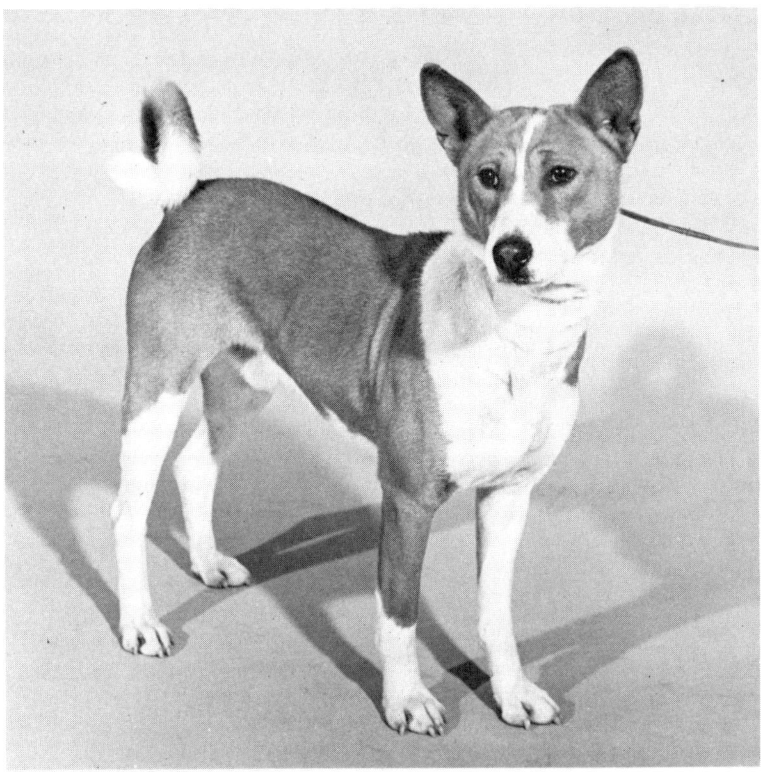

Figure 4.   A basenji dog.   Adults are 16-17 inches in
            height.   Colors are chestnut, black or black and
            tan with white feet, chest and tail tip.

The Basenji breed of dog (Figure 4) originated in the
Sudan. A small number of animals were imported into England
and the United States in the late 1920's. Hereditary non-

spherocytic hemolytic anemia in the breed was documented by
Ewing (1969) and shown to be due to pyruvate kinase deficiency by Searcy Miller and Tasker (1971). As in the human,
the condition is inherited in an autosomal recessive fashion. The condition is common in the breed and presumably
one of the small number of animals imported originally had
the mutation. It is interesting to note that the history
of the breed in England by Tudor Williams (1971) describes
the death of one imported bitch from an enlarged spleen
caused by malaria. Table 1 shows the hematologic data for
normal dogs, heterozygous Basenjis and homozygous affected
Basenjis. The heterozygotes have normal hematological parameters. However, the homozygotes have a considerably
reduced packed red cell volume, reduced red blood cell count
and high reticulocyte counts reflecting the young population
of the cells and the attempt of the reticuloendothelial
system to compensate. Iron 59 studies show that the homozygous dog red cell life span is 10 days compared to a
normal red cell span in the dog of 120 days (Dhindsa et al.
1976). There is, therefore, a very rapid turnover of red
cells in the affected animals.

2,3-Diphosphoglycerate levels are elevated in the homozygous animals and slightly elevated in the heterozygotes
(Dhindsa et al. 1976). There are corresponding changes in
the P_{50} values. Elevated 2,3-diphosphoglycerate levels and
hemoglobin oxygen dissociation curves which are shifted to
the right are also a feature of human pyruvate kinase deficiency. The right shifted curve appears to compensate
partially for the anemia.

The enzyme activity levels in normal, heterozygote and
homozygote are included in Table 1. Heterozygotes have
half normal enzyme activity which is consistent with an
enzyme deficiency state. However, the homozygous animals
have considerably elevated pyruvate kinase activity. This
is contrary to any normal interpretation of an enzyme
deficiency. When a normal dog with anemia induced by
phenylhydrazine injection is used as a control the enzyme
activity in the homozygotes is seen to be within the normal
range for a young population of red cells.

Table 1

Hematologic and enzyme activity comparisons between normal dogs and affected Basenjis.

| | n | Hematologic Data | | Reticulocytes | Pyruvate Kinase Activity |
		PCV (%)	RBC (10^6/cmm)	%	(Units/10^{10} RBC)
Normal	4	45 ± 5	5.7 ± 0.5	>2	1.22 ± 0.15
Heterozygote	5	50 ± 4	5.7 ± 0.5	>2	0.46 ± 0.1
Homozygote	4	19 ± 1	2.2 ± 0.2	18 ± 6	7.98 ± 3.52
Anemic Dog*	1	19	2.8	24	7.14

*Anemia was experimentally induced with phenylhydrazine injection

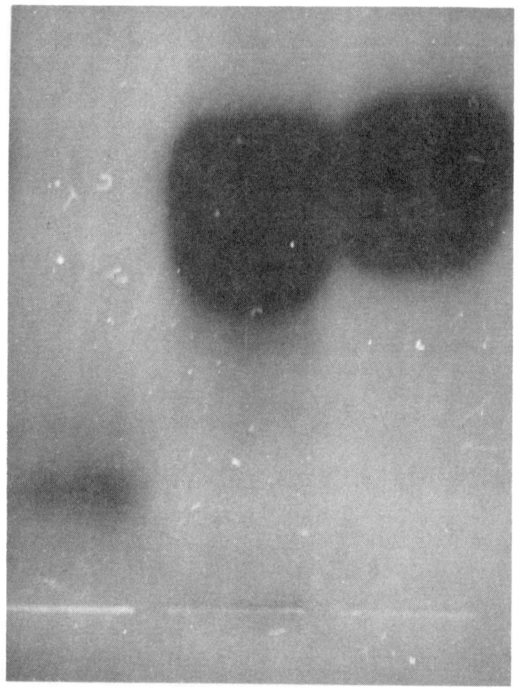

Figure 5. The electrophoretic mobility of erythrocyte pyruvate kinase from a homozygous Basenji (left),
heterozygote (center) and normal dog (right).

Figure 5 shows the electrophoretic mobility of the
enzyme from normal, heterozygote and homozygote. The
heterozygote shows only the normal red cell isozyme. The
homozygote, however, has the M_2 isozyme and there is no
evidence of the red cell isozyme.

Table 2 compares the kinetic parameters of normal
canine erythrocyte pyruvate kinase, the enzyme from homozygous animals and canine M_2 pyruvate kinase. Within the
limits of these determinations the kinetic parameters support the electrophoretic evidence that the homozygous animals contain the M_2 isozyme. In vitro stability studies
show that the enzyme present in the homozygous animals is
considerably less stable than the normal canine erythrocyte
isozyme (Standerfer, Templeton and Black, 1974).

Table 2

The kinetic parameters for normal canine R and M_2 pyruvate kinase isozymes and the enzyme from affected Basenjis.

	Kinetic Parameters	
	$K_{0.5S}^{PEP}$	$K_{0.5S}^{ADP}$
Canine R	1.1 mM	0.025 mM
Heterozygote	0.92 mM	0.052 mM
Homozygote	0.12 mM	0.43 mM
Canine M_2	0.14 mM	0.29 mM

We conclude that the affected Basenjis lack normal erythrocyte pyruvate kinase and contain instead the M_2 isozyme in their red cells. This conclusion is in agreement with the report of Nakashima et al. (1975). The situation is analogous to human classical pyruvate kinase deficiency in which the fetal M_2 isozyme is the only activity detectable in the adult red cells (Miwa et al. 1975, Nakashima et al. 1974). The Basenji dog, therefore, serves as an animal model for these patients who lack functional R pyruvate kinase isozyme. It should be noted, however, that the M_2 activity detected in the affected Basenjis is considerably higher than that usually observed for human patients.

Both examples have similarities to hereditary persistance of fetal hemoglobin (Conley et al. 1963). There may be a defect in the normal developmental transition of gene products or the persistence may represent a response to an acute deficiency of the normal adult form.

Splenectomy has been reported to give a marked improvement in 47% of pyruvate kinase deficient patients where the surgery has been performed (Van Eys and Garms 1971). Splenectomy was carried out on the homozygous animals studied here with no noticable benefits. The hematological parameters remained as they were before splenectomy. This result is consistent with the theory of Nathan et al.

(1968) that there is selective splenic destruction of
reticulocytes in pyruvate kinase deficiency when the deficient cells under the anaerobic conditions of the spleen are
unable to meet the higher ATP requirements of the anabolic
pathways present in these cells and become mis-shapen and
consequently are removed from the circulation. The results
reported above suggest that the reticulocytes in the affected
Basenjis have adequate pyruvate kinase levels and are,
therefore, not subject to this selective destruction process.
The results also suggest that splenectomy may not be
warranted for human patients with classical pyruvate kinase
deficiency.

The higher than normal enzyme activity found in the
red cells of homozygous affected animals presents an interesting problem. This would, at first glance, appear to be
incompatible with the general concept of an enzyme deficiency. The M_2 isozyme may be inherently unstable in the
environment of the adult red blood cell and, therefore,
incompatible with a normal red cell life span. The activity
level of pyruvate kinase in the heterozygous animals, which
is about one-half normal is consistent with this instability
as is the absence of the M_2 isozyme in the heterozygous
erythrocytes on electrophoresis. In vivo instability would,
therefore, be the simplest but not the only explanation.

Since the M_2 and R isozymes have quite different kinetic properties it is also possible that the M_2 isozyme
is kinetically unsuitable for participation in the adult
erythrocyte integrated glycolytic pathway. We offer a
mechanism which is based on the interrelationships present
in Figure 6. Glycolysis in the red cell appears to have
two major functions: a) the production of ATP which must be
necessary for a variety of cellular functions and b) the
maintenance and variation in 2,3-diphosphoglycerate levels
which modulate the function of the hemoglobin in oxygen
transport. In the glycolytic pathway ATP is produced at
the phosphoglycerate kinase step and at the pyruvate kinase
step. Canine R and M_2 pyruvate kinase isozymes have different affinities for ADP with the M_2 isozyme having the higher
affinity. The M_2 isozyme is also relatively unaffected by
ATP whereas the R isozyme is inhibited by this product of
the reaction. We suggest that these different properties
of the M_2 isozyme create an intracellular imbalance in the
erythrocyte between phosphoglycerate kinase and pyruvate
kinase. The higher affinity of the M_2 isozyme for ADP and

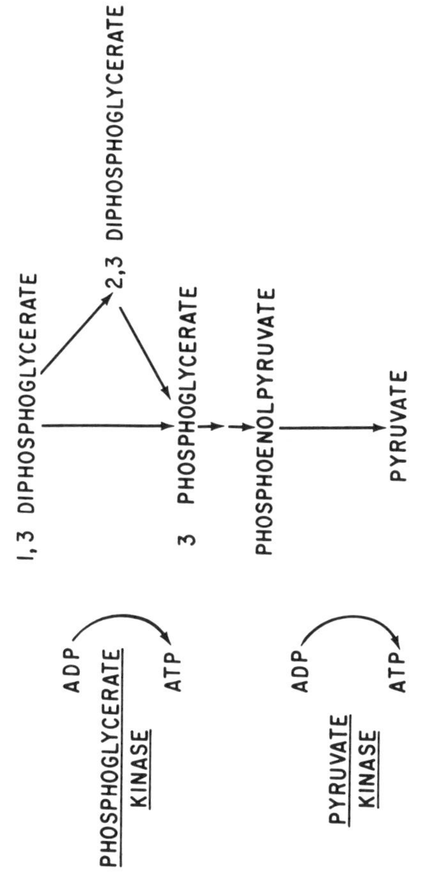

Figure 6. The phosphoglycerate kinase and pyruvate kinase reactions.

the lack of an inhibitory effect with ATP suggests that the
M_2 isozyme will compete better for available ADP. At the
same time the phosphoglycerate kinase step will be at a
competitive disadvantage. The end result will be a defect
in metabolic flow through the phosphoglycerate kinase step
and increased flow through the diphosphoglycerate shunt.
Increased utilization of the diphosphoglycerate shunt
renders glycolysis energetically unproductive since the ATP
produced at the phosphoglycerate kinase level is lost in the
by-pass. This would effectively impair ATP producing capacity and could easily lead to premature cell death. In
support of this argument it should be noted that phosphoglycerate kinase deficiency is associated with hemolytic
anemia (Kraus, Langston and Lynch, 1968, Valentine, 1968,
Konrad et al., 1973).

This more complex mechanism is difficult to examine
experimentally since it involves the competition of two
enzymes for a common substrate. The problem is compounded
by the fact that phosphoglycerate kinase is conventionally
measured in the reverse direction in a linked reaction to
glyceraldehyde-3-phosphate dehydrogenase. Since the mechanism involves the response of the two pyruvate kinase isozymes to changing intracellular ADP and ATP concentrations
we have examined the effect of energy charge on the two
isozymes.

Energy charge has been defined by Atkinson and Walton
(1967) as the ratio (ATP + 1/2ADP)/(ATP + ADP + AMP). When
all of the intracellular nucleotides are in the form of ATP
the energy charge will be 1; when they are all in the form
of AMP the energy charge will be 0. Figure 7 shows the
response of normal canine erythrocyte pyruvate kinase and
the enzyme from a homozygote to energy charge. The energy
charge in canine erythrocytes is around 0.95. In this
region the normal enzyme is relatively unresponsive to
changes in the energy charge while a reduction in ATP and
an increase in ADP concentration giving a reduced energy
charge will have a large effect on the activity of the
enzyme from the homozygote. In the absence of other com-
pensatory effects this increased activity would be at the
expense of the phosphoglycerate kinase reaction. These
results support the concept that the M_2 pyruvate kinase
isozyme is kinetically unsuited to participate in the
integrated glycolytic pathway in the erythrocyte.

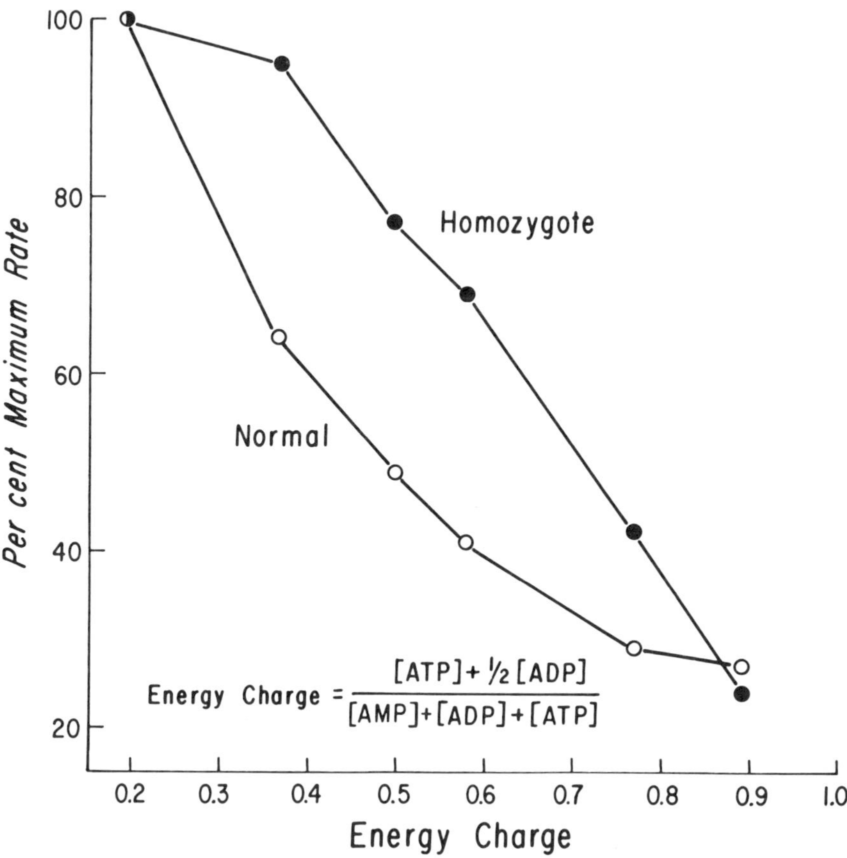

Figure 7. The effect of energy charge on the activities of erythrocyte pyruvate kinase from a normal dog and an affected Basenji

Of these two suggested mechanisms, in vivo instability has the appeal of simplicity and marks the young adult erythrocyte for death rather than the reticulocyte as was previously suggested. This molecular mechanism explains the divergent response of human patients to therapeutic splenectomy.

The second mechanism extends the growing awareness of
the complex metabolic and functional interrelationships
within the red cell and offers a reason for the allosteric
nature of erythrocyte pyruvate kinase. In this model,
however, other mitigating circumstances would be necessary
to give selective destruction of young adult cells rather
than reticulocytes in the affected Basenjis.

Hereditary persistence of fetal erythrocyte pyruvate
kinase in the Basenji dog has provided some insight into
this problem and continued study of this animal model can
be expected to yield information which is relevant to the
human condition.

Summary

Adult canine erythrocytes contain a pyruvate kinase
which is similar in properties to the human erythrocyte
isozyme. Late gestation fetal dog erythrocytes contain the
fetal M_2 isozyme, a small quantity of the adult R isozyme
and two intermediate electrophoretic bands. Immunologic
studies confirm the electrophoretic evidence of a developmental transition from the M_2 to the R isozymes which is
complete at six months of age. Basenji dogs with congenital hemolytic anemia due to pyruvate kinase deficiency have
only M_2 activity in their erythrocytes. The anemia may be
due to the in vivo instability of the M_2 isozyme in the
adult erythrocyte or the kinetic properties of the M_2 isozyme may be incompatible with the requirements of glycolysis
in the adult red cell.

Acknowledgments

Aspects of this work were supported by Research Grant
No. HD 10595 from the National Institute of Health DHEW
and a Clinical Research Grant from the National Foundation
March of Dimes. The expert assistance of Virginia Mansour
is gratefully acknowledged.

References

Atkinson, D.E. and Walton, G.M. (1967) Adenosine triphosphate conservation in metabolic regulation. Rat liver
citrate cleavage enzyme. J. Biol. Chem. 242, 3239-3241.
Black, J.A., Chern, C.J. and Rittenberg, M.B. (1975)
Canine erythrocyte pyruvate kinase I. Properties of the

normal enzyme. Biochem. Genet. 13, 331-339.
Conley, C.L., Weatherall, D.J., Richardson, S.N., Shepard, M.K., and Charache, S. (1963) Hereditary persistence of fetal hemoglobin: a study of 79 affected persons in 15 negro families in Baltimore. Blood 21, 261.
Dhindsa, D.S., Black, J.A., Koler, R.D., Rigas, D.A., Templeton, J.W. and Metcalfe, J. (1976) Respiratory characteristics of blood from Basenji dogs with classical erythrocyte pyruvate kinase deficiency. Resp. Physiol. 26, 65-75.
Ewing, G.O. (1969) Familial nonspherocytic hemolytic anemia of Basenji dogs. J. Am. Vet. Med. Assoc. 154, 503-507.
Imamura, K. and Tanaka, T. (1972) Multimolecular forms of pyruvate kinase from rat and other mammalian species I Electrophoretic studies. J. Biochem. (Tokyo) 71, 1043-1051.
Konrad, P.N., McCarthy, D.J., Mauer, A.M., Valentine, W.N. and Paglia, D.E. (1973) Erythrocyte and leukocyte phosphoglycerate kinase deficiency with neurologic disease. J. Pediat. 82, 456-460.
Kraus, A.P., Langston, M.F. and Lynch, B.L. (1968) Red cell phosphoglycerate kinase deficiency. Biochem. Biophys. Res. Comm. 30, 173-177.
Marie, J., Garreau, H. and Kahn, A. (1977) Evidence for a postsynthetic proteolytic transformation of human erythrocyte pyruvate kinase into L-type enzyme. FEBS Letters 78, 91-94.
Miwa, S., Nakashima, K., Ariyoshi, K., Shinohara, K., Oda, L. and Tanaka, T. (1975) Four new pyruvate kinase (PK) variants and a classical type PK deficiency. Brit. J. Haemat. 29, 135-147.
Nakashima, K. (1974) Further evidence of molecular alteration and aberration of erythrocyte pyruvate kinase. Clin. Chim. Acta 55, 245-254.
Nakashima, K., Miwa, S., Oda, S., Tanaka, T., Imamura, K., Nishina, T. (1974) Electrophoretic and kinetic studies of mutant erythrocyte pyruvate kinases. Blood 43, 537-548.
Nakashima, K., Miwa, S., Shinohara, K., Oda, E., Tajiri, M., Abe, S., Ono, J. and Black, J.A. (1975) Electrophoretic, immunologic and kinetic characterization of erythrocyte pyruvate kinase in the Basenji dog with pyruvate kinase deficiency. Tohoku J. Exp. Med. 117, 179-185.
Nathan, D.G., Oski, F.A., Miller, D.R. and Gardner, F.H. (1968) Life-span and organ sequestration of the red cells in pyruvate kinase deficiency. New Eng. J. Med. 278, 73-81.
Standerfer, R.J., Templeton, J.W. and Black, J.A. (1974)

Anomalous pyruvate kinase deficiency in the Basenji dog.
Am. J. Vet. Res. 35, 1541-1543.
Tudor-Williams, V. (1971) Basenjis. The barkless dogs.
Watmouglis Ltd., London.
Valentine, W.N. (1968) Hereditary hemolytic anemias
associated with specific erythrocyte enzymopathies.
Calif. Med. 108, 280-294.
Van Eys, J. and Garms, P. (1971) Pyruvate kinase defic-
iency hemolytic anemia: a model for correlation of clinical
syndrome and biochemical anomalies. Adv. in Pediatrics
18, 203-229.

DISCUSSION

Dr. Castro: Two questions: Did you measure enzyme activity
before and after splenectomy and found it to be the same?

Dr. Black: Yes.

Dr. Castro: Are these the animals that eventually develop
myelofibrosis and if so, was there any relationship between
the presence of myelofibrosis and enzyme activity?

Dr. Black: Unfortunately, I can't answer that question. My
approach to this problem is from the biochemical viewpoint
and I'm unfamiliar with that medical condition.

Dr. Castro: Thank you.

Dr. Winterbourn: Was hemoglobin F elevated in your homozygotes?

Dr. Black: From the available evidence in the dog, there's
no hemoglobin F. Gary Jones in our lab has looked at the
tryptic peptides of the fetal hemoglobin in the dog and as
far as he is able to determine it's exactly identical to
the adult dog.

Dr. Winterbourn: My reason for asking is that in hereditary
persistence of fetal hemoglobin in humans, certain cells
contained all the hemoglobin F. I wonder if your M_2 enzyme
could be present in only a fraction of the cells that have
been formed as a result of stimulation of erythropoiesis?

Dr. Black: Indeed, that's a good question. There are fundamental differences between canine erythrocytes and adult
human erythrocytes. For instance, we've looked at pyruvic
kinase patterns in cord blood, and we find no evidence for
the similar sort of distribution of isozymes as we find in
the dog. So it may be in this developmental transition occurs
in the dog where there is no transition from fetal hemoglobin
to the adult hemoglobin. Whereas with the human we have a
transition of hemoglobins and there may not be a corresponding transition in the pyruvic kinase isozymes. We can use the
dog as an animal model but one must keep in mind that it is a
model and not the real thing.

Dr. Westhead: Do you have any idea of the mechanism by which,

The Red Cell, pages 291—295

in the case of anemia, you can get a 3 or 4 fold increase in
the activity of pyruvic kinase?

Dr. Black: I don't. It is our observation using phenylhydrazine
injections to induce the anemia. One must always worry, I
think, about what you're doing with phenylhydrazine when you
inject it. But it does perhaps explain, in part, why in the
homozygous dog the enzyme activity is elevated over normal.

Dr. Paglia: Isn't one portion of that in fact that the older
cells are more sensitive to APH hemolysis? This leaves a
select younger population of cells which inherently have a
much higher pyruvic kinase activity. PK is one of those that
is more elevated in reticulocytes and the younger cell population.

Dr. Westhead: Do you know what kind of increase in younger
cell population you would need to get that kind of increase?

Dr. Paglia: Well, just from the data that John presented,
it's well within the range of possibility on this.

Dr. Westhead: So younger cells do have 3 or 4 fold or more?

Dr. Paglia: We've seen 3 or 4 fold elevation in PK as a result
of reticulycytosis and a young mean cell age alone. You can
do a density gradient fractionation on normal peripheral blood
cells and you can also get a 3,4, or 5 fold elevation in PK
in the top 10% or 20% as opposed to the bottom. It's well
within the range. Hexokinase is the one that shows the big-
gest difference, 10 fold or more, but PK is right in behind it.

Dr. Keitt: What was the reticulocyte count running in these
dogs?

Dr. Black: In the homozygotes, the average, I think, was 18.

Dr. Keitt: 18%. It is difficult to interpret glycolytic
intermediate analysis in reticulocytes but you're hypothe-
sizing that there may be competition for ADP. The site of
the block might be reflected in the chain of glycolytic intermediates. Did you measure PEP to see whether in fact the
apparent block was more likely to be immediately proximal to
PK? If PEP was low it might indicate that the PGK step was
blocked instead.

Dr. Black: I have considered this. I think any result you get
will be complicated by the high percentage of young reticulocytes. I think in this anemia, and many others, the cells you
are more interested in are the ones that just died.

Dr. Keitt: Yes.

Dr. Black: They are rather difficult to obtain.

Dr. Keitt: How true, great wisdom. But I would like to know
still that might give you some rough idea. I would be reluctant to take your admonitions against splenectomizing the human
from your biochemical observations, nice ones, in the dog.
In fact, when we look at all the splenectomized cases, it's
true that many of them don't benefit in terms of the hemoglobin.
Some did clearly, but one interesting factor that was pointed
out was that the reticulocyte counts only reached the very
high level in the human after splenectomy. What happened to
your dog's reticulocyte count after splenectomy?

Dr. Black: After splenectomy, there was no elevation as is
sometimes seen in the human. One wonders whether the spleen
is, in fact, trapping reticulocytes and the removal of the
spleen then allows more of them to appear in the general circulation.

Dr. Keitt: In the human you say it doesn't seem to be the
case?

Dr. Black: I'm not suggesting that everyone abandon splenectomy in pyruvate kinase deficiency. I think these observations suggest that since there is a range in the molecular
types of pyruvate kinase deficiency and also in phenotypic
expression that it is worthwhile to try and correlate the
clinical condition with the molecular defect and it may well
be that there is a class of pyruvate kinase deficiencies for
which splenectomy is not beneficial.

Dr. Keitt: One other question: Does the M_2 isoenzyme go up
in a normal dog who has a high retic count as in an induced
hemolytic anemia?

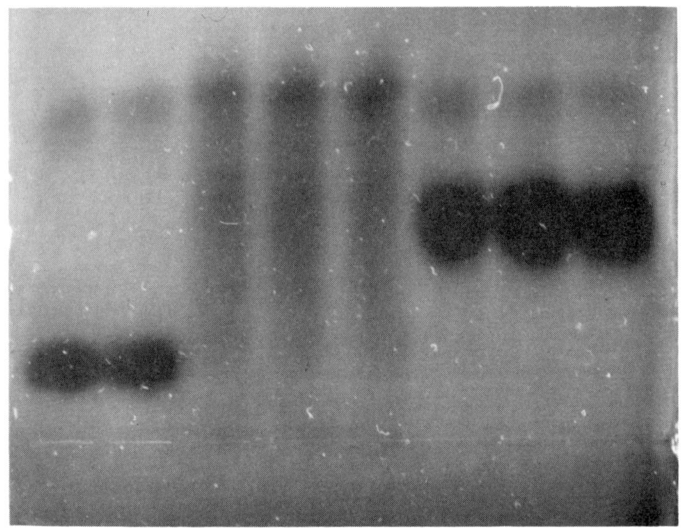

<u>Dr. Black</u>: I'm glad you asked that question. Next slide,
please. We've been interested in just that question, and also
why in the heterozygote the M_2 isozyme is not observed. We
made a normal dog and heterozygote anemic to the same hematocrit as the homozygote by phenylhydrazine injection In the
anemic normal dog there was no evidence of the M_2 isozyme
(3 samples on the right). In the anemic heterozygote, the
separation isn't as clean cut as we would like, but nevertheless there is some evidence of a band corresponding to the
M_2 band (heterozygote - 3 samples in center; homozygote 2
samples on left). So apparently if you make a heterozygote
anemic you can see some of the slow migrating isozymes. It's
possible that if we had been able to get a young enough population of cells in the normal this would also be the case, but
so far we've not observed it.

<u>Dr. Paglia</u>: Thank you, Dr. Black, and in closing this portion
of the session I'd just like to echo John Black's comment
responding to Alan Keitt, that we should recognize, and it's
a point that Bill Valentine frequently emphasizes, that in looking at these kinds of problems we are always dealing with the
population of cells that have survived. It's the only one that
is for you to biopsy by venipuncture, and if Alan is frustrated,
so are we, that we can't look at those that have just gone
beyond the brink. This is not to say, of course, that it's

unimportant to look at glycolytic intermediates and enzyme activities in the surviving population, because this is all we have left to work with, and you must always keep this in mind.

ERYTHROCYTE METABOLISM, CONTROL AND GENETICS

Chairman: D. Harkness

POTENTIAL REGULATORY PROPERTIES OF HUMAN ERYTHROCYTE
PYRUVATE KINASE

John A. Badwey[*] and Edward W. Westhead[**]

*Department of Biological Chemistry, Harvard
Medical School, Boston, Mass. 02115
**Department of Biochemistry, University of
Massachusetts, Amherst, Mass. 01003

Pyruvate kinase (EC 2.7.1.40, ATP-pyruvate phospho-
transferase) occupies a central role in the metabolism of
the human erythrocyte. It catalyzes one of the two ATP
producing reactions, potentially contributes to the control
of NADH levels via production of pyruvate, and is important
in establishing the steady state levels of 2,3-bisphospho-
glycerate (2,3-P_2-glycerate). Both ATP and 2,3-P_2-glycer-
ate are important in regulating the rate of oxygen release
to the tissues because of their preferential binding to
deoxygenated rather than oxygenated hemoglobin as illustrated below (for review of binding constants, see
Hamasaki & Rose 1974).

$$Hb \cdot O_2 + 2,3\text{-}P_2\text{-glycerate} \rightleftharpoons Hb \cdot 2,3\text{-}P_2\text{-glycerate} + O_2$$
$$\text{(or ATP)} \qquad\qquad\qquad \text{(or ATP)}$$

Rose (1970, 1971) has shown that an inverse relationship exists between the activity of pyruvate kinase and the
levels of 2,3-P_2-glycerate. This relationship is the result
of two conditions within the red cell (Rose, I. A. 1970,
1971). First, all of the reactions between fructose-1,6-
bisphosphate (fructose-1,6-P_2) and phosphoenolpyruvate (P-
enolpyruvate) exist in a state of quasi-equilibrium.
Second, pyruvate kinase (PK) operates at a concentration of
P-enolpyruvate well below its K_m. Under such conditions,
an increase in the glycolytic rate or inhibition of the
enzyme results in the P-enolpyruvate levels becoming
elevated in a linear fashion. These increases in the P-
enolpyruvate levels lead to increases in the levels of
1,3-P_2-glycerate (and all other proximal metabolites) and

The Red Cell, pages 299–314

hence to increases in the level of 2,3-P_2-glycerate via the
diphosphoglyceromutase reaction. This relationship is
demonstrated by the frequent occurrence of elevated levels
of 2,3-P_2-glycerate in PK-deficient erythrocytes (Delivoria-
Papadopoulos, et al. 1969, Rose & Warms 1974) and by the
decreased levels of 2,3-P_2-glycerate and P-enolpyruvate
which are observed in erythrocytes containing a PK with
abnormally high activity at low P-enolpyruvate levels
(Brewer et al. 1974).

Because of its critical role in red cell metabolism and
function, the activity of this enzyme must be subject to
strict regulation. During our studies on this enzyme, we
have observed three potential regulatory properties which
we would like to review at this conference; hysteretic responses, allosteric interactions, and chemical modification
(sulfhydryl oxidation). We will also mention recent results
which suggest a possible mode of regulation by hormones.

HYSTERETIC BEHAVIOUR

During routine assays, it was observed that the reaction progress curves of this enzyme were not linear but
rather became steeper over a period of several minutes before maximal activity was achieved. The length of this
activation period (lag phase) was found to be highly dependent upon the treatment of the enzyme prior to assay (Fig.
1). Preincubation of the enzyme with adenine nucleotides
amplified the lag, whereas pretreatment with P-enolpyruvate
diminished it (Badwey & Westhead 1976). This activation
process was first order in enzyme with the pseudo-first
order rate constants being a hyperbolic function of the P-
enolpyruvate concentration (Fig. 2). These results can be
explained by a slow isomerization reaction mediated by PEP
in which an inactive or partially active enzyme species is
converted into an active conformation. Mechanisms which
can account for such slow ligand-mediated isomerization
processes have been developed by Frieden (1970) and Spivey
et al. (1974). The kinetic evidence for different sub-
strate-induced conformational states of PK was buttressed
by chemical modification studies using the irreversible
sulfhydryl inhibitor, N-enthylmaleimide (MalNEt). During
such studies, adenine nucleotides were found to promote
inactivation by MalNEt, whereas P-enolpyruvate protected
against the reagent (Badwey & Westhead 1976).

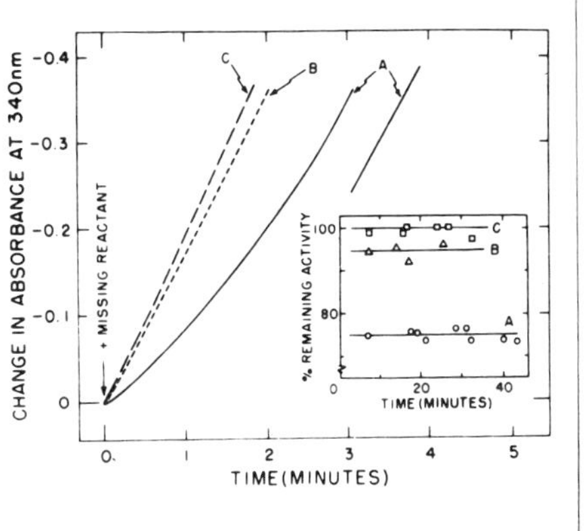

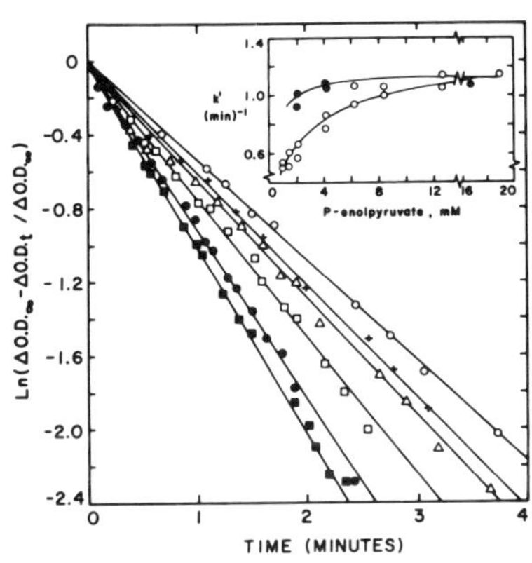

Fig. 1   Fig. 2

Fig. 1. Reaction progress curves for human erythrocyte PK
demonstrating the effects of preincubation conditions on
the lag phase of the reaction. The concentration of P-enolpyruvate was 2.1. The standard reaction mixture was 8.0 mM
P-enolpyruvate, 4.1 mM ADP, 0.38 mM NADH, 5.7 mM $MgCl_2$,
100 mM KCl, 90 mM Hepes buffer (pH 7.4), and 50 units of
lactate dehydrogenase. The variable is the component used
to initiate the reaction. From left to right: C, ADP added
last; B, enzyme added last; A, P-enolpyruvate added last.
Inset, time course of the loss in final activity observed
after preincubation of the enzyme with ADP. Assay mixtures
were preincubated for variable periods of time (ordinate)
before the initiation of the reactions as indicated above
for A, B, and C. The percentages of remaining activities
(abscissa) were determined from the slopes of the final,
fast portions of the progress curve. They are expressed as
the percentage of activity compared to the values obtained
from the assays initiated by ADP (C) which were constant
over the time course.

Fig. 2. Effect of P-enolpyruvate concentration on the lag
phase. The first order plots shown are constructed from the
progress curves obtained at the following representative
concentrations of P-enolpyruvate: O, 1.05 mM; I, 1.47 mM;
Δ, 2.10 mM; □ , 4.20 mM; ●, 6.3 mM; ■ , 8.4 mM. Other assay
conditions are described in Fig. 1. The inset shows the
pseudo first order rate constants versus P-enolpyruvate concentration in the absence (O) and presence (●) of 0.3 mM
fructose 1,6-P_2.

Enzymes which respond slowly to rapid changes in ligand concentrations have been termed "hysteretic" by Frieden (1970). A good example of the potential usefulness of such responses may be provided by human erythrocyte PK. The hysteretic behaviour of this enzyme could conceivably aid in the release of oxygen to the tissues by promoting transient increases in the $2,3-P_2$-glycerate levels as the red cells traverse the capillaries (Badwey & Westhead 1976). The scheme is described below. Deoxygenation in vitro is known to stimulate red cell glycolysis (Asakura et al. 1966, Hamasaki et al. 1970). The major cause of this stimulation is thought to be the following. During anaerobiosis, the level of free $2,3-P_2$-glycerate declines due to increased binding to deoxyhemoglobin. Since $2,3-P_2$-glycerate is an inhibitor of the hexokinase (Dische 1941, Brewer 1969) and the phosphofructokinase (Ponce et al. 1971, Beutler & Guinto 1971) reactions, the glycolytic rate is elevated in response to this decrease. Eaton and Brewer (1968) have suggested that a similar process may also occur in vivo, whereby the normal oxygenation-deoxygenation cycle of the red cell produces oscillations in the glycolytic rate. A hysteretic PK could play a useful role in such a cyclical process. As the erythrocytes move from the lungs into the tissues, the glycolytic flux should increase as described above. If a pronounced lag in PK activity accompanies the increased flux, it would effect a buildup in P-enolpyruvate, $2,3-P_2$-glycerate and all of the other metabolites proximal to PK. This transient buildup of $2,3-P_2$-glycerate could then aid in the release of oxygen to the tissues by its preferential binding to deoxyhemoglobin.

The transient high levels of P-enolpyruvate would then accelerate the conversion of PK to its more active form (Fig. 2). The increased PK activity would help to deplete the high levels of glycolytic intermediates so that the initial levels could be restored and the process repeated. It may be noted here that the half-times for activation of PK under the conditions of our experiments (Fig. 2) are in the range of the resting circulation rate of human erythrocytes (1 cycle/min).

Arguing against such a scheme, however, is the fact that the glycolytic flux, measured in vitro [0.015 - 0.03 μmoles glucose consumed/min/ml cells at 37°C (Rose & Warms 1974)] does not appear to be rapid enough to lead to significant $2,3-P_2$-glycerate synthesis during such short

periods of time in vivo. It is known, however, that the
capacity (V_{max} for hexokinase) does exist for a 5-10 fold
higher rate (Rose 1971), thus making it possible for
different physiological stimuli of unknown origin (perhaps
changes in PH, pyruvate, or other still unsuspected   influences) to effectively augment this rate in vivo.

ALLOSTERIC BEHAVIOUR AND MODIFICATION REACTIONS

The kinetic descriptions of human erythrocyte PK in the
current literature differ widely. Saturation data for P-
enolpyruvate consistent with Michaelis-Menten behaviour
(Campos et al. 1965, Ibsen et al. 1968), positive cooperativity (Kohler and Vanbellinghen 1968, Cartier et al. 1968),
and also negative cooperativity (Boivin et al. 1972) have
been published. Half saturation constants ranging from
0.01 to 4.0 mM have been reported (Ibsen et al. 1968, Campos
et al. 1968). Differences in the assay conditions [buffers
utilized, pH, ADP concentration, etc. (Campos et al. 1965,
Staal et al. 1971, Boivin et al. 1972), storage conditions
(Ibsen et al. 1971, Boivin et al. 1972, Cartier et al.
1968)] and the portion of the reaction progress curve used
in measuring the velocity (Badwey & Westhead 1976) all seem
to contribute to these discrepancies. In addition, this
enzyme also may undergo at least two types of post-translational modification reaction, proteolytic cleavage (Marie
et al. 1977) and oxidation of the enzyme's sulfhydryl groups
(Van Berkel et al. 1973, Badwey & Westhead 1977a).

During our studies on this enzyme, we have been able to
obtain reproducible kinetic constants for different blood
samples only if standard isolation procedures and assay
techniques were strictly observed (Badwey & Westhead, 1976).
The use of ultrapure ammonium sulfate, deionized water and
the addition of EDTA to all of the buffers used in preparing
the enzyme was essential to prevent the occurrence of anoma-
lously shaped saturation curves for P-enolpyruvate. When
such precautions were observed, the freshly prepared enzyme
displayed a slightly sigmoidal saturation curve for P-enolpyruvate (n_H = 1.2 - 1.4) at saturating levels of ADP, with
a $K_{0.5}$ for PEP of approximately 2.5 mM (Fig. 3). Fructose-
1,6-P_2, a positive allosteric effector of this enzyme
(Koler & Vanbellinghen 1968, Cartier et al. 1968) converted
this curve to a normal rectangular hyperbola with a greatly
reduced K_m (Fig. 3). Mannose-1,6-P_2 and glucose-1,6-P_2

were also capable of promoting similar changes in the P-enolpyruvate saturation pattern, the order of effectiveness being fructose- > mannose- > glucose-1,6-P$_2$ (Badwey & Westhead 1977b).

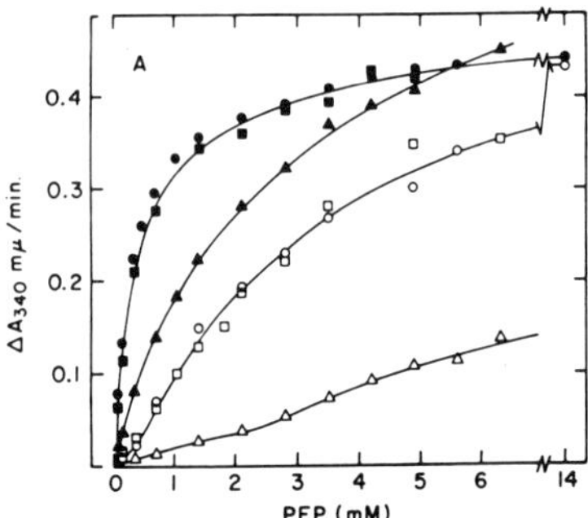

Fig. 3. The P-enolpyruvate (PEP) saturation curves for the freshly isolated enzyme (O), the 48 hr. enzyme sample (Δ) and the 48 hr. enzyme sample incubated in buffer C plus 50 mM DTT for 10 hrs. at 4°C (□). The closed symbols (▲, ●, ■)correspond to the samples described above assayed in the presence of 2.0 mM fructose-1,6-P$_2$. The concentration of ADP was 4.4 mM and all other conditions as described in Fig. 1.

Only hyperbolic saturation curves (n_H = 1.0) were observed for the active substrate complex, Mg·ADP. Even when the concentration of the fixed substrate, P-enolpyruvate, was lowered to 1/10 of its $K_{0.5}$ value (0.2 mM), no evidence of cooperative interactions could be detected. Fructose-1,6-P$_2$ did not appear to <u>directly</u> influence the binding of Mg·ADP to the enzyme (Badwey & Westhead 1977b).

Upon storage, the partially purified enzyme exhibited rapid changes in its saturation kinetics for P-enolpyruvate. An example of one such modified curve is shown in Fig. 3. This sample exhibited reduced activity at all substrate concentrations examined and displayed an elevated $K_{0.5}$ for P-enolpyruvate. Fructose-1,6-P$_2$ converted this anomalous curve to a normal rectangular hyperbola with a slightly higher V_{max} than observed for the freshly prepared enzyme.

Incubating the aged enzyme sample with dithiothreitol
(or mercaptoethanol) largely restored the kinetic properties
observed originally for the freshly prepared enzyme (Fig.3).
This demonstrated that oxidation of the enzyme's sulfhydryl
groups was responsible for the kinetic changes observed.

The ability of the allosteric modifier to overcome the
effects of oxidation of the enzyme and restore maximal
activity is striking, and so far as we are able to discover,
unique among enzymes. We have even observed that enzyme inactivated to the point where no detectable activity could be
observed in the absence of fructose-1,6-P_2 showed a normal
or elevated V_{max} when assayed in the presence of fructose-
1,6-P_2.

In contrast to these changes observed for P-enolpyruvate, storage of the enzyme did not result in any major
changes in the ADP saturation curves (Badwey & Westhead
1977b).

The alterations upon storage occurred only after hemolysis of the cells and did not generally appear during storage
of the intact erythrocytes. The kinetic constants reported
above for the freshly prepared enzyme were the same regardless of whether the blood cells utilized were freshly drawn
or stored (4°C) for periods of 5 days to 8 weeks in acid
citrate dextrose solution prior to use. Paglia and
Valentine (1970) have shown by very careful studies in which
they segregated the youngest and oldest erythrocytes from
fresh blood by centrifugation through density gradients that
the K_m for P-enolpyruvate is elevated upon aging of the intact cells. The changes they observed, however, are much
smaller than the ones we are reporting and would likely go
undetected in the mixed cell populations we are using.
Mechanisms must therefore be present within the red cell
which protect this enzyme from rapid oxidation. We have
previously shown that a number of its positive effectors are
capable of protecting it in vitro (Badwey & Westhead 1975).
Aside from the fact that oxidation of the enzyme can alter
its allosteric characteristics, it is conceivable that
oxidation of this enzyme in vivo may operate as a control
mechanism. We have suggested (Badwey & Westhead 1975) that
reduction of PK activity by oxidation could both increase
production of NADPH via the pentose shunt and spare NADH
for use in the methemoglobin reductase reaction. Thus under
oxidative stress PK oxidation would serve to insure the

maintenance of hemoglobin in its reduced state.

Clinical Significance

An inheritable form of nonspherocytic hemolytic anemia associated with a deficiency in erythrocyte PK was initially reported in 1961 (Valentine et al. 1961). Since then a number of kinetic studies have been performed on this enzyme from a variety of patients and have revealed a complex and heterogenous pattern of defects. Altered enzyme levels and aberrant kinetics both seem to occur (Paglia et al. 1968). In almost all of the cases reported, the abnormal kinetic patterns are associated with the substrate P-enolpyruvate. Saturation curves for ADP showed no abnormal behaviour. Different classes of these defects have been described (Staal et al. 1972, Munro et al. 1970) in terms of the variable kinetic constants for P-enolpyruvate. It was assumed that these defects involved mutations in the structural genes for this enzyme, and this appears to be true in many cases (Kahn et al. 1975).

The general applicability of this assumption was questioned (Van Berkel et al. 1973), however, when it was shown that oxidation of the normal enzyme by GSSG produced a sample which displayed properties identical to those observed in a particular type of PK-deficiency. We (Badwey & Westhead 1977a) have subsequently shown that air-oxidation of the normal enzyme produces similar effects (Fig. 3). In vitro, oxidation is sharply accelerated by traces (0.1 µM) of copper ion. Evidence for the occurrence of oxidative modification in vivo is provided by the existence of PK-deficient patients who also show decreased glutathione reductase activity (Staal et al. 1975, Tajiri 1976). Staal and co-workers (Van Berkel et al. 1974) have also reported two cases of PK-deficiency in which in vitro incubation of the partially purified enzyme with mercaptoenthanol resulted in the conversion of the abnormal kinetic patterns to normal patterns. These results may thus complement the work of Zuelzer and co-workers (1968), whose extensive examination of the genetic problems posed by these anemias has suggested that PK-deficiency may be subordinate to unknown erythrocyte abnormalities such as possible membrane lesions.

It should be remembered, however, that oxidation of the enzyme's sulfhydryl groups could result from either genetic

modifications in the protein itself which may predispose
the enzyme to oxidation with the resulting kinetic changes,
or may be due to inherited alterations [membrane defects ?
(see Nathan et al. 1965)] which produce an internal milieu
in the red cell hostile to PK. More work is obviously
needed to determine the nature of the defects occurring in
this disorder.

Acquired deficiencies in erythrocyte PK have recently
been reported in a number of malignant hematologic disorders (Arnold et al. 1974, Boivin et al. 1975). In a
number of cases, this deficiency appears to be the result
of a dialysable inhibitor present in the plasma (Arnold
et al. 1974, Arnold et al. 1977), the nature of which is
unknown. Whether the other cases might involve an oxidation of the enzyme is presently unexplored. These acquired
defects may offer an excellent opportunity to evaluate the
relationship between the enzyme and its environment.

We would like to take this opportunity to point out a
problem that we have observed in interpreting some of the
kinetic data in the literature. Frequently the most convenient parameter for comparing the normal enzyme with
samples that are abnormal, through disease or in vitro
modification, is the "K_m" value. The "Lineweaver-Burk"
plot in which $1/v$ is plotted against $1/(PEP)$ is widely used
to give a linear presentation of the data points to determine K_m. In principle, only saturation curves which are
rectangular hyperbolas [show Michaelis-Menten kinetics]
when potted as v v.s. (PEP) will produce straight lines
when plotted in the double-reciprocal form. Unfortunately
the latter type of plot is frequently very insensitive to
abnormalities in the saturation behaviour which are readily
apparent in the primary type of plot. The "K_m" determined
in such cases can be a very misleading quantity and obscure
the true complexity of the behaviour observed. A second
and related problem with the double-reciprocal plot is that
a sufficiently limited portion of even a very complex
saturation curve will give an apparently straight line when
the data are plotted as reciprocals. The upper portion of
a sigmoid saturation curve is an example. The extrapolated
K_m values are again highly misleading. Several examples of
misleading linear plots are to be found in the pyruvate
kinase literature, and the data obtained from them must
confuse efforts to discern classes of behaviour among pyruvate kinases observed in disease states. Now that it has

become apparent that this enzyme can show a wide variety of
kinetic behavior, we would plead for the reporting of all
PEP saturation curves in the primary form, even as an insert
to a secondary plot.

Hormonal Effects Possibly Mediated by PK

A possible third mechanism of control of red cell
metabolism through PK is still only in the early stages of
investigation. It has been shown that the pyruvate kinase
from liver, similar in many properties to the erythrocyte
enzyme, is a substrate for a cyclic-AMP-stimulated protein
kinase (Ljungström et al. 1974, Engström et al. 1974).
This phosphorylation results in marked alterations in the
kinetic parameters for P-enolpyruvate (Ekman et al. 1976).
The human erythrocyte has both a c-AMP-dependent protein
kinase (Rubin et al. 1972) and at least a very low level
of adenylate cyclase activity (Rodan et al. 1976).

We have begun to look for evidence of a similar mechanism in the red blood cell. While we have obtained some interesting results, there are aspects of the data that make
us cautious in our interpretation of them. On one hand we
have looked for changes in $2,3-P_2$-glycerate levels in human
erythrocytes incubated in vitro with catecholamines, with
cyclic AMP, and with prostaglandins (Sacco & Westhead 1978).
In the absence of phosphodiesterase inhibitors such as 1-
methyl, 3-isobutyl xanthine or caffeine, no significant
changes in $2,3-P_2$-glycerate levels were found. In the
presence of phosphodiesterase inhibitors, very significant
increases are caused by the above agents. Figure 4 shows
results of incubation with c-AMP and the dibutyryl analogue.
The maximum increase in $2,3-P_2$-glycerate level observed is
100% from the control value. Isoproterenol at 1 mM caused
an increase of 20% above control, with significant increases observed even with 1 μM isoproterenol. Prostaglandin E_2 at 10^{-3} mM raised $2,3-P_2$-glycerate levels 50%
with significant increases at 10^{-3} μM, in accord with an
earlier report (Rörth & Bille-Brahe 1972). In contrast,
prostaglandin E_1 was without effect. The problem with these
data is the time scale on which the changes occur (Fig. 4).
We had expected to find changes occurring in a few minutes
since alterations in oxygenation resulting from stress
(epinephrin secretion) would have to be effected quickly.

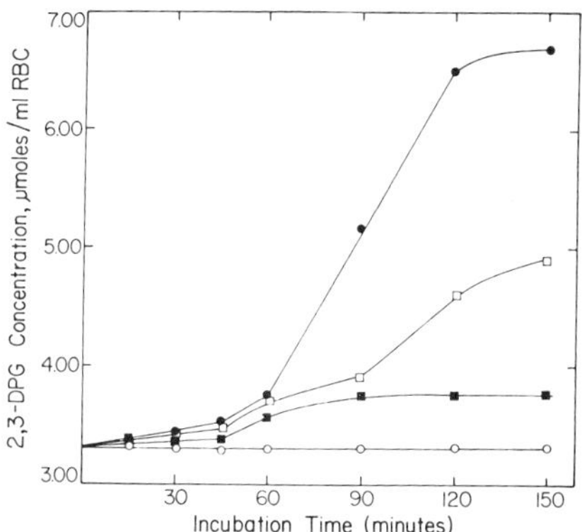

Fig. 4. Human erythrocytes from freshly drawn blood were
incubated with 0.2 mM pyruvate and 5 mM caffeine for 70
minutes. Cyclic AMP and dibutyryl cyclic AMP were added at
70 minutes; which is 0 time on the graph. 0, control, no
additions; ■, -caffeine, +5 mM dibutyryl cyclic AMP; □ ,
+5 mM caffeine, +5 mM cyclic AMP; ●, +5 mM caffeine, +5
mM dibutyryl cyclic AMP.

Our second approach to this problem is to incubate
erythrocytes with radioactive inorganic phosphate and look
for phosphorylation of PK. This work is incomplete but we
are encouraged to find radioactivity accompanying PK through
several steps of purification. Antibodies to the purified
enzyme are being prepared so that separation and analysis
of cross-reacting material can be made quickly using gel
electrophoresis techniques.

PK AND P-GLYCOLATE

Purified PK from both muscle (Kayne 1974) and yeast
(Leblond & Robinson 1976) are capable of catalyzing the
phosphorylation of glycolate as shown below.

$$\text{glycolate} + \text{ATP} \xrightarrow{\text{M}^{++}} \text{P-glycolate} + \text{ADP}$$

Rose (1976) has recently provided evidence that the red cell
enzyme is also capable of catalyzing this reaction _in vitro_.
Normal red cells incubated with glycolate lose $2,3\text{-P}_2\text{-}$

glycerate at a rapid rate, whereas only a slight reduction is observed when PK-deficient cells are utilized. P-glycolate is a powerful activator of $2,3-P_2$-glycerate phosphatase (Rose & Liebowitz 1970).

Whether this reaction is relevant _in vivo_ is presently unknown. However, the ability of P-glycolate to activate $2,3-P_2$-glycerate phosphatase 1,500 fold (Rose & Liebowitz 1970) and the existence of a phosphatase in red cells highly specific for P-glycolate (Badwey 1977) suggest a role for this compound in the regulation $2,3-P_2$-glycerate metabolism.

In summary, human erythrocyte pyruvate kinase exhibits molecular properties that can be imagined to serve as potential control functions. The hysteretic response to increased concentrations of PEP could help to produce cyclic variations in $2,3-P_2$-glycerate. The inactivation by oxidation could be a means of protecting hemoglobin from oxidation. The ability of fructose diphosphate to override oxidative inactivation may be evidence for a complex interlocking of control functions. By analogy with hormonal effects on the liver enzyme we may find that hormonal effects on erythrocyte metabolism are, in part, mediated through phosphorylation of pyruvate kinase. Evaluation of these various possibilities will have to be made as further information on red cell metabolism becomes available. Even the most well established "control" property of PK, its allosteric activation by hexose diphosphates is currently of unknown significance considering the high level of such activators always present in the red cell. Is it possible that these allosteric activators have a significant effect only when (or if) the enzyme is in a state of partial oxidation?

Acknowledgements

These studies were supported by U. S. Public Health Service Grant GM 14945.

Figures 1 and 2 are reprinted with the permission of the _Journal of Biological Chemistry_.

Figure 3 is reprinted with the permission of _Biochemical and Biophysical Research Communications_.

References

Asakura N, Sato Y, Minakami S, Yoshikawa H (1966). Effect
  of deoxygenation of intracellular hemoglobin on red cell
  glycolysis. J Biochem (Tokyo) 59:524.
Arnold H, Blume KG, Löhr GW, Boulard M, Majean Y (1974).
  "Acquired" red cell enzyme defects in hematological
  diseases. Clinica Chimica Acta 57:187.
Arnold H, Blume KG, Löhr GW (1977). Mechanisms for acquired
  red cell enzyme defects. Blood 49:1022.
Badwey JA, Westhead EW (1975). Sulfhydryl oxidation and
  multiple forms of human erythrocyte pyruvate kinase.
  In Markert CL (ed): "Isozymes:I. Molecular Structure"
  New York: Academic Press, p 509.
Badwey, JA, Westhead EW (1976). Hysteretic response of
  human erythrocyte pyruvate kinase to phosphoenolpyruvate.
  J Biol Chem 251:5600.
Badwey JA, Westhead EW (1977a). Post-translational modifi-
  cation of human erythrocyte pyruvate kinase. Biochem
  Biophys Res Commun 74:1326.
Badwey JA, Westhead EW (1977b). Activation of human
  erythrocyte pyruvate kinase by hexose-bisphosphates.
  Biochem Biophys Res Commun 77:275.
Badwey JA (1977). Phosphoglycolate phosphatase in human
  erythrocytes. J Biol Chem 252:2441.
Beutler E, Guinto E (1973). The effect of 2,3-DPG on red
  cell phosphofructokinase. FEBS Lett 37:21.
Boivin P, Galand C, Demartial MC (1972). Études sur la py-
  ruvate kinase erythrocytaire I-quelques propriétés de
  l'enzyme humaine normale. Path Biol 20:583.
Brewer GJ, Oelshlegel FJ, Moore LG, Noble NA (1974). In
  vivo red cell glycolytic control and DPG-ATP levels.
  Ann NY Acad Sci 241(o):513.
Brewer GJ (1972). In Rörth M and Astrup P (eds):"Alfred
  Benzon Symposium, Oxygen Affinity, Hemoglobin, Red Cell
  Acid-Base Status" Munksgaard, Copenhagen, p 609-610.
Brewer GJ (1969).Erythrocyte metabolism and function:
  hexokinase inhibition by 2,3-DPG and interaction with
  ATP and Mg^{+2}. Biochim Biophys Acta 192:157.
Cartier P, Najman A, Leroux JP, Temkine H (1968). Les
  anomalies de la glycolyse au cours de l'anemie hemoly-
  tique par deficit du globule rouge en pyruvate kinase.
  Clin Chim Acta 22:165.
Campos JO, Koler RD, Bigley RH (1965). Kinetic differences
  between human red cell and leukocyte pyruvate kinase.
  Nature 208:194.

Delivoria-Papadopoulos M, Oski FA, Gottlieb AJ (1969).
  Oxygen-Hemoglobin dissociation curves: Effect of
  inherited enzyme defects of the red cell. Science 165:
  601.
Dische Z (1941).Bull Soc Chim Biol 23:1140.
Eaton JW, Brewer GJ (1968).The relationship between red
  cell 2,3-DPG and the levels of hemoglobin in the human.
  Proc Natl Acad Sci USA 61:756.
Ekman P, Dahlquist U, Humble E, Engström L (1976). Compara-
  tive kinetic studies on the L-type pyruvate kinase from
  rat liver and the enzyme phosphorylated by c-AMP stimu-
  lated protein kinase. Biochim Biophys Acta 429:374.
Engström L, Berglund L, Bergström G, Hjelmquist G,
  Ljungstrom O (1974). in Richter D (ed): Lipmann Symposium,
  Energy, Biosynthesis and Regulation in Molecular Biology.
  New York: Walter de Gruyter Inc, p 192.
Frieden C (1970). Kinetic aspects of regulation of metabolic
  processes: The hysteretic enzyme concept. J Biol Chem
  245:5788.
Hamasaki N, Asakura T, Minakami S (1970). Effect of oxygen
  tension on glycolysis in human erythrocytes. J Biochem
  (Tokyo) 68:157.
Hamasaki N, Rose ZB (1974). The binding of phosphorylated
  red cell metabolites to human hemoglobin A. J Biol Chem
  249:7896.
Hatfield GW, Ray WJ, Umbarger HE (1970). Threonine deaminase
  from B subtilis: Pre-steady state kinetic properties.
  J Biol Chem 245:1748.
Ibsen KH, Schiller KW, Venn-Watson EA (1968). Stabilization,
  partial purification, and effects of activating cations,
  ADP and P-enolpyruvate on the reaction rates of an erythrocyte pyruvate kinase. Arch Biochem Biophys 128:583.
Ibsen KH, Schiller KW, Haas TA (1971). Interconvertible
  kinetic and physical forms of human erythrocyte pyruvate
  kinate. J Biol Chem 246:1233.
Kahn A, Marie J, Galand C, Boivin P (1975). Molecular
  mechanisms of pyruvate kinase deficiency. Humangenetik
  29:271.
Koler RD, Vanbellinghen P (1968). The mechanism of precursor
  modulation of human erythrocyte pyruvate kinase I by
  fructose diphosphate. Adv Enzyme Regul 6:127.
Kayne FJ (1974). Pyruvate kinase catalyzed phosphorylation
  of glycolate. Biochem Biophys Res Commun 59:8.
Leblond DJ, Robinson JL (1976). Secondary kinase reactions
  catalyzed by yeast pyruvate kinase. Biochim Biophys Acta
  438:108.

Ljungström O, Hjelmquist G, Engström L (1974). Phosphoryla-
lation of purified rat liver pyruvate kinase by c-AMP-
stimulated protein kinase. Biochim Biophys Acta 358:289.
Marie J, Ganeau H, Kahn A (1977). Evidence for a post-syn-
thetic transformation of human erythrocyte pyruvate
kinase into L-type enzyme. FEBS lett 78:91.
Munro GF, Miller DR (1970). Mechanism of fructose diphosphate activation of a mutant pyruvate kinase from human
red cells. Biochim Biophys Acta 206:87.
Nathan DG, Oski FA, Sidell VW, Diamond LK (1965). Extreme
hemolysis and red cell distortion in erythrocyte pyruvate
kinate deficiency. New Eng J. Med 272:118.
Paglia DE, Valentine WN, Baughan MA, Miller DR, Reed CF,
McIntyre OR (1968). An inherited molecular lesion of
erythrocyte pyruvate kinase. J Clin Invest 47:1929.
Paglia DE, Valentine WN (1970). Evidence for molecular
alteration of pyruvate kinase as a consequence of eryth-
rocyte aging. J Lab Clin Med 76:202.
Ponce J, Roth S, Harkness DR (1971). Kinetic studies on the
inhibition of glycolytic kinases of human erythrocytes by
2,3-P_2-glycerate. Biochim Biophys Acta 250:63.
Rodan SB, Rodan GA, Sha'afi RI (1976). Demonstration of
adenylate cyclase activity in red cell ghosts. Biochim
Biophys Acta 428:509.
Rörth M, BilleBrahe NE (1972) in Rörth N & Astrup P (eds)
Alfred Benzon Symp. IV. Oxygen Affinity, Hemoglobin, and
Red Cell Acid Base Status, Munksgaard, Copenhagen,
p. 692–695.
Rose ZB, Liebowitz J (1970). 2,3-Diphosphoglycerate phos-
phatase from human erythrocytes. J Biol Chem 245:3332.
Rose ZB (1976). A procedure for decreasing the level of
2,3-P_2-glycerate in red cells in vitro. Biochim Biophys
Res Commun 73:1011.
Rose IA, Warms JVB (1970). Control of red cell glycolysis.
J Biol Chem 245:4009.
Rose IA (1971). Regulation of human red cell glycolysis:
A review. Exp Eye Res 118:264.
Rose IA, Warms JVB (1974). Glucose- and Mannose-1,6-P_2 as
activators of phosphofructokinase in red blood cells.
Biochem Biophys Res Commun 59:1333.
Rubin SR, Erlichman J, Rosen OM (1972). c-AMP-dependent
protein kinase of human erythrocyte membranes. J Biol
Chem 247:6135.
Sacco C, Westhead EW (1978). To be published.

Spivey HO, Flory W, Peazon BD, Chandler JP, Koeppe RE
(1974). Kinetics of the activation of rat liver pyruvate
kinase by FDP and methods for characterizing hysteretic
transitions. Biochem J 141:119.
Staal GEJ, Koster JF, Hamp H, Van Milligen-Boersma L,
Veeger C (1971). Human erythrocyte pyruvate kinase, its
purification and some properties. Biochim Biophys Acta
227:86.
Staal GEJ, Koster JF, Nijessen JG (1972). A new variant of
red blood cell pyruvate kinase deficiency. Biochim
Biophys Acta 248:685.
Staal GEJ, Van Berkel ThJC, Nijessen JG, Koster JF,
Van Der Loo A (1975). Normalization of red blood cell
pyruvate kinase in pyruvate kinase deficiency of ribo-
flavin treatment. Clinica Chim Acta 60:323.
Tajiri M (1976). Glutathione reductase deficiency of red
cells in aplastic anemia. Acta Haem Jap 39:263.
Van Berkel ThJC, Koster JF, Staal GEJ (1973). On the molecular basis of pyruvate kinase deficiency. I primary defect
or consequence of increased glutathione disulfide concentration. Biochim Biophys Acta 321:496.
Van Berkel ThJC, Staal GEJ, Koster JF, Nijessen JG (1974).
On the molecular basis of pyruvate kinase deficiency.
II Role of thiol groups in pyruvate kinase from pyruvate
kinase deficient patients. Biochim Biophys Acta 334:361.
Zuelzer WW, Robinson AR, Hsu TH (1968). Erythrocyte pyruvate
kinase deficiency in nonspherocytic hemolytic anemia: A
system of multiple genetic markers. Blood 32:33.

DISCUSSION

Dr. Duhm: I would like to remind you of the reports in which it was claimed that propranolol induces a dramatic increase of the P_{50} and increase of the 2,3-DPG content in human erythrocytes. All these observations have been shown to be an artifact induced by the Ca^{++}-dependent action of the drug on the K^+ **leak** and the resulting intracellular acidification and cell shrinkage. Your 2,3-DPG levels are given in μmoles/ml **cells**. Have the values been corrected for a constant dry weight and hemoglobin content to avoid artifactual results resulting from cell shrinkage? What was the composition of your incubation media and did they contain Ca^{++}?

Dr. Westhead: We have looked at hemoglobin content and found that it was consistent with the cell volume. The red cell volume was determined in the initial incubation mixture and then we took aliquots of the cells so presumably whatever the **size** of the cell volume we had the same number of cells in each sample with time. Do you see what I am saying? We took aliquots of the incubation mixture and measured the total concentration in whatever cells were in that aliquot.

Dr. Duhm: In the formation of 2,3-DPG from glucose one molecule NAD is converted to NADH in the GAPDH reaction for each 2,3-DPG molecule to be synthesized. Do you have any idea concerning the origin of the oxidizing equivalents that are necessary to reoxidize the NADH generated in order to promote a continued 2,3-DPG synthesis? To my knowledge it is not possible to increase the red cell 2,3-DPG content by more than about 1 μmole/ml cells in vitro without adding a substrate to the suspensions promoting oxidation of NADH (or NADPH). Did your media contain added pyruvate?

Dr. Westhead: I hadn't really thought **about** that. We do know that we have to buffer the solution and watch it very carefully. The pH tends to drop in the incubation mixture. We have been using very high concentrations of phosphate which some people have previously used.

Dr. Schoomaker: I am not familiar with the rates of these enzymes but in the normal human with a normal cardiac output the red cells remaining in a deoxygenated state for only 20 or 30 seconds at a time. Is that really an adequate length of time for PK to make major changes in the level of intermediates in the red cell.

The Red Cell, pages 315—317

Dr. Westhead: Rose and one of his co-workers have looked at
the problem of cyclic variance in glycolytic intermediates.
The limiting step, I think, would be the PK step. Flux
is slow and capacity can be increased ten fold under certain
conditions. It would require substantial increase in that
rate to make this scheme plausible.

Dr. Schoomaker: I can understand that if you deoxygenate
patients' blood or put them in a hypoxic state over a long
period of time that hysteresis may serve to change the intermediate levels and would allow better tissue oxygenation.
I do not see that in the brief period of time represented
by in vivo deoxygenation/oxygenation, cyclic variations in
PK activity are going to make that big a difference in the
intermediate levels.

Dr. Westhead: Changes in the levels of venous to arterial
blood have been measured. I believe those results have been
questioned by some other workers. Let me postulate that if
this is a factor, it would fit with the circulation time for
the time constant we see for the conversion of the enzyme
from the less active to the more active form in the order
of a minute, which is close to the time of resting circulation.

Dr. Black: I appreciate your concern over the complicated
nature of the allosteric kinetics. You mentioned the varied
reports on the kinetics with respect to phosphoenol pyruvate
and I should point out, that, the kinetics with respect to
phosphoenol pyruvate do in fact depend on the concentration
of ADP. So in other words, the concentration of the second
substrate is connected to the response you get from the first.
For instance, at high ADP concentrations, you get sigmoidal
kinetics, at low ADP concentration you get curves that approximate to Michaelis-Menton kinetics. Also, at low phosphoenol
pyruvate concentrations as you vary ADP you see negative cooperativity. Taking these complicated relationships into account
it is extremely difficult to determine the actual situation in
vivo.

Dr. Westhead: I certainly agree with the import of your remarks.
But we have found under identical conditions of substrate concentrations that the red cell PK of different workers in the
laboratory, that from one time period to another, the kinetics
of the enzyme seem to change. Have you ever seen anything
like that?

<u>Dr. Black</u>: Unfortunately, yes.

<u>Dr. Brewer</u>: I was quite interested in your results as to the
stimulating effect of catecholamines. The work that Gilroy
and I have published most recently was in the rhesus monkey.
We injected epinephrine and observed an increase in ATP
and glycolytic intermediates of the early part of the pathway.
We did not study these monkeys for an extended period of
time, and we saw no increase in DPG. The DPG increase may
be a late effect, as you have described.

<u>Dr. Westhead</u>: That would be an interesting question. So it
could be manifest first in ATP? Certainly ought to look
at that, thank you.

<u>Dr. Paglia</u>: I just want to raise one point in response to
John's and your comments about the kinetic variability.
I really must say that I have been kind of impressed with
the apparent reproducibility of K_m determinations using
crude hemolysates since we first started doing them over a
decade ago. I don't know the explanation for variability,
but it should be recognized that you can change the kinetics
with very subtle differences in the assay system. Whether
they be in the presence of activators (such as FDP) or the
cation concentrations or the buffer you use or slight variation in the pH. PH may really be the explanation for a lot
of this because you can shift from hyperbolic to allosteric
kinetics just by going across pH 7.5 plus or minus a tad.
So I think pH might be one of the tight things to control to
retain K_m reproducibility.

<u>Dr. Westhead</u>: When we have been in a state of deep bafflemant
about changes in reproducibility , when we have found situations like that we have looked over a pH range, I think it
would be hard to find something we have not looked at.

<u>Dr. Paglia</u>: I am just wondering if all the mutant variants
with abnormal kinetics that we have been reporting simply
reflect irreproducibility?

CONTROL OF RED BLOOD CELL ADENINE
NUCLEOTIDE METABOLISM
STUDIES OF ADENOSINE DEAMINASE

Donald E. Paglia, M.D., William N. Valentine, M.D.
Anthony P. Tartaglia, M.D., Florinda Gilsanz, M.D.
and Robert S. Sparkes, M.D.
Division of Surgical Pathology and the Department
of Medicine, University of California Center for
Health Sciences, Los Angeles, CA 90024, and St.
Peter's Hospital, Albany, N.Y. 12208

It is well established in the lore of hematology that
the mature human erythrocyte is a glycolytically dependent
creature. Like the proverbial child in a candy store, it has
a strong affinity for sugar, and, indeed, its very survival
depends upon a continuously available source of glucose. This
is amply demonstrated by the deleterious effects of the numerous and diverse, hereditary defects of glycolytic enzymes
which have now been defined. These erythroenzymopathies, when
sufficiently severe, impair the generation of essential high-
energy compounds to a degree incompatible with the functional
integrity of the cells, and premature hemolysis results.

It would be an oversimplification, however, to suggest
that erythrocytes are solely or totally dependent upon glucose to maintain an adequately balanced intracellular pool
of high-energy compounds, such as adenosine triphosphate
(ATP). While functional glycolytic mechanisms are necessary
for normal cell longevity, recent observations of other
"experiments of Nature" indicate that certain non-glycolytic
pathways may be equally important. These involve nucleotide
metabolism per se, rather than reactions such as those of
glycolysis that are designed simply to generate energy for
storage in the cells' adenine nucleotide pool.

Intensive investigations into the metabolism of erythrocyte nucleotides was stimulated by the exigencies of blood
banking. In the mid 1950's, it was observed that when blood
was stored in the presence of adenosine or inosine there was
considerable retardation of the usual progressive loss of
intracellular organic phosphates, principally ATP and 2,3-

The Red Cell, pages 319—335

diphosphoglycerate, and that post-transfusion viability of
the stored erythrocytes was substantially improved (reviewed
by Bartlett, 1974). Initially, it was presumed that both of
these nucleosides acted by priming glycolysis (Gabrio and
Huennekens, 1955; Donohue et al., 1956; Gabrio et al., 1956),
since red cells are readily capable of deaminating adenosine
to inosine, cleaving ribose-1-phosphate from the purine base,
and mutating it to ribose-5-phosphate, which can then be catab-
olized through the Embden-Meyerhof pathway via transketolase
and transaldolase (Lowy et al., 1958). Several studies, however, indicated that this too was an oversimplication, since
under certain conditions adenosine was considerably more
effective than inosine in regenerating the ATP of stored blood
(Overgaard-Hansen et al., 1957; Molison and Robinson, 1959;
Shafer and Bartlett, 1962). This enhanced effect eventually
was attributable to direct phosphorylation of adenosine to
AMP via adenosine kinase (Lowy and Williams, 1966; Lerner and
Rubinstein, 1970), an enzyme with less activity than adenosine
deaminase in human erythrocytes, but with greater substrate
affinity (vide infra), so that successful competition for
available adenosine was theoretically possible.

But these were contrived in vitro conditions, and the
possible physiologic significance of adenosine kinase and
deaminase activities in the circulating erythrocyte remained
a subject for speculation. Nonetheless, several groups of
investigators (Meyskens and Williams, 1971; Schrader et al.,
1972; Parks and Brown, 1973; McManus and Lambe, 1973; Snyder
and Henderson, 1973; Lerner and Lowy, 1974) suggested that
the erythrocytes' adenine nucleotide pool might be maintained,
at least in part, by kinase-mediated phosphorylation of endogenous plasma adenosine directly to AMP. Recently we have
had an opportunity to study a unique hereditary erythrocyte
anomally that provides an insight into this interesting and
physiologically important question. Those studies, portions
of which have been reported previously (Paglia et al., 1970;
Paglia et al., 1976; Valentine et al., 1977), constitute the
subject of this report.

CLINICAL SUMMARY

This most unusual "experiment of Nature" occurred in a
New York family of English-Irish ancestry. Half of 24 relatives at risk in three generations were affected, both male
and female, and all the observed defects were transmitted
in a dominant fashion (Figure 1). Signs of a mild, chronic

hemolytic anemia were first detected in the proband in 1968
when he was a young adult in military service (Table 1).
Anemia was so well compensated in the other affected family
members that only one had any known history of a hematologic
abnormality. There was no evidence of unstable or otherwise
abnormal hemoglobin, ovalo- or spherocytosis, paroxysmal
nocturnal hemoglobinuria, antiglobulin reactions, or deficiencies in glucose-6-phosphate dehydrogenase or pyruvate
kinase activities. An abnormal autohemolysis test was noted
on several occasions, however, with only partial correction
by added glucose.

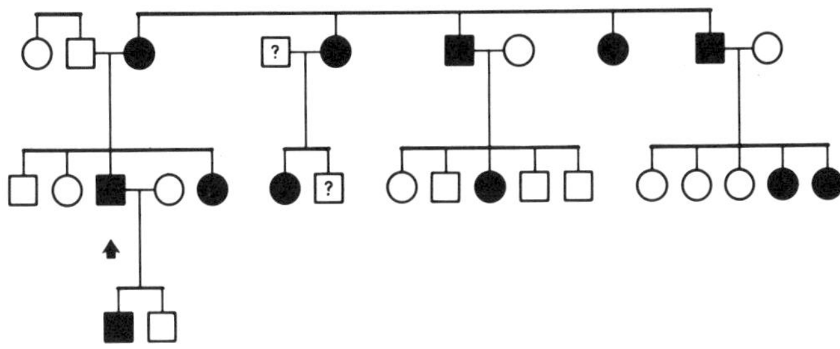

Figure 1. Genealogy of Kindred L.

    An intrinsic erythrocyte defect was subsequently demon-
strated by cross transfusion of chromium labeled cells between the proband and his normal father. Initial studies
in 1970 demonstrated no defects in the enzymes of anaerobic
glycolysis, the hexose monophosphate shunt or glutathione
metabolism nor any abnormal intracellular accumulations of
glycolytic intermediates. Cellular sodium, potassium and
glutathione concentrations were also normal.

Table 1. Mean Proband Values (1970-1976)

Hemoglobin:	12.9 g/dl
Erythrocyte count	$3.95 \times 10^6/\lambda$
Packed cell volume:	37%
Reticulocytes:	11.7% (maximum 21.5%)
Indirect bilirubin	2.7 mg/dl
Haptoglobin	< 50 mg/dl
Cr^{51} survival:	6 days
Autohemolysis:	14% (+ Glucose = 10%)

METHODS & RESULTS

When adenosine phosphates were assayed in neutralized
perchloric acid extracts of venous blood by enzymatic methods
(Minakami et al., 1965), significant reductions below normal
values were obtained in certain family members who also had
mild chronic hemolysis as evidenced by reticulocytosis and/or
lowered erythrocyte values (Table 2). Nucleotide concentrations, summarized in Table 3, ranged from about 25% to 50%
of appropriate control values, taking into account the increased concentrations that normally occur in specimens with
reticulocytosis and younger mean cell ages.

Markedly decreased red cell ATP is known to accompany
certain hemoglobinopathies, but there were no such abnormalities detectable by standard screening tests. Additionally,
Drs. Helen Ranney of the University of California San Diego
and Hermann Lehmann of the University of Cambridge intensively
investigated samples from the proband to rule out the existence of an obscure hemoglobinopathy.

A number of erythrocyte enzymes concerned with nucleotide interconversions, salvage and degradation were assayed
in affected erythrocytes in an attempt to explain the marked
ATP reductions. These included the following, assayed accord-

ing to the cited references: ATPase (Brewer et al., 1968),
adenylate kinase (Halsam and Mills, 1967), adenylate deaminase
(Chaney and Marbach, 1962, as modified by Valentine et al.,
1977), adenosine kinase (Valentine et al., 1977), nucleoside
phosphorylase (Bergmeyer, 1974), ribosephosphate pyrophosphokinase (Valentine and Kurschner, 1972), adenine phosphoribosyl
transferase (Valentine and Kurschner, 1972), phosphatases
(Valentine and Beck, 1951), and nucleoside monophosphate and
diphosphate kinases (Valentine et al., 1974). None was detect-
ably defective.

During the course of these investigations, we discovered
that a nucleotidase existed in normal erythrocytes (Valentine
et al., 1974; Paglia and Valentine, 1975) which differed from
those in other tissues in that it was highly substrate specific
and catalyzed only the dephosphorylation of pyrimidine nucleotides, principally the 5'-analogs:

$$UMP + H_2O \xrightarrow[\text{Nucleotidase}]{\text{Pyrimidine}} Uridine + P_i$$

Cytidine and thymidine monophosphates are somewhat less
effective substrates than uridine, but purine analogs such
as AMP are not hydrolyzed at all.

Table 2. Mean Hematologic Measurements in Kindred L.

Subjects: Number:	Affected 12	Unaffected 12
Erythrocytes ($\times 10^6/\lambda$)	4.18	5.00
Hemoglobin (g/dl)	13.1	13.4
Packed Cell Volume (%)	38.4	40.2
Reticulocytes (%)	6.4	1.2

Table 3. Mean Adenine Nucleotide Concentrations
in Erythrocytes from Kindred L.

Subjects	Number	ATP	ADP	AMP	Total Adenine Nucleotides
		\(m\mu moles/10^{10}\) erythrocytes)			
Affected	12	0.65	0.20	0.03	0.88
Unaffected	12	1.02	0.32	0.05	1.37
Shipped controls	5	1.08	0.28	0.04	1.40
Local controls	22	1.14	0.24	0.05	1.43
High reticulocyte controls (retics = 2.3-22.3% mean = 7.8%)	15	1.39	0.48	0.07	1.94

When assayed as previously described (Valentine et al., 1974; Paglia and Valentine, 1975), pyrimidine nucleotidase activities in affected individuals were prominently elevated and were, in fact, the highest values for this enzyme ever recorded in our laboratory (Table 4). Otherwise the enzyme was in no way demonstrably different from the nucleotidase in normal erythrocytes. Despite its hyperactivity, it could not be shown to dephosphorylate AMP under a variety of conditions and therefore did not appear to constitute an abnormal drain on the cells' adenine nucleotide pool.

The activity of another enzyme, adenosine deaminase, which catalyzes the irreversible deamination of adenosine to inosine, was found to be even more profoundly elevated, whether assayed spectrophotometrically (Beutler, 1975) or by a modification of a technique based on the quantitative measurement of ammonia evolution (Chaney and Marback, 1962) (Table 5). Activity increases of this magnitude, 50- to more than 70-fold, are unprecedented in human erythrocytes, but are reminiscent of the elevations in a similar enzyme (nucleoside deaminase) found in certain genetically anemic mice or in other strains of mice as a result of stress-induced erythropoiesis (Rothman

Table 4. Erythrocyte Pyrimidine Nucleotidase Activities

Subjects	Number	Pyrimidine Nucleotidase (units)[a]	
		Mean	Range
Affected Relatives	10	30.7[b]	18.4 - 40.5
Unaffected Relatives	9	11.1[b]	7.0 - 15.5
Normal controls		8.0 (SD = 1.9)	4.2 - 11.8[c]
Controls with 3-36% reticulocytosis	24	15.0 (SD = 6.5)	2.0 - 28.0[c]

[a] Micromoles of inorganic phosphate liberated per hour per gram hemoglobin at 37°.

[b] Means include all values derived from 2, 6, or 14 determinations performed on each individual.

[c] Range equivalent to mean $\pm$ 2 standard deviations.

Table 5. Erythrocyte Adenosine Deaminase Activities

Subjects	Number	Adenosine Deaminase (units)[a]	
		Mean	Range
Affected Relatives	10	61.3[b]	45.4 - 73.5
Unaffected Relatives	10	0.9[b]	0.6 - 1.5
Normal controls		1.1 (S.D. = 0.52)	0.1 - 2.1[c]
Controls with 4-37% reticulocytosis (mean = 17.5%)	10	1.0	0.6 - 1.4

[a] Micromoles of substrate utilized per minute per gram hemoglobin at 37°.

[b] Means include all values derived from 2 to 6 determinations on each sample.

[c] Range equivalent to mean $\pm$ 2 standard deviations.

et al., 1970; Harrison et al., 1975).

The adenosine deaminase in affected subjects could not be shown to differ from normal in any other way. There were no apparent kinetic or electrophoretic abnormalities accompanying this altered activity, and all of the nine affected individuals thus far tested have exhibited the common ADA 1-1 phenotype (Spencer et al., 1968).

Proband enzyme was purified to homogeneity by affinity chromatography (Rossi et al., 1975) by Dr. William Osborne of the University of Washington, Seattle, and he found no distinction between it and the purified wild enzyme on the basis of starch gel electrophoresis, heat stability, kinetics for adenosine and for guanylurea inhibition, and, most importantly, specific activity. The pronounced hyperactivity therefore seemed ascribable only to an overproduction of normal enzyme protein in the erythrocyte precursors. There has been no demonstrable increase in adenosine deaminase activity in granulated leukocytes or lymphocytes separated by Ficoll-Hypaque discontinuous density gradient fractionation, nor in cultured skin fibroblasts.

DISCUSSION

To summarize briefly, this family harbored an intrinsic erythrocyte defect that was manifested as a mild chronic, non-spherocytic, hemolytic anemia, dominantly transmitted through three generations. The abnormality could not be attributed to any known cause, including hemoglobinopathies, spherocytosis, or established erythroenzymopathies. The only distinct biochemical abnormalities demonstrable were (a) reduction of erythrocyte ATP and total adenine nucleotide concentrations to below 50% of appropriate controls, (b) three- to four-fold increases in activity of red cell pyrimidine nucleotidase, and (c) pronounced hyperactivity of erythrocyte adenosine deaminase. This combination of abnormalities was found in all affected family members, even though most of them had subclinical, well-compensated, chronic hemolysis detectable only by reticulocyte counts and other appropriate laboratory studies. None of these biochemical alterations was evident in unaffected relatives.

Since normal erythrocyte viability is dependent upon sufficient ATP, it is not surprising that cells with less than half normal concentrations have severely shortened lifespans. Inadequate ATP generation presumably causes the premature lysis of cells with any of a number of glycolytic enzyme defects, since mature erythrocytes are incapable of de novo nucleotide synthesis from small precursor molecules.

But the precise cause of reduced adenine nucleotide concentrations remains obscure, and a critical question raised by these studies is whether or not they could be a consequence of the observed enzyme abnormalities, even though the latter were represented not by functional deficiency, but rather by pronounced hyperactivity.

Increased nucleotidase activity could account for reduced adenine nucleotides if the enzyme had been genetically altered so that it had lost its specificity for pyrimidine substrates and therefore could effectively dephosphorylate AMP as well. Even individuals heterozygous for such a mutant isozyme could be affected, thus accounting for the dominant transmission. However, no deviation from the characteristics of the wild enzyme could be demonstrated, and AMP was not degraded by proband nucleotidase under widely varied in vitro conditions.

Hyperactive adenosine deaminase, on the other hand, might account for reduced adenine nucleotide concentrations if the competing reaction mediated by adenosine kinase was physiologically significant in terms of normal nucleotide salvage. Consider the reactions diagramed in Figure 2. The erythrocyte is capable of either incorporating adenosine directly into the adenine nucleotide pool via adenosine kinase (Lowy and Williams, 1966; Ho et al., 1968; Lerner and Rubinstein, 1970; Parker, 1970; Parks and Brown, 1973) or of deaminating it to inosine (Conway and Cooke, 1939; Rubinstein and Denstedt, 1956). In the latter instance, the purine moiety is irretrievably lost, since mechanisms do not exist to divert any of the resultant purine products back into the adenine nucleotide pool (Bishop, 1960; Lowy et al., 1962; Lowy and Williams, 1966).

Under certain conditions adenosine may be preferentially deaminated because the deaminase is considerably more active than the kinase (Parks and Brown, 1973) and also because this enzyme is probably in close physical association with the membrane components responsible for facilitated transport of adenosine (Agarwal and Parks, 1975). At very low adenosine concentrations, however, phosphorylation may predominate because the kinase has a much greater substrate affinity relative to the deaminase: K_m (adenosine) is about 1 μM

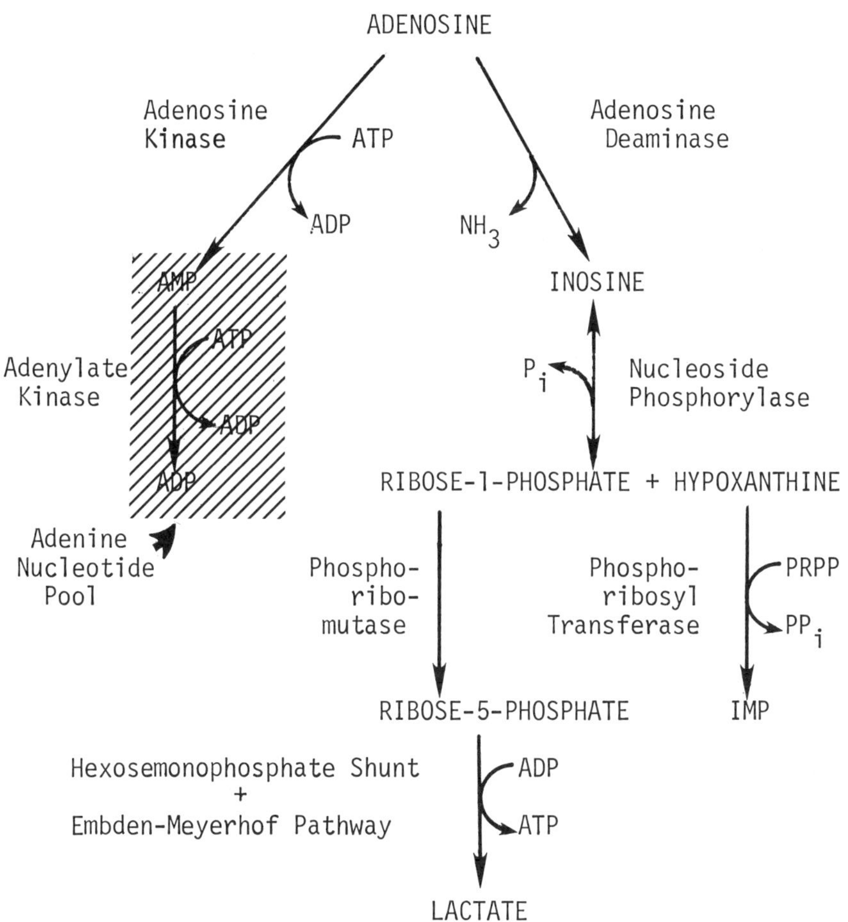

Figure 2. Pathways of Adenosine Utilization in Human Red Cells

(Agarwal et al., 1975) to 2 μM (Meyskens and Williams, 1971)
for adenosine kinase, but values of 15 μM (Agarwal et al., 1973),
25 μM (Agarwal et al., 1975), 30 μM (Osborne and Spencer, 1973;
Siegenbeek van Heukelom, et al., 1976), 40 μM (Meyskens and
Williams, 1971), and 52 μM (Daddona and Kelley, 1977) have been
reported for adenosine deaminase.

It would follow then, that hyperactive adenosine deaminase
could account for reduced concentrations of cellular ATP if the
adenosine kinase pathway was normally necessary for replenishing and maintaining the constancy of the adenine nucleotide
pool by generating AMP. As noted in the introduction, several
groups of investigators have suggested such a possibility, and
the observations in this family study strongly support such an
hypothesis. Deaminase activity in these cells was increased
almost two orders of magnitude, perhaps even more in sub-
populations, and could compete very effectively for ambiently
available adenosine, despite the greater substrate affinity
of adenosine kinase. Deprived of the normal kinase-mediated
salvage pathway, then, the defective cells might not be able
to compensate for random nucleotide losses, for example via
AMP deamination or nonspecific dephosphorylation, and low
concentrations of adenine nucleotides would result.

There is further inferential evidence in support of this
hypothesis. Red cell alterations which are the converse of
those in the present study have been observed in another genetically induced disorder, severe combined immunodeficiency
disease. Certain cases of this syndrome are associated with
absent adenosine deaminase activity, and these exhibit markedly
increased concentrations of cellular ATP and total adenine
nucleotides (Goldblum et al., 1976; Schmalstieg et al,
1976a, 1976b). In this disorder, the absence of deaminase
activity apparently allows an inordinate amount of adenosine
to be converted to AMP (Agarwal et al., 1976), and the cell's
nucleotide pool is expanded. Conversely, in the present cases,
hyperactive adenosine deaminase apparently overwhelms the alternate replenishing pathway, and adenine nucleotide concentrations
fall, presumably to levels incompatible with cell energy needs,
inducing hemolysis. The biochemical abnormalities in these two
distinct genetic anomalies strongly suggest that availability
of adenosine, and a balanced competition for it between adenosine kinase and deaminase, are necessary for the normal maintenance of the adenine nucleotide pool.

These observed consequences of a genetically induced derangement in red cell metabolism provide some interesting insights into normal cellular function, but they also leave many equally interesting questions unanswered. We have speculated previously on possible mechanisms underlying the elevated adenosine deaminase activities in this family (Valentine et al., 1977), but the precise cause remains to be resolved. It is also difficult to account for the apparent restriction of the abnormality to the erythrocyte population. In immunodeficient patients with defective adenosine deaminase, the deficiency is evident in numerous different tissues (Hirschhorn et al., 1973; Chen et al., 1975), yet there was no apparent deaminase abnormality in lymphocytes, granulocytes or fibroblasts from affected individuals in this kindred, and the hyperactive erythrocyte enzyme itself was indistinguishable from normal. While the precise molecular lesion remains un-defined, it might well reside in those genetic control mechan-isms that govern the production of specific enzyme proteins in developing erythroid precursors.

ACKNOWLEDGEMENTS

These studies were supported in part by a grant (HE-12944) from the National Institutes of Health. The authors are grate-ful to J. Brown, R. Brockway, A. Eldatear, S. Gordon and E. Guerque for technical contributions, and to M. Flores for assistance with the manuscript.

REFERENCES

Agarwal RP, Parks RE Jr (1975). A possible association between the nucleoside transport system of human erythrocytes and adenosine deaminase. Biochem Pharmacol 24:547.
Agarwal RP, Sagar SM, Parks RE Jr (1973). Effects of adeno-sine analogs on human erythrocytic adenosine deaminase. Fed Proc 32:512.
Agarwal RP, Sagar SM, Parks RE Jr (1975). Adenosine deami-nase from human erythrocytes. Biochem Pharmacol 24:693.
Agarwal RP, Crabtree GW, Parks RE Jr, Nelson JA, Keightley R, Parkman R, Rosen FS, Stern RC, and Polmar SH (1976). Purine nucleoside metabolism in the erythrocytes of patients with adenosine deaminase deficiency and severe combined immunodeficiency. J Clin Invest 57:1025.

Bartlett GR (1974). Red cell metabolism: Review highlighting changes during storage. "The Human Red Cell In Vitro." Greenwalt TJ, Jamieson GA (eds). New York: Grune and Stratton, p 5.

Bergmeyer HU (1974). "Methods of Enzymatic Analysis." New York: Academic Press, vol 1, p 490.

Beutler E (1975). "A Manual of Biochemical Methods." New York: Grune and Stratton, p 85.

Bishop C (1960). Purine metabolism in human and chicken blood, in vitro. J Biol Chem 235:3228.

Brewer GJ, Eaton JW, Beck CC, Feitler L, Shreffler DC (1968). Sodium-potassium stimulated ATPase activity of mammalian hemolysates: Clinical observations and dominance of ATPase deficiency in the potassium polymorphism of sheep. J Lab Clin Med 71:744.

Chaney AL, Marbach EP (1962). Modified reagents for determination of urea and ammonia. Clin Chem 8:130.

Chen SH, Scott CR, Swedberg KR (1975). Heterogeneity for adenosine deaminase deficiency: Expression of the enzyme in cultured skin fibroblasts and amniotic fluid cells. Am J Hum Genet 27:46.

Conway EJ, Cooke R (1939). The deaminases of adenosine and adenylic acid in blood and tissues. Biochem J 33:479.

Daddona PE, Kelley WN (1977). Human adenosine deaminase. Purification and subunit structure. J Biol Chem 252:110.

Donohue DM, Finch CA, Gabrio BW (1956). Erythrocyte preservation. VI. The storage of blood with purine nucleosides. J Clin Invest 35:562.

Gabrio BW, Finch CA, Huennekens FM (1956). Erythrocyte preservation: A topic in molecular biochemistry. Blood 11:103.

Gabrio BW, Huennekens FM (1955). Nucleoside metabolism of stored erythrocyte. Fed Proc 14:217.

Goldblum RM, Schmalstieg FC, Nelson A, Monahan T, Mills G (1976). Elevated levels of lymphocyte adenine nucleotides in adenosine deaminase deficiency. Clin Res 24:68A.

Halsam RJ, Mills DCB (1967). The adenylate kinase of human plasma, erythrocytes and platelets in relation to the degradation of adenosine diphosphate in plasma. Biochem J 103:773.

Harrison DE, Malathi VG, Silber R (1975). Elevated erythrocyte nucleoside deaminase levels in genetically anemic W/W^v and Sl/Sl^d mice. Blood Cells 1:605.

Hirschhorn R, Levytska V, Pollara B, Meuwissen HJ (1973).
  Evidence for control of several different tissue-specific
  isozymes of adenosine deaminase by a single genetic locus.
  Nature (New Biol) 246:200.
Ho DHW, Luce JK, Frie E III (1968). Distribution of purine
  ribonucleoside kinase and selective toxicity of 6-methyl-
  thiopurine ribonucleoside. Biochem Pharmacol 17:1025.
Lerner MH, Lowy BA (1974). The formation of adenosine in
  rabbit liver and its possible role as a direct precursor
  of erythrocyte adenine nucleotides. J Biol Chem 249:959.
Lerner MH, Rubinstein D (1970). The role of adenine and
  adenosine as precursors for adenine nucleotide synthesis
  by fresh and preserved human erythrocytes. Biochim Biophys
  Acta 224:301.
Lowy BA, Jaffé ER, Vanderhoff GA, Crook L, London IM (1958).
  Metabolism of purine nucleosides by the human erythrocyte
  in vitro. J Biol Chem 230:409.
Lowy BA, Williams MK (1966). Studies on the metabolism of
  adenosine and adenine in stored and fresh human erythrocytes.
  Blood 27:623.
Lowy BA, Williams MK, London IM (1962). Enzymatic deficiencies
  of purine nucleotide synthesis in the human erythrocyte.
  J Biol Chem 237:1622.
McManus TJ, Lambe C (1973). Species differences in nucleoside
  metabolism of red cells. "Erythrocytes, Thrombocytes, Leuko-
  cytes. Recent Advances in Membrane and Metabolic Research"
  Gerlach E, Moser K, Deutsch E, Wilmanns W, (eds): Stuttgart:
  Georg Thieme, p 135.
Meyskens FL, Williams HE (1971). Adenosine metabolism in
  human erythrocytes. Biochim Biophys Acta 240:170.
Minakami S, Suzuki C, Saito T, Yoshikawa H (1965). Studies
  on erythrocyte glycolysis. I. Determination of glycolytic
  intermediates in human erythrocytes. J Biochem 58:543.
Mollison PL, Robinson MA (1959). Observations on the effects
  of purine nucleosides on red-cell preservation. Brit J
  Haematol 5:331.
Osborne WRA, Spencer N (1973). Partial purification and properties of the common inherited forms of adenosine deaminase
  from human erythrocytes. Biochem J 133:117.
Overgaard-Hansen K, Jørgensen S, Praetorius E (1957). Rephos-
  phorylation produced by inosine and adenosine of adenosine
  monophosphate and adenosine diphosphate in human erythrocytes.
  Nature 179:152.
Paglia DE, Valentine WN (1975). Characteristics of a pyrimidine-
  specific 5'-nucleotidase in human erythrocytes. J Biol Chem
  250:7973.

Paglia DE, Valentine WN, Tartaglia AP, Gilsanz F (1976). Perturbations in erythrocyte adenine nucleotide metabolism: A dominantly inherited hemolytic disorder with implications regarding normal mechanisms of adenine nucleotide preservation. Blood 48:959.

Paglia DE, Valentine WN, Tartaglia AP, Konrad PN (1970) Adenine nucleotide reductions associated with a dominantly transmitted form of nonspherocytic hemolytic anemia. Blood 36:837.

Parker JC (1970). Metabolism of external adenine nucleotides by human red blood cells. Am J Physiol 218:1568.

Parks RE Jr, Brown PR (1973). Incorporation of nucleosides into the nucleotide pools of human erythrocytes. Adenosine and its analogs. Biochem 12:3294.

Rossi CA, Lucacchini A, Montali U, Ronca G (1975). A general method of purification of adenosine deaminase by affinity chromatography. Int J Pept Protein Res 7:81.

Rothman IK, Zanjani ED, Gordon AS, Silber R (1970). Nucleoside deaminase: An enzymatic marker for stress erythropoiesis in the mouse. J Clin Invest 49:2051.

Rubinstein D, Denstedt OF (1956). The metabolism of the erythrocyte. Canad J Biochem Physiol 34:927.

Schmalstieg FC, Goldman AS, Mills GC, Monahan TM, Nelson JA, Goldblum RM (1976). Nucleotide metabolism in adenosine deaminase deficiency. Ped Res 10:393.

Schmalstieg FC, Mills G, Goldblum RM (1976). Purine and pyrimidine metabolism in adenosine deaminase deficiency. Clin Res 24:69A.

Schrader J, Berne RM, Rubio R (1972). Uptake and metabolism of adenosine by human erythrocyte ghosts. Am J Physiol 223:159.

Shafer AW, Bartlett GR (1962). Phosphorylated carbohydrate intermediates of the human erythrocyte during storage in acid citrate dextrose. III. Effect of incubation at $37^{\circ}C$ with inosine, inosine plus adenine, and adenosine after storage for 6, 10, 14, and 18 weeks. J Clin Invest 41:690.

Siegenbeek van Heukelom LH, Boom A, Bartstra HA, Staal GEJ (1976). Characterization of adenosine deaminase isozymes from normal human erythrocytes. Clin Chim Acta 72:109.

Snyder FF, Henderson JF (1973). Alternative pathways of deoxyadenosine and adenosine metabolism. J Biol Chem 248:5899.

Spencer N, Hopkinson DA, Harris H (1968). Adenosine deaminase polymorphism in man. Ann Hum Genet (London) 32:9.

Valentine WN, Beck WS (1951). Biochemical studies on leucocytes. I. Phosphatase activity in health, leucocytosis, and myelocytic leucemia. J Lab Clin Med 38:39.

Valentine WN, Fink K, Paglia DE, Harris SR, Adams WS (1974).
  Hereditary hemolytic anemia with human erythrocyte pyrimidine 5'-nucleotidase deficiency. J Clin Invest 54:866.
Valentine WN, Kürschner KK (1972). Studies on human erythrocyte
  nucleotide metabolism. I. Nonisotopic methodologies. Blood
  39:666.
Valentine WN, Paglia DE, Tartaglia AP, Gilsanz F (1977). Hereditary hemolytic anemia with increased red cell adenosine
  deaminase (45- to 70-fold) and decreased adenosine triphosphate. Science 195:783.

DISCUSSION

<u>Dr. Smith</u>: Do you get accumulation of any bases or nucleosides?

<u>Dr. Paglia</u>: No, the free bases and nucleosides are freely diffusible. Only the phosphorylated nucleotides remain entrapped within the cell.

<u>Dr. Smith</u>: Have you done anything in vitro with the cell, for instance to see if the ATP level would drop faster than in a normal cell?

<u>Dr. Paglia</u>: Yes. That was one of the first things we attempted after discovering the marked reductions in cellular ATP. In various experiments, we incubated cells with adenosine, inosine and adenine as well as glucose, alone and in various combinations, and we could never demonstrate any significant abnormality in rates of reconstitution of the adenine nucleotide pool or in ATP stability. These people have intact adenosine kinase activity as well as an intact salvage pathway via ribosephosphate pyrophosphokinase and adenine phosphoribosyl transferase. The only enzyme alterations apparent were the two that I indicated, and those of course were not deficient, but hyperactive.

<u>Dr. Mitchell</u>: One of the most convincing demonstrations that this is a regulatory defect would be the demonstration of increased amounts of immunologically reactive enzyme in these cells. I wondered if you'd looked at that?

<u>Dr. Paglia</u>: I believe Bill Osborne has also been working on that aspect, but I don't have anything to report on it yet. One thing I forgot to point out is that decreased ATP concentrations have been reported in association with certain hemoglobinopathies, for example, one that I recall by Cartier. We checked this with routine heat stability and denaturation tests but could find no abnormality. Then Dr. Valentine convinced Dr. Lehmann that he should look at it to rule out an obscure hemoglobin defect, which he graciously did for us. What Dr. Lehmann doesn't know is that we also shipped off a specimen to Dr. Helen Ranney in San Diego to make sure that Dr. Lehmann was being straight with us, so I think we can accept their confirmation that no hemoglobinopathy was present.

The Red Cell, Pages 337—338
© 1978 Alan R. Liss, Inc., New York, New York

Dr. Rosa: Two small questions: First, what is the level of the 2,3,-DPG in your patient's red cells and second, have you measured the activity of the ADA in the young and old red cells in this patient?

Dr. Paglia: Yes. In answer to the first question: We did not find any obvious abnormalities in any of the glycolytic intermediates including 2,3,-DPG. In answer to the second question, we were unable to demonstrate any deviation from normal controls in terms of relative amounts of enzyme in young and old cells separated by buoyant density gradients in bovine serum albumin. The decay rate was the same, the stabilities appeared the same.

Dr. Krivit: Did I understand you to say that the enzyme has been measured and the ATP looked at in the fibroblasts and in the lymphocytes, and just the red cells are involved?

Dr. Paglia: What I said was that the enzyme activity in cultured skin fibroblasts, in granulated leukocytes and in lymphocytes was the same in the proband as it was in the normal controls. There was no hyperactivity of adenosine deaminase in any of those three tissues, only in the erythrocyte population.

Dr. Krivit: Has the ATP level and adenosine deaminase activity been measured in platelets?

Dr. Paglia: No, we have not. We would like to get to that though, because that's also a non-nucleated cell and it would be a very important one to look at. We have the problem, of course, of dealing with specimens that are being shipped from Albany, New York, and getting adequate separations on shipped specimens has been kind of a problem.

Dr. Harkness: Next time you have a vacancy in your lab, you might try to hire one of the family members.

ASSOCIATION OF GENETICALLY DETERMINED RED CELL
2,3 DIPHOSPHOGLYCERATE LEVELS WITH BETA GLOBIN
POLYMORPHISM IN LONG-EVANS HOODED RATS

George J. Brewer, Nancy A. Noble, John G. Gilman,
Virginia L. Crews, and Walter C. Kruckeberg
Departments of Human Genetics and Internal
Medicine, University of Michigan Medical School
Ann Arbor, Michigan   48109

INTRODUCTION

It is well established that 2,3-diphosphoglycerate (DPG)
and hemoglobin are functionally related. The oxygen affinity
of hemoglobin of many mammalian species including man, rat,
and mouse is largely determined and also finely tuned by
levels of DPG.

Our interests in the quantitative genetics of DPG levels
stem from an interest in possible genetic effects on oxygenation in mammalian organisms. Oxygenation is a very basic
process, vital to mammals, yet there is considerable variability in the levels of DPG within populations of man, rat,
and mouse, and this DPG variability presumably results in
variability in oxygenation. Specifically, we are interested
in the following questions:

1). Are levels of DPG partly inherited in various
     mammalian species?

2). Does genetically determined variation in red cell
     glycolysis, since DPG is a product of glycolysis,
     account for some of the DPG and oxygenation
     variability?

3). If inheritance is playing a role in determining DPG
     and oxygenation variability, what are the selec-
     tive mechanisms which operate to maintain this
     considerable variability over such widely diver-
     gent mammalian species?

The Red Cell, pages 339–357

Concerning the question of genetic factors influencing red cell glycolysis, ATP levels, and DPG levels, Brewer (1967) has shown that the levels of red cell ATP are partly inherited in the human, and Noble and Brewer (1972 and 1977) have shown that the levels of DPG are under genetic influence in the rat. Studies reported in this volume by Gilroy et al (1978) and Moll et al (1978) indicate partial genetic control of a number of glycolytic intermediates in the human. Thus, it is now established that genetic influences on glycolytic, ATP, and DPG variability exist. At this point we can only speculate on selective mechanisms which might operate to maintain this variability, but we hope the data and hypotheses to be presented in this paper will throw fresh fuel on such speculation.

It is our purpose in this paper to provide evidence that DPG levels and β hemoglobin type are genetically related, at least in the population of hooded Long-Evans rats which we have studied. After presenting this evidence in the rat, we will then discuss preliminary studies in mouse and man, and then try to generalize in our discussion of these results.

In previous publication Noble and Brewer (1972 and 1977) have described genetic variation in DPG levels in Long-Evans hooded rats obtained from the random bred population of Simonsen Laboratories, Gilroy, California. Genetic selection was used to develop a High-DPG and a Low-DPG line. Appropriate genetic crosses established that the major difference in DPG was due to the operation of a single gene with two alleles (Noble and Brewer, 1977). These alleles have been termed D for High-DPG and d for the Low-DPG allele. Studies of the intermediates of glycolysis in these rat strains (Noble and Brewer, 1972) have suggested a difference in in vivo activity of phosphofructokinase (PFK). That is, the glycolytic intermediate patterns in the High-DPG animals, relative to the Low-DPG animals, show lower levels of glucose-6-phosphate and fructose-6-phosphate, and higher levels of fructose-diphosphate and succeeding intermediates. This "PFK crossover pattern" is quite typical of High-DPG animals versus Low-DPG animals.

Subsequently we established that these hooded rats also showed genetically determined electrophoretic variation in their hemoglobin patterns. This type of genetic variation has been previously reported by a number of workers, and the variation observed in our rats corresponded closely to that previously reported (French and Roberts, 1965; Brdicka, 1967;

Marinkovic et al, 1967; Martinovic et al, 1970; Travnicek et al, 1971; and French et al, 1971). Previous studies have indicated that this electrophoretic variation in hemoglobin is due to a single-locus, two allele-system (French and Roberts, 1965; Martinovic et al, 1970). The rat has two α and three β chains. The electrophoretic variation is due to variation in one of the β chains called $^{III}\beta$ (Garrick et al, 1975). In conformity with the nomenclature of earlier workers we will refer to the two alleles of this hemoglobin polymorphism as Hbb$\underline{^a}$ and Hbb$\underline{^b}$ (Brdicka, 1967; Travnicek et al, 1971; French et al, 1971). In the present paper we have studied the relationship between the DPG polymorphism and the hemoglobin polymorphism in these rats. The data show a clear association between hemoglobin and DPG types and are interpreted as a marked linkage disequilibrium in the base population.

METHODS

Blood was obtained from rats and mice by intracardiac puncture at the age of six and eight weeks, respectively. Red cell DPG concentration was determined by modification of the method of Keitt (1971) on tricholoracetic acid extracts. Results are expressed as μmoles per gram of hemoglobin. This is a reasonable frame of reference for contrasts between types of animals and in particular for evaluating physiological effects of DPG which depend upon the molar ratio of DPG to hemoglobin. However it must be kept in mind that DPG/hemoglobin is a ratio, and variability in this ratio can arise from variation in hemoglobin as well as from variation in DPG. Variability in this present study involves primarily variability in DPG, and not in hemoglobin. The one partial exception to this statement will be pointed out in the text at the appropriate point. Electrophoretic hemoglobin typing of rats was carried out using starch gel electrophoresis at pH 8.6, with 0.045M-tris, 0.02M-boric acid, 0.001M-EDTA (Smithies, 1965).

RESULTS

<u>Hemoglobin Types</u>. Figure 1 shows the starch gel electrophoretic patterns we have observed in the hooded Long-Evans rats. The patterns are similar to those previously reported by others with other strains of rats. Our genetic studies, confirming those carried out by others, indicate that the pattern in slots 1 and 2 (left hand side of Figure 1),

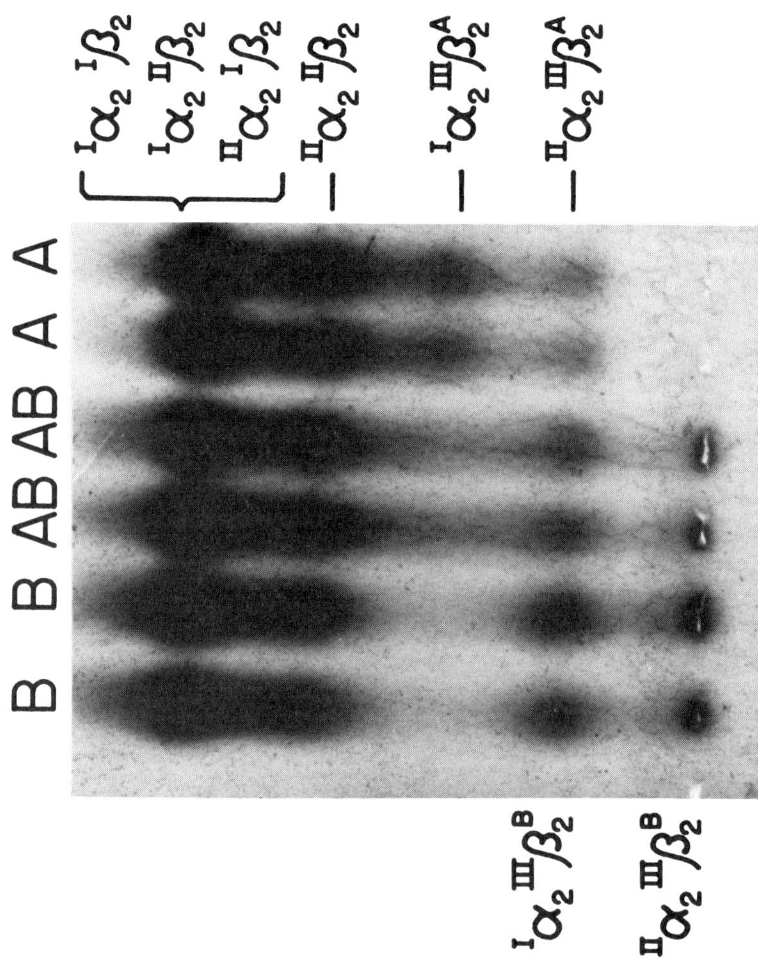

Fig. 1. The three hemoglobin phenotypes as shown by starch gel electrophoresis.

is one homozygote type termed phenotype B, slots 5 and 6 contain the other homozygote type termed phenotype A, and the heterozygote phenotype pattern AB is in the middle two slots. This nomenclature is in keeping with that of Brdicka (1967) and Travnicek et al (1971). These three patterns correspond to types III, I, II respectively of Marinkovic et al (1967) and Martinovic et al (1970).

It was soon apparent that only hemoglobin phenotype B was present in the High-DPG line and that only hemoglobin type A was present in the Low-DPG line. This stimulated us to initiate a genetic study of the possible association between hemoglobin and DPG types.

Genetic Studies. Three types of matings were initially constructed and the result with respect to hemoglobin and DPG types are shown in Table 1. The first incross, involving animals of the High-DPG line, produced progeny all of which are, of course, High-DPG and B hemoglobin type. DPG concentrations ranged from 27.05 to 34.69 μmoles. The second incross involved animals of only the Low-DPG line and all of the progeny were Low DPG in type and all were A hemoglobin type. DPG levels ranged from 18.52 μmoles to 23.83 μmoles (Table 1). The third cross was between animals of the high line and animals of the low line and as expected all F_1 progeny were hemoglobin genotype AB. The DPG levels ranged from 25.8 to 30.97 μmoles. The range of DPG levels in the heterozygotes is closer to that of the high homozygotes than to that of the low homozygotes as previously reported by Noble and Brewer (1977).

We next intercrossed the F_1 progeny, to produce an F2 and the results are shown in Table 2. The classification of the DPG levels in the F_2 progeny are based upon the levels observed with the three classes of animals in Table 1. The numbers of hemoglobin phenotypes A, AB, and B in the 70 F2 progeny were 13, 37, and 20 respectively, which was not significantly different than the expectation of 17.5, 35, and 17.5, for a one-locus, two-allele system. With respect to the DPG classification of the F_2 animals in Table 2 there is a clear association between hemoglobin phenotype and DPG levels. Ten of the 13 hemoglobin A animals had DPG levels in the dd range. Sixteen of 20 hemoglobin B animals had DPG levels within the DD range. Thirty-two of 37 hemoglobin AB animals had DPG levels within the Dd range (Table 2).

TABLE 1

Cross	PHENOTYPES DPG	Hb	PROPOSED GENOTYPES DPG	Hb	Number of Matings	Total Number of Progeny	PHENOTYPES DPG Mean	DPG Range	Hb	PROPOSED GENOTYPES DPG	Hb
I	High X High	B B	$\underline{DD}$ X $\underline{DD}$	$\underline{bb}$ $\underline{bb}$	9	66	30.69	27.05–34.69	All B	All $\underline{DD}$	All $\underline{bb}$
II	Low X Low	A A	$\underline{dd}$ X $\underline{dd}$	$\underline{aa}$ $\underline{aa}$	14	90	21.52	18.52–23.83	All A	All $\underline{dd}$	All $\underline{aa}$
III	High X Low	B A	$\underline{DD}$ X $\underline{dd}$	$\underline{bb}$ $\underline{aa}$	6	40 (F_1)	28.79	25.8–30.97	All AB	All $\underline{Dd}$	All $\underline{ab}$

TABLE 2

DPG Classification of F$_2$ Progeny

Hemoglobin Phenotypes of F$_2$ Progeny			Low Homozygote (dd) Only Range 18.5-23.8	Gap 23.8-25.8	Heterozygote (Dd) Only Range 25.8-27.0	Dd and DD Overlap Range 27.0-30.9	High Homozygote (DD) Only Range 30.9-34.6
Hb Type	Observed N	Expected N					
A	13	17.5	10	2	1		
B	20	17.5			4	13	3
AB	37	35		5	12	20	

All the F_2 animals of Table 2 who did not fit into the
appropriate DPG classification based upon their hemoglobin
type were progeny tested. With the exception of one animal,
the progeny from the various mating showed DPG levels consistent with the hemoglobin type, and thus did not provide evidence for recombination. The likely explanation for most of
these animals exceeding the ranges expected on the basis of
their hemoglobin phenotype is an increased variance of DPG
values in the F_2 of the intercrosses as compared to the
values in the High DPG and Low DPG lines. This is because
the lines are somewhat inbred (F about 0.3) which tends to
reduce their variance.

One animal of A hemoglobin type with a DPG level of 26.6
in the Dd range is more interesting. This animal was mated
to a Low DPG animal of A hemoglobin type. Of the seven progeny,
all of A hemoglobin type, two support the possibility of a
recombinant event having occurred in the F_2 parent, with
DPG levels of 28.3 and 30.2. The other five progeny had DPG
levels in the dd or "gap" range. The possible F_2 recombinant
and her two offspring showing the recombinant phenotype all
have "PFK type patterns" of their glycolytic intermediates,
indicative of a more active PFK, as would be expected if they
were of Dd heterozygous type.

Base Population Study. Ninety-six hooded Long-Evans
rats purchased directly from Simonsen Laboratories were studied for the possible association of hemoglobin and DPG types
in the random-bred base population. Table 3 summarizes the
results. The distribution of observed hemoglobin phenotypes
fits the expected Hardy-Weinberg values quite well. The
allele frequency for A in this sample is 0.25. A clear association between DPG levels and hemoglobin types is also seen
in this random sample of the base population. That is, all
hemoglobin A animals had Low DPG levels, 52 out of 55 hemoglobin B animals had high DPG levels, and 29 out of 34 AB
hemoglobin animals had DPG levels in the heterozygous range.
None of the possible exceptions have been progeny tested.

Inbred Rat Line Study. Results of hemoglobin and DPG
studies on 22 inbred lines obtained from Dr. Carl Hansen of
NIH are shown in Figure 2. Two types of hemoglobin patterns
were seen, corresponding precisely to those observed in our
hooded Long-Evans strains shown in Figure 1. Animals from
9 of the lines were of B hemoglobin type and of 13 of the
lines were A hemoglobin type; thus this genetically

TABLE 3

Hemoglobin Phenotypes of Random Sample			DPG Classification of Random Sample				
Hb Type	Observed N	Expected N	Low Homozygote (dd) Only Range 18.5–23.8	Gap 23.8–25.8	Heterozygote (Dd) Only Range 25.8–27.0	Dd and DD Overlap Range 27.0–30.9	High Homozygote (DD) Only Range 30.9–34.6
A	7	6	7				
B	55	54		2	1	25	27
AB	34	36	1	4	2	24	3

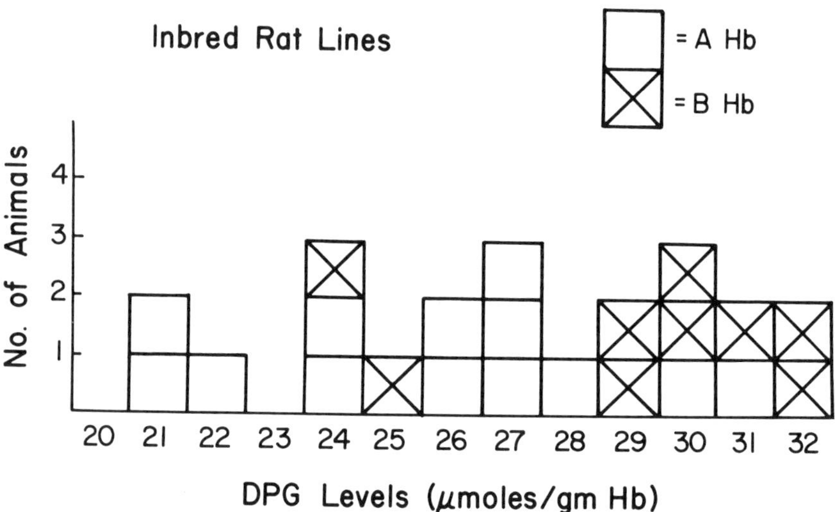

Fig. 2. The distributions of DPG levels in inbred lines of
rats with hemoglobin phenotype A or B, as indicated. Each
square represents the mean for one line, as determined from
assays on four rats per line.

determined variation in hemoglobin types is widespread
across inbred rat lines. The mean DPG levels of each strain
(4 animals each strain) are plotted in Figure 2. The DPG
levels of the A hemoglobin type animals vary considerably
among the strains, while the B hemoglobin type animals tend
to have high DPG levels. The mean DPG level for A hemoglobin
type lines is 25.7 μmoles per gram of hemoglobin, while it is
29.1 μmoles in the lines with B hemoglobin, about 13 per cent
higher. The means of the DPG of the two hemoglobin type animals are significantly different by Student's t test ($p <$
0.05). However, in this particular case, about half of this
difference in DPG levels/gram hemoglobin may be contributed by
hemoglobin differences, since the A hemoglobin type animals
average about 7 per cent higher hemoglobin level than the B
hemoglobin type animals.

Inbred Mouse Line Study. Inbred mouse lines show
hemoglobin electrophoretic variation among the lines also due
to variation in a β globin locus. One type of pattern is
called "single" with s as the gene symbol and the other pattern is called "diffuse" with d as the gene symbol. Inbred
mouse lines available at the Jackson Laboratory, Bar Harbor,
Maine, have been typed for hemoglobin and that information
is available in the literature (Staats, 1976). The mean
DPG levels of each line (5 animals each line) of 26 inbred
mouse lines are shown in Figure 3. While there is overlap,
it is clear that animals with diffuse hemoglobin tend to have
a lower DPG than animals with single hemoglobin. The mean
DPG level for diffuse hemoglobin lines is 30.7 μmoles per
gram of hemoglobin, while it is 33.6 μmoles in the lines with
single hemoglobin. These means are significantly different

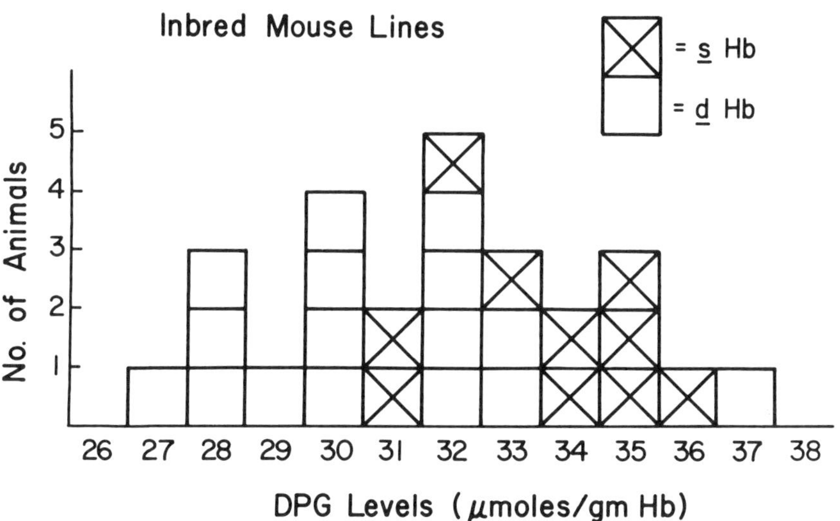

Fig. 3. The distribution of DPG levels in inbred lines of
mice with hemoglobin phenotypes single or diffuse, as indicated. Each square represents the mean for one line, as
determined from assays on five mice per line.

at the 0.01 level by Student's t test. The mean quantitative
hemoglobin levels are similar in the two groups of mice.
This preliminary work on the mouse will be published in more
detail at a later date by Brewer, Bernstein, Whitney, and
Russell.

DISCUSSION

The components of rat hemoglobin involved in the
hemoglobin polymorphism are the slower migrating components
labeled c, d, and e in Figure 1 which comprise about 20 per
cent of the total hemoglobin in adult rats (Travnicek and
Sulc, 1967; Garrick et al, 1975). The faster migrating
major components have been monomorphic in all our studies.
Rat hemoglobins appear to be comprised of five globin chains,
two of α type, $^{I}\alpha$ and $^{II}\alpha$, and three of β type, $^{I}\beta$, $^{II}\beta$, and
$^{III}\beta$ (Travnicek et al, 1971; Garrick et al, 1975). The
polymorphism in rat hemoglobins involves the $^{III}\beta$ chain as
described by Garrick et al (1975) which comprises about 20%
of the β chains. Components c and d (Figure 1) of Type A
rats probably share $^{III}\beta$ but have differing α chains based
on the work of Garrick et al (1975).

Noble and Brewer (1977) have previously described a locus
responsible for variation in DPG concentration in the blood of
Long-Evans hooded rats. Two lines were generated by selection,
one homozygous for the High-DPG gene (genotype DD) and the
other homozygous for the low DPG gene (dd). The difference
in the DPG concentrations in the red cells of High-DPG and
Low-DPG rats causes a difference in oxygen affinity. On the
average, the p50 of High-DPG rats is about 6 mm higher than
that of Low-DPG rats (Brewer et al, 1972).

Surprisingly, we have found that the High-DPG line animals
are homozygous for the b hemoglobin allele and the Low-DPG
line animals are homozygous for the a hemoglobin allele. Our
breeding studies show conclusively that the association of the
D allele with b and of d with a is a genetic association.
Further, this association is present in the random-bred Long-
Evans hooded rat base population of Simonsen Laboratories from
which our High- and Low-DPG lines were derived. All of the a
hemoglobin type animals had low DPG levels and almost all of
the b hemoglobin type animals had high DPG levels.

Two possible hypotheses may be considered for this
association. One is that we are dealing with one locus,

namely the hemoglobin locus, and that the two different
hemoglobin alleles cause variation in DPG levels. The best
evidence against this is that we have identified one probable
genetic recombinant who has given birth to two recombinant type
offspring, and all three of these animals show not only DPG
levels in the Dd range with A hemoglobin phenotype, but
"active PFK type" glycolytic intermediate patterns. The
second hypothesis, and our working hypothesis, is that we
are dealing with two loci, closely linked, one determining
hemoglobin type and the other DPG levels, with marked linkage
disequilibrium in the Simonsen population. According to
personal communications, we believe that the Simonsen population has been in existence about 200 generations. If this is
the case, linkage disequilibrium could only be maintained by
two general mechanisms. One would be a very low recombination
frequency, of the order of 0.001, either due to extremely
close linkage or recombination suppression. The second
general mechanism would be selection against certain linkage
types. Since we have observed one recombinant in fairly
limited breeding studies, we suspect that the genes are not
extremely closely linked, and thus we postulate that certain
linkage phases are under differential selection. Of course,
even if this is so, selection might not be operating on the
genes we are studying. The DPG and $^{III}\beta$ globin loci may be
marking the chromosome, but selection could be operating on
the linkage phases of other close-by genes. Of course, it is
much more exciting if selection for certain linkage phases is
operating on the genes under study, because one can then go
on to study mechanisms. Three facts provide some hope that
the linkage phases of the DPG and $^{III}\beta$ globin loci themselves
might be under selection. These are, first, the functional
relationship between the products of the two loci, second, the
fundamental importance of oxygenation to life, and third, the
apparent non-random relationship between β globin type and
levels of DPG in another species, the mouse.

Assuming that a favorable relationship between D and b,
and d and a, has been maintained in the Long-Evans hooded
populations by selection against the alternate linkage phases,
or other genetic mechanisms, the question of the possible physiologic advantage of these relationships must be considered.
It is of interest that the hemoglobin components involved,
while comprising only 20 per cent of adult hemoglobins, are
the predominant hemoglobins synthesized in the anemic period
after bleeding (Travnicek et al, 1967; Travnicek and Sulc,
1967; Travnickova and Sulc, 1970; Sulc et al, 1976). These

components are also predominant during fetal and early neonatal
life (Brdicka, 1966; Travnicek et al, 1966; Travnicek and Sulc,
1967; Travnickova and Sulc, 1970). It may be that in hypoxia,
and in early life, the hemoglobins containing $^{III}\beta$ globin are
the most important hemoglobin components and that, at least
in the Long-Evans hooded population, a very special relationship with DPG levels exists.

It might be noted in passing that the $^{III}\beta$ globin gene of
the rat may be an interesting gene to study from the standpoint
of gene switching. Most of this work involving animals has
involved sheep of A hemoglobin type, who switch to hemoglobin
C synthesis during hypoxia. Three considerations make the rat
system of interest. First, the rat is a much more convenient
laboratory animal than the sheep. Second, the shift in hemoglobin type with bleeding is rather marked, perhaps making
this a suitable model. The third is that rats are very responsive to hypoxia in terms of erythrocyte production and thus
signaling mechanisms for switching may be sharper than in
larger animals.

Finally, we would like to call attention to a very
interesting linkage homology between the rat and the mouse
involving the β globin locus, and possibly involving the DPG
locus as well. This linkage homology is illustrated in Figure
4 and was first pointed out by French et al (1971). French
et al (1971) have shown linkage in the rat of the albinism
locus, designated c, with the Hbb locus determining the $^{III}\beta$
globin chain, with a recombination frequency of 5. Additional
data (Greaves, 1970), show that these two loci are linked at
a recombination distance of 19 with a locus called "pink eye
dilution" for which the gene designator is p. In the mouse,
this same linkage group is intact with a map distance of 14
between p and c and 6 between c and Hbb (Figure 4). In the
rat, our work puts a DPG locus somewhere in the region of the
Hbb locus. We now postulate, in view of the association between DPG levels and hemoglobin type in the mouse, that the
linkage homology will be extended to a DPG determining locus
in the region of the Hbb locus in the mouse. This postulate
is now under study. If this study is positive, it suggests
the possibility that a linkage relationship between a DPG
determining locus and a β globin locus has been maintained
during evolution of these quite divergent species. Further,
if the mouse follows the rat example, the two loci involved
are highly polymorphic, with non-random relationships between
alleles at the two loci. If the rat and mouse do turn out

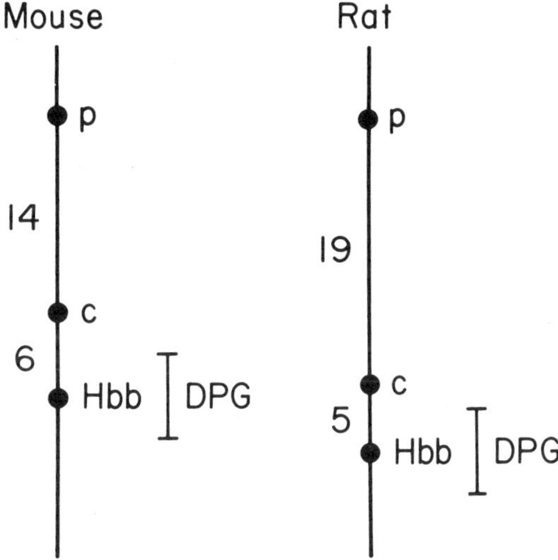

Fig. 4. The linkage homologies involving the beta globin
locus in mice and rats. See text for explanation of gene
symbols.

to be parallel cases, we might speculate that many mammalian
species which depend upon DPG for modulation of hemoglobin
function will show a similar linkage relationship. As a
matter of fact, Sing, Brewer, and Whitten (In preparation)
have already found evidence of linkage between a DPG determining locus and the β globin locus in the human.

We believe the implications of this work are quite
exciting. If a gene determining a major effect on DPG levels
is linked to the β globin structural locus, and this linkage
relationship has been maintained through a wide span of
evolution, it suggests that it might be worthwhile to search
rather intensively for the functional mechanisms underlying
this linkage relationship. Further, the maintenance of
preferential linkage relationships between certain alleles, as
illustrated most dramatically by the presence of severe linkage disequilibrium in the Simonsen hooded rat population ,
suggests that certain combinations of alleles may have
functional advantage.

SUMMARY

It is well established that 2,3-diphosphoglycerate (DPG)
and hemoglobin are functionally related. The oxygen affinity
of hemoglobin of many mammalian species including man, rat,
and mouse is largely determined and also finely tuned by
levels of DPG. Our interests in the quantitative genetics of
DPG levels stem from an interest in possible genetic effects
on oxygenation in mammalian organisms. Oxygenation is a very
basic process, absolutely vital to mammals, yet there is considerable variability in the levels of DPG within populations
of man, rat, and mouse, and this DPG variability presumably
results in variability in oxygenation. Specifically, we are
interested in the following questions: (1) Are levels of DPG
partly inherited in various mammalian species? (2) Does genetically determined variation in red cell glycolysis, since DPG
is a product of glycolysis, account for some of the DPG and
oxygenation variability? (3) If inheritance is playing a
role in determining DPG and oxygenation variability, what are
the selective mechanisms which operate to maintain this considerable variability over such widely divergent mammalian
species?

A commercially available, random-bred, Long-Evans hooded
rat population has previously been used for genetic selection
studies and two sub-lines developed which have widely differing levels of erythrocyte 2,3 diphosphoglycerate (DPG) (Noble
and Brewer, 1972 and 1977). Previous work demonstrated that
the major difference in DPG was due to the operation of a
single gene with two alleles. In the present work we demonstrate that these hooded rats also show genetically determined
electrophoretic variation in their hemoglobin patterns. This
variation involves two alleles of the $III\beta$ globin chain locus.
This type of genetic variation observed in our rats corresponds precisely to that previously reported.

Of most interest in the present work, particular
hemoglobin types have been found to be strongly associated
with certain DPG types, not only in the High-DPG and Low-DPG
lines, but in the F_2 resulting from crosses made from the two
lines. Further work established that this association also
is present in the commercial rat base population. Based upon
additional evidence discussed, the most likely explanation
for this association is that two loci, one determining

hemoglobin β globin type, and the other determining DPG levels, are closely linked and in linkage disequilibrium.

Additional studies on inbred lines of rats and inbred lines of mice indicate that lines homozygous for particular β globin alleles have statistically significant differences in levels of DPG compared to lines homozygous for alternate β globin alleles. Our working hypothesis is that in mice, as well as rats, linkage of a DPG determining locus with the β globin locus, with preferential linkage relationships between certain β globin and DPG alleles, is responsible for the observed quantitative differences in DPG levels. Most recently, Sing, Brewer, and Whitten (in preparation) have obtained evidence of a linkage relationship between the β globin locus of man, and a DPG level-influencing locus, using families ascertained because of the presence of sickle cell anemia.

Finally, we speculate that if a gene determining a quantitative effect on DPG levels is linked to the β globin structural locus, and that this linkage relationship has been maintained through a wide span of evolution, important functional mechanisms underlying this linkage relationship are likely and should be sought. Further, the maintenance of preferential linkage relationships between certain alleles, as illustrated most dramatically by the presence of severe linkage disequilibrium in the hooded rat population, suggests functional relationships between specific alleles of the two loci.

ACKNOWLEDGEMENTS

This work was supported in part by a Michigan Heart Association Grant, The Meyers Foundation, and by NIH Training Grant (5 T01-GM-0071).

REFERENCES

Brdicka R (1966). Zur ontogenese der rattenhamoglobine. Acta Biol Med German 16.617.
Brdicka R (1967). On the ontogenesis and genetics of rat hemoglobins. Thesis 1967.
Brewer GJ (1967). Genetic and population studies of quantitative levels of adenosine triphosphate in human erythrocytes. Biochem Gen 1:25.

Brewer GJ, Oelshlegel FJ Jr, and Eaton JW (1972). Oxygen
  Affinity of Hemoglobin and Red Cell Acid Base Status. In
  Rorth M, Astrup P (eds): "Alfred Benzon Symposium IV,"
  New York: Academic Press, p 539.
French EA and Roberts KB (1965). The multiple haemoglobins
  of the rat. Proceedings of the physiological society
  22:16P.
French EA, Roberts KB, and Searle AG (1971). Linkage between
  a hemoglobin locus and albinism in the norway rat. Biochem
  Gen 5:397.
Garrick L, Sharma VS, McDonald MJ, and Ranny HM (1975). Rat
  haemoglobin heterogeneity. Biochem J 149:245.
Gilroy T, Brewer GJ, and Sing C (1978). Quantitative genetics
  of human RBC glycolytic intermediate concentrations.
  Proceedings this meeting.
Greaves JH (1970). Personal communication cited in French et al.
Keitt AS (1971). Reduced nicotinamide adenine dinucleotide-
  linked analysis of 2,3-diphosphoglyceric acid: spectro-
  photometric and fluorometric procedures. J Lab Clin Med
  77:470.
Marinkovic D, Martinovic J, Kanazir D (1967). Electrophore-
  tic haemoglobin patterns in one random bred and two inbred
  strains of laboratory rats. Nature 1:819.
Martinovic J, Marinkovic DV, Kanazir DT, and Martinovitch
  PN (1970). Inheritable differences in the electrophoretic
  pattern of hemoglobin revealed in a local random-bred
  colony of albino rats. Blood 35:447.
Noble NA and Brewer GJ (1972). Studies of the Metabolic
  Basis of the ATP-DPG Differences in Genetically Selected
  High and Low ATP-DPG Rat Strains. In Brewer GJ (ed):
  "Hemoglobin and Red Cell Structure and Function," New York:
  Plenum Press, p 155.
Noble NA and Brewer GJ (1977). Identification of a major
  locus contributing to erythrocyte 2,3-diphosphoglycerate
  variability in hooded (Long-Evans) rats. Genetics 85:669.
Moll G, Brewer GJ, Gilroy T, and Sing C (1978). Multivariate
  analysis of the genetic effects on RBC glycolysis. Proceed-
  ings this meeting.
Sing C, Brewer GJ, and Whitten C (in preparation).
Smithies O (1965). Proc Congr Int Soc Blood Transf. 10th
  Stockholm 1964 p 1175.
Staats J (1976). Standard nomenclature for inbred strains of
  mice: sixth listing. Cancer Res 36.
Sulc K, Travnicek T, Neuwirt J, and Radikovska E (1976).
  Haemoglobin types in peripheral blood and bone marrow cells
  in rats after a single blood loss. Physiol Bohemoslov 25:
  345.

Travnicek T, Travnickova E, Sulc K (1966). Changes in Hb
  fractions separated on CM-Sephadex in normal newborn
  rats and in newborn rats after repeated blood losses.
  Physiol Bohemoslov 15:75.
Travnicek T, Sulc K, and Travnickova E (1967). Changes in
  haemoglobin separation on CM-Sephadex in adult rats after
  blood loss. Physiol Bohemoslov 16:160.
Travnicek T, Borova J, and Sulc K (1971). Subunit composition
  of polymorphic rat haemoglobins. Physiol Bohemoslov 20:27.
Travnicek T and Sulc K (1967). A comparison of the separation of rat haemoglobin on starch-gel electrophoresis
  and on CM-Sephadex. Physiol Bohemoslov 16:330.
Travnickova E and Sulc K (1970). Effect of repeated blood
  loss on haemoglobin synthesis in young rats. Physiol
  Bohemoslov 19:243.

<u>Dr. Harkness</u>: You indicated that there is a 7% difference in the hemoglobins in the different inbred rat strains that you looked at; was that also true of the high and low DPG rats which you selected for?

<u>Dr. Brewer</u>: In the high and low DPG strains the difference in hemoglobins is about 5% whereas the difference in DPG is about 35%.

<u>Dr. Harkness</u>: Have you looked to see whether there is any differential effect of DPG upon these different separated hemoglobins after they have been stripped?

<u>Dr. Brewer</u>: I haven't. I think Nancy Noble has been doing some work on that, but I don't know if she wishes to say anything at this point.

<u>Dr. Russell</u>: Seldon Bernstein gave you C57B1/6 carrying Hbb-d or Hbb-p to test?

<u>Dr. Brewer</u>: Yes, we have received these mice and we have recently measured them. I haven't had time to analyze the results. I would like you to take a look at these results before you leave.

<u>Dr. Beuzard</u>: Did you find a difference in the hematological data of the <u>a</u> and <u>b</u> strain?

<u>Dr. Brewer</u>: The hemoglobin levels are about 5% lower in the high DPG line. They haven't really been looked at extensively with regard to mean cell size, mean cell volume and that kind of thing. We do know their electrolyte levels and so forth, and nothing was very abnormal. The magnesium levels were high probably on the basis of a high ATP level.

<u>Dr. Beuzard</u>: My second question is do you know if those minor hemoglobins are stable or unstable?

<u>Dr. Brewer</u>: I really don't know. Maybe Nancy Noble has information on that. Do you have another question while she is coming to the microphone?

<u>Dr. Beuzard</u>: What is the oxygen affinity of the different hemoglobins with and without 2,3,-DPG?

The Red Cell, pages 359—361

<u>Dr. Brewer</u>: There is no comparative information on the different hemoglobins.

<u>Dr. Noble</u>: I have looked at the stripped Hb p50s in solutions with all six adult hemoglobins present and they appear not to differ in the high-DPG and low-DPG rat strains. The p50 response to DPG is still somewhat uncertain, but it looks like the two strains are going to be the same. I have been able to show no difference in heat stability in solutions with all six hemoglobins.

<u>Dr. Beuzard</u>: Because in the human, Labie and Huehns have shown for Hb Hammersmith, when you measure the level of 2,3-DPG as a function of hemoglobin concentration, there is a high 2,3,-DPG level and low oxygen affinity in intact cells. But the purified abnormal hemoglobin has a higher oxygen affinity than the normal hemoglobin in humans.

<u>Dr. Cameron</u>: Do you have any information as to what maintains the high or low DPG in these hooded rat strains? What other factors in the cell are involved in this? In other words what would explain the maintenance of the high DPG level.

<u>Dr. Brewer</u>: If I understand your question, you want to know the glycolytic mechanism. There is probably a difference in PFK activity. Whether there is a structural difference in PFK or differences in factors which activate PFK, we do not know. I suspect that there is a structural difference in PFK.

<u>Dr. Button</u>: Dr. Brewer these experiments recall a report given at your conference about four years ago when some exercise studies of rats transfused with high DPG blood were compared with those with low DPG blood. No difference in the effect of DPG level was demonstrated and these data were in contradiction to those described in other unpublished studies by Huggins who showed that quite the contrary was true in his rat model. Have you had an opportunity to measure the effect of exercise after transfusion of your high DPG rats?

<u>Dr. Brewer</u>: No, we haven't done transfusions. I think you are referring to the studies of Woodson on exercise tolerance of rats that were transfused with high DPG and low DPG blood? Those studies did not show any effect; however, subsequent work by others, and I think Collins will be talking about this tomorrow, indicates that under some conditions DPG levels are

important. We have subjected our untransfused rats to a
number of physiological tests. Swimming to exhaustion and
running on a treadmill revealed no differences with the
strains. In an altitude study at 25-30,000 feet, the low
DPG animals retained consciousness longer than high DPG
animals. This is explained by what Eaton has done, that if
you give animals cyanate and take them to extremely high
altitudes it is better to be left-shifted than right-shifted.
I think that in the long run we are going to find that the
position of the curve is important in the everyday biology
of the organism in many ways.

Dr. Button: I think it also proves that you must really
select your animal model very carefully.

Dr. Friedman: I wonder if you can say a little bit more
about humans and high and low levels of DPG. You mentioned
something about the associational linkage with beta S and
maybe you have some data. There are many delta chain abnormalities to which this can also be linked if this is appli-
cable.

Dr. Brewer: Yes. With respect to DPG levels in the human,
they are extremely variable, just as they are in the rat population that we have discussed. As far as the linkage study
is concerned, that has been done by Dr. Sing who will be
giving the second paper after this. That question might be
directed to him.It is a very recent finding. I think that
if the linkage is established, then any hemoglobin variability which is linked to the beta such as the delta would be
fair game for looking at the same relationship.

Dr. Lehman: This work reminds one of the old work on two
sheep populations with different oxygen affinity and in
that case it could be related to the geographical altitude
distribution of different sheep. Has any research been done
on the geographical distribution of these rats and the frequency of high and low affinity hemoglobins in relation to
these distributions?

Dr. Brewer: I think that would be a very interesting area of
investigation. Nothing has been done so far. I think that
the selective mechanisms which have caused and maintained
variation in these rat populations is something well worth
looking at and the geographical approach would be a good
one.

QUANTITATIVE GENETICS OF HUMAN ERYTHROCYTE GLYCOLYTIC
INTERMEDIATE CONCENTRATIONS*

Thomas E. Gilroy, George J. Brewer, and Charles
F. Sing
Department of Human Genetics, University of
Michigan Medical School
Ann Arbor, Michigan   48109

INTRODUCTION

In human populations continuous variation among
individuals exists for several aspects of erythrocyte
glycolysis, such as glycolytic rate, maximal catalytic
capacity of glycolytic enzymes, intracellular pH, as well
as the concentration of glycolytic intermediates, adenine
nucleotides, inorganic orthophosphate, Mg^{2+} and K^{+} (Brewer,
1974). This variation is probably determined by the joint
action of unknown genetic and environmental influences.
The relative magnitude of genetic control of specific
traits associated with human red cell glycolysis is the
subject of this report. While the regulation of mammalian
erythrocyte glycolysis has been the subject of considerable
research (Rapoport, 1968; Yoshikawa and Minakami, 1968;
Rose, 1971), there has been little quantitative genetics
work directed toward the elucidation of the magnitude of

*Abbreviations used in this paper: Hb, blood hemoglobin
level; Hct, hematocrit; MCHC, mean cellular hemoglobin concentration; ESC, erythropoietin sensitive cell; G6P, glucose
6-phosphate; F6P, fructose 6-phosphate; FDP, fructose 1,6-
diphosphate; DHAP, dihydroxyacetone phosphate; GAP, glyceraldehyde 3-phosphate; DPG, 2,3-diphosphoglycerate; 3PG, 3-
phosphoglycerate; 2PG, 2-phosphoglycerate; PEP, phosphoenolpyruvate; PYR, pyruvate; AMP, adenosine monophosphate; ADP,
adenosine diphosphate; ATP, adenosine triphosphate; HK,
hexokinase; PFK, phosphofructokinase; PK, pyruvate kinase;
AK, adenylate kinase; Vmax, maximal catalytic capacity; MAR,
mass action ratio (for indicated enzymatic reaction).

The Red Cell, pages 363—381

genetic control of normal variation in mammalian red cell glycolysis. Erythrocyte glycolysis is closely related to oxygen transport and red cell viability through the influence of 2,3-diphosphoglycerate (DPG) and ATP, respectively. The mammalian erythrocyte is well suited for studies of glycolysis because it lacks some of the metabolic pathways which interact with glycolysis and complicate interpretations of this pathway in nucleated cells.

We have chosen the _in vivo_ concentrations of glycolytic intermediates and adenine nucleotides in the cytosol of the human erythrocyte as traits for investigation in this study. These concentrations are the best available measures of the functional status of glycolysis and glycolytic enzymes _in vivo_ and thus presumably of the genes which specify these enzymes. Heritability was estimated for each of the measures of glycolysis to answer the basic question regarding the extent of genetic control of continuous glycolytic variation among normal individuals. In a previous study, a familial aggregation of human red cell ATP level suggested this trait might have a genetic component (Brewer, 1967). The response to selection of red cell DPG level in an outbred population of hooded rats (Noble and Brewer, 1972) suggested an important role for genes in determining normal phenotypic variability of DPG. In this study, we have obtained statistically significant heritability estimates for the concentration of human erythrocyte G6P, F6P, 3PG, 2PG, and ATP.

MATERIALS AND METHODS

Population Sampled and Sampling Design

Volunteer subjects between the ages of 11 and 25 years were ascertained by mailing letters to all students at one of the Ann Arbor high schools. Respondents were screened to determine that they had the appropriate relatives available for the study. The 172 sampled individuals, 84 males and 88 females, were healthy Caucasians residing in southeastern Michigan.

The sampling scheme employed for this genetic analysis is a "family set" design (Chakraborty, et al., 1977). Each family set in this study consists of an index case (I), his or her full sibling (S), their first cousin (C), and an

unrelated individual. All four members are of the same sex
and the maximum allowable age difference between members
was 10 years. The unrelated member serves as a control for
environmental effects, such as age, sex, and any effects
associated with residence in southeastern Michigan which
are shared by the relatives in the family set. This family
set design provides three degrees of genetic relationship
(1/2, 1/8, and 0). Forty-three family sets, 21 male and
22 female, were studied.

Blood Sampling and Assay Procedures

Most blood samples were taken in the homes of the
participants. Aliquots were precipitated into perchloric
acid or trichloroacetic acid, as previously described, for
assays of glycolytic intermediates and adenine nucleotides.
These acid-treated homogenates were immediately frozen on
dry ice and subsequently transferred to a -70°C Revco
freezer until assay.

Blood hemoglobin level (Hb) was measured by the
cyanmethemoglobin technique. Hematocrit (Hct) was
measured by the standard microhematocrit procedure. ATP
and DPG levels were determined according to the published
procedures of Brewer and Powell (1966) and Keitt (1971),
respectively. GAP, DHAP, and FDP were assayed by the
fluorometric procedure described by Neissner and Beutler
(1973) on an Eppendorf Model 1101M fluorometer. The remainder of the glycolytic intermediates, as well as AMP
and ADP, were assayed by the procedures of Minakami, et
al. (1965), as modified by Oelshlegel, et al. (1972).
Erythrocyte PK Vmax was assayed in hemolysates made from
cells which were stored in acid-citrate-dextrose solution
for no more than two weeks. The assay was carried out by
the method of Tanaka, et al. (1962), except that 0.17 $\underline{M}$
tris buffer pH 8.0 was used instead of triethanolamine
buffer and the concentration of KCl and $MgSO_4$ were 0.1 M
and 0.01 M, respectively. The intracellular concentration
of each phosphorylated glycolytic intermediate and adenine
nucleotide was calculated as follows:

$$\mu moles/liter\ red\ cell\ cytosol = \frac{(\mu moles/liter\ whole\ blood)\ (100)}{Hct - Hb}$$

PK Vmax is expressed as μmoles PEP consumed/min/liter of red cell cytosol.

Statistical Analysis

The first step in the analysis of these data was to identify the extraneous concomitant sources of variation which tend to inflate the estimate of total phenotypic variation and thus lead to an underestimate of the true role of genetic compared to environmental causes of variation among individuals. Both analytical and biological types of concomitant variation were considered. The effect of sample storage time in the freezer was one source of analytical variation which was considered. The assayed quantities of GAP, PEP, pyruvate, AMP, and ADP were found to correlate significantly with sample storage time and these storage effects were removed by standard linear regression techniques. The next step was to statistically describe each trait and tabulate the descriptive statistics (Table 1). Next, the biological concomitant effects were removed from each trait by computing each individual's deviation from the phenotypic mean of his or her sex. Effects of age, Hb and Hct were removed from each trait by employing a standard multiple regression approach. This step was performed separately in the two sexes. Since skewness in the frequency distribution of phenotypic values can bias heritability estimation, traits for which significant skewness persisted (even after the data standardization described next) were transformed to eliminate skew by applying the appropriate power transformation. The traits so transformed and their associated powers are FDP (0.6), GAP (0.2), PYR (0.1), ADP (0.8), PFK MAR (0.1), and [ATP]/[ADP] (0.1). Since differences among the four family set member populations for phenotypic means and/or variances of a trait can bias family set heritability estimation, these differences were removed by standardizing the data so that each family set member had a mean of zero and a variance of one. Next, for each standardized trait, we regressed the phenotypic values of all three relatives, taken as a group (I, S, and C), on that of their matched, unrelated individual. This generated residual deviations for I, S, and C which are free of common environmental associations measured by the unrelated case. Next, the heritability estimate was computed, using the method of Chakraborty, et al. (1977). The estimator is

Table 1. Descriptive statistics on glycolytic[a] and hematologic[b] traits of 172 normal individuals (84 males and 88 females). Variation attributable to the indicated concomitant effects was removed.

| Trait | Mean | Standard Deviation | | | Fraction of Total Measured Variance Attrib. to Assay Error |
| | | Concomitant Effect Removed | | | |
		None	Sex, Age	Sex, Age Hb and Hct	
Age	16.3	2.41	---	---	---
Hb	13.9	1.26	0.855	---	---
Hct	41.4	3.66	2.71	---	---
MCHC	33.6	0.99	0.933	---	---
G6P	44.5	9.08	8.96	8.81	0.028
F6P	13.2	3.12	3.12	3.02	0.107
FDP[c]	3.68	0.86	.39	.39	0.718
DHAP	17.7	4.09	4.04	3.99	0.434
GAP[c]	1.09	0.416	.74	.23	0.441
DPG	6630.0	567.0	552.0	540.11	0.112
3PG	105.0	17.2	16.6	15.98	0.145
2PG	8.88	2.80	2.72	2.54	0.356
PEP	20.1	4.62	4.37	4.00	0.150
PYR[c]	54.8	16.0	.39	---	0.125
AMP	55.4	8.19	7.82	5.84	0.834
ADP[c]	327.0	53.2	16.06	14.84	0.166
ATP	2020.0	216.0	207.0	195.73	0.136

[a]All glycolytic intermediates, except pyruvate, and adenine nucleotides are expressed as μmolar concentration in the red cell cytosol. Pyruvate is expressed as μmolar concentration in whole blood.

[b]Units are: Hb in grams/100 ml whole blood; Hct in volume percent; and MCHC in grams/100 ml packed cells.

[c]Power transformation applied after concomitant effect removal.

$$\hat{h}^2 = \frac{\frac{4}{3}\left[\frac{S^2_{(P_I-P_C)} + S^2_{(P_S-P_C)}}{2} - S^2_{(P_I-P_S)}\right]}{S^2_p}$$

where S^2_p is the mean phenotypic variance derived from the four family set members and $S^2_{(P_I-P_C)}$ is the sample variance of the differences (P_I-P_C) between the phenotypic values of index cases and their corresponding first cousins (one difference per family set). $S^2_{(P_S-P_C)}$ and $S^2_{(P_I-P_S)}$ have analogous definitions for sibling-cousin and index-sibling differences, respectively.

In order to reduce a trait-specific depression of the heritability estimate caused by assay error and to standardize comparisons between heritability estimates on different traits, we adjusted the heritability estimate on each trait in accordance with the estimated assay error associated with the trait. This was accomplished by dividing each heritability estimate by one minus the estimated fraction of total variance which is attributable to assay error. Assay error was estimated using a sample of blood from each of 10 volunteers from the main study, precipitating this blood immediately in duplicate and then assaying the duplicates a few days later. The two samples in each duplicate pair were assayed on separate days spaced one week apart. An estimate of the fraction of total variance attributable to assay error effects was made using the one-way analysis of variance, assuming individuals and duplicates are random effects.

The variance of the heritability estimator is given by Chakraborty, et al. (1977), as

$$V_{\hat{h}^2} = \frac{1}{n}\left[\frac{64}{3} - \frac{32}{3}h^2 + \frac{5}{4}(h^2)^3\right]$$

where n is the number of family sets. An approximate one-tailed t-test of size α with n-1 degrees of freedom of the form

$$t_{\alpha,\ n-1} = \frac{\hat{h}^2}{S_{\hat{h}^2}}$$

was used to test the hypothesis of zero heritability. In
this study of 43 family sets, the smallest heritability
estimates to achieve statistical significance at the
α = 0.05 and 0.10 level of probability are 0.91 and 0.75,
respectively.

RESULTS

Statistics which describe the traits of interest are
presented in Table 1. The phenotypic means of the total
sample, the standard deviations after removing various
sources of extraneous variability, and the fraction of
total variance which is attributable to assay errors are
presented for the distribution of concentrations of each
variable studied. The fraction of phenotypic variation
in GAP, PEP, pyruvate, AMP, and ADP which was attributable
to the effects of sample storage in the freezer was statistically significant and was removed by regression before
any of the descriptive statistics in Table 1 were computed.
There were no significant freezer storage effects on the
other metabolites. Descriptions of the distributions of
age, Hb, Hct, and MCHC are also presented in Table 1. The
µmolar concentrations of the different glycolytic intermediates and adenine nucleotides have quite different
means and standard deviations. The standard deviations
contain biological and non-biological components. The
non-biological sources of phenotypic variance in the data
arise from unexplained random sources of error associated
with the assay procedure, and any temporal variation which
might occur in some part(s) of the overall measurement
process. Non-biological variation can cause a false
depression of the heritability estimate.

While the two sexes did not have statistically signifi-
cent differences in their mean concentrations of glycolytic
intermediates or adenine nucleotides in their erythrocytes,

the small sex differences which were observed were removed,
by computing each individual's deviation from his or her
sex mean, in order to avoid the inflation of total phenotypic variance relative to additive genetic variance. In
the female sample, ATP concentration was the only trait
which had a significant linear regression on age at the
0.05 probability level. In the males, Hb, Hct, DPG, 3PG,
PEP, PYR, AMP, ADP, and ATP concentrations had significant
linear regressions on age and a significant quadratic
effect was also present for Hb and Hct. Only the linear
effects of age, whether significant or not, were removed
from the traits except for the instances of Hb and Hct in
males in which the quadratic effects were also removed.
The standard deviations of most of the traits decreased
only slightly when the effects of sex and age were removed
(Table 1). However, the standard deviation of Hb decreased
considerably from 1.26 grams % to 0.85 gram %, and that of
Hct decreased from 3.66% to 2.71%.

Hb and Hct have heritability estimates of 0.77 and
0.60, respectively. MCHC has a heritability estimate of
0.74. The estimate for Hb is significantly greater than
zero at the 0.1 level of probability. Hb and Hct are both
used to calculate the concentration of metabolites in the
erythrocyte cytosol. Hct minus Hb is a direct measure of
the amount of erythrocyte cytosol an individual has per
unit volume of blood. Some of the metabolite concentrations
under investigation in this study have significant
($P < 0.01$) negative correlations with Hb and Hct (data not
shown). A consideration of these facts along with the
heritability estimates obtained for Hb and Hct caused us
to ask whether or not part of estimated heritability for
glycolytic traits might be due to inheritance of Hb and/or
Hct. We approached this question by adjusting by regression for the variation in each metabolite concentration
which was attributable to variation in Hb and Hct. The
effects of these sources of variation are reduced in these
data by doing a multiple regression of each sex-adjusted
metabolite concentration on age, Hb and Hct. This regression was done separately in the two sexes. For each
glycolytic trait, the residual deviations from the regression model, which are uncorrelated with age and the
hematologic traits, were used to estimate heritability.
The standard deviation of each trait after removal of the
variation attributable to hematologic variation is shown
in Table 1.

Heritability is a function of both the additive genetic variance and the total phenotypic variance. Adjustment of heritability estimates for assay error (given in Table 1) resulted in the adjusted estimates given in Figure 1.

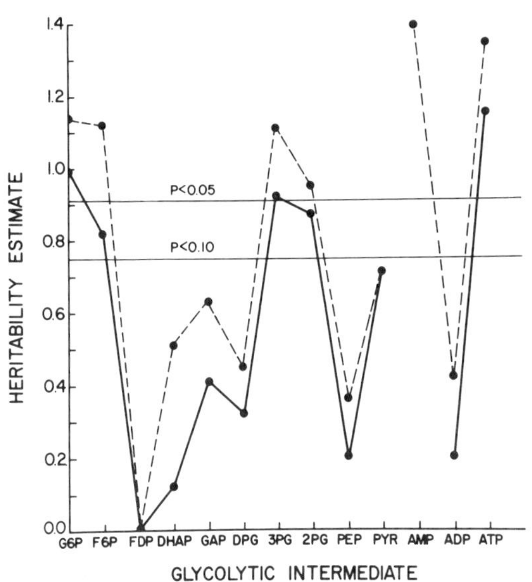

Figure 1. Heritability estimates for the concentration of glycolytic intermediates and adenine nucleotides in human erythrocytes. Traits have been adjusted for the effects of sex, age, and assay error (●----●) or sex, age, Hb, Hct, and assay error (●——●).

The heritability estimates are slightly higher after adjustment for error, than before adjustment (data not shown) but the change was relatively minor. The AMP heritability estimate is a notable exception to this statement since it had a large assay error which caused a major increase in the heritability estimate upon adjustment.

The effect of adjusting the linear associations with the hematologic traits can be seen by the differences between the two heritability estimate patterns in Figure 1. The broken line is data not adjusted for Hb and Hct, while the solid line is data which has been adjusted. Adjustment for these hematologic traits decreases the heritability estimate for each glycolytic trait to a certain degree.

Turning now to the heritability estimates on traits adjusted for hematologic variation (solid line in Figure 1), we notice considerable variation in the point estimates. We should point out that there is a relatively large standard error of each heritability estimate because of the relatively small sample of 43 family sets. Thus, even relatively high point estimates for heritability may not be significantly greater than zero. However, at the moment, these estimates are the best available of the presence of heritability in the population.

The heritability estimates for G6P and F6P are both high and significantly greater than zero at the 0.05 and 0.10 probability levels, respectively (Figure 1). The four glycolytic intermediates which occur immediately after F6P in the pathway, namely, FDP through DPG sequence, have considerably lower heritability estimates than the two hexose 6-phosphates. In fact, with the exception of 3PG and 2PG, all of the phosphorylated glycolytic intermediates have considerably lower heritability estimates. The heritability estimates for DPG, 3PG, and 2PG are 0.32, 0.92, and 0.87, respectively. The estimates for 3PG and 2PG are significant at probability levels of 0.05 and 0.1, respectively. After this point in the pathway, heritability estimates are lower for PEP and PYR. The heritability estimates for ADP and ATP are 0.20 and 1.15, respectively. The ATP heritability estimate is significant at the 0.025 level of probability.

After finding significant heritability estimates for some of the individual glycolytic intermediates and adenine nucleotides, we decided to turn to heritability studies of enzyme activities _in vivo_. To approach this question, we

computed the mass action ratios for the regulatory glycolytic
kinases and adenylate kinase. Descriptive statistics on
these mass action ratios and two other traits are presented
in Table 2. The heritability estimates for these traits are
presented in Table 3. The heritability estimate for the
PFK mass action ratio (PFK MAR) is significantly greater
than zero at the 0.05 probability level.

Table 2. Descriptive statistics on glycolytic traits of
172 normal individuals (84 males and 88 females).
Variation attributable to the indicated concomitant effect was removed.

| | | Standard Deviation | | |
| | | Concomitant Effects Removed | | |
Trait[a]	Mean	None	Sex, Age	Sex, Age, Hb & Hct
HK MAR[b]	7.20	1.75	1.72	1.68
PFK MAR[c]	0.047	0.0156	0.0232	0.0228
PK MAR[c]	18.7	10.1	0.0600	0.0571
AK MAR	0.973	0.230	0.229	0.226
[ATP]/[ADP][c]	6.32	1.07	0.0193	0.0189
PK Vmax[d]	1130.0	.9987	.9574	.9384

[a]Each individual's phenotypic value was calculated by employing the μmolar concentration of the appropriate
glycolytic intermediates and adenine nucleotides in the
red cell cytosol. Blood pyruvate concentration was used
to calculate PK MAR.

[b]The hexokinase mass action ratio (HK MAR) does not include
glucose concentration in its calculation.

[c]Power transformation applied after concomitant effect
removal.

[d]PK Vmax is expressed as μmoles per minute per liter of red
cell cytosol.

Table 3. Heritability estimates on glycolytic traits.
Effects of sex, age, blood hemoglobin level,
and hematocrit on the trait were removed where
indicated.

| | Concomitant Effects Removed | |
Trait	Sex, Age	Sex, Age, Hb & Hct
HK MAR	0.67	0.51
PFK MAR	1.05*	0.96*
PK MAR	0.26	0.26
AK MAR	-0.14	-0.08
[ATP]/[ADP]	-0.14	-0.16
PK Vmax	0.56	0.41

*Significantly greater than zero at the 0.05 level of
probability.

DISCUSSION

The heritability estimates for human erythrocyte
glycolytic traits which have been statistically adjusted
for the effects of Hb and Hct have been presented along
with those for their corresponding traits which have not
been adjusted for hematologic variation. Some of the
latter traits have the negative correlation with Hb and
Hct originally observed by Eaton and Brewer (1968). The
heritability of both types of glycolytic trait, and of
hematologic traits, is of interest because the hematologic
traits are potentially heritable and they interact with
at least some of the glycolytic traits. Some of the heritability of certain glycolytic intermediates and adenine
nucleotides may derive from heritability of the hematologic
traits. Adjusting the concentration of glycolytic intermediates and adenine nucleotides for hematologic variation
should considerably reduce the influence of Hb and Hct on
heritability estimates for the glycolytic traits. This
approach assumes that variation in the hematologic traits
causes variation in the concentration of glycolytic inter-

mediates and adenine nucleotides. However, the reverse
could be true, and it should be noted that either direction
of causality could produce the observed negative associations
between red cell metabolite concentrations and the hematologic traits. Thus, the converse approach might be meaningful: One could study the heritability of Hb and Hct after
they have been adjusted for the concentration of one or more
red cell metabolites, such as ATP. The modest reduction
of heritability (Figure 1 and Table 3) after linear adjustment for Hb and Hct effects did not appreciably affect the
main inferences to be drawn from this study.

The statistically significant heritability estimates
for G6P and F6P imply that there is a considerable amount
of genetic control over these two hexose-6-phosphates at
the beginning of the glycolytic pathway. There are at
least two reasonable biochemical explanations for such a
finding. The first involves hexokinase (HK) and phosphofructokinase (PFK), which are both regulatory enzymes and
each is thought to limit glycolytic rate with the relative
importance of each in rate limitation depending somewhat
on intracellular conditions. Thus, HK and PFK constitute
a regulatory complex or system with HK influencing PFK
through the concentration of F6P, and PFK influencing HK
through the concentration of G6P. Considering the very
interesting kinetic properties of HK (Rose, et al., 1964;
Rose and O'Connell, 1964; Rose, 1971, Brewer, 1969; Ponce,
et al., 1971) and PFK (Passonneau and Lowry, 1962; Tsuboi
and Fukunaya, 1965; Rapoport, 1968; Ponce, et al., 1971),
the finding of considerable genetic control over G6P and
F6P seems quite reasonable and might be mediated through
allelic differences in the structures of HK and/or PFK, or
through genetic control of enzyme concentration. It is
also entirely possible that this genetic control is mediated through effects of the genotype on any of a number of
traits which ultimately affect the immediate environment
of red cell HK and/or PFK. There might be genetic control
over intracellular pH, phosphate concentration, Mg^{2+} concentration or other factors which would influence the
activity of HK and/or PFK <u>in vivo</u>. Our finding of a
significant heritability estimate for the PFK mass action
ratio and the fact that this estimate is somewhat larger
than that for the HK mass action ratio provides some
support for the hypothesis that the heritability of the
hexose 6-phosphates is more dependent on inheritance of
PFK activity than it is on inheritance of HK activity.

The second biochemical explanation for high heritability of G6P and F6P relates to the adenine nucleotide system. There is a very high heritability of ATP concentration. It is possible that the adenine nucleotide synthesis pathway might be the predominant inherited feature and that ATP has a major subsequent influence on the concentration of G6P and F6P. It should be noted that the concentrations of G6P and ATP in the red cell have a significant positive correlation (0.53, P < 0.01), and it is possible that this correlation is the result of causal influences of ATP. Red cell hexokinase is thought to be subsaturated with respect to ATP and thus the enzyme may be stimulated in vivo by any increase in ATP concentration and this would increase the concentration of G6P and F6P. The actions of ATP are, of course, quite complex. ATP is also an effective inhibitor of PFK activity in vivo under most circumstances, and by this mechanism exerts feedback control over its own rate of production. Also added to this complexity are the roles of ADP and AMP which are known to be stimulators of PFK activity in many tissues.

The reasons for the high and statistically significant heritability estimate for 3PG and 2PG are not clear at this time. One possibility is that genetic control of monophosphoglycerates is a reflection of genetic control of DPG phosphatase activity in vivo. DPG phosphatase has a very low activity in vitro (Harkness, et al., 1969) and its product, 3PG, is a competitive inhibitor of its substrate, DPG (Rapoport and Luebring, 1951). It is conceivable that genetic control of DPG phosphatase activity would have more impact on the heritability of 3PG and 2PG concentration than on that of DPG concentration if the latter is buffered through the action of other enzyme activities such as DPG mutase. Another possible explanation for the genetic control of 3PG and 2PG concentrations in the red cell relates to the fact that the phosphoglycerate kinase (PGK) reaction is near equilibrium (Minakami and Yoshikawa, 1966). The quasi-equilibrium condition means that ATP, ADP, 3PG, and 1,3-DPG all have an important mass action effect on the PGK reaction. Furthermore, ATP is an inhibitor of PGK. These facts mean that the concentration of ATP in the red cell can have an influence on the concentration of 3PG. Hence, the heritability of ATP (Figure 1) might be a cause of the 3PG and 2PG heritabilities. However, the very low correlation between ATP and 3PG (-0.13) argues against this mechanism of monophosphoglycerate heritability.

Since pyruvate readily crosses the membranes of red cells and other cells in the body, its concentration in the blood is a function of the metabolic activity of many cells. Hence, if there is heritability of blood pyruvate concentration in the population, it probably reflects genetic control over glycolysis and other metabolic pathways in various cell types and tissues of the body.

The adenine nucleotides represent a very interesting group of metabolites since ATP is the primary energy source of the cell, and since ADP and AMP metabolism is so closely related to that of ATP. A large number of different enzymes, and thus genes, are involved with ATP metabolism. All of the glycolytic kinases are directly involved with ATP production or consumption and, of course, the net result of glycolysis and all of its enzymes is the production of ATP. ATP levels show a very high and significant heritability (Figure 1).

The discussion of the biohcemical mechanisms for the high heritability of ATP is a continuation of the discussion of the high heritability of the hexose 6-phosphates. Are the genetic influences exerted primarily through the adenine nucleotide synthesis pathway, or are they exerted on the production of ATP from ADP in the glycolytic pathway? Either explanation is plausible, and they are not mutually exclusive. However, our working hypothesis at the moment is the glycolytic explanation. The adenine nucleotide synthesis hypothesis suffers a little from the low heritability of ADP (the AMP heritability is uninterpretable in our judgment). The use of a path model (Moll, et al. - following paper in these proceedings) suggests that the heritability of G6P accounts for a greater fraction of the ATP variability than does ADP. This finding is compatible with the glycolytic hypothesis.

Thus, our working hypothesis is that part of the genetic control of erythrocyte ATP levels derives from genetic control over ATP production from ADP through the glycolytic mechanism. Since the rate of glycolysis, and thus the rate of ATP production, is primarily controlled by the regulatory enzymes, HK and PFK, it would be quite reasonable for genetic control of ATP production rate and concentration to reside in genetic control of HK and/or

PFK. This concept is supported by the highly significant heritability estimates for G6P and F6P, the concentrations of which are tightly regulated by HK and PFK, and from the significant heritability estimate for the PFK mass action ratio.

It is important to keep in mind the fact that multiple ATPases in, or on, the red cell membrane are involved with the breakdown of ATP. Also, ATP is utilized in the synthesis of purine and pyridine nucleotides, which are of great importance in glycolytic regulation. Part of the genetic control of ATP concentration might reside in genetic control of the rate of ATP breakdown in the red cell. However, this concept implies that normal variation in the rate of red cell ATP consumption in the population is partly responsible for the normal variation in intracellular ATP concentration. While this situation is not entirely impossible, ATP consumption rate probably has little or no long-term effect on ATP concentration because PFK is stimulated by any transient decrease in ATP concentration. Thus glycolysis has a substantial reserve capacity for the production of ATP and this capacity is normally held under tight constraint through the inhibition of PFK by this important nucleotide. Of course, ATP consumption rate might have important short-term effects on ATP concentration in the red cell.

With the involvement of such a large number of genes in ATP metabolism it is not very surprising that heritability of ATP concentration has been detected in this sample. The implication is that one or more of the enzymes of ATP metabolism either show allelic structural variation, genetically controlled enzyme concentrations, or genetically controlled enzyme modulation. Genetic control over Mg^{2+} concentration or enzyme modulators such as pH or the intracellular concentration of inorganic orthophosphate, which are known to have effects on HK and PFK <u>in vitro</u>, might be one mechanism for genetic effects on HK and/or PFK activity <u>in vivo</u>.

The phylogeny of red cell ATP concentration provides some hints that this metabolite might be inherited. Evolution of the red cell is marked by a loss of the nucleus, decreased carbohydrate metabolism, and a decreased ATP concentration. An analysis of red cell ATP levels in fish, amphibians and mammals has demonstrated a phylogenetic

decrease in this important nucleotide (Brewer, 1974). This
decrease in red cell ATP concentration might represent an
evolutionary adjustment which has been made to provide the
red cell with a metabolism which is less favorable for
malaria, and perhaps other forms of intra red cell parasitism.
The change in red cell ATP concentration with evolution
indicates that genetic variation in this important
metabolite existed in the past because genetic variation
is the basis for evolution. The results of the present
investigation indicate that genetic variation exists in
the red cell ATP concentration of modern man, at least
those residing in southeast Michigan.

In light of the very interesting oxygen transport
function of hemoglobin, its heritability is quite exciting
and might even imply there is genetic control of the level
of blood oxygen transport and tissue oxygenation through
this mechanism. It is quite possible that some aspect(s)
of erythropoiesis regulation has genetic variation in the
normal population: There might be genetic control of
erythropoietin synthesis, release, activation, degradation
or some other factor(s) which might be responsible for
maintaining the titer of this hormone in the vicinity of
erythropoietin sensitive cells (ESC) in the bone marrow.
Also, the rate of proliferation and differentiation of the
ESC to hemoglobin-producing erythroid cells may be dependent on the genotype of the ESC. Finally, there might be
genetic control of the reticuloendothelial system with
respect to its removal of senescent erythrocytes from the
circulation.

SUMMARY

We have studied the heritability of the concentration
of each glycolytic intermediate and adenine nucleotide in
the cytosol of human erythrocytes obtained from apparently
healthy young individuals. Preliminary to our analysis
of heritability, each trait was statistically described
and the effects of sex and age variability among the
individuals were removed. Heritability was estimated
using the family set method. This method removes covari-
ances between the index, sib, and cousin, due to those
environmental determinants of the phenotypic values which
were shared with an unrelated member of the family set.
Heritability was estimated by employing the fact that the

variance of differences between first cousins minus the
variance of differences between full siblings estimates
three-fourths of the additive genetic variance.

The heritability estimates obtained for ATP concentration was found to be significantly greater than zero
at the 0.025 level of probability. The heritability
estimates obtained for G6P and F6P are also high and
significantly greater than zero. The inheritance of the
concentration of these two hexose 6-phosphates is likely
attributable to the inheritance of in vivo activity of
HK and/or PFK, because the concentrations of G6P and F6P
are tightly regulated by these two enzymes. Our finding
of a statistically significant heritability estimate for
the PFK mass action ration supports an important role for
inheritance of PFK activity. Genetic control of one or
both of these important regulatory enzymes could derive
from allelic differences in their structures of genetic
control over enzyme concentration or Mg^{2+} concentration.
It could also derive from genetic control over such enzyme
effectors as pH and inorganic orthophosphate concentration.

We speculate in this paper that part of the genetic
control of ATP concentration probably derives from genetic
control of the rate and regulation of ATP production via
glycolysis. Thus, inheritance of the hexose 6-phosphates
and ATP may derive from the same cause, namely, genetic
control of the activity of HK and/or PFK in vivo. However, alternative explanations, such as an important
genetic influence on adenine nucleotide synthesis, are
also quite plausible.

ACKNOWLEDGMENT

This work was supported in part by the National
Institutes of Health Training Grant No. ST01-GM-0071.

REFERENCES

Brewer GJ (1967). Biochem Genet 1:25.
Brewer GJ (1969). Biochem Biophys Acta 192:157.
Brewer GJ (1974). In Surgenor DM (ed). "The Red Blood
  Cell," New York: Academic Press.
Brewer GJ and Powell RD (1966). J Lab Clin Med 67:726.

Chakraborty R, Schull WJ, Harburg E, Schork MA and Roeper
  P (1977 - accepted for publication). Heritability
  estimates. J Chron Dis, paper V.
Eaton JW and Brewer GJ (1968). The relationship between
  red cell 2,3-diphosphoglycerate and levels of hemoglobin
  in the human. Proc Nat Acad Sci 61:756.
Harkness DR, Ponce J and Grayson V (1969). Comp Biochem
  Physiol 28:129.
Keitt AS (1971). J Lab Clin Med 77:470.
Minakami S, Suzuki C, Saito T and Yoshikawa H (1965). J
  Biochem 58:543.
Minakami S and Yoshikawa H (1966a). J Biochem 59:139.
Niessner H and Beutler E (1973). Experientia 29:268.
Noble NA and Brewer GJ (1972). In Brewer GJ (ed):
  "Hemoglobin and Red Cell Structure and Function," New
  York: Plenum Press, p. 155.
Oelshlegel FJ Jr, Brewer GJ, Penner JA and Schoomaker EB
  (1972). In Brewer GJ (ed): "Hemoglobin and Red Cell
  Structure and Function," New York: Plenum Press, p. 377.
Passonneau JV and Lowry OH (1962). Biochem Biophys Res
  Commun 7:10.
Ponce J, Roth S and Harkness DR (1971). Biochem Biophys
  Acta 250:63.
Rapoport S (1968). Essays in Biochem 4:69.
Rapoport S and Luebring J (1951). J Biol Chem 189:683.
Rose IA (1971). Exp Eye Res 11:264.
Rose IA and O'Connell EL (1964). J Biol Chem 239:12.
Rose IA, Warms JVB and O'Connell EL (1964). Biochem Biophys
  Res Commun 15:33.
Tanaka K, Valentine WN and Miwa S (1962). Blood 19:267.
Tsuboi KK and Fukunaga K (1965). J Biol Chem 240:2806.
Yoshikawa H and Minakami S (1968). Folia Haematol 89:357.

DISCUSSION

<u>Ms. Mansfield</u>: Have you looked at the levels of these meta-
bolites in G6PD deficient cells to compare the heritability
estimates in the G6PD deficient group with the estimates you
get in this control population?

<u>Dr. Gilroy</u>: No, that hasn't been done. It could be interest-
ing. It might help winnow out any effects that might be coming
in from the pentose phosphate pathway.

<u>Ms. Mansfield</u>: I should think that it would also show how
reliable your heritability estimates are because there you
are directly looking at changes due to a known genetic alteration.

<u>Dr. Gilroy</u>: It would probably be a very interesting study to
do.

MULTIVARIATE ANALYSIS OF THE GENETIC EFFECTS ON RED BLOOD
CELL GLYCOLYSIS

Patricia P. Moll, Charles F. Sing, George J.
Brewer, and Thomas E. Gilroy*
Department of Human Genetics, University of
Michigan Medical School

INTRODUCTION

Continuously varying differences among individuals in
the human population have been observed for most measures
of health. Common diseases such as diabetes, gout, hypertension and atherosclerosis are clinically defined by the
extremes of the continuous range of phenotype values of
those traits which reflect the complex multifactorial determination of health. Levels of insulin, blood sugar, uric
acid and blood pressure are but a few of the intervening
quantitative variables which are measures of health. Evaluating the contribution of genes to such quantitatively
varying phenotypes in order to understand the common diseases of man is great because the costs to society are so
high. However, the genetic analyses of such measures of
health requires complex statistical procedures not widely
used in human genetics to identify gene effects. We must

*Department of Pediatrics, Baylor College of Medicine,
Houston, Texas   77030

This work was supported in part by N.I.H. Postdoctoral
Fellowship 1 F 32 HL 05293, ERDA Contract E-(2828), Public
Health Service Training Grant (5-T01-GM-0071) and the
Michigan Heart Association Grant.

The Red Cell, pages 385—405

rely on statistical analyses of the quantitative variation
to sort out those components of the disease system that are
likely under the control of genetic variation.

Red blood cell glycolysis is an ideal biological model
for developing strategies for the analysis of complex disease systems which are under genetic control. A number of
special features of this system, combined with knowledge of
its function, serve as advantages in developing the multivariate analytic techniques which may be used to sort out
the genetic causations of the continuous variability of the
elements of a complex system. The tissue is easily accessible, metabolism of the red blood cell is simplified, laboratory assays of glycolytic intermediates and adenine
nucleotides have been developed and there is considerable
information about the biochemistry of the enzymes which control the system.

The general goal of our research is to understand how
genetic variation in the enzymes of glycolysis is translated into variability in glycolytic intermediates and then
how that variability contributes to determining oxygen
transport and ATP production. Our initial effort, reported
here, is to estimate the extent to which genetic differences
among individuals determines quantitative variability in a
subset of measures of glycolysis. Glycolysis of the red
blood cell represents a highly integrated system of interrelated variables which each show continuous variability
among members of the population. The levels of an individual's red blood cell glycolytic intermediates and adenine
nucleotides are determined by his unique combination of
environmental conditions and inherited enzyme characteristics. Our understanding of the relationships among the
elements of the system and of the role that genetic variation plays in determining the variability of the system as
a whole has been limited to inferences from separate analyses of each variable or the correlations between pairs of
variables. The intent of this presentation is to illustrate
how a path analysis of a set of correlations can 1) give insight into the relationships among certain variables of the
glycolytic system and 2) can be used to determine the role
of gene effects in determining variability of the system as
a whole.

The example used here will focus on the determination
by a subset of measures of glycolysis of adenosine triphos-

phate (ATP) levels. Glycolysis provides the energy for various red cell functions through the net synthesis of two
molecules of ATP from adenosine diphosphate (ADP) for each
molecule of glucose passing through the pathway. ATP is
known to play a number of important roles in red cell structure and function. In the mature red cell ATP is involved
in maintaining cell shape and deformability, transporting
sodium, potassium, and calcium, and modifying the oxygen
affinity of hemoglobin and regulating glycolysis by allosteric inhibition of phosphofructokinase (Brewer, 1974).
Statistically significant ATP variation among both normal
individuals and sickle cell anemia patients has been reported by Oelshlegel, Brewer, and Sing (1977). Genetic analyses
of related individuals suggest that the observed variability
of ATP may be due in part to genetic differences (Gilroy et
al, 1978). We have conducted a multivariate statistical
analysis to determine the contributions of hemoglobin (HB),
glucose-6-phosphate (G6P), and ADP to the physiological and
and genetic determination of individual variability in ATP.
HB, G6P, and ADP each measure a separate kind of influence
on the levels of ATP. Hemoglobin may be thought of as a
measure of the environment within the red blood cell, G-6-P
as an indicator of variability in the glycolytic process,
and ADP a measure of adenine nucleotide metabolism. From
previous studies using a variety of data samples (Oelshlegel
et al, 1977; Moll et al, 1978, Sing et al, 1978) we know
that HB relates differently to each glycolytic intermediate
and that G6P, probably because of the role hexokinase plays
in controlling glycolysis, is the most informative measure
of the highly significant differences among individuals
which have been observed for the front half of the pathway.
These same studies have also suggested that G6P variation
has a major influence on the variability of ADP and ATP
among individuals.

The degree to which deviations in each of these variables contributes to variability in each of the other variables was estimated from correlations between variables
using a sample of unrelated individuals. Correlations between full sibs were used to simultaneously estimate the
inheritance of the four variables. These estimates of
heritability were combined with the estimates of the physiological relationships to subdivide an individual's ATP variability into the fractions attributable to genetic and non-
genetic variability in HB, G6P, and ADP and variability in
genetic and non-genetic factors acting on ATP alone. This

work represents a first attempt to apply multivariate techniques to the genetic analysis of variables which are measures of red cell glycolysis.

METHODS

THE SAMPLE

The data for this study were assays of blood samples collected by Gilroy (1977) in family sets (Schull et al, 1970) for estimating genetic control of glycolysis in human erythrocytes. Each family set consisted of an index (I), a full sib (S), a first cousin (C) and one unrelated individual (U) who was matched to the three relatives for readily observable environmental determinants of the trait. All four members of the set were chosen to be of the same sex and within 10 years of the same age. The sample included 21 male and 22 female sets, all from southeastern Michigan. The 172 individuals were all Caucasians and ranged between 11 and 25 years of age.

METHODS OF ASSAY AND DEFINITION OF MEASUREMENT

The methods of assay are the same as reported by Oelshlegel, et al (1977) and described in detail by Gilroy (1977). These methods were modified from the methods of Minakami and Yoshikawa (1966). The levels of G6P, ADP, and ADP were measured by end-point analysis of a perchloric acid extract of homogenized red blood cells. The change in optical density per ml of a whole blood extract in the presence of an excess of enzyme was measured and then converted to u moles per 100 ml whole blood. This measure, rather than u mol/gm HB or the concentration per liter cell water was chosen so that the role of individual variability in HB in defining variability in G6P, ADP, and ATP could be estimated separately.

ANALYSIS OF DATA

The data were first adjusted by polynomial regression within each of the four groups (I, S, C, U) for the concomitant variables which accounted for a statistically significant portion of the variability (Li, 1964). Then, within each group, HB, G6P, ADP and ATP were each standardized so as to have a mean of zero and a standard deviation of one.

The adjusted values of the indexes and unrelated individuals were used to compute correlations between HB, G6P, ADP, and ATP. These correlations were used in a path analysis to estimate the strength of the influences of variability of each variable on the variability of the other variables being considered. The objective of a path analysis is to obtain an interpretation of the set of correlations in terms of hypothesized paths of causation. The hypothesized paths of causation are defined by a path diagram (the model). Such a model represents directional paths as standardized partial linear regression coefficients (the path coefficients) and bidirectional paths as correlation coefficients. The path model used in this analysis is shown in Figure 1.

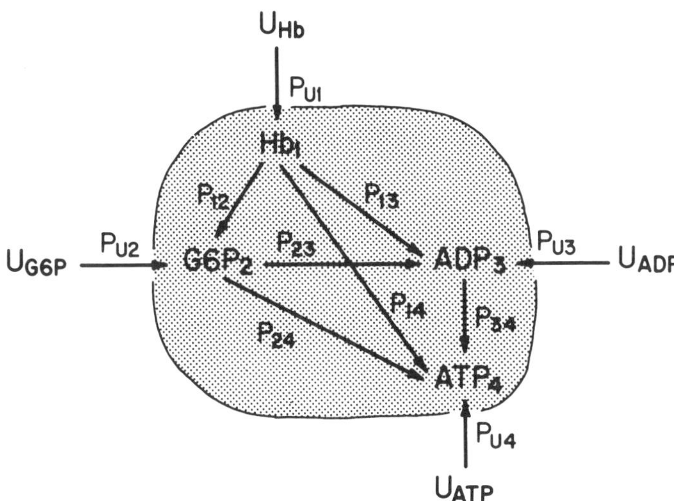

Figure 1. The path model of the hypothesized relationships among HB, G6P, ADP and ATP. Pij is the path coefficient from variable i to variable j.

This model assumes that HB influences G6P, ADP and ATP; G6P influences ADP and ATP; and ADP influences ATP. An analysis of this path model partitions the separate contributions of variability in HB, G6P and ADP and their joint contributions to determination of the variability of ATP among individuals. The apriori assumptions of the causal relationships stated by this path model are based on the postulated roles of glycolytic intermediates and adenine nucleotides in the Embden-Meyerhof pathway. The U variables represent the unmeasured factors which influence the model. They include both environment and measurement error.

Expansion of the path model to include an individual and his sibling (Figure 2) provides a basis for the simultaneous estimation of the influence of gene variation on these four variables. The genetic model assumes that the quantitative traits (HB, G6P, ADP, and ATP levels) are under the control of four separate sets of unlinked loci. The square of the estimated path ($G_i \rightarrow X_i = h_i$) is an estimate of the proportion of variability in X due to the variability in average effects of alleles, among individuals, which influence X. We assume that there is no linkage or epistasis between any of the pairs of loci which contribute to the determination of the variability of the four traits. A detailed explanation of this "narrow sense" definition of heritability is presented by Falconer (1960).

The mathematics of the path model and the statistical strategy for applications of path analysis to a path model are discussed in great detail elsewhere (Wright, 1968; Kempthorne, 1969; Li, 1975; Li, 1976; Morton, 1974; Rao et al, 1974). The objective of the statistical analysis is to use correlation statistics to estimate the path coefficients suggested by the path model. The likelihood (expected value as a function of the path coefficients) for each correlation between variables measured on an individual and between variables measured on sibs are given in Appendix A and B, respectively. The logarithm of the joint likelihood of the bias corrected Z transformations (Fisher, 1954) of each set of correlations is distributed approximately as $-\chi^2/2$. The chi-square measures the goodness-of-fit of the transformed correlations to their expected values. The estimates of path coefficients were taken to be those values which maximized the likelihood (equivalent to minimizing the chi-square fit of expectations to the data). The Newton Raphson iteration procedure and the Fisher scoring principle utilized

by the modified MAXLIK computer program (Fisher, 1958;
Reed and Schull, 1968) were used to search the parameter
space for the maximum likelihood estimates.

RESULTS

CONCOMITANTS

The sex of an individual, the number of days his blood
sample was stored at -70°C, and the date of assay of the
sample (both linear and quadratic) are all statistically
significant sources of variability among individuals for the
four variables studied. After adjustment for individual
differences in these concomitants, the effects of age, height,
and weight were not a statistically significant source of
variability. Table 1 gives the proportion of variability
explained by fitting the concomitants. Adjustments for concomitants and removal of the differences among the group
means of the I,S,C, and U accounted for between 8% and 50%
of individual variability. The remaining variability, represented by the adjusted variables, was used in the path
analyses.

PHYSIOLOGICAL CONTRIBUTIONS

Table 2 presents the partial correlations between the
four variables in the top half of the table. All these
correlations, except between HB and G6P, are statistically
significant. For comparison, the bottom half of the table
presents the total correlations based on the I and U individuals before adjustment of the data for the concomitants.
All of these correlations are significant. The expectations
for these correlations given the path model is true (Figure
1) are in Appendix A.

Figure 3 presents the path model with the estimates of
the path coefficients, Positive paths imply a positive deviation in a causal variable will cause a positive deviation
in the affected variable. For example, an individual who is
one standard deviation above the mean for his G6P is expected
to have an ATP level which is .41 standard deviations above
the ATP mean. A comparison of these scale-free path coefficients reveals that HB has a larger relative influence on
ADP and ATP deviations than on G6P deviations. G6P has a
larger effect on ATP than on ADP.

Table 1

Percent Variability Explained by Concomitants

Variable	Concomitants (sex, storage time, dat assayed, dat assayed squared, differences among I,S,C,U, means)	Residual variability after adjustment for concomitants
HB	29.22**	70.78
G6P	8.17*	91.83
ADP	50.31**	49.69
ATP	18.43**	81.57

* statistically significant at the .05 level of probability.

** statistically significant at the .01 level of probability.

The total variance of an affected variable in the network is partitioned using the concept of degree of determination. The degree of determination due to a single causal variable is the square of the path leading from that variable of concern. The joint effects of causal variables on the degree of determination is twice the product of the connecting paths and correlations which lead away and back to the variable of interest without passing through the same variable twice. Table 3 presents the degree of determination by single and joint effects. HB singly accounts for 14.3% of ADP and 13.59% of ATP variability. G6P singly accounts for 17.0% of ATP variability but only 4.9% of ADP variability. ADP accounts for 4.5% of ATP variability. HB and G6P jointly account for 5.9% of ATP variability (twice the product of the paths from HB and G6P to ATP and the path between HB and G6P). Overall the proportion of contributions to variability explained by the model ranges from 1.4 to 49.6% for G6P and ATP, respectively. A path analysis of the hypothesized network of variables considered here suggests that HB and G6P account for a major portion of the variability in ATP. To summarize, the path coefficients indicate influence on deviations and coefficients of determination measure the contribution to variance of hypothesized causal variables on hypothesized affected variables. Because they are scale-

Table 2

Correlation coefficients[1] computed on 86 unrelated individuals.

HB	1.0000	.1193	.4047 **	.5033**
G6P	-.2405*	1.0000	.2657	.5123**
ADP	-.2807**	.2595*	1.000	.4699**
ATP	-.2176	.5601**	.2362*	1.0000

[1]The total correlations below the diagonal were calculated
on the unadjusted data. The partial correlations above the
diagonal were calculated after the variability attributable
to sex, storage time, date assayed, date assayed squared
and differences among the group means has been removed.

*Statistically significant at the .05 level of probability.

**Statistically significant at the .01 level of probability.

free measures, the path coefficients can be compared among
different causal variables as can coefficients of determination.

GENETIC CONTRIBUTIONS

The inclusion of siblings in the analysis of the path
model allows us to partition the variability of each variable into three components: the influence of genes on that
variable alone, the influence of the environment on that
variable alone, and the influence of other variables in the
model. This analysis is based on the analysis of the correlations presented in Table 4 according to the set of
equations (Appendix B) which define the path model given in
Figure 2. For HB, 98.5% of the variability is due to genes
for HB while 1.5% is due to the environment. Genes acting
directly on G6P contribute 70.7%, environment contributes
27.9% and HB contributes 1.4% to G6P variability. Genes
acting on ADP alone contribute 75.0%, the environment con-

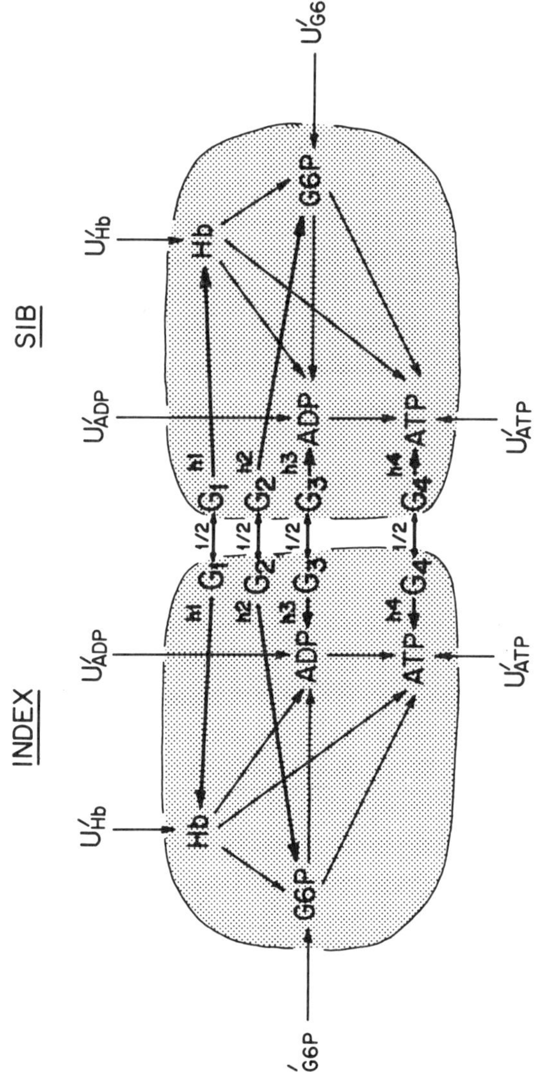

Figure 2. The path model including an individual and his sibling. h_i is the path coefficient from the alleles at the loci which influence i.

Figure 3

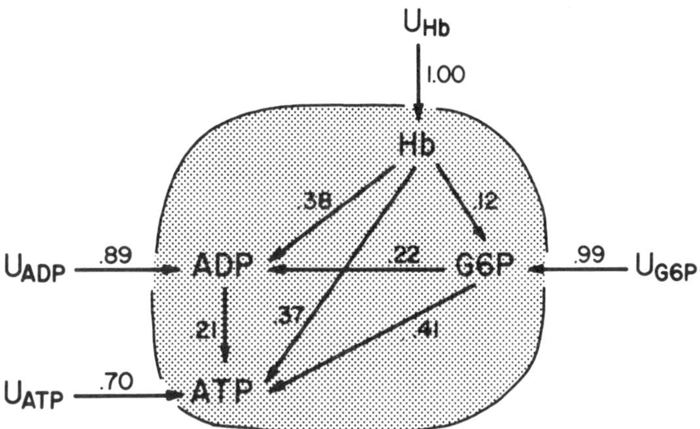

Figure 3.   The path model of hypothesized relationships among HB, G6P, ADP and ATP with estimated path coefficients.

tributes 3.8% while HB and G6P contribute 21.2% to ADP variability. Finally, gene effects on ATP alone contribute 34.8%, the environment 15.6% and the other variables in the model 49.6%. All gene effects in this model are statistically significant.

The 49.6% of ATP variability can be further partitioned into the contributions of the genetic and environmental effects acting on other variables in the system. A summary of these effects is presented in Table 5. The genes for HB, G6P and ADP contribute 39.7% to ATP variability. Environmental effects on HB, G6P and ADP contribute 6.7% to ATP variability. The remaining 3.2% of ATP variability may be assigned to the genes for some of the casual variables acting jointly with the environmental influences on the other causal variables to influence ATP. Therefore, approximately 50% of the large genetic component of ATP variability (74.5%) may be accounted for by the direct influence of genes on ATP while approximately 50% is assigned to the direct effects of genetic variation in HB, G6P, and ADP.

Table 3

Partition of variation according to path analysis of correlations between variables using a sample of unrelated individuals.

Causation	Percent Determination of Variation[1] in		
	G6P	ADP	ATP
Singular Effects of			
HB	1.42	14.32	13.59***
G6P		4.87	16.99***
ADP			4.46*
Joint Effects of			
HB-G6P		1.99	3.63
HB-ADP			5.89
G6P-ADP			3.84
Hb-G6P-ADP			1.20
Total Due to Model	1.42	21.18	49.60
Unexplained	98.58	78.82	50.40
Total	100.00	100.00	100.00

[1] After adjustment by regression for concomitant variability, table 1.

* Statistically significant at the 0.05 level of probability.

*** Statistically significant at the 0.001 level of probability.

Table 4

The correlations between 43 index and sib pairs.

		Index Variable		
Sib Variable	HB	G6P	ADP	ATP
HB	.5823**	-.1299	.1141	.1462
G6P	.0091	.4059**	-.0695	.1773
ADP	.2968	-.0937	.5314**	.1769
ATP	.3207*	.2641	.1911	.4068**

* Statistically significant at the .05 level of probability.

** Statistically significant at the .01 level of probability.

DISCUSSION

The role of the concomitants in determining variability
was different for each of the measures of glycolysis considered here. A comparison of the two sets of correlations
in Table 2 (before and after adjustment for concomitant
variability) gives a measure of the differential effect of
adjustment on the data used to estimate the physiological
relationshsips. HB has a significant negative correlation
with G6P, ADP, and ATP before adjustment. After adjustment
of the data, these correlations were all significant and
positive. The ADP-ATP correlation was twice as high after
adjustment. If the concomitant sources of variability had
been ignored in calculating these correlations the results
of the path analysis and our interpretation of the sources
of variability which influence ATP would have been quite
different. The role of uncontrolled sources of variation
in biasing inferences about glycolysis which are made from
correlations may be great.

The differential influence of HB on variability of G6P,
ADP, and ATP (Table 3) was also reported by Moll et al (1977)

Table 5

Percent contribution to ATP variability of genetic and environmental variability in HB, G6P and ADP.

		Source		
			Joint	
	Genetic	Environment	G and E	Total
Singular Effects of				
HB	13.38	.21		13.59***
G6P	12.02	4.97		16.99***
ADP	3.34	1.12		4.46*
Joint Effects of				
HB–G6P	3.00	.02	.60	3.63
HB–ADP	5.03	.17	.69	5.89
G6P–ADP	2.35	.08	1.41	3.84
HB–G6P–ADP	.57	.08	.55	1.20
Total due to Model	39.69	6.66	3.25	49.60
ATP	34.81	15.59	–	50.40
Grand Total	74.50	22.25	3.25	100.00

*Statistically significant at the 0.05 level of probability.
***Statistically significant at the 0.001 level of probability.

for sickle cell anemia patients. These findings have major implications for the choice of scale of measurement to study the variability of the glycolytic system among individuals. Expression of adenine nucleotides and glycolytic intermediate levels as concentrations per unit hemoglobin or cell water confounds this differential effect of HB variability with variation attributable solely to G6P, ADP, or ATP. The observed difference in hemoglobin effect and the highly significant correlation between HB and hematocrit suggests

that the relative size of the red blood cell, the water content of the cell, and the spacing between HB molecules may
influence the function of certain enzymes and the production
of glycolytic intermediates and/or adenine nucleotides in
the pathway. Failure to properly consider the variability
of HB among individuals and between variables can lead to
misinterpretation of the meaning of glycolytic variability.
The HB contribution to the variability in G6P, ADP and ATP
is probably a minimum estimate since there may be biological
interactions between HB and the glycolytic intermediates
and adenine nucleotides which dampen variability. Such a
feedback relationship has been suggested from earlier studies
of 2,3-diphosphoglycerate and HB (Eaton and Brewer, 1968).

The observation that G6P plays a major role in determining ADP and ATP variability is consistent with the finding
in sickle cell anemia patients by Moll et al (1978) that, of
the eight glycolytic intermediates considered, G6P variation
was the single most important influence on ATP variability.
A strong G6P influence is consistent with the hypothesis
that the rate limiting enzyme hexokinase (HK) is a regulating factor in red cell glycolysis (Rapoport, 1968; Yoshikawa
and Minakami, 1968). It is important to realize, however,
that inferences made from these results are only valid for
the path model studied. Comparisons among alternative models
which might explain ATP variability are beyond the scope of
this presentation. We have considered a simplified model
which represents only one-way causal relationships to ex-
emplify path analysis. A feedback mechanism may exist in
the red cell whereby increasing ATP levels could activate
HK and thus cause G6P levels to increase. Similarly, ATP
may have an influence on both HB and ADP variability that
is not included in this model. An extension of the model
might also include DPG, an important glycolytic intermediate
which is highly associated with ATP variability. Also, because path analysis deals only with linear relationships
among variables, any significant higher order relationships
are ignored.

The path analysis of sibling correlations indicates
that each of the variables in this study are under separate
genetic control. The large contribution of genes to HB
variability may be due to any one of the several of the
mechanisms suggested by Gilroy (1977). These include control over the sensitivity of erythropoietin-producing cells
to the oxygen tension within these cells or their immediate

environment. Genetic control over HB may also be due to
the genetic control over the rate of erythropoietin synthesis,
release, activation, degradation or other factors which might
be responsible for maintaining the titer of this hormone
in the vicinity of erythropoietin sensitive cell (ESC) which
reside in the bone marrow. The genotype of the ESC may control the rate of proliferation and differentiation of the ESC
to hemoglobin producing erythroid cells. Finally, genes could
control how aggressively the reticulendothelial system removes
senescent erythrocytes from circulation. Due to the oxygen
transport function of hemoglobin, the high heritability
suggests the possibility that one source of genetic control
over the level of tissue oxygenation may be influencing the
level of hemoglobin.

The large contribution of genes to G6P variability is
probably due to inherited variation in HK and possibly phosphofructokinase (PFK). Both are regulatory enzymes and are
thought to contribute to limiting the glycolytic rate (Rapoport,
1968; Yoshikawa and Minakami, 1968). The genetic control over
G6P could be through allelic differences in the structures of
HK and/or PFK or through genetic control of enzyme concentrations. Genetic control of intracellular pH, phosphate concentration, Mg2+ concentration or other factors may also
influence the activity of HK and/or PFK in vivo.

The contribution to variability in ADP and ATP (74.9 and
34.8%) by the genes which directly control these two variables is probably due to the large number of enzymes involved
in ADP and ATP metabolism. These data imply that one or
more of the enzymes of ADP and ATP metabolism either show
allelic structural variation, genetically controlled enzyme
modulation, or genetically controlled enzyme concentrations.

The study by Gilroy et al (1978) using traditional measures
to estimate the heritability of individual quantitative traits
showed that ATP has a high heritability. We have combined information about the relationship of HB, G6P and ADP with ATP
with information on relatives to estimate the role of genes
which affect each of these variables in determining ATP variation among individuals. By analyzing ATP as part of a system we have found genes contribute 74.5% to ATP variability.
While 34.8% of ATP variability is due to the genes controlling
ATP, we found that genes for HB, G6P and ADP contribute a
total of 39.7% to ATP variability. Therefore, of the total
genetic component of ATP variability over one half is due

to genes for other variables. Since these other variables
are so involved with ATP variability and together the variables all act within the same system, it is not surprising
that they contribute to the determination of ATP levels.

The strategy used in analyzing these data should be help-
ful in determining the genetic contributions to variability
in other systems of variables. Several steps are involved in
the strategy. First, all variables in the system under
study should be adjusted for the relevant concomitant variables. Next, the appropriate model which defines the
physiological relationships among the variables in the system must be selected. Thirdly, the estimates of the physiological relationships among the variables of the system are
computed on unrelated individuals. Lastly, the genetic analysis of the system, assuming the physiological model, is
carried out using the correlations between relatives. This
strategy enables us to go a step beyond the identification
of a general genetic factor to identify the relative roles
of the variables of the system. The study reported here
results in directing our attention to the study of the
genetics of HB and G6P to understand the genetics of ATP.
Such information encourages us to invest in studies of enzymes
such as hexokinase which are related to G6P. This study
illustrates a fruitful interaction between qualitative biochemistry and mathematical genetics to understand the quantitative variability of a multifactorial system.

SUMMARY

A multivariate analysis of the variability and covariability
of HB, G6P, ADP and ATP was performed to estimate the degree
to which individual variability in ATP is attributable to the
genetic and environmental variability of the other variables.

The path model for an individual assumes that HB influences
G6P, ADP and ATP; G6P influences ADP and ATP; and ADP influences
ATP levels. A sample of unrelated individuals was used to
estimate the physiological influences of HB, G6P and ADP on
ATP while correlations between relatives was used to estimate
the influence of genes on the four variables. The functional
relationships among variables estimated by the paths of causation hypothesized by the path model showed that HB singly
accounts for 14.3%, 13.6% and 1.3% of ADP, ATP and G6P vari-

ability. ADP contributes only 4.5% to ATP variability. The joint contributions of Hb, G6P, and ADP account for 14% of the observed variability in ATP.

Extension of the path model to include siblings provided the basis for simultaneously estimating heritability of the four variables while taking into account the physiological relationships among them estimated from unrelated individuals. The effect of genes acting on the system of variables accounts for 74% of the ATP variability (35% due to genetic variability acting on ATP alone, 29% due to the effects of genetic variation of HB, G6P, and ADP acting independently and 11% due to genes acting jointly). Sixteen percent of the remaining 26% of the variability in ATP may be assigned to the variability of environmental factors operating on ATP alone and 6% may be assigned to variability of environmental factors operating on HB, G6P and ADP. The remaining 4% of ATP variability is due to the joint influence of genes and environmental effects of causal variables affecting ATP variability.

This research represents a departure from classical heritability analysis of a single quantitative trait. A multivariate approach to the analysis of a system of variables which represent red blood cell glycolysis provides greater insight into the genetic and environmental influences on a system than separate univariate analyses. The inclusion of a model of relationship between variables enables one to subdivide the heritability of a trait into the contribution of genes controlling those variables which influence the trait. The example presented here reveals that 50% of the heritability of ATP levels may be assigned to genes controlling HB, G6P and ADP.

APPENDIX A

These equations are based on the path model in Figure 1.

Product Moment[1]

Correlation	Expectation

$$r_{12} = P_{12}$$

$$r_{13} = P_{13} + R_{12}P_{23}$$

[1] Between variables on unrelated individuals. HB, G6P, ADP and ATP are denoted as subscripts 1, 2, 3, and 4 respectively.

$$r_{14} = P_{14} + P_{12}P_{24} + P_{13}P_{34} + P_{12}P_{23}P_{34}$$

$$r_{23} = P_{23} + P_{21}P_{13}$$

$$r_{24} = P_{24} + P_{21}P_{14} + P_{21}P_{13}P_{34} + P_{23}P_{34}$$

$$r_{34} = P_{34} + P_{31}P_{14} + P_{32}P_{24} + P_{31}P_{12}P_{24} + P_{41}P_{12}P_{23}$$

$$r_{22} = 1 = P_{12}^2 + P_{U1}^2$$

$$r_{33} = 1 = P_{13}^2 + P_{23}^2 + P_{U2}^2 + 2P_{31}P_{12}P_{23}$$

$$r_{44} = 1 = P_{14}^2 + P_{24}^2 + P_{34}^2 + P_{U4}^2 + 2P_{43}P_{31}P_{12}P_{24}$$
$$+ 2P_{43}P_{31}P_{14} + 2P_{43}P_{32}P_{24} + 2P_{41}P_{12}P_{24}$$
$$+ 2P_{43}P_{32}P_{21}P_{14}$$

APPENDIX B

The equations are based on the path model in Figure 2.

Product Moment
   Correlation
<u>r(Index,Sib)</u>[1]   Expectation

$$r_{11} = \frac{1}{2} h_1^2$$

$$r_{22} = \frac{1}{2} [h_2^2 + h_1^2 P_{12}^2]$$

$$r_{33} = \frac{1}{2} [h_3^2 + h_2^2 P_{23}^2 + h_1^2 (P_{13}^2 + P_{12}^2 P_{23}^2)]$$
$$+ P_{31} h_1^2 P_{12} P_{23}$$

$$r_{44} = \frac{1}{2} [h_4^2 + h_3^2 P_{34}^2 + h_2^2 (P_{24}^2 + P_{23}^2 P_{34}^2)] + h_1^2 (P_{14}^2 +$$
$$P_{12}^2 P_{24}^2 + P_{13}^2 P_{34}^2 + P_{12}^2 P_{23}^2 P_{34}^2)]$$
$$+ P_{42} h_2^2 P_{23} P_{34} + h_1^2 [P_{41} P_{12} P_{24} + P_{41} P_{13} P_{34} + P_{41} P_{12} P_{23} P_{34}$$
$$+ P_{42} P_{21} P_{13} P_{34} + P_{42} P_{21} P_{12} P_{23} P_{34} + P_{43} P_{31} P_{12} P_{23} P_{34}]$$

1 Between variables on index and sib. HB, G6P, ADP and
ATP are denoted as subscripts 1, 2, **3**, and 4
respectively.

$$r_{12} = r_{21} = \frac{1}{2} H_1^2 P_{12}$$

$$r_{13} = r_{31} = \frac{1}{2} h_1^2 [P_{13} + P_{12}P_{23}]$$

$$r_{14} = r_{41} = \frac{1}{2} h_1^2 [P_{14} + P_{13}P_{34} + P_{12}P_{24} + P_{12}P_{23}P_{34}]$$

$$r_{23} = r_{32} = \frac{1}{2} [h_1^2 (P_{21}P_{13} + P_{21}P_{12}P_{23}) + h_2^2 P_{23}]$$

$$r_{24} = r_{42} = \frac{1}{2} [h_1^2 (P_{21}P_{14} + P_{21}P_{12}P_{24} + P_{21}P_{13}P_{34} + P_{21}P_{12}P_{23}P_{34}) + h_2^2 (P_{24} + P_{23}P_{34})]$$

$$r_{34} = r_{43} = \frac{1}{2} [h_1^2 (P_{31}P_{14} + P_{31}P_{13}P_{34} + P_{31}P_{12}P_{23}P_{34} + P_{32}P_{21}P_{14} + P_{32}P_{21}P_{13}P_{34} + P_{32}P_{21}P_{12}P_{24} + P_{32}P_{21}P_{12}P_{23}P_{34}) + h_2^2 (P_{32}P_{24} + P_{32}P_{23}P_{34}) + h_3^2 P_{34}]$$

REFERENCES

Brewer GJ (1974). Red cell metabolism and function. In: Surgenor NM (ed):"The Red Blood Cell," New York: Academic Press, p 473.

Eaton JW, Brewer GJ (1968). The relationship between 2,3 diphosphoglycerate and levels of hemoglobin in the human. PNAS 61: 756.

Falconer DS (1960). "Quantitative Genetics." New York: Ronald Press.

Fisher RA (1958). "Statistical Methods for Research Workers." New York: Hafner.

Gilroy TE (1977). Genetic Control of Glycolysis in Human Erythrocytes. PhD Dissertation, University of Michigan.

Gilroy TE, Brewer GJ, and Sing CF (1977). Quantitative genetics of human red blood cell glycolytic intermediate concentrations. Proceedings of this conference.

Kempthorne O (1957). "An Introduction to Genetic Statistics." New York: John Wiley.

Li CC (1975). "Path Analysis - a primer." Pacific Grove, California: Boxwood Press.

Li CC (1976) "First Course in Population Genetics." Pacific
Grove, California: Boxwood Press.

Li JRC (1964). "Statistical Inference." Ann Arbor: Edward
Brothers. Vol. 2

Minakami S and Yoshikawa H (1966). Free energy changes and
rate limiting steps in erythrocyte glycolysis. J Biochem
59: 139.

Moll PP, Sing CF, and Brewer GJ (1978). A path analysis
of the causal relationships between red cell glycolytic
intermediates, ADP and ATP in sickle cell anemia.
BioSystems, in press.

Morton NE (1974). Analysis of family resemblance. I. Introduction. Am J Hum Genet 26: 318.

Oelshlegel FJ, Brewer GJ, and Sing CF (1977). Patterns of
red cell glycolytic intermediates in sickle cell anemia.
I. Values and first analysis. J Mol Med 2:51.

Rao DC, Morton NE and Yee S (1974). Analysis of family
resemblance. II. A linear model for familial correlation. Am J Hum Genet 26: 331.

Rapoport S (1968). The regulation of glycolysis in mammalian
erythrocytes. In: Campbell PN, Grenville GD (eds):
"Essays in Biochemistry." New York: Academic Press, p 69.

Reed TE and Schull WJ (1968). A general maximum likelihood
estimation program. Am J Hum Genet 20: 579.

Schull WJ, Harburg E, Erfunt JC, Schork M, and Rise R (1970).
A family set method for estimating heredity and stress.
II. J Chron Dis 23: 83.

Sing CF, Gilroy TE, Brewer GJ and Moll PP. A path analysis of
the causal relationships between red cell glycolytic
intermediates in a normal population. In preparation.

Wright S (1968). "Evolution and the Genetics of Populations."
Chicago: University of Chicago Press. Vol 1, p 299.

Yoshikawa H and Minakami S (1968). Regulation of glycolysis
in human red cells. Folia Haemat 89: 357.

DISCUSSION

<u>Dr. Schoomaker</u>: If I understand path analyses, there's no
real good way of testing exactly which of a number of apriori
models is the better in a statistical sense, except by trying
to chisel away more and more of that unexplained variability,
is that not true? If so, have you been able to look at a
more complete array of variables that you think influence
ATP to see if you can account for even more than 50% of the
total variability in ATP that you see?

<u>Dr. Sing</u>: In general, the answer to each of your questions
is yes. The report given here today is our first attempt at
this sort of analysis. You must recognize that all statistical
analyses are model dependent. There is no way to use a set
of data to simultaneously tell us the causal relationships
among variables and the strength of those relationships.
Factor analysis or stepwise regression can be used to find
the set of variables which gives the best explanation of
the variability but no attempt is made in such an approach
to incorporate apriori knowledge about causation. The
causation hypothesis fit to data by path analysis must be
generated apriori from other studies. Data can be used to
estimate parameters in a model and test hypotheses about
these parameters. Model testing is not intended in the
presentation given here. We have tested the strengths of
the path relationships in the path model but I must empha-
size that those relationships were established from apriori
judgments using other sources of information. I should also
point out that if we are simply interested in reducing the
unexplained variability it is possible to add variables
(even biologically ridiculous variables) to account for a
greater percent of the variability of ATP.

<u>Dr. Schoomaker</u>: Regardless of whether they have biological
significance?

<u>Dr. Sing</u>: If our concern was to accurately predict ATP it
would be reasonable to include that set of predictors which
accounted for the greatest amount of variability. However,
we are more interested here in explaining the biological
basis of ATP variability. The variables chosen and the
direction of influences included in the path model that we
consider are based on our apriori knowledge of biological
information gleaned from other studies. We are interested

The Red Cell, pages 407—409

in bringing together this apriori information on hemoglobin, G-6-P and ADP to determine their relative influence on ATP determination.

Dr. Meyers: In Dr. Gilroy's discussion, as well as in yours, the term "environment" is brought in as an important contribution to heritability and variability. Could you define it as used in this context?

Dr. Sing: The environment is a difficult entity to define. For our purposes the environment includes all those influences on the variability of the trait that are not accounted for by genetic variation. Included in that definition is the residual unexplained variability which may be simply due to a measurement error.

Dr. Meyers: Does a positive correlation carry with it an implication of a beneficial effect?

Dr. Sing: A positive correlation does not imply a good benefit or a bad benefit. I remind you that correlation is a statistical evaluation of the relationship between two random variables. The analysis here is a statistical analysis. No statistic that I am aware of has an implied social value. Statistical analyses are meant to give insights into the relationships among variables which may be used as an aid in the process of decision-making. One uses his accumulated scientific experience to interpret the biological meaning of statistics derived from data which is collected on a relevant biological problem which may or may not have implied social connotations.

Dr. Cameron: I have several questions in terms of the use of this kind of model analysis. First, in terms of expanding the model, does this technique allow a process somewhat like factor analysis; that is, bring in another factor and remove it if it doesn't reduce the variance sufficiently? In this sense you could build a model which, while not necessarily designed on the basis of your apriori knowledge, at least partitions out those factors which mathematically give you the greatest contribution to variance?

Dr. Sing: Yes, we have some experience with this sort of statistical procedure. Our work with sickle cell patients follows this line of reasoning. We found that for sickle cell anemia patients certain variables of the glycolytic

system are better indicators than others of the variability
of the entire system. This seems to hold true in the data
set discussed here today. For example, G-6-P is a very good
indicator of the total variability of the first four glycolytic intermediates considered, i.e., G-6-P, F-6-P, FDP,
and DHAP. So in the factor analysis sense G-6-P is a very
important factor in predicting the behavior of the glycolytic
system. The reason why factor analysis was not used for
the analysis just presented is that it does not incorporate
the apriori knowledge that is available about the glycolytic
system. We now have enough experience with the glycolytic
system to enable us to go one step beyond the fishing expedition which is characteristic of a factor analysis.

Dr. Cameron: One technical question which interests me: If
you add a variable, does the model allow you to include
specific two-way variances with the new variable or do you
have to include all two-way variances in your analysis?

Dr. Sing: Yes. It is our intent to expand our model to
include reciprocal relationships between variables in the
system. We have begun to analyze a path model which accounts
for a reciprocal relationship between hemoglobin and ATP.

Dr. Cameron: Do any of your samples include twins or have
you considered the use of twins for these kinds of studies?

Dr. Sing: We chose the family set method because it is not
affected by the kinds of environmental bias which are typical
of the twin sampling designs.

ERYTHROCYTE MEMBRANES

Chairman: T. Steck

ULTRASTRUCTURAL CHARACTERIZATION OF PROTEINS AT THE NATURAL
SURFACES OF THE RED CELL MEMBRANE

R.S. Weinstein, J.K. Khodadad and T.L. Steck

Department of Pathology, Rush Medical College
and Departments of Biochemistry and Medicine,
The University of Chicago, Chicago, Il.

INTRODUCTION

A major goal in modern biology is to delineate the
molecular organization of the cell periphery. In recent
years, particular attention has been focused on the human
red cell membrane as an object for study since red cells
are readily available in large quantities, are relatively
homogeneous, and may serve as models for the study of
certain properties of more complex cells. Considerable
progress has been made in the elucidation of red cell
membrane structure by electron microscopy and protein
analysis but the integration of ultrastructural and
biochemical approaches has been difficult. Our present
studies address this goal.

Proteins comprise approximately 60 percent of the isolated red cell membrane mass. Approximately 10 percent of
this fraction is bound carbohydrate in the form of glycoproteins. The individual polypeptide species in the isolated
ghost membrane are best resolved by polyacrylamide gel
electrophoresis (PAGE) in the detergent, sodium dodecylsul-
fate (SDS), as shown in Figure 1, gel 1. The disposition
of these polypeptides, and a complementary group of glycoproteins visualized after staining with periodic acid-Schiff
(PAS) for carbohydrates (not illustrated) has been mapped
in several studies (see Steck 1974a; Marchesi et al., 1976
for recent reviews).

The Red Cell, pages 413—427

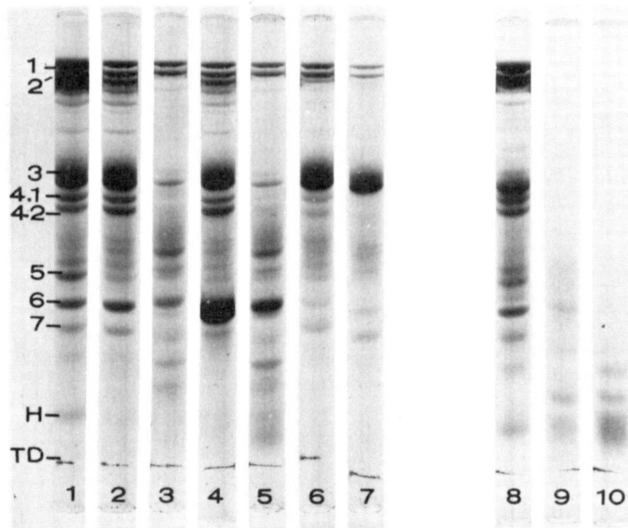

Figure 1. Polyacrylamide gel electrophoresis in SDS (Fairbanks
et al., 1971; Steck and Yu, 1973) of the polypeptides of membrane preparations examined by freeze-fracture electron
microscopy in this study. Left: selective elution, digestion and decoration of inside-out (IO) vesicle proteins.
Gel 1: Ghosts. Gel 2: IO vesicles (88% pure) (Steck, 1974b).
Most of the spectrin (bands 1 and 2) and actin (band 5) have
been eluted. Gel 3: IO vesicles digested with trypsin (5 ug/
ml in 5 mM sodium phosphate buffer, pH 8, for 60 minutes at
0°C) and washed; see Steck et al., 1976. Gel 4: IO vesicles
decorated with rabbit muscle G3PD (2 mg/ml for 30 minutes
at 0°C in 5 mM phosphate buffer, pH 7) and washed; see Yu
and Steck, 1975. Note the dramatic increase in band 6 (G3PD)
associated with the membranes. Gel 5: Trypsin-treated IO
vesicles decorated with G3PD. Gel 6: IO vesicles stripped
of peripheral proteins with 5mM para-chloromercuribenzene-
sulfonate (pCMBS) as in Steck and Yu (1973). Gel 7: IO
 vesicles stripped of their peripheral proteins with 2 mg/ml
dimethylmaleicanhydride (DMMA) as in Steck and Yu (1973).
Right: chymotrypsin digestion of human red cell ghosts.
Ghosts were digested at 37°C for four hours in 50 mM NH_4HCO_3,
pH 7.8, the enzyme was inhibited with DFP and the membranes
were washed as in Steck et al., 1976. Gel 8: Untreated ghosts.
Gel 9: 0.1 mg/ml chymotrypsin. Gel 10: 1.0 mg/ml chymotrypsin. H represents the globin chains of hemoglobin and
TD, the tracking dye.

A current formulation of the disposition of the major
membrane proteins is illustrated schematically in Figure 2.
Implicit in this figure are the following concepts: (1) An
absolute asymmetry exists between the protein constituents
at the two natural surfaces of the membrane, presumably
reflecting their functional anisotropy. (2) There are two
modes of association between the proteins and the membrane
lipid bilayer, i.e. strong and weak. Proteins which are
strongly associated are designated integral proteins and
those which are weakly associated are peripheral proteins
(Singer, 1974). The strongly bound proteins, representing
about half of the membrane protein mass, are believed to
penetrate into the apolar core of the membrane where they
are anchored by hydrophobic contacts. These proteins cannot
be solubilized without disruption of the lipid bilayer in
which they are integrated. The remaining half of the protein
mass is in the form of weakly bound polypeptides which can
be solubilized without membrane dissolution. Various treat-
ments of graded severity solubilize certain of these
components selectively (Steck and Yu, 1973; Steck, 1974a).
Weakly bound proteins are confined to the cytoplasmic surface of the membrane while all of the outer surface species
are integral glycoproteins. (3) Some, and perhaps all, of

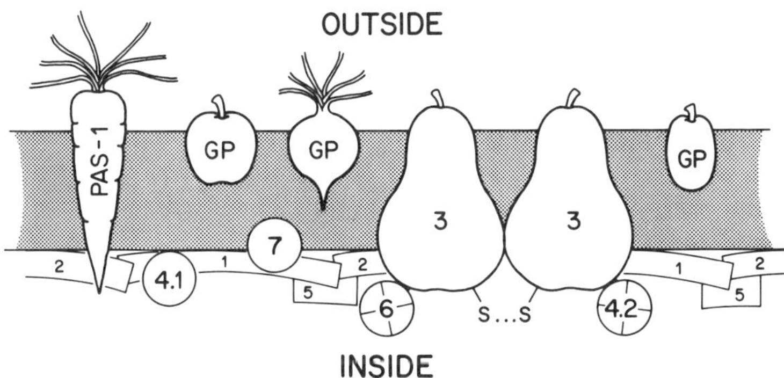

<u>Figure 2.</u> A schematic representation of the distribution of
the major red cell membrane proteins. From Steck, 1974a with
permission of the publisher.

the integral proteins span the membrane asymmetrically. This
is particularly well documented for the red cell protein
called "band 3", and the sialoglycoprotein called "PAS-1"
or "glycophorin." (cf. Steck, 1974a; Marchesi et al., 1976).
(4) Many of the membrane polypeptides are probably organi-
zed into homo-oligomers and homopolymers. Bands 1 and 2
(spectrin) form homo- and heterodimers and higher aggregates.
Band 3 forms homodimers and band 4.2 forms homotetramers
(Steck, 1972; Peters and Richards, 1977). Furthermore,
band 6 is known to be the protomer of the tetramer, glyceralde-
hyde-3-P dehydrogenase (G3PD) (Steck, 1974a).

It is widely held that some of the membrane proteins
associate to form supramolecular ensembles. For example,
spectrin and actin may contribute to a filamentous reticulum
which appears to be in close proximity to the cytoplasmic
surface of the cell membrane (cf. Steck, 1974a; Kirkpatrick,
1976; Marchesi et al., 1976; Hainfeld and Steck, 1977).
Band 3 dimers have specific binding sites for the glycolytic
enzymes, G3PD and aldolase (Yu and Steck, 1975; Strapazon
and Steck, 1977). While there is a sufficient amount of
band 3 in the membrane to bind the entire cellular comple-
ments of both these enzymes, the extent of their association
in vivo is unknown. Band 4.2 protein also appears to bind
to band 3 (Yu and Steck, 1975).

Recent advances in our understanding of membrane ultrastructure have come from studies using freeze-fracture electron microscopy. The freeze-fracturing process hemisects
lipid bilayers, creating two complementary fracture faces
which reflect a cleavage plane in the interior of the cell
membrane (Branton, 1966; Weinstein et al., 1970). A plati-
num-carbon replica is cast of the fracture faces which can
then be examined by transmission electron microscopy. Water
adjacent to the membrane may be sublimed away by deep-
etching, making the natural surfaces accessible for replication. Current conventions for describing the various surfaces of the red cell membrane revealed by freeze-fracture
electron microscopy are schematically illustrated in Figure 3.

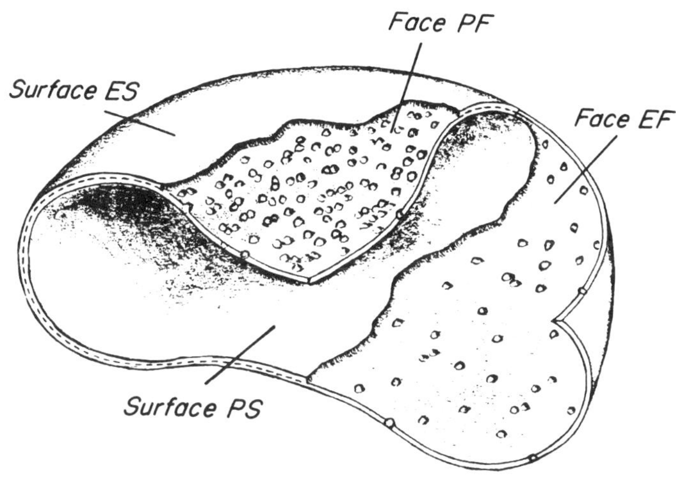

Figure 3. Nomenclature for the natural surfaces (ES and PS)
and internal faces (EF and PF) of the red cell membrane.
Adapted from Branton et al., 1975.

The two fracture faces of membranes bear different
populations of intramembrane particles (IMP) designated IMP_E
on the EF face and IMP_P on the PF face (Weinstein, 1976).
The IMP_P are many times more abundant than IMP_E in red cells
(Weinstein and McNutt, 1970). This asymmetrical distribution
of the IMP on the two fracture faces persists when membranes
are fragmented into right-side out and inside-out vesicles
and thus serves as a useful marker of membrane orientation
(Steck et al., 1970). Some IMP appear to span the full
thickness of the red cell membrane (Weinstein and McNutt,
1970).

Despite the fact that all of the proteins in the red
cell membrane are accessible to chemical and biochemical
probes at one or both of the membrane's natural surfaces,
freeze-etch studies of these surfaces have heretofore been
rather uninformative. The outer surface (ES) of red cells
appears smooth or finely granular. Rugae have been described

at the outer surface (Pinto da Silva et al., 1973) but discrete particles which might correspond to the glycoproteins envisaged by Winzler (1969, 1970) are not apparent (Weinstein, 1974). The cytoplasmic face (i.e. protoplasmic surface, PS) has not been visualized in intact red cells because hemoglobin interferes with deep-etching. The PS surface of isolated membranes, however, shows substructure (Lessin, 1973). While generally smooth, the cytoplasmic surface bears elevated regions or rugae which correspond in distribution to IMP following the induction of IMP aggregation (Pinto daSilva et al., 1973; Seeman and Iles, 1973).

It has been repeatedly suggested that band 3 may be represented in the IMP of red cell membranes. It is also possible that the poles of band 3 projecting from the membrane surfaces contribute to the etched profiles. Nevertheless, the contribution of this protein to freeze-etch images of the natural surfaces of the membrane has not been established.

Therefore, we have examined the natural surfaces of the red cell membrane. In addition, we depleted red cell membranes of specific proteins by selective solubilization and examined the consequences by electron microscopy. Furthermore, the ultrastructural changes accompanying proteolysis were documented. Finally, the specific decoration of band 3, with G3PD, permitted its identification at the cytoplasmic surface.

MATERIALS AND METHODS

Blood was obtained by venipuncture from a single human donor (TLS) and washed 3 times with 150 mM NaCl in 5 mM sodium phosphate buffer (pH 8). The results of some experiments were confirmed on outdated blood from the blood bank. Unless otherwise stated, experimental procedures were performed at 0-5°C. Details of these procedures are described in the figure legends. Standard methods were used to prepare freeze-fracture replicas with a Balzers Model BAF 301 freeze-etch unit.

RESULTS AND DISCUSSION

Ultrastructure of Intramembrane Particles

The ultrastructure of the IMP in intact red cells and isolated membranes was examined following protease digestion. Vigorous proteolysis of unsealed ghosts with chymotrypsin, trypsin or pronase released 50-80 percent of the protein (as estimated according to Lowry et al., 1951) and cleaved all of the membrane polypeptides to small segments (Fig. 1, gels 8-10). However, the IMP_P (compare Figs. 4 and 5) and IMP_E (not illustrated) remained morphologically intact. Clearly, if the IMP are proteins, their retention under these conditions demonstrates a behavior unlike the bulk of the (released) membrane protein.

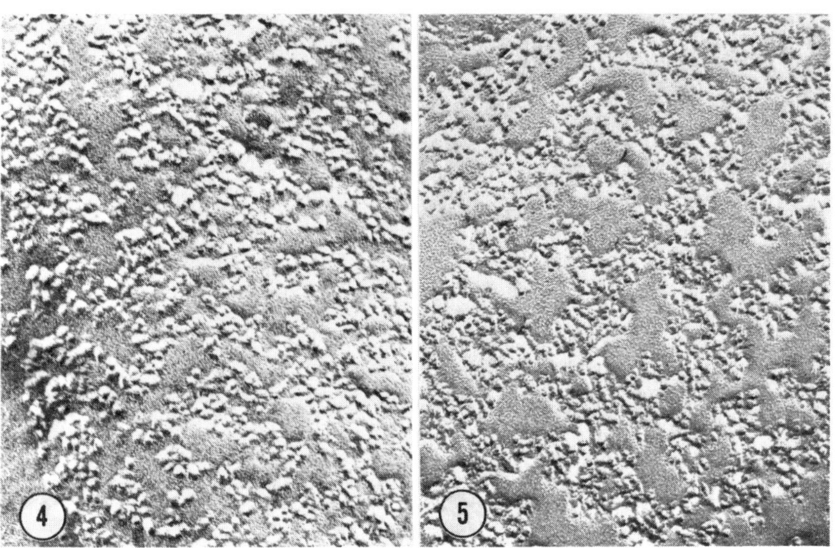

Figure 4 (left) and Figure 5 (right). Effect of proteolysis on IMP_P. Ghosts were incubated with no enzyme (left) or 1 mg/ml chymotrypsin (right). The reaction was terminated with 4mM diisopropylfluorophosphate (DFP) on ice and the samples were then incubated another hour at 23°C. The ultra-structure of the IMP_P was unaltered although PAGE electro-phoresis showed extensive digestion of all proteins (see Fig. 1, gel 10). x 104,000.

Undigested membranes showed minimal clustering of IMP at 0°C; more clustering was seen after incubation at 23°C or 37°C. Prior proteolysis greatly enhanced this temperature dependent process. Vigorous proteolysis led to marked IMP clustering even at 0°C. Since particle redistribution was not observed when proteolysis was performed on sealed ghosts or intact cells, the protease induced redistribution must have been mediated by events at the cytoplasmic surface.

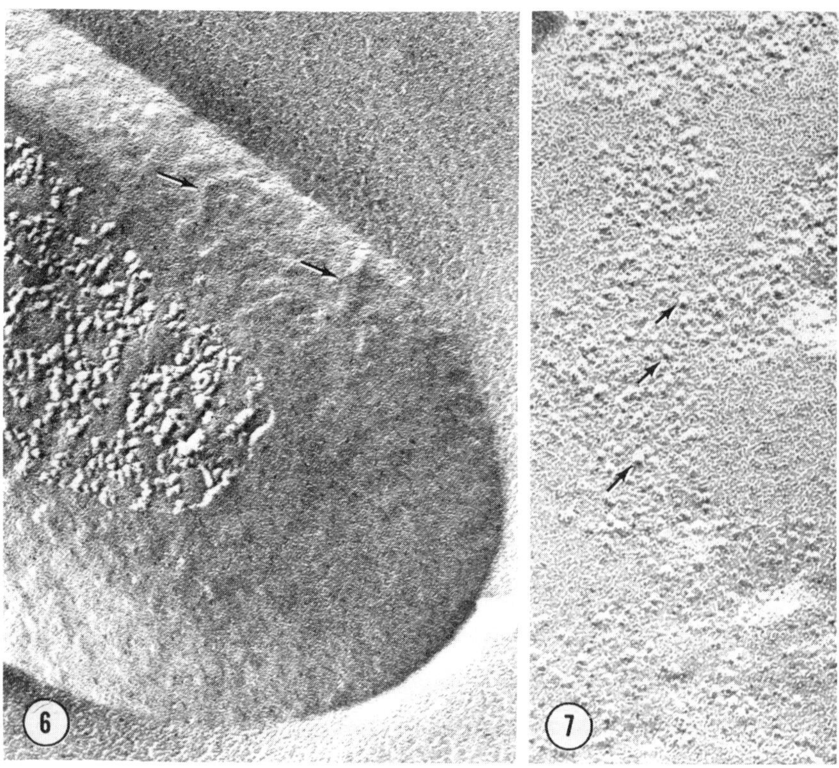

Figure 6. Freeze-etched isolated red cell membrane. There are amorphous mounds at the ES surface (arrows). IMPp are mildly clustered. x 102,000. Figure 7. Freeze-etched extracellular surface (ES) of ghosts following proteolysis. Ghosts were incubated with 1 mg/ml pronase for four hours at 0°C. As a result, there are many 30–50 Å particles at the ES surface (arrows). x 178,000.

Ultrastructure of the True Extracellular Surface

The effects of proteolysis on the natural outer surface of the membrane were striking. The freeze-etched, undigested extracellular surface appeared flat and barren, except for the presence of low mounds or rugae lacking substructure (Fig. 6). However, following proteolysis, a population of discrete 30-50 Å diameter particles was revealed at this surface corresponding to the distribution of the ES mounds (Fig. 7).

Ultrastructure of the Cytoplasmic Surface of Ghosts

The etched cytoplasmic surface of ghosts bore an irregular coarse meshwork which roughly corresponded in distribution to the IMP_P (Fig. 8a). Mild to moderate proteolysis of unsealed ghosts removed most of the meshwork leaving a discrete population of 90 Å globular particles (Fig. 8b). The 90 Å particles were only ablated by prolonged digestion with pronase at 37°C (not shown). The prevalence and the topological distribution of the 90 Å PS particles closely resembled that of the IMP_E population, raising the possibility that freeze-etching is revealing the cytoplasmic surface poles of these intramembrane particles.

Demonstration of Band 3 Protein at the Cytoplasmic Surface.

The PS surface of IO vesicles appeared significantly different from that of ghosts, due to loss of material from a coarse meshwork. This change may be due to the selective loss of spectrin and actin (band 1, 2 and 5) during vesiculation (Steck, 1974b; Marchesi et al., 1976) (compare Figs. 8a and 9). The PS surface of IO vesicles bore an irregular array containing both granulofibrillar material, and discrete 90 Å globular particles (PS particles). These particles were indistinguishable from the PS particles revealed in ghosts by proteolysis. Both of these elements persisted in IO vesicles (Fig. 1, gel 2), even when stripped of nearly all peripheral proteins by extraction with pCMBS or DMMA (Fig. 1, gels 6 and 7). This led us to theorize that the cytoplasmic poles of membrane-integrated proteins, and band 3 in particular, might be major components of the PS array.

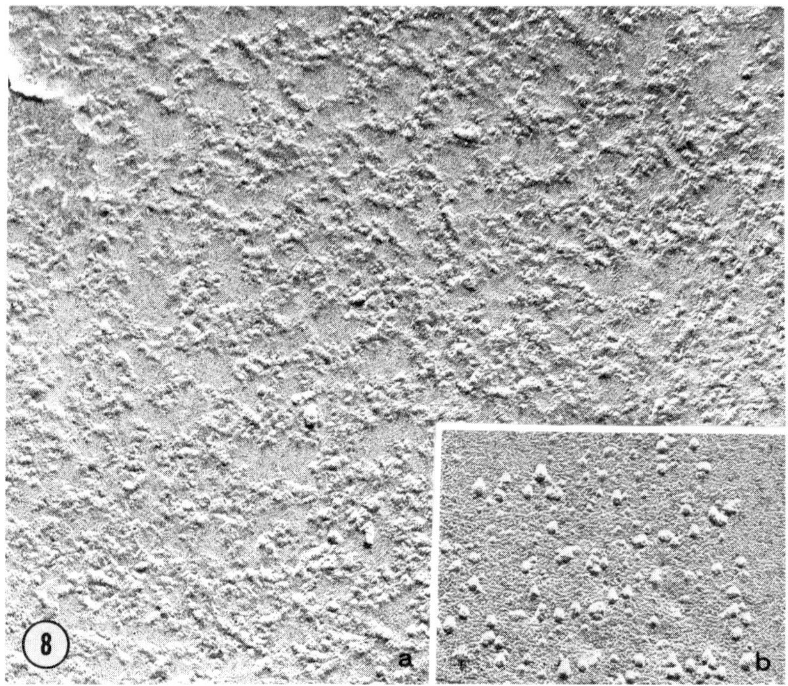

<u>Figure 8a.</u> The cytoplasmic surface (PS) of a ghost membrane.
An irregular coarse meshwork covers this surface. Areas of
membrane within the interstices of the meshwork are smooth.
x 104,000. <u>Figure 8b.</u> The cytoplasmic surface (PS) of unsealed ghosts following proteolysis. Ghosts were incubated
in 50 mM NH_4HCO_3 (pH 7.8) with 0.1 mg/ml chymotrypsin at $37\,^{\circ}C$
for four hours. The enzyme was then inactivated with 1 mM
DFP. Note the appearance of PS particles. x 151,000.

     Further evidence that the cytoplasmic domain of band 3
protein is present in the PS granulofibrillar array was obtained from decoration experiments. Since G3PD binds exclusively to the cytoplasmic domain of band 3 (Yu and Steck,
1975), we used this enzyme to decorate band 3 for ultrastructural studies. After saturating IO vesicles with rabbit
muscle G3PD, many new coarse globular particles were seen
on the granulofibrillar elements of the PS array (Fig. 10).

In contrast, G3PD did not decorate trypsinized IO vesicles from which the G3PD binding domain of band 3 protein had been cleaved (Yu and Steck, 1975; Steck et al., 1976).

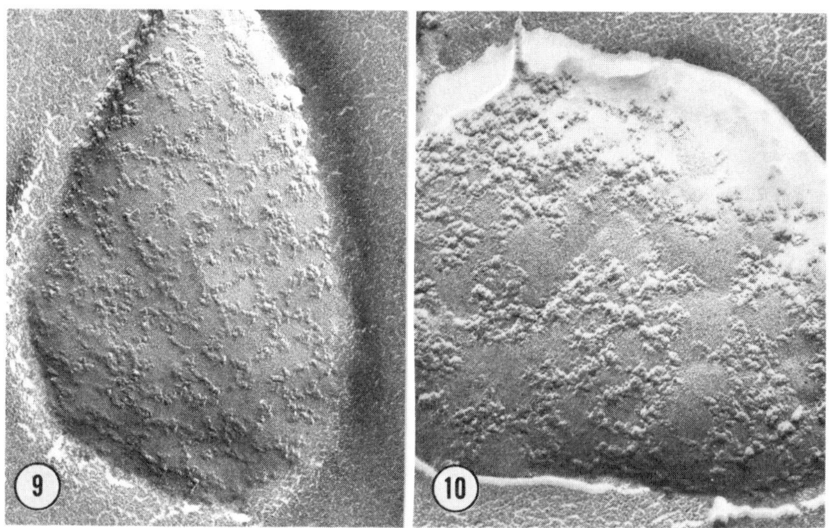

Figure 9. Inside-out (IO) vesicle control (see Fig. 1, gel 2). A granulofibrillar array is present at the surface of the vesicle. x 83,000. Figure 10. IO vesicle decorated with rabbit muscle G3PD as in Fig. 1, gel 4. x 83,000.

ANALYSIS AND CONCLUSIONS

We interpret our data to indicate that the red cell membrane protein, band 3, is represented morphologically in: (a) the outer surface (ES) ridges or mounds of undigested membranes and the novel ES particles seen after protease digestion of that surface; (b) the IMP visualized by freeze-fracture electron microscopy; and (c) the granulofibrillar material found on the etched cytoplasmic face of the membrane. Our reasoning is as follows.

Band 3 is the predominant red cell membrane polypeptide, accounting for roughly 25% of its protein mass (Steck, 1974a). It exists as a dimer in the membrane (Steck, 1972; Yu and Steck, 1975; Peters and Richards, 1977).

Since the protomer has a mass of 90,000 daltons, it has
been suggested that the dimer could account for the entire
mass of an IMP (Steck, 1974a). Another observation which
relates band 3 to the IMP is that there are approximately
600,000 band 3 dimers per ghost (Steck, 1974a) and a similar
number of IMP per human red cell (Weinstein, 1974).

Band 3 is a glycoprotein which spans the membrane
asymmetrically (Fig. 2). It can be proteolytically dissec-
ted into large subfragments representing outer surface,
transmembrane, and inner surface regions of the molecule
(Steck et al., 1976). These studies have suggested that much
of the band 3 molecule is not confined to the lipid bilayer
but projects into the aqueous compartments.

The major glycopeptide fragment generated at the outer
surface has an apparent molecular weight of 38,000, is hydrophobic, and apparently intercalates into the lipid bilayer,
since this segment remains firmly embedded in the membrane
after proteolysis (Steck et al., 1976). This finding suggests a mechanism for the persistence of the ES particles
at the outer surface of the red cell membrane following
proteolysis; that is, the 38,000 dalton domain of the molecule, although nicked, is retained in the membrane, perhaps
still non-covalently bound to the hydrophobic core of the
band 3 molecule.

How ES mounds are converted to particles by proteolysis
is unknown. Intramolecular rearrangements of partially
digested band 3 molecules could be involved. Also, proteolysis may release extracellular surface projections of certain
other proteins (e.g., the proteolytically sensitive sialo-
glycoproteins), but leave in place, although nicked, species
such as band 3. The latter alternative is supported by the
observation that the overall distribution of the mounds in
control preparations is conserved by the ES particles following proteolysis. Quantitative comparison of IMP_p and ES
particle numbers is consistent with this suggestion
(Weinstein, Khodadad and Steck, unpublished data). Digestion of the membrane surface may thus be thinning out a
forest of projecting glycoproteins, unmasking the more stable
structures such as the outer surface region of band 3.

We have presented evidence that the granulofibrillar component of the PS array consists primarily of the cytoplasmic surface extensions of band 3 molecules. This is suggested by: (a) the persistence of both band 3 and the granulofibrillar array after removal of all peripheral proteins from the IO vesicles with DMMA or pCMBS; (b) the exquisite sensitivity of both the band 3 polypeptide (Steck et al., 1976) and the granulofibrillar component to proteolysis; (c) the binding of G3PD to band 3 (Yu and Steck, 1975) and to the granulofibrillar component of the PS array; and (d) the similarity of the topographical distribution of the PS array to that of the IMP_P.

Finally, we have identified a novel population of 90 Å PS particles at the cytoplasmic surface which resists proteolytic digestion and, in other respects, does not correspond to band 3 protein. Based on their topological distribution and quantitation (Weinstein, Khodadad, and Steck, to be published), we suggest that these particles may be the cytoplasmic tips of the IMP_E.

ACKNOWLEDGEMENTS

This work was supported in part by the Office of Naval Research Contract NR 207-002, and American Cancer Society Grant BC-95E. We take pleasure in thanking Elaine Olson, William Leonard, and Benita Ramos for their excellent technical assistance.

REFERENCES:

Branton D (1966). Fracture faces of frozen membranes. Proc Natl Acad Sci USA 55:1048.

Branton D, Bullivant S, Gilula NB, Karnovsky MJ, Moor H, Muhlethaler K, Northcolte DH, Packer L, Satir B, Satir P, Speth V, Staehlin LA, Steere RL, Weinstein RS (1975). Freeze-etching nomenclature. Science (Wash DC) 190:54.

Fairbanks G, Steck TL, Wallach DFP (1971). Electrophoretic analysis of the major polypeptides of the human erythrocyte membrane. Biochemistry 10:2606.

Hainfeld J, Steck TL (1977). The sub-membrane reticulum of the human erythrocyte: a scanning electron microscope study. J Supermol Struct, In press.

Kirkpatrick FH (1976). Spectrin: current understanding of its physical, biochemical and functional properties. Life Sciences 19:1.

Lessin LS (1973). Membrane ultrastructure of normal, sickled and Heinz-body erythrocytes by freeze-etching. In Bessie M, Weed RI, Leblond PF (eds): "Red Cell Shape," New York; Springer-Verlag, p 151.

Lowry OH, Rosebrough NJ, Farr AL, Randall J (1951). Protein measurements with the Folin Phenol reagent. J Biol Chem 193:265.

Marchesi VT, Furthmayer H, Tomita M (1976). The red cell membrane. Annu Rev Biochem 45:667.

Peters K, Richards FM (1977). Chemical cross-linking: reagents and problems in studies of membrane structure. Annu Rev Biochem 46:523.

Pinto da Silva P, Moss PS, Fudenberg HH (1973). Anionic sites on the membrane intercalated particles of human erythrocyte ghost membranes. Freeze etch localization. Exp Cell Res 81:127.

Seeman P, Iles GH (1973). Pits in the freeze-cleavage plane of normal erythrocyte membranes and ultrastructure of membrane lesions in immune lysis. In Bessie M, Weed RI, Leblond PF (eds): "Red Cell Shape," New York: Springer-Verlag, p 169.

Singer SJ (1974). The molecular organization of membranes. Annu Rev Biochem 43:805.

Steck TL (1972). Cross-linking the major proteins of the isolated erythrocyte membrane. J Mol Biol 66:295.

Steck TL (1974a). The organization of proteins in the human red blood cell membrane. J Cell Biol 62:1.

Steck TL (1974b). Preparation of impermeable inside-out and right-side out vesicles from erythrocyte membranes. In Korn ED (ed): "Methods in Membrane Biology," New York: Plenum Press, p 245.

Steck TL, Ramos B, Strapazon E (1976). Proteolytic dissection of band 3, the predominant polypeptide of the human erythrocyte membrane. Biochemistry 15:1154.

Steck TL, Weinstein RS, Straus JM, Wallach DFH (1970). Inside-out red cell membrane vesicles: preparation and purification. Science (Wash DC) 168:255.

Steck TL, Yu J (1973). Selective solubilization of proteins from red blood cell membranes by protein perturbants. J Supramol Struct 1:220.

Strapazon E, Steck TL (1977). Interaction of the aldolase and the membrane of human erythrocytes. Biochemistry 16:2966.

Weinstein RS (1974). Morphology of adult red blood cells. In
   Surgenor DMacN (ed): "The Red Blood Cell," New York:
   Academic Press, p 213.
Weinstein RS (1976). Changes in plasma membrane structure
   associated with malignant transformation in human urinary
   bladder epithelium. Cancer Res 36:2518.
Weinstein RS, Clowes AW, McNutt NS (1970). Unique cleavage
   planes in frozen red cell membranes. Proc Soc Exp Biol
   Med 134:1195.
Weinstein RS, McNutt NS (1970). Electron microscopy of red
   cell membranes. Semin Hemat 7:259.
Winzler RJ (1969). The association of a glycoprotein com-
   ponent of erythrocyte stroma with the cell membrane. In
   Smith RT, Good RA (eds): "Cellular Recognition,"
   New York: Appleton-Century-Crofts, p 11.
Winzler RJ (1970). Carbohydrates in cell surfaces. Int Rev
   Cytol 29:77.
Yu J, Steck TL (1975). Associations of band 3, the pre-
   dominant polypeptide of the human erythrocyte membrane.
   J Biol Chem 250:9176.

DISCUSSION

<u>Dr. Rittenhouse</u>: I gathered from your model of the red cell membrane that the terminal portion of the band 3 glycoprotein loops back into the membrane exposing two regions of the protein to the exterior environment. According to your model, trypsin treatment cleaves the most terminal portion of band 3 leaving the loop region and consequently a portion of the protein oligosaccharide.

<u>Dr. Steck</u>: That's been demonstrated.

<u>Dr. Rittenhouse</u>: Is there a significant amount of carbohydrate in red cell ghosts after trypsin treatment?

<u>Dr. Steck</u>: Yes, chemical analysis of ghosts demonstrate that not all of the carbohydrate is removed from the membrane after trypsin treatment. Several years ago, Shrier, Hoffman Green and others found that several glycolytic enzymes bound to the membrane in vitro and suggested that these could provide a proximal source of energy for transport functions. However, I feel no need to speculate on this matter until we know the state of G3PD in situ. We **are** now studying that problem by both cytochemical and immunoferritin labeling.

<u>Dr. Meyers</u>: We often hear the statement that the membrane is fifty per cent lipid and fifty per cent protein. In your studies, have you taken these factors into account, or the methods for the identification of lipids in the membrane.

<u>Dr. Weinstein</u>: Yes, we have done quantitative **studies** of the membranes. It is generally held that the smooth areas represent the lipid and the particulate areas represent the protein going through the membrane. Now, of course, the hydrophobic segments of the protein which go through the membrane represent a very small percentage of the total protein of the membrane, so we know that the vast majority of protein should be in the surface.

THE ATP-DEPENDENT RED CELL MEMBRANE SHAPE CHANGE:
A MOLECULAR EXPLANATION

Michael P. Sheetz, David Sawyer and Suzanne
Jackowski
Physiology Department
University of Connecticut Health Center
Farmington, Connecticut 06032

SUMMARY

In dissecting the intact erythrocyte membrane with nonionic detergents, we have found spectrin, actin, a distinct
portion of bands 3 (3') and band 4 associated in a proteolipid shell of the erythrocyte. All these components are
resistant to proteolysis when in the intact erythrocyte.
Upon incubation of the proteolipid shells in isotonic media
the electrophoretic mobility of band 4 on sds gels changes
such that component 4.1 moves to the position of 4.2 and
component 3' coalesces into a sharper band. Spectrin is
selectively solubilized from the shells in isotonic media
with divalent cations (isotonic spectrin). The isotonic
spectrin does not differ in molecular weight from spectrin
normally associated with the erythrocyte membrane and does
not retain bound detergent. However, the solubilization of
isotonic spectrin correlates with dephosphorylation of the
protein. Our studies of the ATP-dependent shape change of
erythrocyte ghosts reveal that the rate of the echinocyte
to disc transformation is modified by lectin binding in con-
junction with the membrane ATPase activity. The ATPase
activity was measured in the presence of ouabain, EGTA and
Mg^{+2} and is therefore a membrane-associated Mg^{+2}-ATPase.
When taken together, these results suggest a molecule explanation of the ATP-dependent shape change. The model is
based upon (1) an interaction between lipid-associated proteins and a spectrin-actin complex;(2) a complete submem-
branous network formed by the spectrin-actin complex, and
(3) a Mg^{+2}-ATPase which creates tension in the network
which in turn is translated into a surface area change and

The Red Cell, pages 431—450

concomitant shape change by the lipid-associated proteins.
Detailed proposals are made for future experimental testing.

INTRODUCTION

The shape changes of the human erythrocyte membrane
are of interest since they are similar to the shape changes
of other cells and since an altered erythrocyte morphology
is associated with several disease states. In 1960 Nakao
and coworkers described the crenation of intact erythrocytes upon ATP depletion. Crenation was later related to
the deformability characteristics of the membrane (Weed et
al, 1969) and related to the relative surface areas of the
halves of the membrane bilayer (Sheetz and Singer 1974).
From studies of the ATP-dependent crenation in the intact
cell it is deduced that proteins most likely cause the
shape change directly (Sheetz, et al, 1976). We have been
characterizing the ATP-dependent shape alteration of
erythrocyte ghosts rather than intact cells, however,
because of the practical difficulties in studying the molecular basis of this process in intact cells, e.g., the
problems of controlling cofactor pools and ionic environment. The conversion from an echinocyte to a disc in whole
cells differs from the same conversion in ghosts in that
the ghost membrane will continue the shape change beyond
the biconcave disc-like form to a stomatocyte with endocy-
totic vesicles (Penniston and Green 1968). Other than the
implied absence of some shape regulatory factor, the ATP-
dependent alteration of ghost morphology is very likely the
same as that which occurs in intact cells. There are
probably other mechanisms whereby the erythrocyte can alter
its own shape such as by lipase activation (Allen and
Michell, 1976) but we will not consider them here.

We have recently shown that a bivalent antibody to
spectrin component 1 doubles the rate of transformation of
shape at a ratio of one antibody molecule to 5 to 10
spectrin molecules; a monovalent derivative of the same
antibody does not affect the rate (Sheetz and Singer, 1977).
Antibodies tested thus far to the other membrane proteins
(bands 3 and 4) do not accelerate the transformation (M.
Sheetz, unpublished results), and so the crosslinking of
spectrin probably has a unique and important role in the
shape change process. Given that there are no rigid
structures such as microtubules and microfilament bundles

in the erythrocyte and that the membrane proteins can diffuse laterally (Fowler and Branton, 1977), an attractive molecular explanation of the mechanism involved in the transformation can be proposed, a spectrin network provides the internal structure through which mechanical work can be done.

There is disagreement between Birchmeier and Singer (1977) and Sheetz et al (1977) concerning the role of ATP in the shape change and the development of tension in the spectrin network. Birchmeier and Singer suggest that a kinase activity is active in the phosphorylation of spectrin. This in turn causes spectrin aggregation and this aggregation is the driving force behind the shape change. This conclusion is based on evidence that phosphatase activity inhibits the conversion from echinocyte to disc and that spectrin is phosphorylated when the ghost is crenated prior to the transformation. We will show that spectrin dephosphorylation produces disaggregation of spectrin in accord with the suggestion of Birchmeier and Singer. However, we will also demonstrate that a membrane ATPase rather than a spectrin kinase activity correlates with the rate of transformation (Sheetz et al, 1977). To explain these data, we propose that the shape change depends upon the integrity of the spectrin complex as well as an ATPase which produces tension in that complex.

It is generally agreed that the conversion from a crenated to a biconcave ghost requires the relative expansion of the internal surface of membrane. In terms of the bilayer couple hypothesis (Sheetz and Singer, 1974), oriented proteins hydrolyze ATP to produce an asymmetric change in the membrane surfaces. The means whereby the spectrin complex and the ATPase are attached to the membrane surface, i.e., via lipid or protein interaction, is obviously of interest. We will present evidence that supports the contention that spectrin is bound to discrete lipophyllic proteins. We have devised a method of dissecting the intact erythrocyte with nonionic detergents yielding a complex of spectrin, actin, a portion of band 3 (component 3') and band 4. The elution of spectrin from this complex in isotonic solutions correlates with spectrin dephosphorylation. From a related study of the membrane ATPase, we have found that the modulation of the ATPase activity caused correlates with regulation of the rate of shape change.

MATERIALS AND METHODS

Blood was drawn from healthy donors in a citrate anti-coagulant and used within 2-3 days. Cells were washed (3x by centrifugation at 600g for 10 min) with 146 mM NaCl, 20 mM Tris pH 7.4 (isotris) to remove plasma and the buffy coat. Concanavalin A (Sigma) was purified further by affinity absorption onto Sephadex G-75 in 1M NaCl, 0.5 mM $MnCl_2$, 0.5 mM $CaCl_2$ and 20 mM Tris pH 7.4 and was eluted by 0.1 M α-methylmannoside. All chemicals were reagent grade or better.

Proteolipid Shell Preparation

A washed cell pellet was resuspended at 20% hematocrit in isotris and 6.0 ml of this suspension was mixed with 6.0 ml of a Triton extraction buffer: double the final concentration of Triton X-114 (with [^{3}H]-Triton X-100 added in some cases), 140 mM KCl, 24 mM n-2-hydroxyethylpiperazine-N'-2-ethane sulfonic acid (HEPES), 5 mM reduced glutathione, 1 mM ethyleneglycol-bis (β-aminoethyl ether)-N,N, N',N'-tetraacetate (EGTA), pH 7.0 at 4°C. Ionic conditions were altered in certain experiments where noted. The cells were stirred on ice for 2 to 10 minutes and the total mixture was layered on a 25 ml linear sucrose density gradient (10-50% sucrose) containing 140 mM KCl, 24 mM HEPES, 0.2 mM dithiothreitol (DTT), and 0.5 mM EGTA (pH 7.0). The gradients were centrifuged 120,000g for 2 hours in a SW27 rotor. Protein concentrations were determined by the method of Lowry <u>et al</u>. (1951) and SDS-polyacrylamide gel electrophoresis was performed according to the method of Fairbanks <u>et al</u>. (1971).

Shape Change Assay

The washed cell pellet was diluted to 50% hematocrit and lysed 1:100 in 10 mM Tris, pH 7.4 at 4°C. White ghosts were obtained after two washes in the lysing buffer. Normally 20λ of ghosts diluted 1:1 were added to 100-150λ of H_2O (such that the final volume was 200λ) with 20λ of 10 mM $MgCl_2$, 10 mM ATP, 2 mM EGTA (pH 7.0) with 20λ of 1 4 M KCl, 0.25 M Na HEPES and with 10 mM of the competing sugar where noted. An aliquot of the lectin stock solution was then added on ice and the sample was incubated at 37°C.

Portion (50λ) of the membrane suspension were drawn at
various times and mixed with an equal volume of 2% glutaraldehyde in 140 mM KCL, 10 mM PO_4 (pH 7.0). After 1 hour
samples were viewed in a dark-field light microscope and at
least 250 ghosts were counted as either echinocytes or
disc-like membranes. ATPase activity was assayed by the
method of Lin and Morales (1976).

Spectrin Phosphorylation

Cells were preincubated for 2 hr. in a modified HEPES-
Ringer solution and after washing in isotrix 2x the shells
were prepared. The procedure of Sheetz and Singer (1977)
was used to determine the specific activity of spectrin
component 2 in the various samples.

RESULTS

Proteolipid Shells

Intact erythrocytes were extracted with 0.5% Triton
X-114 in a medium containing 0.14 M KCl, 0.024 M HEPES and
0.5 mM EGTA (pH 7.0), layered on a sucrose gradient and
centrifuged for 2 hr at 120,000g. After centrifugation two
light-scattering bands are evident on the gradient and are
shown in Figure 1. Band I, which has a density of 1.10-
1.15 gm/ml, is not prominent and the amount of light scattering there is variable. When run on SDS-polyacrylamide
electrophoresis gels, the band I materials has two Coomassie blue staining proteins which are portions of components
3 and 4 and has no PAS (Periodic Acid-Schiff reagent)
staining components. The band II material, which we will
refer to as the proteolipid shell, has a density of 1.18-
1.21 gm/ml and it is composed of spectrin, actin, and components 3 and 4. From 1.2 ml of packed cells (∿6.8 mg of
membrane protein) we obtain 2.0-2.5 mg of protein in band
II that is 50-70% spectrin as determined by densitometer
scans of Coomassie blue stained SDS-polyacrylamide gels.

If the concentration of Triton X-114 is varied, then
the density of the proteolipid shell is directly affected
as shown in Table I. An increased detergent concentration
causes an increased density and a decreased phosphate to

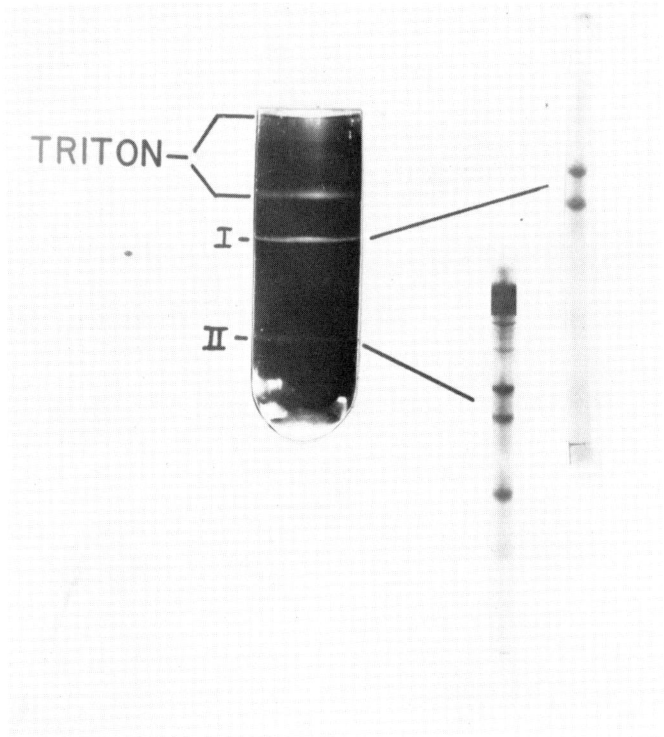

FIG. 1. Isolation of Proteolipid Shells on Sucrose Density
Gradient. Linear sucrose density gradient after preparation of proteolipid shells and SDS-polyacrylamide gel electrophoreses of material in two light-scattering bands.
Intact red cells were extracted with 0.5% Triton, layered
on 10-50% sucrose density gradient, and centrifuged 120,000g
for 2 hr. Gradient shows localization of Triton, light-
scattering Band 1 and Band II material. Polyacrylamide gels
(5.6%) were run on the isolated fractions and stained with
Coomassie blue.

protein ratio of the band II material. Thus a higher concentration of detergent removes more lipid from the band II
proteins. Over the range from 0.2% to 5% Triton X-114 there
is no change in the protein composition of band II as determined by SDS-polyacrylamide gel analysis.

TABLE 1

Effect of Triton Concentration on Proteolipid Shell

Concentration of Triton X-114 in Extraction (%)	Density of Proteolipid Shell (g/ml)	Phosphate/Protein of Proteolipid Shell (μmole/mg)
0.2	1.156	1.00
0.4	1.183	0.60
0.8	1.230	0.24
1.0	1.258	0.10
2.5	1.274	0.04
5.0	1.270	0.04

The shell contains a protein which electrophoreses in the region of the major integral membrane protein of the erythrocyte, Band 3. Knowing that Band 3 is chymotrypsin-sensitive, we treated intact cells with proteases prior to extraction to characterize the protein. As seen in Figure 2 the portion of component 3 in the proteolipid shell is not altered by chymotrypsin nor by a nonspecific bacterial protease. We will call this protease insensitive portion of component 3, component 3'. In addition, density of the shells is not altered by the protease treatment of the intact erythrocytes.

For a long time we puzzled over the fact that the SDS-polyacrylamide gels of the proteolipid shells show variable staining patterns in the component 3' and 4 region. We found that upon overnight dialysis in isotonic salt solutions at 4°C, the material representing component 4.1 moves to the position of 4.2 and component 3' coalesces into a sharper band as seen in figure 3. There is no change in the relative amount of Coomassie blue staining in either the component 3' or 4 region with this conversion. The process, however, is not reversible by dialysis against low

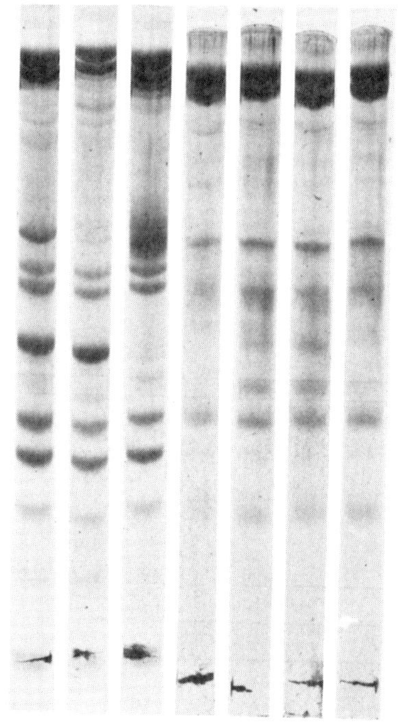

FIG. 2. Proteolipid Shells and White Ghosts of Red Cells Pretreated with Proteases. Intact red cells were pretreated with proteases (200 µg/ml for 1 hr at 37°C) and then washed. White ghosts and proteolipid shells were prepared as described in the text. SDS-polyacrylamide gels were run on the following samples and stained with Coomassie blue:

a) ghosts prepared from chymotrypsinized cells
b) ghosts from bacterial protease treated cells
c) ghosts from control cells
d) proteolipid shells from trypsinized cells
e) proteolipid shells from chymotrypsinized cells
f) proteolipid shells from bacterial protease treated cells
g) proteolipid shells from control cells

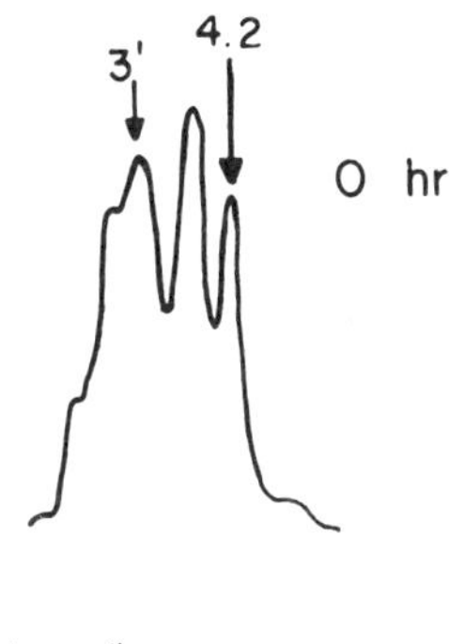

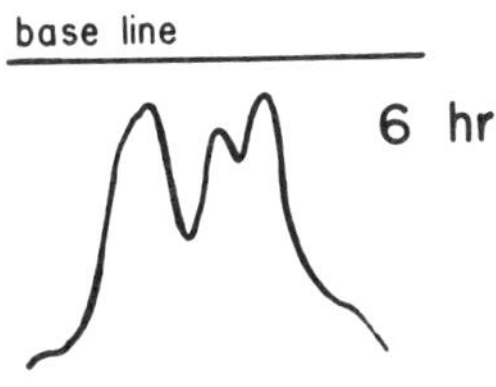

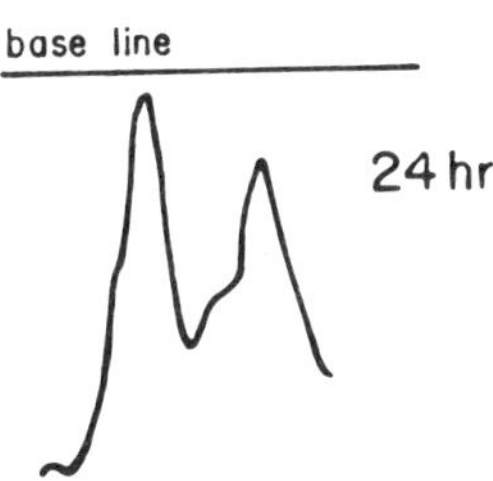

FIG. 3. Conversion of Band 4.1 to 4.2 and Coalescing of Band 3'. Gel scans (OD 550) of portions of SDS-polyacrylamide gel electrophoreses stained with Coomassie blue. Proteolipid shells obtained under hypotonic Triton extraction were adjusted to isotonic salt conditions and incubated at 4°C. Aliquots were removed and 5.6% polyacrylamide gels were run at 0 hr, 6 hr, and 24 hr. Figure shows only the band 3 and band 4 region of the gels.

ionic strength media although proteolipid shells kept in 10 mM HEPES, pH 7.0, do not exhibit any change in their gel staining pattern.

Dialysis of the shells against 0.2 mM Tris, 0.2 mM ATP, 0.2 mM DTT, 0.2 mM EGTA, pH 8.2, results in the solubilization of spectrin and actin. The remaining shells contain a lipoprotein complex including components 3' and 4.2 that appears to be very similar to the Band I material off the sucrose density gradients.

Isotonic Spectrin Solubilization

Spectrin alone is selectively solubilized from the proteolipid shells upon overnight dialysis against isotonic salt solutions containing Mg^{+2} or Ca^{+2}. When the shells are prepared with 0.5% Triton X-114 in 5 mM Mg^{+2} and later dialyzed against isotris plus 0.2 mM DTT and 0.5 mM Mg^{+2}, 45% ± 10% (n = 9) of the shell protein is extracted. The soluble protein is 80-90% spectrin which comigrates on 3.25% SDS-acrylamide gels with spectrin prepared by hypotonic elution from ghosts. (In this electrophoretic system spectrin components 1 and 2 can be separated by 0.7 cm.) When purified by velocity sedimentation, the spectrin isolated under isotonic conditions ("isotonic spectrin") contains less than 1 mole of Triton per mole of spectrin dimer. Gel scans are presented in figure 4.

The solubilization of spectrin from the shells is correlated with spectrin dephosphorylation. In Table 2 we show that the kinetics of spectrin dephosphorylation and solubilization are related. The amount of spectrin released from the shells is dependent upon the presence of Mg^{+2} -- more spectrin is released upon incubation with Mg^{+2} than upon incubation without this cation. In addition, more phosphate is released from the shells in the presence of Mg^{+2} and this fact is supportive of the positive correlation between spectrin solubilization and dephosphorylation. The maximal specific activity of spectrin solubilized from the shell is 50% of that of spectrin in the shell prior to solubilization or spectrin in Tris ghosts of the same cells.

In figure 5 electron micrographs of the negative stained shells before and after spectrin solubilization demonstrate the presence of filaments the size of actin filaments; the negative stained isotonic spectrin definitely lacks filaments and appears almost amorphous. These qualitative observations concur with our biochemical evidence that isotonic spectrin is selectively solubilized from actin and the other protein components in the proteolipid shells.

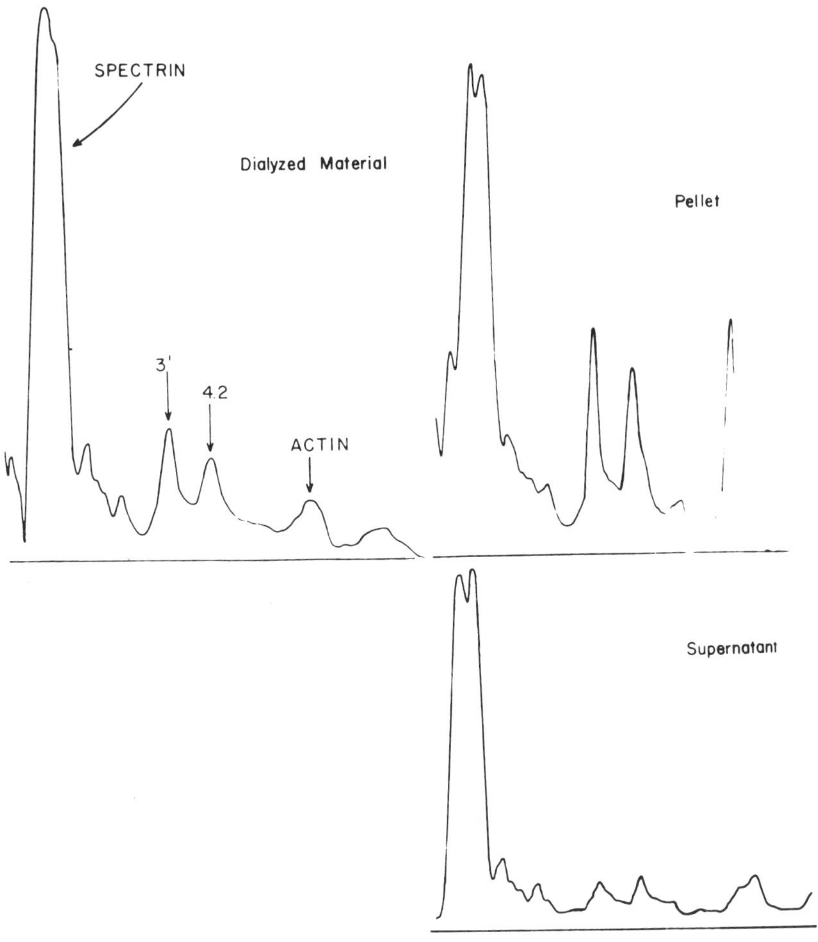

FIG. 4. Proteolipid Shells and Isotonic Spectrin Solubilization. Gel scans (QD 550) of SDS-polyacrylamide gel electrophoreses stained with Coomassie blue. Proteolipid
shells dialyzed overnight at 4°C; pellet and supernatant
obtained from 20 min spin of proteolipid shells at 140,000g.

Correlation of the Shape Change with Membrane ATPase
Activity

The plant lectins, Concanavalin A (Con A) and Anti-H
lectin (<u>Ulex europeus</u>), alter the rate of the ATP-dependent

TABLE 2

Solubilization and Dephosphorylation of Spectrin

Time at 25°C (hr)	Solubilization of Protein (%)[a]	Specific Activity of [^{32}P]-Labelled Spectrin
0	0	1.00[b]
1	18	0.50
2	30	0.38
4	41	0.25

[a]Amount protein solubilized relative to total present in proteolipid shell.

[b]Specific activity of spectrin component 2 in the proteolipid shell before solubilization defined as 1.00; other values denote relative specific activities of solubilized spectrin component 2.

shape change and the membrane ATPase activity of erythrocyte ghosts (Sheetz et al., 1977) Con A inhibits both processes whereas Anti-H lectin stimulates them. These lectin effects are saturated at low levels of bound lectin (less than 10,000 molecules per cell) whether the lectins are added exogenously to the assay mixture containing ghosts, or the lectins are bound to intact red cells prior to ghost preparation. [There are approximately 10^6 binding sites for Con A per ghost (Rehfeld et al., 1975; Phillips et al., 1974).] The lectin effects are not detectable when 10 mM of the competing sugar (α-methylmannoside in the case

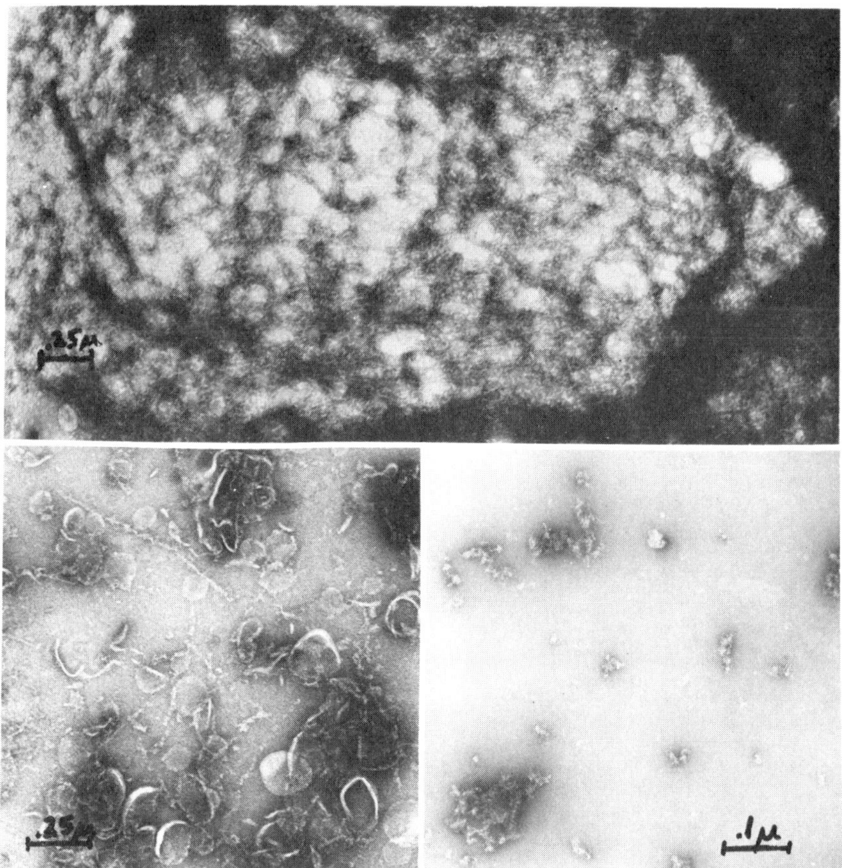

FIG. 5. Electron Microscopy of Proteolipid Shells. Top: proteolipid shell, negative stained; Bottom left: proteolipid shell after removal of spectrin, negative stained; Bottom Right: spectrin after elution from shell, negative stained.

of Con A and fucose in the case of Anti-H lectin) is added to the assay mixture. Trypsinization of intact red cells with 50 µg/ml for 15 minutes at 37°C prior to ghost preparation also abrogates the lectin effects on the shape change and the ATPase. Table 3 shows the inhibition of the echinocyte to disc transformation as well as the ATPase activity. It also includes the results obtained after

TABLE 3

Correlation of Shape Change and ATPase Activity

Ghost Assay Mixture	Shape Change-Disc-Shaped Ghosts*		ATPase Activity*	
	Absolute %	Fraction Relative to control	$\left(\dfrac{\mu\text{moles PO}_4}{\text{mg prot/hr}}\right)$	Fraction Relative to control
Control	74.6	1.00	0.250	1.00
Ouabain (5×10^{-4}M)	76.9	1.03	0.244	0.98
Con A -10 ug/ml	60.1	0.81	0.235	0.90
-50 ug/ml	56.7	0.76	0.215	0.86
Con A (pretreated 100 ug/ml)[a]				
prep I[b]	62.3	0.83	0.178	0.71
II	47.7	0.64	0.161	0.64
III	33.4	0.45	0.123	0.49
Trypsin (pretreated 50 ug/ml)[c]	69.7	0.93	0.219	0.88
Trypsin (pretreated 50 ug/ml)+	68.4	0.92	0.229	0.92
Con A -10 ug/ml	72.3	0.97	0.216	0.86
-50 ug/ml	69.5	0.93	0.232	0.93

*After incubation for 15 min at 37°C.

[a]Con A incubated with intact RBC's 30 min at 37°C before ghost preparation.

[b]Representative of variations among Con A preparations.

[c]Trypsin incubated with intact RBC's 10 min at 37°C before ghost preparation.

trypsinization and when ouabain, 5×10^{-4} molar, is added to the mixture. Ouabain has no effect on either the shape change or the ATPase activity and, recalling that the assay mixture contains 0.2 mM EGTA, we conclude that the ATPase involved in the shape change is a Mg^{+2}-ATPase.

DISCUSSION

We have already discussed these data in a critical fashion in three other manuscripts presently in press (Sawyer and Sheetz, 1977, Sheetz and Sawyer, 1977; Sheetz et.al; 1977). Here we propose a molecular mechanism for the ATP-dependent shape change of erythrocyte ghosts that is derived from the existing data and easily lends itself to further experimentation. The model is put forth as a possibility and remains to be tested.

We propose that the four proteins in the proteolipid shells are the basis of the shape change complex. Other molecules can and do interact with these proteins to effect or alter the shape transformation. Our understanding of the system suggests that there are three main requirements for the ATP-dependent process:
1. Lipid-associated proteins must bind the spectrin-actin complex to the membrane.
2. The spectrin-actin complex must form an integrated two-dimensional network beneath the membrane.
3. A membrane ATPase must do work to create tension in the spectrin-actin complex. This tension development is converted into a asymmetric surface area change via the proteins linking the spectrin-actin complex to the membrane.

Assuming that the above conditions must be satisfied for the alteration of shape to occur, several factors present themselves as points of control. Namely, the rate of transition from the echinocyte to the disc-like ghost would be influenced by (1) the membrane ATPase activity, and (2) the binding affinity of the lipid-associated proteins for the spectrin-actin complex, which both depend upon the ionic and cofactor concentrations. The regulation of the biconcave shape of the intact cell probably involves additional proteins. As an example, the disease state of hereditary spherocytosis which represents a defect in shape regulation could result from an alteration of any of the proteins in the shape change complex and/or accessory regulatory proteins.

There has been considerable interest in the interaction of spectrin with the erythrocyte membrane; both lipids (Juliano et al., 1971; Sweet and Zull, 1970) and proteins (Bennett and Branton, 1977) have been proposed as anchoring sites on the membrane. Spectrin prepared under hypotonic conditions is capable of interacting with lipids but intramolecular electrostatic repulsions generated by hypotonic preparation may partially denature the protein. Thus, the lipid affinity may not be physiologically relevant. Indeed, the binding of hypotonically prepared spectrin to inside-out vesicles is clearly dependent upon the presence of membrane protein (Bennett and Branton, 1977). Also, the isotonic spectrin solubilized from proteolipid shells does not show any lipophyllic character. High detergent concentrations remove nearly all of the lipid from the shell and the solubilized spectrin has no detergent associated with it. Protein components 3' and 4, in contrast to the lipid, remain attached to the spectrin-actin complex over a wide range of detergent concentrations. The evidence of other investigators also indicates that component 4 interacts with spectrin. This work entailed analyses of Triton extracted ghosts (Steck and Yu, 1973) and the proteins crosslinked by a Ca^{+2}-activated transglutaminase (Lorand et al., 1976). Taking these data together, we suggest that component 4 forms a stable association with spectrin and provides the membrane attachment site for the spectrin-actin network. It is uncertain whether components 4.1 and 4.2 are different proteins or are, in fact, different forms of the same protein so we will not differentiate between them at this time. Component 3' may also bind to spectrin or it may associate with component 4 but it has not been studied in detail as a protein distinct from the majority of band 3.

Many investigators have proposed that a spectrin network lies beneath the erythrocyte membrane (for review see Kirkpatrick, 1976) and that the spectrin network is responsible for controlling shape, deformability and surface protein distribution in the erythrocyte. In the micrographs of the negatively stained shells there are very distinct filamentous structures of the size of actin filaments. This suggests that filamentous actin, in addition to spectrin, plays an important role in forming the network.

Although electron microscopic observations of filaments in shells do not prove their existence in vivo, we have confirmed that hypotonic spectrin extracts from fresh erythrocytes promote actin polymerization (M. Sheetz unpublished results) as have others (D. Birchmeier and Singer, S. Lux, and Shotten and Taylor unpublished results). The contrary observation was made with a hypotonic spectrin extract made over a relatively long time from outdated material (Tilney and Detmers, 1975). We propose that the spectrin and filamentous actin network forms a structural base of the erythrocyte membrane. Proteolipid shells prepared in hypotonic salt solutions contain decreased amounts of components 3' and 4. Because the majority of the spectrin and actin still sediments as a proteolipid shell even when the amounts of components 3' and 4 are decreased, the spectrin-actin network as a unit appears to encompass the inner surface of erythrocyte membrane without being linked together by components 3' and 4.

Spectrin solubilization from the spectrin-actin complex in isotonic media is correlated with spectrin dephosphorylation. The phosphatase inhibition of the membrane shape change (Birchmeier and Singer, 1977) was also interpreted as an effect of dephosphorylation on spectrin aggregation. We propose that the hydrolysis of one of spectrin's phosphate moieties causes it to be released from the network but not from spectrin's membrane attachment site. In this way the cell could alter the network structure to adjust to deformations and spectrin would remain concentrated at the membrane interface during the process.

Although ATP hydrolysis is generally thought to be required for the shape change, there is disagreement about whether a spectrin kinase (Birchmeier and Singer, 1977) or membrane ATPase (Sheetz et al., 1977) drives the transformation. The inhibition of the shape change by phosphatases (Birchmeier and Singer, 1977) can be explained as a disruption of the spectrin-actin network resulting from dephosphorylation of the spectrin molecule; the effect need not imply that phosphorylation drives the shape change. On the contrary, we find that alteration of the rate of the ATP-dependent shape change in the presence of lectins always correlates with alteration of the Mg^{+2}-ATPase activity rather than with the spectrin kinase activity. The Mg^{+2}-ATPase and shape change are assayed under conditions where there is no detectable ouabain-sensitive

ATPase activity and where the Ca^{+2} concentration is less than 10^{-8} molar, thereby excluding the direct involvement of either a Na^+, K^+-ATPase or a Ca^{+2}-activated ATPase. Higher Ca^{+2} concentrations, in fact, inhibit the shape change. This inhibition of the shape transformation by Ca^{++} is probably the result of depletion of the substrate utilized by both the Ca^{+2}-activated and the Mg^{+2}-ATPase. We propose that a myosin-like ATPase, Mg^{+2}-rather than Ca^{+2}-activated, drives the shape change by creating tension in the spectrin-actin network. Experiments are underway to isolate the ATPase involved in the shape change.

We feel that the explanations presented here are consistent with the current data on the ATP-dependent shape change of erythrocyte ghosts. As with many other biological processes, cell shape alterations appear to depend upon a number of proteins. We have identified four proteins as components of the shape change complex in ghosts presume that there are more proteins involved. Only by examining in more detail all the components of the complex can we hope to understand the mechanism whereby the biconcave shape is maintained.

ACKNOWLEDGEMENTS

We thank Dr. Phillip Stritmatter for his gift of $[^3H]$-Triton. This research was supported by NIH grant #HL 18317.

REFERENCES

Allan D, Watts R, Michell R (1976). Production of 1,2-diacylglycerol and phosphatidate in human erythrocytes treated with calcium ions and ionophore A 23187. Biochem J 156:225.

Bennet, Branton D (1977). Selective association of spectrin with the cytoplasmic surface of human erythrocyte plasma membranes. J Biol Chem 252:2753.

Birchmeier W, Singer SJ (1977). On the mechanism of ATP-induced shape changes in human erythrocyte membranes. II The role of ATP. J Cell Biol 73:647.

Fairbanks G, Steck TL, Wallach DFH (1971). Electrophoretic analysis of the major polypeptides of the human erythrocyte membrane. Biochem 10:2606.

Fowler V, Branton D (1977). Lateral mobility of human
   erythrocyte integral membrane proteins. Nature 268:23.
Juliano RL, Kimelberg HK, Papahadjopoulos D (1971). Syner-
   gistic effects of a membrane protein (spectrin) and Ca^{2+}
   on the Na^+ permeability of phospholipid vesicles.
   Biochim Biophys Acta 241: 894.
Kirkpatrick FH (1976). Spectrin: Current understanding of
   its physical, biochemical, and functional properties.
   Life Sci 19:1.
Lin TI, Morales MF (1977). Application of a one step procedure for measuring inorganic phosphate in the presence
   of proteins: the actomyosin ATPase system. Anal Biochem
   71:10.
Lorand L, Weissmann LB, Epel DL, Lorand JB (1976). Role of
   the intrinsic transglutaminase in the Ca^{2+}-mediated
   crosslinking of erythrocyte proteins. Proc Natl Acad
   Sci USA 73:4479.
Lowry OH, Rosebrough NJ, Farr AL Randall RJ (1951). Protein
   measurements with the Folin phenol reagent. J Biol Chem
   193:265.
Nakao M, Nakao T, Yamazoe S (1960). Adenoside triphosphate and maintenance of shape of the human red cells.
   Nature 187:945.
Penniston JT, Green DE (1968). The conformational basis of
   energy transformations in membrane systems. IV Energized
   states and pinocytosis in erythrocyte ghosts. Arch
   Biochem Biophys 128:339.
Phillips PG, Furmanski P, Lubin M (1974). The interaction
   of albumin and concanavalin A with normal and sickle
   human erythrocytes. Biochem Biophys Res Comm 66:586.
Sawyer D, Sheetz MP (1977). Proteolipid shells from intact
   erythrocytes. Submitted.
Sheetz MP, Jackowski S, Sawyer D (1977). On the transmembrane control of ATP induced shape changes in human
   erythrocyte membranes. I Correlation with membrane
   ATPase activity. Submitted.
Sheetz MP, Painter RG, Singer SJ (1976). The contractile
   proteins of erythrocyte membranes and erythrocyte shape
   changes. In Pollard TD, Rosenbaum J (eds): "Cell
   Motility," New York: Cold Spring Harbor Laboratory,
   p 651.
Sheetz MP, Sawyer D (1977). Isotonic spectrin I. Solubilization. Submitted.
Sheetz MP, Singer SJ (1974). Biological membranes as
   bilayer couples A molecular mechanism of drug-erythro-
   cyte interactions. Proc Natl Acad Sci USA 71:4457.

Sheetz MP, Singer SJ (1977). On the mechanism of ATP-
    induced shape changes in human erythrocyte membranes. I
    the role of the spectrin complex. J Cell Biol 73:638.
Sweet C, Zull JE (1970). Interaction of the erythrocyte-
    membrane protein, spectrin, with model membrane systems.
    Biochem Biophys Res Comm 41:135.
Tilney LG, Detmers P (1975). Actin in erythrocyte ghosts
    and its association with spectrin. J Cell Biol 66:508.
Weed RI, LaCelle PL, Merrill EW (1969). Metabolic depen-
    dence of red cell deformability. J Clin Invest 48:795.
Yu J, Fischman D, Steck T (1973). Selective solubilization
    of proteins and phospholipids from red blood cell mem-
    branes by nonionic detergents. J Supramol Struct 1:233.

<u>Unidentified speaker</u>: You may have two, three, or four slightly different proteins. Have you tried doing three-dimensional gel electrophoresis on these to see if in fact you are dealing with a version of the same thing or whether they are slightly different, both the spectrin and the band III proteins?

<u>Dr. Sheetz</u>: We have not done that but other people have done spectrin on two-dimensional iso electric focusing and second-dimension SDS gels and have found that it seems to be a single feature. And we isolated here at least 50% of the spectrin from that expected to be in the intact erythrocyte as this isotonic structure, and we have no reason to believe that this represents a sub-population of the structure.

<u>Dr. Greenquist</u>: Have you looked at the effect of alkaline, phosphatase on release of spectrin from the shells?

<u>Dr. Sheetz</u>: We have tried some preliminary experiments. The activity of alkaline phosphatase that we added has not been sufficient to cause any change in the dephosphorylation rate. We are afraid of adding proteases with the alkaline phosphatase since they are very often contaminated with proteases.

<u>Dr. Greenquist</u>: Can you comment on the possibility that shells that are produced in 0.2% Triton may be an artifact induced by that concentration of Triton?

<u>Dr. Sheetz</u>: That's a possibility. We have tried to check by preparing a mixture of erythrocytes and putting them on a sucrose layer. We have a second sucrose layer underneath that initial sucrose layer so that we are now sedimenting the intact erythrocytes into a Triton layer, so that they are not in the Triton any longer than the time it takes them to sediment into the layer. And in those cases we find the same proteins are associated in the isolated shells. There is always the possibility that Triton is causing a change in conformation of the components 2.9 and 4, which causes them to bind to spectrin or actin.

<u>Dr. Fung</u>: Do you have NaCl in the SDS gel and in the sucrose

The Red Cell, pages 451–452

gradient experiments?

Dr. Sheetz: The sucrose gradient we try to make isotonic, to mimic the KCl environment of the cell, and it contains 0.14M KCl.

Dr. Roses: With regards to spectrin being a single component, have you done two-dimensional electrophoresis? We have found several components of spectrin on isoelectric focusing gels.

Dr. Sheetz: I think there are a lot of people who look with some skepticism on the isoelectric focusing experiments, and I don't think the story is complete. What I am saying is that we have no indications from our work that spectrin is not a single species.

EFFECTS OF HEAT AND METABOLIC DEPLETION ON ERYTHROCYTE
DEFORMABILITY, SPECTRIN EXTRACTABILITY AND PHOSPHORYLATION

Narla Mohandas, Alfred C. Greenquist,
and Stephen B. Shohet
Departments of Laboratory Medicine and
Medicine, Cancer Research Institute,
University of California San Francisco, CA 94143

SUMMARY

Both heating and metabolic depletion result in a
reduction of erythrocyte deformability and spectrin
extractability from membranes. Heated erythrocytes also
show a temperature-dependent reduction in spectrin
phosphorylation measured in isolated membranes. During
metabolic depletion when ATP drops to about 15% of normal,
spectrin begins to rapidly dephosphorylate to about 50%
of the initial labelling value. Possibly as a consequence
of spectrin rearrangement, no further dephosphorylation
occurs. During dephosphorylation initial echinocyte shape
changes take place; a progressive increase of first echinocytes I, II, and then III appear. The spheroechinocytes
appear at a later time.

Results of the various experiments suggest that
deformability and spectrin extractability are interrelated.
Both heating at 47° and metabolic depletion cause an
equivalent alteration in both properties. Extended incubation
with Ca^{++} during metabolic depletion or heating at 50° leads
to a secondary transition in both properties producing an
undeformable cell and unextractable spectrin. These results
support the hypothesis that spectrin is involved in the
regulation of erythrocyte membrane deformability.

INTRODUCTION

Identifying the biochemical determinants in cellular

The Red Cell, pages 453–472

deformability and shape control is an intriguing problem.
For the red cell, adequate deformability is a prerequisite
for passage through restricted areas of the microvasculature;
altered deformability may be a common pathway for a number
of diseases which cause hemolytic anemia. Cell deformability may also be important in controlling release of
reticulocytes from the bone marrow (Leblond et al., 1971).

In the erythrocyte, cell shape and deformability are
influenced by both structural and dynamic components. The
essential structural components for shape and deformability
control appear to be contained within the membrane since
isolated membranes can retain the biconcave shape (Ponder,
1971), and possess deformability properties similar to
those of the intact cell (LaCelle and Weed, 1969). One of
the membrane components favored as a possible structural
entity is spectrin, which consists of Bands 1 and 2 on an
SDS - polyacrylamide gel of electrophoresed membrane
proteins. These bands make up about 25% of the membrane
protein (Fairbanks et al., 1971) and they may contain
multiple components (Fuller et al., 1974). The involvement
of spectrin in cell shape is suggested by the observation
that isolated membranes rapidly fragment (Steck et al.,
1971, Hoogeveen et al., 1970) under conditions which
release spectrin (but also erythrocyte actin). Further,
spectrin appears to weakly cross react with an anti-human
uterine myosin (Painter et al., 1975), suggesting a
possible contractile mechanism for spectrin in the regulation of cell shape. In mice with the genetic trait
sph/sph, spectrin is virtually absent and the red cells
are profoundly spheroidal. They are also anisocytic and
possess numbers of microcytic forms which probably arise from
the release of exocytic vesicles. Membranes isolated from
these cells are unstable and rapidly fragment (Greenquist
and Shohet, 1975b).

The dynamic component of cell shape and deformability
control is evidenced by sensitivity of the cell to metabolic
depletion. The metabolically depleted erythrocyte is
transferred from a biconcave disc to a spheroidal form,
the spheroechinocyte (Nakao and Nakao, 1960; Weed et al.,
1969), with reduced deformability (Weed et al., 1969). This
transformation can be reversed by reincubation with adenosine.
The transformation has often been considered to be closely
linked to ATP levels in the cells (Weed et al., 1969). The

linkage cannot be direct, however, since cells devoid of ATP by incubation with iodoacetate can maintain normal morphology and deformability for nearly two hours (Feo and Mohandas, 1977).

Spectrin is also a substrate for phosphorylation by membrane bound protein kinases (Guthrow et al., 1972; Rubin et al., 1972; Roses and Appel, 1973). Intact cells incubated with $^{32}P_i$ show incorporation of label into spectrin band 2 (Palmer and Verpoorte, 1971; Greenquist and Shohet, 1975a, 1976; Shapiro and Marchesi, 1977). The labelled erythrocyte can exhibit reversible spectrin phosphorylation and dephosphorylation depending upon the metabolic state of the cells (Greenquist and Shohet, 1975a, 1976).

In the current study changes in erythrocyte morphology and deformability induced by heat or metabolic depletion are compared to changes in spectrin extractability from membranes and to the spectrin phosphorylation reaction.

METHODS

Preparation of Erythrocyte and Erythrocyte Membranes

Blood was collected in heparinized tubes from normal donors and passed over cotton to remove white cells (Beutler 1975), then washed 3 times in 5 volumes of isotonic phosphate buffered (0.01M, pH 7.4) saline (PBS). Isolated membranes were prepared by hypotonic hemolysis, repeated centrifugation, and washings with .01M sodium phosphate, pH 8.0.

Heating and Spectrin Extraction

Aliquots of an erythrocyte suspension were added to PBS prewarmed to the specified temperature + 0.05°. The hematocrit was 10%. At the end of the incubation the cell suspension was transferred to ice. The cells were centrifuged and membranes were isolated as above. For extraction isolated membranes were suspended in 40 volumes of 0.1 mM EDTA, pH 8.0 and heated to 37° for 15 min. This suspension was centrifuged at 39,100 x g for 45 min. The "extract pellet" was stored frozen before analysis.

Sodium Dodecyl Sulfate - Polyacrylamide Gel Electrophoresis
(SDS PAGE)

SDS-PAGE was performed as previously described (Weber
and Osborn, 1969) on membranes using 5% polyacrylamide
gels. For analyses requiring solubilization of gel segments,
7.5% gels were prepared using N, N diallyl tartardiamide
as a crosslinker and 2% periodic acid as a solubilizing
agent (Anker, 1970). Staining was done with Coomasie
Brilliant Blue (Fairbanks et al., 1971) either overnight
or at 60° for 2 hrs with equivalent results. Spectrin
extractability was evaluated by scanning the SDS-PAGE gels
of extract pellets and determining the ratio of spectrin:
Band 3 by densitometry.

Deformability

Measurements of deformability were made using an
Ektacytometer as previously described (Bessis and Mohandas,
1975; Allard et al., 1977). A 75 μl aliquot of cell
suspension was transferred to 5 ml of a phosphate buffered
dextran solution (25 g of dextran, average m.w. 40,000, in
100 ml of .01M sodium phosphate, pH 7.4, made to 285 mOsm
with NaCl). Measurements were made on photographic negatives
of the diffraction pattern produced by the deformed cells
at a shear stress of 500 dynes/cm^2.

Phosphorylation Reactions

For casein kinase activity 50 μg of ghost membrane
protein were assayed in 200 μl final volume containing
.025 M imadazole HCl, pH 7.0, 10 mg/ml casein, 10 mM MgCl$_2$,
2 mM γ-^{32}P-ATP ($\sim$4 x 10^5 cpm), 0.5 mM EGTA, ImM DTT incubated
at 37° for 5 or 10 min. Endogenous phosphorylation in
isolated membranes were run as previously described
(Greenquist and Shohet, 1974).

Whole cell phosphorylation was performed at 37° at
10% hematocrit in .025 M imidazole.HCl, pH 7.4, made isotonic
with NaCl, .015 M glucose, 250 units/ml of penicillin, and
250 mg/ml of streptomycin containing about 2 x 10^8 cpm of
^{32}P$_i$ per ml of suspension. For metabolic depletion studies,
after labelling for 10-20 hrs cells were washed 3 times
in PBS, pH 7.4, and resuspended to 10% hematocrit in PBS

containing penicillin/streptomycin as above. For analysis
of spectrin phosphorylation the reaction was stopped by
the addition of 100 μl of a solution containing 10% SDS,
25% sucrose, 50 mM DTT, 25 mM EDTA to 100 μl of cell
suspension. Frozen aliquots of the suspension were stored
and the analysis of spectrin ^{32}P made after SDS PAGE.

Other Procedures

ATP was measured using a luciferin-luciferase assay
(Beutler, 1971). Morphology was examined by phase
microscopy after fixation in 0.2% glutaraldehyde in Isoton
(Coulter Diagnostics). Tryptic digestion of isolated
membranes of heat treated cells was performed as previously
described (Greenquist and Shohet, 1974).

RESULTS

Heat Effects

<u>Heat Effects on Erythrocyte Morphology and Deformability.</u>
Erythrocytes exposed to elevated temperatures up to 49° showed
no change in cell shape. No changes were observed in cellular
ATP or in mean cell volumes when analyzed in a Coulter model
Z_H particle size analyzer (not shown). At 50°, however, cells
began to rapidly sphere and fragment as shown in Figure 1.

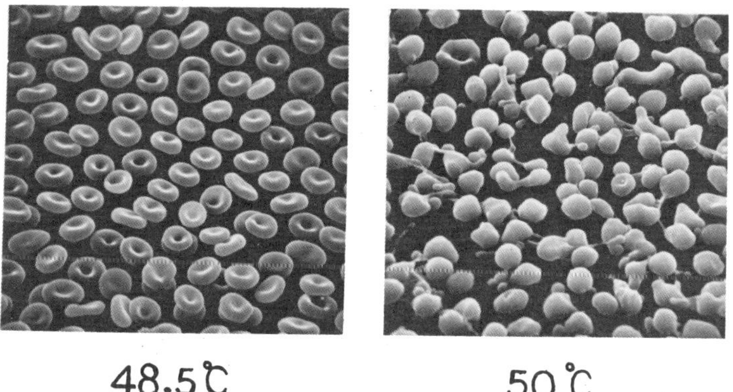

Figure 1. Scanning electron micrographs of erythrocytes
heated to 48.5° and 50° for 10 min.

The effects of elevated temperature on red cell deformability as measured by the Ektacytometer are shown in Figure
2. Up to 46°, heating erythrocytes for 10 min produced
no change in cellular deformability. Above 46°, red cells
showed a progressive time- and temperature-dependent decrease
in deformability and at 50°, they became undeformable.

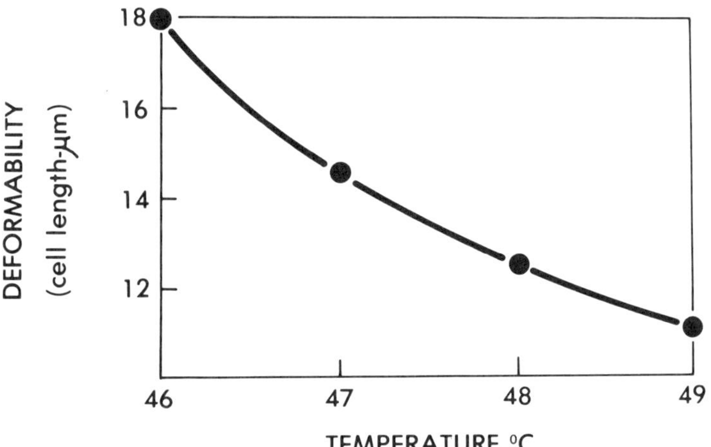

Figure 2. The effect of heating for 4 min at various
temperatures on the deformability of erythrocytes.

The change in deformability at any temperature is time
dependent as shown in Figure 3. At 47° a progressive
decrease in deformability occurred up to 6 min. No further
change in deformability occurred for at least 1 hr.

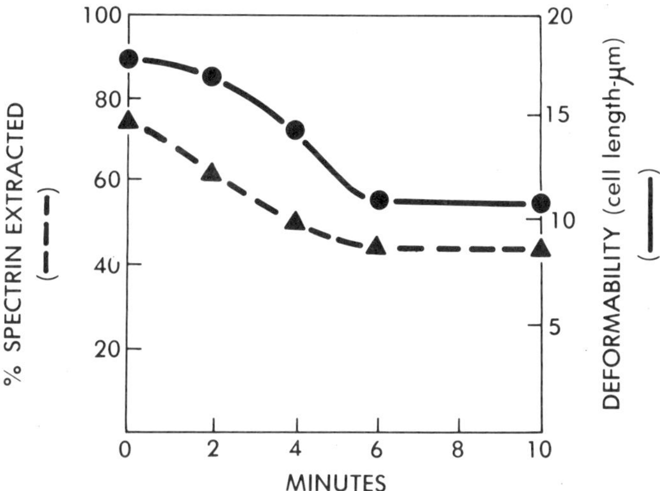

Figure 3. The effect of heating as a function of time at
47° on the deformability (0-0) and spectrin extractability
(Δ - Δ) of erythrocytes.

Heat Effects on the Extractability of Spectrin from
Membranes. The exposure of isolated erythrocyte membranes
to very low ionic strength media produced a rapid release of
several membrane polypeptides. Band 1 and 2 (spectrin) and
Band 5 (actin) were released. The kinetics of the release
reaction at 37° for spectrin in the presence of 0.1 mM EDTA,
pH 8.0 are shown in Figure 4. Most of the spectrin
extraction from both unheated and 48° heated cells occurred
within 15 min. About 70% of the material in the spectrin
position was released from membranes of unheated cells.
Most of the unextracted residual material was found in the
Band 2 component of spectrin.

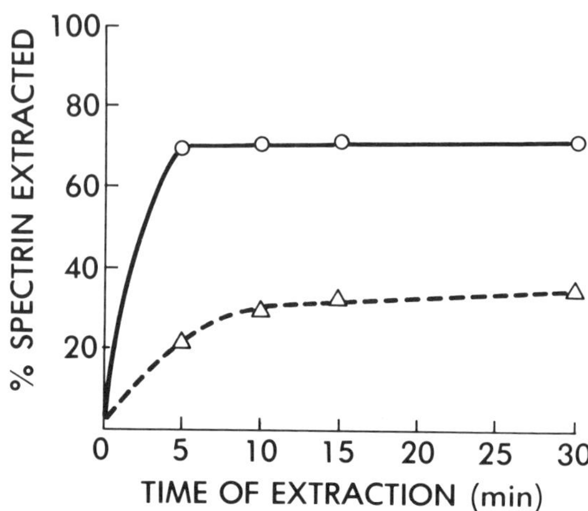

Figure 4. The rate of release of spectrin from membranes of unheated erythrocytes (0-0) and erythrocytes heated to 48° (Δ -Δ).

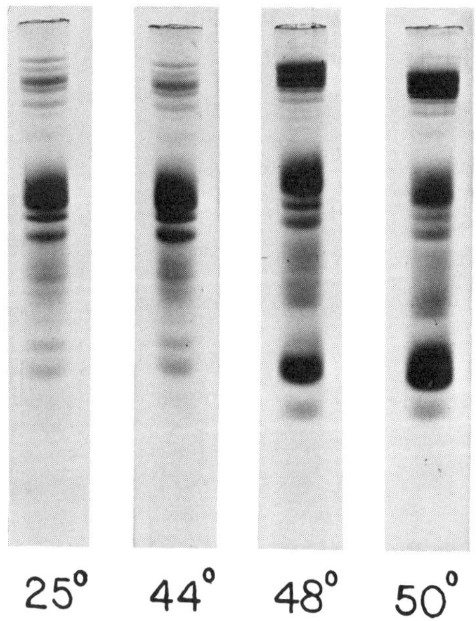

Figure 5. SDS polyacrylamide gel electrophoresis of extract pellets from membranes of erythrocytes heated for 10 min at the specified temperatures.

The analysis of spectrin extractability was made by densitometric examination of the ratio of spectrin to Band 3 in the SDS-PAGE gels of the extract pellet obtained after extraction with low ionic strength media. Figure 5 shows the polypeptide patterns of the unextracted membrane polypeptides in the extracted pellets of red cells heated to the specified temperature for 10 min. It can be seen that heating to 44° had no effect, while heating to 48° caused a marked increase in spectrin retention and at 50° spectrin became unextractable. Heating cells caused the adherence of cytoplasmic protein, including hemoglobin, to isolated membranes. Hemoglobin was largely released by the extraction procedure but other polypeptides can be seen in Figure 5 which are not generally associated with the membrane.

The effects of heating erythrocytes at various temperatures on the extractability of spectrin from membranes are shown in Figure 6. The first appreciable effect was observed when the temperature increased from 46° to 47°. A progressive decrease in extractability with increasing temperature occurred until spectrin became unextractable at 50°.

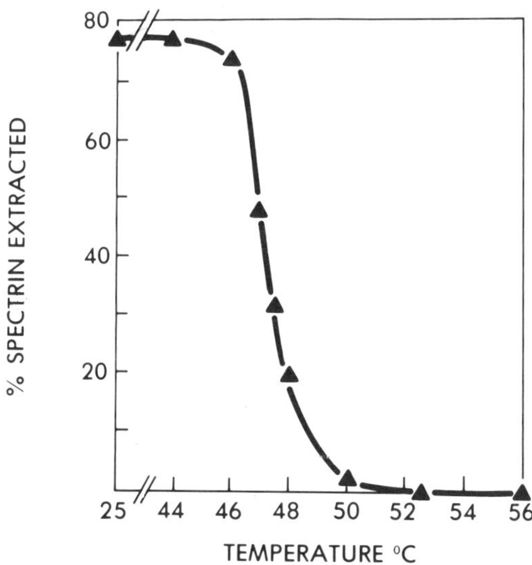

Figure 6. The extent of spectrin extraction from membranes of erythrocytes exposed for 10 min at the indicated temperatures.

The change in spectrin extractability of membranes from
heated erythrocytes was also time dependent at 47° as shown
in Figure 3. Spectrin extractability progressively decreased
for 6 min after which no additional changes occurred (recent
results show no further change in extractability after heating
erythrocytes up to 1 hr at 47°).

Heat Effects on the Erythrocyte Membrane Protein
Phosphorylation Reaction. Membranes from erythrocytes heated
to 50° showed a marked decrease in the endogenous phosphorylation of spectrin, as shown in Figure 7.

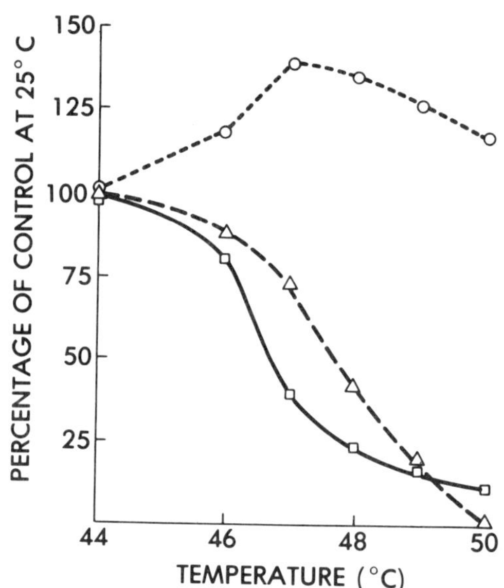

Figure 7. The effect of temperature on phosphorylation
reactions and spectrin extractability of the membrane of
erythrocytes exposed for 10 min at the indicated temperatures.
(0-0) casein kinase in isolated membranes; (□-□) phosphorylation of spectrin in isolated membranes and (△-△)
spectrin extractability.

A progressive temperature-dependent decrease in spectrin
phosphorylation measured in isolated membranes from heated
cells began at 47° and paralleled the decrease observed in

spectrin extractability. Enzyme inactivation did not appear
to produce this effect, since the protein kinase activity
measured with an exogenous substrate, casein, was not inhibited by heating cells up to 50°. The increase in activity
with heat may have reflected adherence of cytoplasmic protein
kinase to isolated membranes. Spectrin was labelled with
^{32}P by prior incubation of cells with ^{32}P$_i$. Heating the
labelled cells up to 50° for 10 min did not alter the ^{32}P
label in spectrin. This indicated that heating did not
produce a rapid phosphorylation (thereby depleting potential
labelling sites in the isolated membrane) or dephosphorylation
in the intact cell.

Metabolic Effects

Incubating erythrocytes in the absence of metabolites
causes alteration in shape and deformability. The following
studies examined changes in spectrin extractability and
membrane protein phosphorylation that occurred under these
conditions:

Metabolic Depletion Effects on Erythrocyte Morphology
and Deformability. The effects of metabolic depletion on
erythrocyte morphology have been well characterized. Cells
are transformed from biconcave discs to spiculated discs
(echinocytes) and finally to smooth spheroidal forms
(spheroechinocytes).

The effects of metabolic depletion on erythrocyte
deformability were measured by the Ektacytometer. The change
in deformability during metabolic depletion in the presence of
1 mM EDTA is shown in Figure 8. Up to 10 hrs, no decrease in
deformability was observed. Between 10 to 40 hrs a progressive decrease in deformability occurred which reached
a plateau at 40 hrs. The plateau for deformability change
observed during metabolic depletion was very similar to that
produced by heating at 47° (see Figure 9 and Figure 3).
However, different results were obtained when the incubations
were carried out in buffer media without EDTA or in media
containing 0.1 mM Ca^{++}. In the media without EDTA the
changes in deformability were similar to those described
above up to 36 hrs, but beginning at 36 hrs a second
population of completely undeformable cells appeared. The
percentage of these undeformable cells increased with time,
becoming completely undeformable at 72 hrs. In contrast,

cells in incubation with 0.1 mM Ca^{++}, the cells were completely undeformable at 44 hrs.

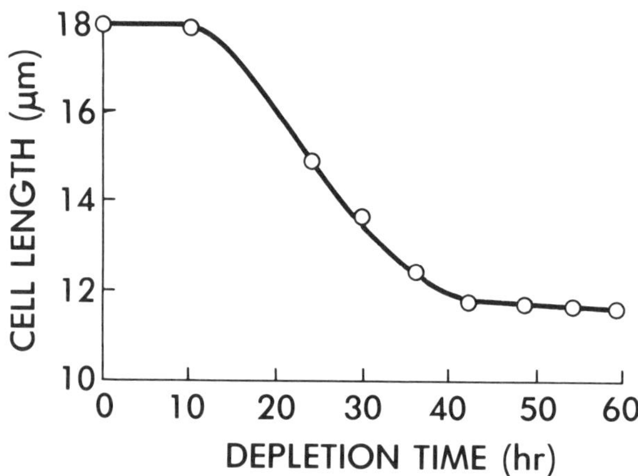

Figure 8. The effect of metabolic depletion in the presence of EDTA on the deformability of erythrocytes.

Metabolic Depletion Effects on the Extractability of Spectrin from Membranes.

The change in extractability of spectrin from membranes during metabolic depletion is shown in Figure 9. Spectrin extractability had decreased from 72% to 54% by 30 hrs. This level of extractability remained unaltered until 36 hrs when a second component in the extractability began, causing a large time-dependent decrease in spectrin extract-ability. As with deformability, the second component in the extractability change was eliminated by the presence of 1 mM EDTA and the limiting value for extractability in the presence of EDTA was similar to the value obtained by heating cells at 47°.

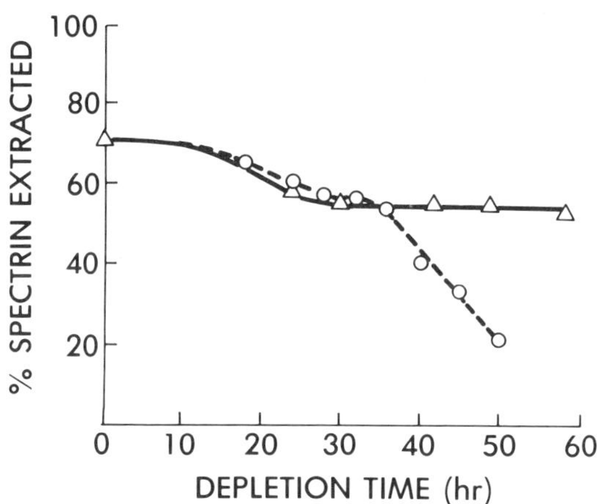

Figure 9. The effect of metabolic depletion time on the
extractability of spectrin from isolated membranes. ($\Delta-\Delta$)
with EDTA; (0-0) without EDTA.

Metabolic Depletion Effects on the Phosphorylation of
Spectrin.

Incubation of erythrocytes in the presence of glucose
and $^{32}P_i$ resulted in the incorporation of $^{32}P_i$ into spectrin
Band 2 and polypeptide(s) in the Band 3 position (Palmer and
Verpoorte, 1971; Greenquist and Shohet, 1975a, 1976; Shapiro
and Marchesi, 1977) as the predominant sites of membrane
protein labelling. Under the conditions of labelling described
here, erythrocytes incorporated approximately 50 dpm into
spectrin/ml RBC/hour/10^6 dpm of $^{32}P_i$ added. The incorporation
of label into spectrin in the presence of glucose continued
linearly for at least 30 hrs.

Cells and spectrin were prelabelled with $^{32}P_i$ and then
washed free of extracellular glucose for reincubation at
37° under conditions of metabolic depletion. The results
are shown in Figure 10.

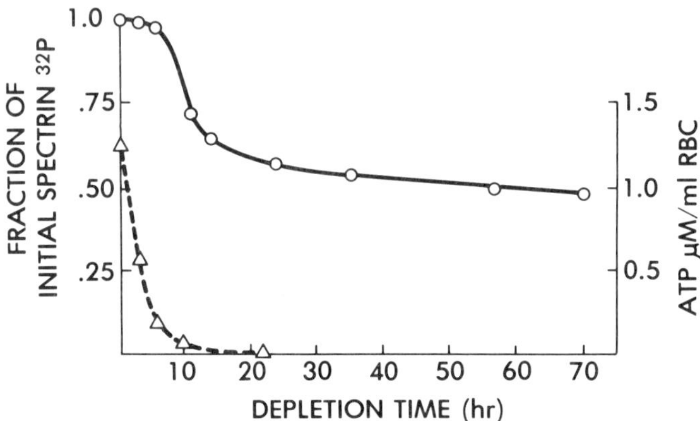

Figure 10: The effect of metabolic depletion time on the levels of ^{32}P-spectrin in erythrocytes preincubated with ^{32}P$_i$. (0-0) ^{32}P-spectrin; (Δ-Δ) ATP.

The total change in ^{32}P-spectrin is about 50% and occurred in less than 4 hrs between 6 and 10 hrs of depletion time. Release of label began rapidly after the ATP dropped to about 15% of the initial level. After 10 hrs there was negligible further depletion of ^{32}P-spectrin up to 60 hrs of incubation. This depletion was not affected by extracellular EDTA. After 3 hrs of depletion, the cells were >95% biconcave discs. By 6 hrs, early morphologic changes were apparent (i.e., some echinocyte I cells were present). There was a progressive transition with time and at 10 hrs most of the cells were echinocytes I and II. Transformation to spheroechinocytes began at 18 hrs.

DISCUSSION

Previous studies have shown that red cells heated to 50° are transformed into spherocytes and begin to fragment (Ham et al., 1948), while temperatures between 45° and 50° produce changes in deformability and negligible morphological changes (Rakow and Hochmuth, 1975; Mohandas et al., 1976). In the present study, the heat effects on deformability have been

compared to two spectrin-related properties: spectrin
extractability and spectrin phosphorylation. The decrease
in deformability was sensitive to both the temperature
during incubation and the time of incubation. Spectrin
extractability from membranes was also sensitive to both
the temperature and the time of incubation. The coin-
cidental onset and termination of changes in deformability
and spectrin extractability with incubation further
support the hypothesis that the two properties may be
related. The mechanism associated with spectrin release
from membranes is not known, nor have the processes that
inhibit this release been extensively studied. The loss
of extractability with heat does not appear to result
from a resealing of the membrane, since trypsin has ready
access to the ghost membrane interior and adherent hemoglobin is released during the extraction. However, spectrin
is much larger than these proteins, and its size could limit
its release from the membrane interior. Based on analyses
of membranes by SDS-PAGE in the absence of reducing agent,
spectrin does not appear to be involved in the formation of
disulfide-induced aggregates during heating.

Erythrocyte membranes showed thermal transitions,
measured by differential heat capacity calorimetry, which
began around 40°, with a first peak at 50° which appeared
to be related to protein denaturation (Jackson et al., 1973).
Obviously it would be desirable to determine if these events
are related to the altered state of spectrin extractability.

We had previously found that spectrin phosphorylation
in isolated membranes was markedly inhibited as the temperature was increased from 45° to 50° (Greenquist and Shohet,
1975a). This inhibition could have been due to enzyme
inactivation, impaired interaction of the enzyme with spectrin
in the membranes, and/or alteraton in the spectrin substrate
itself. As shown here, the activity of the membrane casein
kinase [which appears to be spectrin kinase (Avruch and
Fairbanks, 1974; Fairbanks and Avruch, 1974)] actually increased when cells wcre heated to 50°. This increase in activity could be due to the adherence of this cytoplasmic enzyme
to the membranes as a result of heating. [It should be noted,
however, that heating isolated membranes or membrane casein
kinase extracted with 0.5M NaCl (Avruch and Fairbanks, 1974)
leads to rapid inactivation of the enzyme at 50°]. The
inactivation of the phosphorylation reaction in membranes
from heated cells showed a temperature sensitivity that was

similar to the change in spectrin extractability and cellular deformability . It is interesting that in the human disease hereditary spherocytosis, in which erythrocytes exhibit impaired deformability (Allard et al, 1977; Smith et al., 1975), there is also an alteration in the spectrin phosphorylation reaction in isolated membranes (Greenquist and Shohet, 1974, 1976).

The second subject of this study deals with changes in deformability, spectrin extractability, and the spectrin phosphorylation reaction during metabolic depletion. The events which follow metabolic depletion in the erythrocyte have been of considerable interest. Changes in morphology (Nakao and Nakao, 1960; Weed et al., 1969) and deformability (Weed et al., 1969) occur in a reversible manner, and an intimate role for ATP, Ca^{++}, and Mg^{++} has been suggested for these changes (Weed et al., 1969). However, erythrocytes depleted of ATP by exposure to indoacetate persist for some time with normal morphology and deformability (Feo and Mohandas, 1977). Changes in erythrocyte deformability and spectrin extractability from membranes occurred at the same stage of metabolic depletion. The changes appeared to reflect both intrinsic membrane changes and an extracellular Ca^{++} effect. In the absence of EDTA and after extensive depletion, both extractability and deformability showed a further parallel decrease and support the view that deformability and spectrin extractability are interdependent phenomena. The change after 36 hrs most likely represented the slow influx of trace amounts of Ca^{++} to a critical level. Events prior to 36 hrs appeared to be independent of low concentrations of extracellular Ca^{++}. It is also interesting that deformability and extractability changes reached similar plateaus upon heating to 47° or with metabolic depletion in the presence of EDTA. The close correspondence of these plateaus suggests common underlying molecular events produced by heating or metabolic depletion; for example, a partial rearangement of spectrin into a second metastable structure as a consequence of a thermal transition or dephosphorylation. A further transition to the undeformable cell with Ca^{++} and metabolic depletion or heating at 50° may result from a more drastic denaturation of spectrin. The latter transition corresponds closely to the thermal transition peak observed in differential heat capacity measurements and also to the temperature at which cells begin to sphere and fragment. The application of a spectrin extractability procedure to metabolically depleted erythrocytes was first described by

Lux and John (Lux and John, 1974). These authors found a
large decrease in spectrin extractability with metabolic
depletion. The conditions for extraction used by these
authors differed considerably in time and temperature from
the conditions described here. However, they did not observe
a Ca^{++} dependent effect up to 33 hrs of depletion. This
result is consistent with that described here.

The effect of metabolic depletion on the spectrin
reaction is particularly interesting since this protein is
one of the potential loci for both structural and dynamic
contributions to cell shape and deformability. Phosphorylation of spectrin in the intact cell occurs on a limited
region of the molecule demonstrated by the release of a
single ^{32}P-labelled peptide (m.w. $\sim$4800) after tryptic
digestion of radiolabelled spectrin (Wyatt et al., 1977).
Phosphorylation or dephosphorylation of spectrin occurs
depending upon the metabolic state of the cell (Greenquist
and Shohet, 1975a). As shown here, dephosphorylation began
when ATP levels dropped to about 15% of their initial value.
It was surprising that after a rapid decline in labelling,
the reaction virtually stopped within 3.5 hours, and negligible release was observed for 60 hrs. A sudden inhibition
of a protein phosphatase could have produced this effect.
Alternatively, rearrangement of spectrin induced by conditions
of metabolic depletion may also have accounted for termination
of the reaction if the phosphorylation site became inacces-
sible to protein phosphatase. The extractability data during
depletion indicate that metabolic depletion had induced
some alteration in spectrin. It must be noted that the final
shape transformation to a spheroechinocyte was not coincident
with the achievement of the plateau for phosphorylated
spectrin. It will be important to determine whether the
events which occur subsequent to dephosphorylation of spectrin
are a consequence of dephosphorylation or reflect other events
resulting from metabolic depletion.

In conclusion these results demonstrate the possible
interrelationship between spectrin extractability, level of
phosphorylation, and membrane deformability.

ACKNOWLEDGEMENTS

The authors wish to acknowledge the excellent technical assistance of Mrs. Mary Rossi. This work was supported by USPHS Grants AM16095 and HL07100 from the National Institutes of Health, and by a career development award to one of us (SBS: AM37237).

REFERENCES

Allard C, Mohandas N, Bessis M (1977). Red cell deformability changes in hemolytic anemias. Blood Cells 3:209.

Anker HS (1970). A solubilizable acrylamide gel for electrophoresis. FEBS Letters 7:293.

Avruch J, Fairbanks G (1974). Phosphorylation of endogenous substrates by erythrocyte membrane protein kinases. I. A monovalent cation-stimulated reaction. Biochemistry 13:5507.

Bessis M, Mohandas N (1975). A diffractometric method for the measurement of cellular deformability. Blood Cells 1:307.

Beutler E (1971). "Red cell metabolism. A manual of biochemical methods." New York: Grune & Stratton, p. 92.

Beutler E (1975). Op. cit., second edition, p. 10.

Beutler E, Guinto E, Johnson C (1976). Human red cell protein kinase in normal subjects and patients with hereditary spherocytosis, sickle cell disease and autoimmune hemolytic anemia. Blood 48:887.

Fairbanks G, Steck T, Wallach D (1971). Electrophoretic analysis of the major polypeptides of the human erythrocyte membrane. Biochemistry 10:2606.

Fairbanks G, Avruch J (1974). Phosphorylation of endogenous substrate by erythrocyte membrane protein kinase. II. Cyclic adenosine monophosphate-stimulated reactions. Biochemistry 13:5514.

Feo C, Mohandas N (1977). Clarification of the role of ATP in red cell morphology and function. Nature 265:166.

Fuller GM, Boughter JM, Morazzani M (1974). Evidence for multiple polypeptide chains in the membrane protein spectrin. Biochemistry 13:3036.

Greenquist AC, Shohet SB (1974). Defective protein phosphorylation in membranes of hereditary spherocytosis erythrocytes. FEBS Letters 48:134.

Greenquist AC, Shohet SB (1975a). Phosphorylation and dephosphorylation in the erythrocyte membrane. In Brewer G (ed.):
  "Erythrocyte structure and function", New York: Alan R. Liss,
  p 515.
Greenquist AC, Shohet SB (1975b). Abnormal erythrocyte
  membrane properties of hereditary spherocytosis in mice.
  Blood 46:1005.
Greenquist AC, Shohet SB (1976). Phosphorylation in
  erythrocyte membranes from abnormally shaped cells. Blood
  48:877.
Guthrow CE Jr, Allen JE, Rasmussen H (1972). Phosphorylation
  of an endogenous membrane protein by an endogenous
  membrane-associated cyclic adenosine 3',5'-monophosphate
  dependent protein kinase in human erythrocyte ghosts.
  J Biol Chem 247:8145.
Ham TH, Shen S, Fleming E, Castla W (1948). Studies on the
  destruction of red cells. IV. Blood 3:373.
Hoogeveen J Th, Juliano R, Coleman J, Rothstein A (1970).
  Water soluble proteins of the human red cell membrane.
  J Memb Biol 3:156.
Jackson W, Kostyla J, Nordin J, Brandts J (1973).
  Calorimetric study of protein transitions in human
  erythrocyte ghosts. Biochemistry 12:3663.
LaCelle PL, Weed RI (1969). Reversibility of abnormal
  deformability and permeability of the hereditary spherocyte.
  Blood 34:858.
Leblond PF, LaCelle PL, Weed RI (1971). Cellular deform-
  ability: A possible determinant of the normal release of
  maturing erythrocytes from the bone marrow. Blood 37:
  40.
Lux SE, John KM (1974). Alteration of the physical state
  of spectrin in ATP-depleted red cells. Blood 44:909.
Mohandas N, Greenquist AC, Shohet SB (1976). Red cell
  deformability and spectrin. Blood 48:991.
Nakao M, Nakao T (1960). Adenosine triphosphate and maintenance of shape of human red cells. Nature 187:945.
Painter RG, Sheetz M, Singer SJ (1975). Detection and
  ultrastructural localization of human smooth muscle
  myosin-like molecules in human non-muscle cells by specific
  antibodies. Proc Nat Acad Sci USA 72:1359.
Palmer FB, Verpoorte JA (1971). The phosphorus components
  of solubilized erythrocyte membrane protein. Can J Biochem
  49:337.
Ponder E (1971). "Hemolysis and related phenomena." New
  York: Grune & Stratton.

Rakow AL, Hochmuth RM (1975). Effect of heat treatment on the elasticity of human erythrocyte membrane. Biophys J 15:1095.

Roses AD, Appel SH (1973). Erythrocyte protein phosphorylation. J Biol Chem 248:1408.

Rubin CS, Erlichman J, Rosen OM (1972). Cyclic adenosine 3',5'-monophosphate-dependent protein kinase of human erythrocyte membrane. J Biol Chem 247:6135.

Shapiro D, Marchesi V (1977). Phosphorylation in membranes of intact human erythrocytes. J Biol Chem 252:508.

Smith BD, LaCelle PT, LaCelle PL (1975). Time-dependent fragmentation/failure of normal erythrocytes and hereditary spherocyte membranes. Blood 46:1005.

Steck TL, Fairbanks G, Wallach D (1971). Disposition of the major proteins in the isolated erythrocyte membrane. Proteolytic dissection. Biochemistry 10:2617.

Weber K, Osborn M (1969). The reliability of molecular weight determinations by dodecyl-sulfate-polyacrylamide gel electrophoresis. J Biol Chem 244:4406.

Weed RI, LaCelle PL, Merrill EW (1969). Metabolic dependence of red cell deformability. J Clin Invest 48:795.

Wyatt JL, Greenquist AC, Shohet SB (1977). A single phosphorylated tryptic peptide from spectrin of human erythrocyte membranes. Fed Proc 36:640.

DISCUSSION

Dr. Fairbanks: Al, I wonder if you'd like to comment on the possible role of disulfide cross-linking in forming aggregates of spectrin that might restrict membrane deformability? The studies of Jiri Palek, in particular, suggest that you get a reorganization of spectrin but you prevent the cross-linking if you do the depletion under nitrogen. So I wonder if you've compared deformability with metabolic depletion under anaerobic and aerobic conditions?

Dr. Greenquist: No, that would be an interesting thing to do. But we have looked at whether there are disulfide cross-linked aggregates that are formed as a consequence of heating to see if that would potentially rationalize what's happening to deformability and it does not appear that there are such aggregates being formed. We have looked at SDS polyacrymide gels of membranes from cells after metabolic depletion and have seen the same thing Palek has described, that these disulfide cross-linked aggregates are being formed. I think that disulfide linkage per se is not critical for the rearrangements that occur; Palek has also shown that under anaerobic conditions he can demonstrate susceptibility to cross-linking by other agents which implies that the rearrangements has occurred even though disulfide cross-linking hasn't occurred, so that there is a rearrangement that's not directly related to the cross-linking process. I think that event is the event that we'd be interested in trying to follow to determine whether it was related to deformability, spectrin extractability or to the spectrin dephosphorylation process.

Dr. Fairbanks: Right, well the question would be whether it is the reorganization, or the cross-linking that's expressed in a change of deformability?

Dr. Greenquist: I don't think anyone has answered that yet.

Dr. Fairbanks: But I wondered if you know what happens to glutathione in these cells over this temperature range?

Dr. Greenquist: I really don't know. I'm sure it's dropping during metabolic depletion, but we've never really looked at glutathione after heating.

The Red Cell, pages 473—477

Dr. Fairbanks: It would be interesting to know if there's
even blockage of spectrin sulfhydryls.

Dr. Greenquist: I know ATP doesn't drop at all in the time
course that we're doing the heating experiment - that is,
ten minutes. I have a feeling that glutathione also doesn't
drop significantly. One of the things that surprised us in
the dephosphorylation reaction with spectrin was that it
really essentially stopped after about four hours after initiation of dephosphosphorylation. It could be inactivation of
phosphatase under those circumstances, but I think it would
be surprising to see such a sudden rapid inactivation and
another interesting possibility is that as a consequence of
this initial dephosphorylation there has been some rearrangement of spectrin which makes it no longer accessible to
the protein phosphatase.

Dr. Levander: I couldn't help but be extremely stimulated
by your paper and this afternoon we're going to be talking
about the effects of experimental vitamin E deficiency on
deformability changes in erythrocytes from rats. We find
that this is also extremely temperature-dependent and is
presumably related to lipid peroxidation. In effect you can
protect against these deformability changes by incubating
the cells at 0°. My question to you is related to the previous comment. Since this apparently is related to lipid
peroxidation this again might invoke glutathione dependent
disulfide formation.

Dr. Greenquist: It's hard for me to imagine that change
of lipid in the membrane by themselves would be sufficient
to change the deformability of the red cell and even though
peroxidation events maybe going on, I think that some modification other than the lipids themselves would have to be involved in that situation.

Dr. Levander: Right, my point was that the lipid peroxidation would just be an indication of a general oxidative
stress on the cells which might then lead to disulfide
formation.

Dr. Morse: Another possible way of thinking of the interaction of spectrin that could cause these deformability changes
would be to think that spectrin not only changes its relationship with the proteins and lipids on the inside of the membrane, but it somehow affects bound water associated with

the membrane. We've done electron spin resonance studies
that show that in the temperature ranges that you studied
the internal viscosity of both intact and hemoglobin-free
cells goes up considerably, especially between about 48°
and 50°. These seem to be long range effects and it makes
me think that there is probably an extremely complex sort
of thing going on that may affect water as well as protein
and lipid associated with the membrane.

Dr. Greenquist: I imagine the bound water changes that you
are looking at would be a way of monitoring changes in protein conformation at the membrane interface.

Dr. Sheetz: Don't you think you're doing more than just
modifying the metabolic enzymes by treating with iodoacetic
acid and might you not be involving some of the membrane
shape changing proteins, etc.?

Dr. Greenquist: That could be true, but the important point
is the iodoacetate treatment doesn't- at least in the initial hour- produce any shape change and it takes another
hour before you actually see initiation of shape changes.
But that is a real limitation on the application of iodoacetate.

Dr. Kurantsin-Mills: Three questions: first of all, under
what conditions do you heat the cells? In their autologous
plasma, or in buffer?

Dr. Greenquist: We incubate in phosphate buffered saline.
We preheat the phosphate buffered saline and add red cell
suspensions to that and that's the starting point of our
incubation.

Dr. Kurantsin-Mills: The cells are washed?

Dr. Greenquist: We pass cells over cotton fiber to remove
white cells as described by Beutler and wash three times
in phosphate buffered saline.

Dr. Kurantsin-Mills: The second question is, you don't
have calcium in your phosphate procedure, I suspect?

Dr. Greenquist: In the absence of EDTA we have trace amounts
of calcium. We have done studies with and without EDTA
to see what effect that has.

Dr. Kurantsin-Mills: Have you looked at the role of calcium in spectrin extractability and deformability?

Dr. Greenquist: We have added calcium and gone through a prolonged incubation to 44 hours and done extractability and deformability studies. In the absence of added calcium the cells are mixed, a portion are undeformable and there's a group that are deformable. In the presence of calcium after 44 hours they're all undeformable and the spectrin is unextractable. We haven't done a detailed kinetic course in the presence of added calcium.

Dr. Kurantsin-Mills: My third question is, if you look at your graphs for deformability, the ranges are from about 18 to 13, or 15, or 12, thereabouts. What is the range of sensitivity of the ektacytomate and therefore what is the range of the cell shape changes you are measuring in microns?

Dr. Greenquist: Fully deformable fresh red cell distend to about 18 microns. The undeformable cell is 8 microns so we would measure from 8 to 18 microns.

Dr. Kurantsin-Mills: What is the standard deviation?

Dr. Greenquist: It's about plus or minus 5% on each set of determinations termination.

Dr. Kurantsin-Mills: Thank you.

Dr. Greenquist: It is interesting that both metabolic depletion and heating effects, heating at 47°, leads to a cell that has the same limiting value for spectrin extractability and deformability . It is as if there's a transformation to a new type of cell that has similar deformability and extractability properties and that if we further perturb it by the addition of Ca^{++} to the metabolically depleted cell or by heating to 50° there's a new transition to the totally undeformable cell and unextractable spectrin.

Dr. Cameron: Are there effects of calcium in the early phase of spectrin dephosphorylation?

Dr. Greenquist: Trace amounts of calcium have no influence on spectrin dephosphorylation through the whole kinetic course that we studied; even at 36 hours of depletion when

we found that deformability and extractability changes
with traces of calcium, there's no effect on the dephosphorylation reaction. We haven't added calcium to see if
that would affect the initial dephosphorylation.

Dr. Fairbanks: Just to add a little potential complexity
to this, do these cells that you heated become dehydrated
at all, Al?

Dr. Greenquist: We've done   particle size analyses of
heated cells followed by fixation and they have no change in mean
cell volume, so I don't think so.

Dr. Fung: Have you done any similar experiments on sickle
cells?

Dr. Greenquist: We've done a few sickle cell studies to see
if there was any change in the sensitivity to deformability
and extractability and it looked like it shifted slightly
to the left, that is changes begin to occur at slightly
lower temperatures. We've also done some studies on a red
cell disease called pyropoikilocytosis in which there are
abnormally shaped red cells that have an unusual heat sensitivity and these show an even greater shift- all these effects
start to happen at lower temperatures and are completed at
lower temperatures.

Dr. Steck: Before we break for coffee, I want to thank Dr.
Greenquist for filling in for Dr. Shohet, who was originally
scheduled on our program. I also want to point out that
Dr. Lux was not able to attend this meeting and Dr. Lessin
will be presenting an over-view on sickle cell ultrastructure
in his place.

ALTERED COMPONENT a PHOSPHORYLATION IN ERYTHROCYTE
MEMBRANES IN MYOTONIC MUSCULAR DYSTROPHY

Pierre Wong and Allen D. Roses
Department of Medicine
Division of Neurology
Duke University Medical Center
Durham, North Carolina

This symposium provides an opportunity to update and
summarize some of the erythrocyte membrane protein phosphorylation studies in myotonic muscular dystrophy. This
work spans a period of seven years and has been reported
in the literature intermittently, but a concise summary
has never been published (Roses and Appel, 1973; Butterfield et al., 1974; Roses and Appel, 1975; Miller et al.,
1976; Roses, 1976). The data provide insights into the
heterogeniety of membrane proteins as well as to suggest
a testable model for the biochemical defect in MyD (Roses,
1976; Hull and Roses, 1975). Since MyD is inherited as
an autosomal dominant trait these studies have obvious
significance in the broader area of human biochemical
genetics.

In 1973 we reported decreased phosphorylation of MyD
membrane proteins when the membranes were stored at $-20°C$
for one week. We viewed these data as support for our
suggestion that MyD was a disease involving the function
of cellular membranes (Roses and Appel, 1973). We chose
to follow up these observations by studying the erythrocyte
ghost membranes under freshly prepared conditions rather
than to investigate effects of freezing, storage, etc.
After experimenting with many techniques for ghosting red
cells, we found·that there was a specific decrease in the
endogenous phosphorylation of Band 3 (apparent molecular
weight 90-100,000 daltons) in MyD membranes when assays
were performed under initial rate conditions using freshly
prepared ghosts (Fairbanks et al., 1971; Roses and Appel,
1975). When protein and glycoprotein fractions of Band 3

The Red Cell, pages 479–488

were separated, the difference in phosphorylation was present only in the glycoprotein or Component a fraction. The Component a fraction could be separated as SDS-polyacrylamide gels from the major sialoglycoprotein of erythrocyte membrane. No difference in phosphorylation was present in the major sialoglycoprotein (Roses and Appel, 1975).

For the past three years our laboratory has attempted to purify the particular species of MyD Component a glycoprotein that demonstrates decreased phosphorylation. We have used affinity chromatography methods to fractionate Component a glycoproteins. Concanavalen A (Con-A) affinity chromatography of solubilized erythrocyte ghosts can be used to purify approximately one third of the Band 3 material (Findlay, 1974; Roses, 1976) but this fraction was only minimally phosphorylated by the endogenous protein kinase reaction and no differences were noted in MyD. The difference in phosphorylation between controls and MyD was present in the Con-A unretained fraction of Band 3 proteins and glycoproteins. This study demonstrated that the apoprotein portion of Component a glycoproteins differ with respect to their ability to accept transfer of $[\gamma-^{32}P]$ATP into phosphoserine and phosphothreonine ester linkages. They demonstrated apoprotein heterogeneity in addition to their carbohydrate heterogeneity (Roses, 1976). Using a number of lectin affinity labels and a variety of detergents we have described several heterogenous fractions of Component a glycoproteins (Wong and Roses, submitted for publication). We have isolated a highly purified minor glycoprotein component of Band 3 that represents approximately 0.3% total membrane protein but contains the decreased phosphorylation in MyD.

METHOD

Fresh erythrocyte ghosts are prepared by the method of Fairbanks, et al. (1971) with pronase inhibitor added to the lysis step. Endogenous membrane protein kinase reactions are performed as previously described (Roses and Appel, 1977). For these studies the incubation time is 30 min. Following spectrin extraction the membranes are solubilized in 0.1% Triton X-100 and applied to a Ricinus Communis 1 (RC-1)-Sepharose 4B Column. Sequential elution with variable salt and specific lectin (D-galactose)

concentrations of non-retained, non-specifically retained and
D-gal specific retained fractions are analyzed in detail by
SDS-polyacrylamide gel electrophoresis and scintillation
spectroscopy of individual protein and glycoprotein bands
(Wong and Roses, submitted for publication). Each experiment includes ghosts from a MyD patient and an age, sex, and
race matched control. Blood type is not controlled except
that all patients and controls in these experiments are RH
positive.

RESULTS

There are no differences in the Coomassie blue and
periodic acid Schiff staining patterns of MyD or control[1]
ghosts in any of the nine sequentially eluted fractions.
Figure 1 illustrates the 0.1% Triton X-100 solubilized

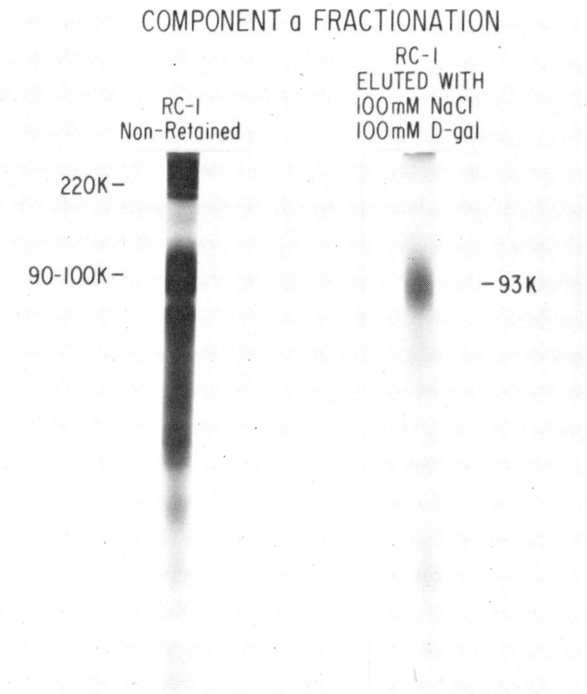

[1]Space does not permit delineation of the complete
methodology including solubilization and affinity chromatography sequential elution fractionation. The details of
these procedures are to be published (Wong and Roses, submitted for publication).

erythrocyte membrane fraction specifically eluted by 100mM
NaCl, 100mM D-gal. Duplicate gels are cut and each band
counted. In this fraction, the 93K band (species of
Component a) is the major (>90%) polypeptide in overloaded
gels and the only polypeptide labeled with [32]P.

The total RC-1 specific Component a fraction represents
0.7% of the total membrane protein in both MyD and controls,
and demonstrates approximately 70% of the Component a radioactivity. The sequential elution step using 100mM NaCl,
100mM D-gal represents approximately 0.3% of the total
membrane protein and approximately 30% of the total Component a radioactivity. In several experiments the total
Band 3 phosphorylation at 30 minutes was increased (not
initial rate conditions) in the MyD membranes yet the

TABLE 1

COMPARISON OF COMPONENT a PURIFICATION TECHNIQUES

	Radioactivity cpm	mg Protein	% Total Protein	cpm/mg
Band 3	144,000	25,500	30	5.65
Component a (LIS extraction)[1]	114,000	16,600	20	6.87
Con-A Retarded Fraction (93K)[2]	12,000	6,800	8	1.76
RC-1 Retarded Fraction (93K)[3]				
10mM NaCl, 100mM D-gal	48,700	360	.42	135
100mM NaCl, 100mM D-gal	34,300	230	.27	149

(Legend) Data are derived from one experiment using the same ghost and
[γ-^{32}P]ATP preparations. These data are characteristic of the
purification techniques on each experiment.

Methods
1. Steck & Yu, 1973; Roses & Appel, 1975.
2. Findlay, 1974; Roses, 1975.
3. Wong & Roses (submitted for publication).

phosphorylation of the 100mM NaCl, 100mM D-gal RC-1 specific Component a was still decreased. The yield of the 93K polypeptide was the same in experiments using erythrocytes from patients with Duchenne muscular dystrophy and congential myotonia but no consistent differences from controls in any RC-1 fraction could be demonstrated in these genetic diseases (Wong and Roses, in preparation).

TABLE 2

EXPERIMENT	CONTROL pmoles/mg prot(93K)	MYOTONIC DYSTROPHY pmoles/mg prot(93K)	RATIO* C/M
1	5.8	1.9	3.2
2	6.6	2.5	2.6
3	4.6	2.5	1.8
4	4.6	4.1	1.1
5	5.3	3.1	1.7
6	13.0	7.2	1.8
7	5.0	2.6	1.9
Mean	6.41	3.41	1.99
SD	2.99	1.80	0.63
SEM	1.13	0.68	
P	$< .025$ [1]	$< .005$ [2]	

*In each experiment the glycoprotein content of the fractions eluted with 100mM NaCl, 100mM D-gal were identical for control and MyD patient. While some variation may be reflected in the computation of the specific phosphorylation, the ratio of the counts per minute per mg total protein is derived directly from raw data. The 93K component of this fraction is the only phosphorylated band.

Table 2 presents the data from seven consecutive experiments. Each experiment demonstrates decreased phosphorylation of MyD Component a sequentially eluted by 100mM NaCl, 100mM D-gal from the RC-1 Sepharose column. The levels of phosphorylation compares with previously reported differences. This contrasts with the data from other sequentially eluted fractions from RC-1 Sepharose (such as 10mM NaCl, 100mM D-gal) as well as experiments using other lectins in which no consistent differences between MyD and control are found. (Table 3)

[1]Student's t test.

[2]Paired t test.

TABLE 3

PHOSPHORYLATION OF RC-1 SEPHAROSE 4B SPECIFIC
COMPONENT a FRACTION

ELUTED STEP	CONTROL	MYOTONIC DYSTROPHY	p[1]
	(picomoles/mg 93K protein)		
10mM NaCl 100mM D-galactose	10.2 ±2.6	11.1 ±3.4	NS
100mM NaCl 100mM D-galactose	6.41 ±1.18	3.41 ±0.68	< .005

LEGEND: Data are derived from the same seven experiments
reported in Table 2.
[1]Paired t tests.

DISCUSSION

Each of the experiments demonstrate decreased phosphorylation of the 100mM NaCl, 100mM D-gal RC-1 Sepharose
Component a fraction. Experiment 4 is of particular interest
since the control and patient are almost equal (Table 2).
The MyD patient in this experiment is unusual. Unlike the
other patients who represent classical pedigrees, this
patient has myotonia, diabetes mellitus with elevated insulin levels, mature cataracts, and decreased IgG levels
but neither he nor any of the four affected members of his
family have any evidence of dystrophy. In fact, this
pedigree may represent an unusual and different genetic
disease, presently best classified as MyD. The other six
patients have MyD of varying severity but all have at least
one relative with classical MyD in their pedigrees.

We believe we have isolated and partially purified
the species of Component a that is less phosphorylated
during the endogenous membrane protein kinase reaction in
MyD. Further technical modifications are necessary to
isolate the 93K Component completely free of contamination.
It is still unclear whether the difference represents a
primary sequence alteration or whether the identical glycoprotein exists in a less phosphorylated state in control
membranes and can accept the transfer of more ^{32}P from
$[\gamma-^{32}P]ATP$. Peptide mapping of the purified phosphorylation

glycoproteins may clarify these points.

There is no *a priori* reason to assume that an altered primary sequence abnormality would be identical in each pedigree. In fact MyD may be due to a number of mutations each affecting the same molecule. Thus if an altered peptide can be demonstrated in mapping experiments it need not be identical in each pedigree but should be identical for every affected member within each pedigree. The hemoglobinopathies provide a precedent for mutation of a non-enzymatic protein causing disease.

We have previously reported an alteration in the stoichiometry of the ouabain sensitive Na^+K^+ ATP-ase (Hull and Roses, 1975). Several groups have demonstrated that the acyl-phosphorylate and Na^+K^+ ATP-ase migrates with Band 3 of the erythrocyte membrane (Avruch and Fairbanks, 1972; Knauf et al., 1974). Previous studies have demonstrated no alteration in the amount of acyl-phosphorylation of MyD Band 3 (Roses and Appel, 1975). It is intriguing to speculate that the defect in MyD may be a structural mutation of the Na^+K^+ ATP-ase, not affecting acyl-phosphorylation or the energy utilizing mechanism, but affecting the function of the molecule. This hypothesis forms the basis of our current investigation and is testable by existing techniques.

Our laboratories have also reported decreased Ca^{++} stimulated K^+ efflux and altered membrane fluidity as measured by electron spin resonance spectroscopy in MyD erythrocytes (Gardos, 1958; Appel and Roses, 1976; Butterfield et al, 1976). The molecular machinery for the Ca^{++} stimulated K^+ efflux is unknown but other investigators have suggested that the ouabain sensitive Na^+K^+ ATP-ase "channel" may be involved (Knauf et al., 1974). A difference in charge (phosphorylation) of an intrinsic membrane protein such as Component a could affect the electron spin resonance spectra obtained with either inter-calculated lipid nitroxide labels or proteins specific nitroxide labels.

The question of whether similar alterations are present in muscle, lens, and other affected tissues remains to be answered. Red cells were used because of the lack of availability and controllability of other involved tissues. Experiments using skin fibroblast tissue culture

and isolated intact human muscle cells from intercostal
muscle biopsies are designed to test the data derived
from erythrocyte studies. Should a specific abnormal peptide be isolated from MyD red cells, antibodies to that
peptide may be useful in detecting and localizing abnormal
proteins in other affected MyD tissues.

Although recent literature has suggested that Component
a glycoproteins are broadly similar with respect to cleavage by pronase treatment (Steck and Fairbanks, 1971), it
is possible that a wide range of molecular microheterogeneity
exists. Microheterogeneity of structure may be translated
into heterogeneity of function. It is possible that
sequential elution lectin affinity chromatography could be
useful in dissecting specific transport proteins from the
Component a group. Experiments designed to label the
Na^+K^+ ATP-ase specifically, as well as other transport
proteins, and to further evaluate these purification methods
are currently in progress.

ACKNOWLEDGEMENTS

This work was supported by a Basil O'Conner Starter
Research Grant from the National Foundation March of Dimes,
N.I.N.C.D.S. Program Project Grant NS-12213-01, and N.I.N.
C.D.S. Grant NS-13455-01A1. During the course of this
work Allen D. Roses was the recipient of a Research Career
Development Award of the N.I.N.C.D.S. Pierre Wong is a
Fellow of the Muscular Dystrophy Association of America.
Allen D. Roses is an Investigator of the Howard Hughes
Medical Institute.

REFERENCES

Appel SH, Roses AD (1976). Membrane biochemical studies in
     myotonic muscular dystrophy. In Bolis L, Hoffman JF,
     Leaf A (eds) "Membranes and Disease," New York: Raven,
     p.183.
Avruch J, Fairbanks G. (1972). Demonstration of a phospho-
     peptide intermediate in the Mg^{++}-dependent, Na^+K^+-
     stimulated adenosine triphosphatase reaction of the
     erythrocyte membrane. Proc Nat Acad Sci U.S.A.
     69:1216.

Butterfield DA, Chesnut DB, Roses AD, Appel SH (1976).
    Erythrocyte membrane fluidity in myotonic and Duchenne
    muscular dystrophy and congenital myotonia: a spin
    study. Nature 263:159.
Butterfield DA, Roses AD, Chesnut DB, Appel SH (1974).
    Electron spin resonance studies of erythrocyte from
    patients with myotonic muscular dystrophy. Pro Nat
    Acad Sci U.S.A. 71:909.
Butterfield DA, Roses AD, Chesnut DB, Appel SH (1976).
    Electron spin resonance studies of membrane proteins
    in erythrocytes in myotonic dystrophy. Arch Biochem
    Biophys 177:226.
Fairbanks G, Steck TL, Wallach DFH (1971). Erythrophoretic
    analysis of the major polypeptide of the human erythro-
    cyte membrane. Biochem 10:2620.
Findlay JBC (1974). The receptor proteins for concanavalin
    a lens culinaris phytohemagglutinin in membrane of
    the human erythrocyte. J Bio Chem 249:4398.
Gardos G (1958). The function of calcium in the potassium
    permeability of human erythrocytes. Biochem Biophys
    Acta 30:653.
Hull KL, Roses AD (1976). Stoichiometry of sodium and
    potassium transport in erythrocytes from patients with
    myotonic muscular dystrophy. J Physiol 254:169.
Knauf PA, Proverbio F, Hoffman JF (1974). Chemical character-
    ization and pronase susceptibility of the Na:K pump-
    associated phosphoprotein of human red blood cells.
    J Gen Physiol 69:305.
Miller SE, Roses AD, Appel SH (1976). Scanning electron
    microscopy studies in muscular dystrophy. Arch
    Neurol 33:172.
Roses AD (1976). Substrate Heterogeneity of Component a of
    of the human erythrocyte membrane. J Supramol Struct
    4:481.
Roses AD, Appel SH (1973). Erythrocyte protein phosphory-
    lation. J Bio Chem 248:1408.
Roses AD, Appel SH (1976). Erythrocyte spectrin peak II
    phosphorylation in Duchenne muscular dystrophy.
    J Neuro Sci 29:185.
Roses AD, Appel SH (1975). Phosphorylation of component a
    of the human erythrocyte membrane in myotonic muscular
    dystrophy. J Membr Biol 20:51.
Steck TL, Fairbanks G, Wallach DFH (1971). Disposition of
    the major protein in the isolated erythrocyte membrane.
    Proteolytic dissection. Biochem 10:2617.

Steck TL, Yu J (1973). Selective solubilization of proteins from red blood cell membranes by protein perturbants. J Supramol Struct 1:220.

DISCUSSION

Dr. Steck: I share with you the hypothesis that band 3 is heterogenous, as Mike Sheetz, you, and others have indicated. However, the glucose transport polypeptide no longer seems to be associated with this material. Furthermore, we have been struck by how much homogeneity there is in the polypeptide portion of this conspicuously polydisperse glycoprotein. We think that most of the diffuseness is due to carbohydrate heterogeneity and not the polypeptide portion. I think your work is consistent with that. I would be willing to call this component bands 3 and not band 3, if I thought that would lessen the confusion.

Dr. Roses: I really don't think there's that much confusion. It is a difficult field to follow closely. However, I think the operational definition that you're giving to band 3 is valid. We find that we get the same results, though in terms of separating further fractions by affinity chromatography we can pick up apoprotein heterogeneity as indicated by the differences in phosphorylation and, when we do the peptide mapping on high pressure ion exchange chromatography, heterogeneity is definitely there.

Dr. Fairbanks: Going back to the first part of the talk, it's clear that ionic strength plays some role in the selective elution of this peptide from your ricin column. Can you exclude the possibility that phosphorylation itself is changing the yield of the polypeptide, the phosphoprotein from the column and thereby introducing artifactually the differences that you see?

Dr. Roses: The yield is not different, the yield is exactly the same, and the relative specific phosphorylation in the fraction myotonic is one half that of the control. When we measure incorporation of ^{32}P we are not seeing the total phosphorylation of the protein. In fact we are only able to add ^{32}P to available serine or threonine residues. What we're talking about is the amount of phosphate that may be able to be put on these proteins in an in vitro reaction and I don't know whether, for instance, the defect in myotonic dystrophy may be a protein that is already more phosphorylated so that new phosphate cannot be added so that total phosphorylation would be the same.

The Red Cell, pages 489—491

Dr. Fairbanks: Yes, there are at least three ways to
generate the result: One is an altered acceptor capacity
due to variations in the phosphorylation as you get it; a
second is a membrane reorganization that changes the relationship between the kinase and the acceptor; the third is
a difference in the amount of kinase activity in the membrane.

Dr. Roses: Absolutely.

Dr. Fairbanks: In relation to the last, I'd like to suggest
that the phosphorylation in band 3 area is cyclic AMP independent and you wouldn't see the enzyme activity with histone
or protamine as substrate; if you want to look for that, the
thing to use is casein as a substrate.

Dr. Roses: We never found any differences using casein as
a substrate nor any differences in myotonic dystrophy membranes using F2C histone as a substrate. As a matter of
fact, we have been working on this one small shred of specific
difference which is only a small part of the Band 3 phosphorylation. The difference has never been there in any of the
other lectin affinity columns that we've used. The RC-1
data represents over 3 years of work and is the only method
so far that has separated a fraction of decreased relative
specific phosphorylation in myotonic dystrophy.

Dr. Forman: You mentioned that there were very little hematological manifestations in the myotonic syndrome. I wondered on the basis of the experiment showing the difference
of efflux of sodium from the cell whether there would in
fact be any morphological changes or changes in the MCV of
red cells as a function of that sodium remaining within the
cell itself.

Dr. Roses: There doesn't appear to be in measurements that
one could make. I'm sure you are all familiar with the
flurry of excitement over muscular dystrophy having echinocytes. It reached the front pages of both Nature and Science
and since we had done those experiments previously and never
found those results, we repeated them in a very, very careful
fashion. We found that the myotonic dystrophy red cells as
well as those from a number of other genetic diseases tend
to form stomatocytes easier under certain conditions of fixation. Trying to relate changes in the NaK ATPase to this
phenomenon is a futile exercise. Investigators have estimated
approximately 150-300 molecules of the Na,K ATPase per cell

and it probably has little effect. Ion leaks probably account
for more flux.

Dr. Lehman: You did not mention on your list the lowered IgG
in these patients, did you?

Dr. Roses: Yes, it's on there. The IgG is lowered in many
patients. There is a hypercatabolism of IgG such that the
IgG levels are lowered in myotonic patients. Nobody has
ever really explained this phenomenon in molecular terms but
it appears to be a hypercatabolism of normal IgG. Myotonic
dystrophy patients have all sorts of things that are abnormal;
you can make a list five times greater. One of the most
interesting abnormalities that they have is a unique kind
of cataract. It's a scintillating cataract close to the
rear part of the lens, and it's almost diagnostic in human
disease for myotonic dystrophy. The only other disease that
it's been seen in is a form of mouse hereditary cataracts.
Iwata studied the membranes from the cataract of this mouse
and found a difference in the activity of the Na,K ATPase.

CHRONIC GRANULOMATOUS DISEASE, Kx ANTIGEN AND THE KELL BLOOD GROUPS

W. Laurence Marsh

Immunohematology Laboratory
Lindsley F. Kimball Research Institute of The
New York Blood Center, 310 East 67th Street
New York, New York 10021

The Kell blood group of red cells was discovered by
Coombs, Mourant and Race[6] in 1946. As with most blood
groups, subsequent studies have revealed a complex system
which at present includes about 20 different antigens.
The blood group is inherited in a straightforward manner
as an autosomal dominant characteristic. A rare null
phenotype, in which all Kell antigens are missing, was
described by Chown et al.[5] and named K_O. Family studies
indicate that it arises by inheritance of silent K^O genes
at the Kell locus from both parents. Another rare variant, in which the red cells show very weak antigenicity
in the Kell system, was found by Allen et al.[1] and named
McLeod after the propositus. Family studies were at first
uninformative in establishing the manner of inheritance
of the McLeod phenotype.

Blood group notation has many inconsistencies and
Allen and Rosenfield[2] have proposed a numerical system
for the Kell blood group in an attempt to establish uni-
formity. The numerical terminology has been extended as
new specificities have been recognized.

In 1969 a boy with X-linked chronic granulomatous
disease (CGD) was found to possess a rare red-cell variant in the Kell blood group system.[15] Other CGD cases
involving variant Kell blood groups were described by
Giblett et al.[9] who pointed out that blood transfusions
given to these children often provoke an antibody that
reacts with virtually all random donor bloods. Early
studies suggested that the Kell variant found may be
either the K_O or the McLeod types, but differentiation
between these two closely similar phenotypes is difficult

The Red Cell, pages 493—507

© **1978 Alan R. Liss, Inc., New York, New York**

to make without certain rare Kell system antisera. Recent
investigations indicate that the variant seen is invariably that of the McLeod type. Only one person in N.
America[1] and two in New Zealand[36] are known to have the
McLeod phenotype without CGD and the findings in CGD cannot be due to coincidence.

CHRONIC GRANULOMATOUS DISEASE

Chronic granulomatous disease is a disorder in which
the main feature is high susceptibility to infection by
low-grade bacterial pathogens.[4] The disease is characterized pathologically by sterile granulomata containing
lipid-laden macrophages. A family incidence to the disease was noted in early reports and the condition was
believed to have an X-linked recessive mode of inheritance.
Reports of female patients with CGD raised doubts concerning the genetic background of the condition,[3] but it is
now clear that at least one other defect may cause the
same clinical syndrome. In the majority of cases the
disease affects male children and is inherited as an
X-linked condition from the carrier mother.[42] Affected
boys show no evidence of any immunodeficiency disorder
but have normal delayed hypersensitivity responses[36,4]
and hypergammaglobulinemia.[13] The finding that immune
mechanisms in these patients were normal prompted critical studies of their phagocytic leukocyte function. Lyso-
zyme activity of the cells proved to be normal and they
possessed normal phagocytic capability. The important
finding was that although phagocytosis was normal certain
intracellular metabolic changes which should accompany it
did not occur,[12] and the leukocytes had impaired *in vitro*
killing power against several pathogenic and non-patho-
genic organisms.[28] The clinical entity of X-linked chronic granulomatous disease, in which a defect in bactericidal activity of monocytes and neutrophil leukocytes
allows repeated, and sometimes overwhelming, infections
thus became firmly established. Metabolic studies on
leukocytes from these children show impairment in oxidative metabolism, hexosemonophosphate shunt activation and
in generation of superoxide and hydrogen peroxide during
phagocytosis. Phagocytosis by normal leukocytes is accompanied by a burst of cell oxidative enzyme activity which
is largely responsible for the cell bacterial killing
power.[14] Early studies on leukocytes from CGD patients

suggested that deficiency of oxidative enzymes might be
responsible for the functional abnormality. Studies on
separated cell components of neutrophil leukocytes have
now confirmed the involvement of oxidative enzymes and
localized the abnormality to a defect in activation of an
NADH-dehydrogenase present in the plasma membrane.[34]
The precise nature of the biochemical lesion that causes
the defect, however, is still unknown. As with many
inherited diseases the severity in different individuals
varies, but within a single family affected members show
somewhat comparable degrees of disability. In the most
severe form of CGD boys die from an infection in the first
years of life.

KELL BLOOD GROUP RELATIONSHIPS BETWEEN RED CELLS AND
LEUKOCYTES

Initial aspects of our investigation were aimed at
establishing the relationship between the red cell Kell
autosomal blood group and the X-linked functional defect
of the phagocytic leukocytes. In these studies it was
essential to distinguish accurately between K_O and McLeod,
the two important Kell-variant phenotypes. One antibody
that helps make this differentiation is anti-Ku. This
is found in the serum of immunized K_O people and is compatible only with other examples of the K_O type.[5] A
second informative antibody was found by van der Hart
et al.[10] in 1968, and named anti-KL. This antibody occurred in the serum of a boy whose red cells possessed
weak antigens in the Kell system. He suffered from
repeated infections and died subsequently from what, in
retrospect, was probably chronic granulomatous disease.
Red cells of common Kell types and K_O cells were all
reactive with anti-KL, but McLeod type red cells were
compatible. The investigation by van der Hart et al.[10]
included antibody absorption studies using K_O red cells,
with results which suggested that anti-KL serum may
contain more than one component. The observation that
two antibodies might be present was confirmed by Marsh
et al.[18] who separated an example of anti-KL into two
antibody fractions. The name anti-Kx (anti-K15 in
numerical notation) was proposed for an antibody component that reacts strongly with K_O red cells but extremely weakly with red cells of common Kell type. The second
fraction, anti-KL, reacts strongly with red cells of

common Kell type but is non-reactive with K_o cells.
Anti-Kx makes a clear distinction between the McLeod and
the K_o red cell types, for McLeod cells lack Kx, while
K_o cells possess greatly increased amounts of the antigen.

Kx ANTIGEN

The link between the red cell Kell blood group system
and the X-linked defect of the phagocytic leukocytes
proved to be Kx antigen. Marsh et al.[18] were unable to
detect the Kell antigens K, k, Kp[b], Js[b], K12, K13 or Ku
on normal leukocytes, but demonstrated strong Kx using
an antibody absorption technique. Tests on separated
cell types from buffy-coat preparations showed Kx antigen
on normal neutrophil leukocytes and monocytes,[19] the two
cell types that are functionally defective in CGD.[28,7]
Absorption of unprocessed anti-KL+Kx serum with normal
leukocytes removed the anti-Kx component but left anti-KL,
an experiment which confirmed the presence of Kx on leukocytes.[18] Investigation of defective leukocytes from boys
with CGD then established that these cells lack Kx antigen. Leukocytes from 50 normals were all Kx positive but
9 patients with X-linked CGD all had Kx negative leukocytes.[22] The probability that this association would
occur by chance is 7.95×10^{-11} (Fisher's exact method).
The case for a direct association between lack of leukocyte Kx and the defect in bactericidal function is thus
overwhelming. The 50 normal tests establish that the
Kx positive white cell phenotype has a minimum frequency
of 0.94 (confidence level 95%) but it seems probable that
the antigen is a fundamental property of normal phagocytic
leukocytes. The biochemical nature of Kx is as yet unknown. The functional defect of CGD leukocytes is believed to result from a failure to activate NADH-dehydrogenase in the cell membrane. Marsh et al.[22] have suggested
that the membrane structure that has Kx antigenicity may
be a trigger mechanism involved in activation of this
oxidative enzyme. Other leukocyte antigens are normal in
CGD patients and the functional abnormality is associated
specifically with the absence of Kx.

THE GENETICS OF Kx

There is now good evidence to show that Kx is

produced by an X-linked gene. The observation that K_O red cells have strong Kx allows the conclusion that the antigen cannot be produced by the Kell autosomal gene, for K_O cells are homozygous for silent Kell alleles. The most reasonable explanation assigns Kx to the role of a precursor in the Kell biosynthetic pathway. Inheritance of silent Kell genes causes the K_O phenotype and leaves a great excess of unconverted Kx as the only Kell-related antigen on the red-cell membrane.

More individuals of McLeod type have been found and all are males. The absence of the phenotype in females and the finding that the McLeod-producing locus is inactivated by Lyon effect all indicate an X-borne mode of transmission. The weak Kell antigens of McLeod individuals differ qualitatively as well as quantitatively from the Kell antigens of other people.[18,20] All of these findings indicate that lack of Kx precursor substance modifies expression of a normal Kell gene to produce the McLeod phenotype. Inheritance of the McLeod type thus reflects the genetics of Kx.

THE KELL BIOSYNTHETIC PATHWAY

Race and Sanger[31] have proposed that more than one locus might be involved in production of Kell antigens and that the McLeod phenotype might result from a defect in a Kell precursor. Subsequent studies have confirmed this proposal of genetic complexity. The Kell phenotype of normal red cells must arise by interaction between products of two independent genes. One, named X^1k, is X-linked and controls synthesis of the precursor-like substance named Kx.[18] The Kell autosomal gene utilizes Kx substance in production of Kell antigens.

Both normal leukocytes and normal red cells possess Kx antigen. Red cells of common Kell type have only a small amount of residual Kx, which probably remains through incomplete conversion in the Kell pathway. Absence of the antigen in either cell type is a rare event and the finding in some boys that both cell types lack Kx cannot be a result of coincidence and must be evidence that synthesis in both cell lines is ordered by the same structural gene. Most CGD boys with Kx negative leukocytes, however, have Kx positive red cells and common Kell phenotypes. Three males are known who have Kx negative (McLeod) red cells but do not have the leukocyte dysfunction that causes CGD. Leukocytes from one of

these have been examined and are Kx positive.[18] In all
of these cases family studies indicate an X-linked mode
of inheritance. It appears, therefore, that the common
allele called X^1k orders synthesis of Kx by phagocytic
leukocytes and red cells in healthy people. Each of
three rare variants named X^2k, X^3k, and X^4k, at the same
X-linked locus allows a different permutation of Kx synthesis between the two cell types. Absence of leukocyte
Kx is associated with a defect in bactericidal activity
and CGD, while lack of red cell Kx results in the McLeod
phenotype. Table 1 summarizes these antigenic and
functional relationships.

Table 1   Phenotypic and Clinical Effects
              Associated with Variant *Xk* Alleles

Kx antigen	Xk allele			
	X^1k	X^2k	X^3k	X^4k
Red cells:	present	absent	present	absent
Leukocytes:	present	absent	absent	present
Clinical effects:	None	CGD & McLeod Syndrome	CGD with normal red cells	Normal leuko-cytes & McLeod Syndrome

REGULATORY CHANGES AFFECTING THE Xk LOCUS

In a general sense variant alleles at the Xk locus
may be viewed as modifying genes of the Kell blood group
system. The antigenic pattern which results from hemizygous inheritance of a variant *Xk* allele must result from
a regulatory change in the gene. Normal Kx synthesis in
either leukocytes or red cells presumably requires the
structural gene and aberrant synthesis in either cell type
must reflect a change in regulation. This effect cannot
be caused by inheritance of an independent modifying
gene, for affected members of a single family always have
the same pattern of Kx antigen synthesis. The variant
allele must, therefore, be at the Xk locus. The human
blood groups offer precedents for such inherited cell-
specific modifications of structural gene activity. The
A_m and B_m phenotypes in the ABO blood group, for example,

are characterized by strong secretion of A or B blood
group substances in saliva, which must require an A or B
structural gene, but aberrant production of the antigen
in red cells. Family studies establish that the phenotype
may be inherited through an allele at the ABO locus.[30]
In this situation, also, it must be assumed that the modified permutation of antigenicity between secretory
tissues and red cells is caused by a tissue-specific
change in gene regulation.

HEMATOLOGICAL CHANGES ASSOCIATED WITH THE McLEOD
PHENOTYPE

Although blood group characteristics of the McLeod
phenotype were recognized by Allen et al.[1] in 1961, not
until 1975 was it realized that the phenotype was associated with profound changes in red cell morphology and
a hemolytic condition. Wimer et al.[41] found that red
cells from the first known McLeod person showed aniso-
cytosis and marked acanthocytosis, and that the donor,
although apparently healthy, had an enlarged spleen,
reticulocytosis, reduced serum haptoglobin, and a compensated hemolytic state. The cell morphological changes
are readily discernable by light microscopy and are even
more striking by scanning electron microscopy. Marsh
et al.[20] found the same acanthocytic red cell changes in
5 other examples of the McLeod phenotype and Taswell
et al.[39] have reported a CGD boy with the McLeod phenotype, acanthocytic red cell morphology, and hemolytic
anemia. The red cell anomalies arise by lack of Kx
antigen and not through deficiency of Kell antigens.
K_O red cells, which have strong Kx but lack Kell system
antigens, are morphologically normal. Leukocytes from
K_O donors are also normal, both in their bactericidal
function[9] and Kx antigenicity.[18] Individuals of McLeod
type do not have abetalipoproteinemia[24] and their red-cell
lipid composition is normal.[26]
The i antigen strength of red cells is known to
increase during hyperactive red cell production.[11] Tests
for i antigenicity on red cells from two CGD boys with
McLeod phenotype by Marsh et al.[22] showed enhanced activity, suggesting they had increased erythropoiesis. CGD
boys with McLeod type red cells frequently require blood
transfusions, but the need for transfusion is rare in
CGD boys whose red cells are of common Kell type. The

previous clinical impression has been that the anemia in
CGD was an effect of chronic sepsis but it seems probable
that it results, in part at least, from abnormal survival
of morphologically atypical red cells.

TYPE I AND TYPE II CGD

Absence of leukocyte Kx antigen in X-linked CGD is
not a secondary change caused by the disease, and the
cell-membrane structure that carries the Kx antigenic
marker appears to be one of profound biologic importance.
Marsh et al.[22] have divided X-linked CGD into two categories based on the distribution of Kx antigen. Type I
CGD has Kx deficiency which is restricted to the leukocytes,
and red cell morphology in this case is normal. Type II
CGD has Kx deficiency in both leukocytes and red cells
and as a consequence the granulomatous disease is accompanied by the McLeod phenotype, acanthocytic changes in
red cell morphology, and hemolytic anemia. The Xk genes
responsible for Type I and Type II CGD are X^3k and X^2k,
respectively, the majority of cases being of Type I. For
those wishing to commit details to memory, it is convenient to remember that X^2k produces Type II CGD and is
characterized by Kx deficiency in both cell lines.

THE McLEOD SYNDROME

Hemizygous inheritance of X^4k allows normal leukocyte Kx antigenicity but results in McLeod phenotype red
cells with the associated clinical and hematological
complications. It seems appropriate to call the interrelated consequences of red-cell Kx deficiency that arise
through inheritance of X^2k or X^4k the McLeod Syndrome.
Only two families are known in which some male members
have McLeod Syndrome without CGD. Shepherd and Marsh[36]
have studied a New Zealand family in which two males
have McLeod Syndrome with moderately severe hematological
effects, and two other male members have died from unexplained anemia at ages of 3 years and 19 years. It
appears possible that clinical manifestation of the McLeod
Syndrome may range from abnormal red-cell morphology with
a compensated hemolytic state, to a fatal hemolytic condition.

Xk VARIANT ALLELES IN CARRIER FEMALES

Windhorst et al.[42] have reported that phagocytic
leukocytes from mothers of boys with X-linked CGD comprise
a double population of functional and non-functional cells.
Marsh et al.[19] found that carrier females have leukocytes
with an intermediate level of Kx antigenicity, a finding
that is consistent with a dual Kx positive and Kx negative
cell population.

Swanson et al.[38] demonstrated by quantitative studies
that red cells from mothers of McLeod boys had weak k and
Kp^b antigens. Marsh et al.[21] subsequently found that
these female carriers were blood group mosaics, having a
mixture of common Kell and McLeod type red cells. The
mosaicism is also detectable hematologically, for blood
smears from carrier females show a mixture of normal red
cells and acanthocytes. Meticulous blood group studies
are necessary to demonstrate the mosaicism in female
carriers who have relatively few McLeod type red cells.
In these cases the double cell population may be recognized more easily by identifying acanthocytes in a stained
blood smear. In each of 7 females who were carriers of
variant *Xk* alleles Marsh et al.[23] found that the population of red cells having common Kell type and normal morphology greatly outnumbered the abnormal cells that were
of McLeod type. The bias that favors normal red cells is
unlikely to be a chance phenomenon and probably arises
because the cells of common Kell type have normal survival in the peripheral circulation while the abnormal
McLeod cells are prematurely eliminated.

LYONIZATION OF THE *Xk* LOCUS

The leukocyte and/or red cell mosaicism seen in
females who are carriers of variant *Xk* alleles is attributed to the Lyon phenomenon of X-chromosome inactivation,[17] and the finding provides convincing support for
assignment of the Xk locus to the X-chromosome. The
mosaicism also proves that Kx is a property of the red
cells themselves and is not acquired by passive absorption from the plasma.

In man not all X-borne genes are inactivated by
Lyon effect. The X-linked Xg^a blood group provided
significant information in this respect. It might have
been expected that *Xg^{a}Xg* females would have a double

population of Xg(a+) and Xg(a-) red cells. Because of
technical difficulties it was some time after recognition
of Xg[a] before Race,[29] in 1971, could conclude that females
who are heterozygous at the Xg locus do not have a mixed
Xg[a] population of red cells and that the Xg locus is not
inactivated by Lyon effect. Wimer et al.[41] and Marsh
et al.[23] have studied bloods from *Xg[a]Xg* female carriers
of variant *Xk* alleles, whose sons had the McLeod Syndrome.
All red cells in the double population present in the female bloods were Xg(a+). Furthermore, when the normal red
cells were removed by agglutination with anti-Kx serum the
remaining Kx negative (McLeod) cells could still be typed
as Xg(a+). It appears, therefore, that a lyonized X
chromosome has an inactive Xk locus but a functional Xg
locus that can order production of Xg[a].

In 1975 Marsh[20] compared antigenic strength in the
Kell system of red cells taken from normal males and females to determine whether the homozygous female produces
more Kx and therefore has stronger Kell antigens. The
study showed no significant difference between the sexes,
a finding that would be expected in the light of the more
recent discovery that one Xk locus in females is inactivated by Lyon effect.

LINKAGE OF THE Xg AND Xk LOCI

Red cells of boys with CGD may be Xg(a+) or Xg(a-).
Marsh et al.[18] were unable to detect Xg[a] on normal leukocytes. Although there is no evidence of any functional
relationship between the products of the *Xg* and *Xk* genes,
recent data have established that the two loci are closely
linked. Race and Sanger[33] mention two Xg non-recombinant
CGD children who hint at possible linkage between the
loci, and more non-recombinants were added to the list
through a CGD family study by Marsh et al.[19] Analysis
of other informative families has now established the
linkage ($\theta = 0.00$ with a lod score of 3.426).[26] If
there is no linkage disequilibrium, about 45 percent of
Xk carrier mothers will also be heterozygous at the Xg
locus and potentially informative in using Xg[a] to trace
transmission of the variant *Xk* gene. The fathers, of
course, do not have to be considered in studies on boys
suspected to have X-linked CGD. In those informative
families where the father is Xg(a-) it may also be possible
to use Xg[a] typing to identify daughters who are probable

carriers of *Xk* variant alleles.

THE RELATIONSHIP BETWEEN KELL AND Kx

Little is known of the biochemical nature of antigenic determinants in the Kell system. Extraction of red
cell membranes with *n*-butanol at 0°C leaves inhibitory
activity for anti-k (and anti-K if the cells are K positive) in the aqueous phase of the extraction.[23] This
suggests that some Kell activity is present as glycoprotein. But whether the carbohydrate or the protein moiety
of the glycoprotein carries the specific determinant is
not known. Discovery that a coliform organism, which
caused infantile enterocolitis, produces a metabolite
with Kell-like antigenicity allows some speculation. Infection with the organism stimulated production of apparent naturally-occuring anti-K in the patient.[25] Characterization of the bacterial K-like substance is in progress but preliminary results indicate that it is poly-
saccharide.[23] If the antigens of the Kell system result
from immuno-dominant sugars the Kell gene product must
be transferase enzymes. Kx antigen may, therefore, be a
marker on a structural protein to which the Kell specific
sugars are attached. The limited information available
concerning the biological importance of blood group antigens indicates that loss of carbohydrate antigens, such as
ABH, does not alter red cell shape or survival[35,17] but
absence of an antigen which marks a membrane protein, such
as Rh, causes changes in red cell shape and decreased cell
survival[16,37]. The proposed Kx-Kell relationship is in
accord with these general characteristics, and would
explain why K_O cells, which may lack only Kell-specific
sugars, have normal appearance and appear to have normal
in vivo survival, while McLeod cells, which lack Kx, a
possible structural protein, have changes in shape and
reduced survival.

NON X-LINKED GRANULOMATOUS DISEASE

On rare occasions, granulomatous disease affects
girls.[3] In these cases blood group anomalies in the
Kell system are not involved and the leukocytes do not
lack Kx.[22] The disease in these cases is inherited as
an autosomal recessive condition. A boy with this type

of CGD studied by Marsh et al.[24] had Kx positive leukocytes. Although the clinical findings and leukocyte
functional studies are similar, it appears probable that
autosomal-recessive CGD is a different disease.

CONCLUSION

Despite 70 years of blood group studies only
recently has it been possible to assign a biologic function to certain antigens. Absence of Rh antigens changes
red cell shape,[37] and the Duffy antigen has been identified as the membrane receptor used for invasion of the
red cell by the parasite of benign tertian malaria.[27]
Although chronic granulomatous disease and the McLeod
phenotype are rare conditions they are important, for
their investigation has revealed that the Kx blood group
antigen plays a vital functional role in red cells and
leukocytes. Synthesis of Kx is ordered by an X-linked
gene and the fundamental defect in X-linked CGD must be
failure to inherit $X^l k$. The enzymatic and functional
disorders of the phagocytic leukocytes, the structural
changes in the red cells, and the infections and hemolytic anemia in the patients, are consequences which
follow. Perhaps one of the most exciting aspects of these
investigations has been the discovery that the Xg and Xk
loci are closely linked. Xg[a] has been detected on red
cells from fetuses aged less than 20 weeks[40] although the
antigen increases greatly in strength later in fetal
life.[32] For purposes of counselling, in about half of
CGD families Xg[a] red cell typing will allow recognition
at birth of sons who have probably inherited the variant
Xk gene. It is also possible that tests for Xg[a] on fetal
cells may allow the same recognition prior to birth.
The wonderful complexity of the human blood groups
astounds the imagination. The challenge to discover
functional roles for other cellular antigenic structures
lies before us.

Acknowledgements

I am grateful to Ms. M.E. Nichols and Ms. R. Øyen
who between them have been responsible for all of the
technical work in this investigation. The cooperation
of many clinicians and blood bankers who have referred
CGD cases to our laboratory for investigation, is

gratefully acknowledged.

References

1. Allen FH, Krabbe SMR, Corcoran PA (1961). A new
      phenotype (McLeod) in the Kell blood group system.
      Vox Sang 6:555
2. Allen FH, Rosenfield RE (1961). Notation for the
      Kell blood group system. Transfusion 1:305.
3. Azimi PH, Bodenbender JG, Hintz RL, Kontras SB (1968).
      Chronic granulomatous disease in three female
      siblings. JAMA 206:2865.
4. Bridges RA, Berendes H, Good RA (1959). A fatal
      granulomatous disease of childhood. Am J Dis
      Children 97:387.
5. Chown B, Lewis M, Kaita H (1957). A 'new' Kell blood
      group phenotype. Nature 180:711.
6. Coombs RRA, Mourant AE, Race RR (1946). In-vivo
      isosensitization of red cells in babies with hae-
      molytic disease. Lancet i:264.
7. Davis WC, Huber H, Douglas SD, Fudenberg HH (1968).
      A defect in circulating mononuclear phagocytes in
      chronic granulomatous disease of childhood.
      J Immunol 101:1093.
8. Galey WR, Evan AP, Van Nice PS, Dail WG, Wimer B,
      Cooper RA (in press). Morphology and physiology
      of the McLeod phenotype erythrocyte: I. scanning
      electron micorscopy and electrolyte and water
      transport properties. Blood.
9. Giblett ER, Klebanoff SJ, Pincus SH, Swanson J,
      Park BH, McCullough J (1971). Kell phenotypes
      in chronic granulomatous disease: a potential
      transfusion hazard. Lancet i:1235.
10. Hart Mvd, Szaloky A, van Loghem JJ (1968). A 'new'
      antibody associated with the Kell blood group
      system. Vox Sang 15:456.
11. Hillman RS, Giblett ER (1965). Red cell membrane
      alteration associated with marrow stress. J Clin
      Invest 44:1730.
12. Holmes B, Quie PG, Windhorst DB, Good RA (1966).
      Fatal granulomatous disease of childhood: An
      inborn abnormality of phagocytic function.
      Lancet i:1225.

13. Janeway CA, Craig J, Davidson M, Downey W, Gitlan D
    (1954). Hypergammaglobulinemia associated with
    severe recurrent and chronic non-specific infection.
    Am J Dis Child 88:388.
14. Klebanoff SJ, Clem WH, Leubke RD (1966). The perox-
    idase-thiocyanate-hydrogen peroxide anti-microbial
    system. Biochem Biophys Acta 117:63.
15. Klebanoff SJ, White LR (1969). Iodination defect in
    the leukocytes of a patient with chronic granulo-
    matous disease of childhood. New Eng J Med 280:460.
16. Levine P, Tripodi D, Struck J, Zmijewski CM, Pollack
    W (1973). Hemolytic anemia associated with Rh_{null}
    disease. Vox Sang 23:182.
17. Lyon MF(1961). Genetic factors on the X chromosome.
    Lancet ii:434.
18. Marsh WL, Øyen R, Nichols ME, Allen FH (1975).
    Chronic granulomatous disease and the Kell blood
    groups. Brit J Haematol 29:247.
19. Marsh WL, Uretsky SC, Douglas SD (1975). Antigens
    of the Kell blood group system on neutrophils and
    monocytes: their relation to chronic granulomatous
    disease J Pediat 87:1117.
20. Marsh WL (1975). Studies on the Kell blood group
    system. Med Lab Tech 32:1.
21. Marsh WL, Taswell HF, Øyen R, Nichols ME, Vergara MS,
    Pineda AA: Kx antigen of the Kell system and its
    relationship to chronic granulomatous disease.
    Evidence that the *Kx* gene is X-linked. Transfusion
    15:527.
22. Marsh WL, Øyen R, Nichols ME (1976). Kx antigen,
    the McLeod phenotype, and chronic granulomatous
    disease: further studies. Vox Sang 31:356.
23. Marsh WL, Øyen R, Nichols ME (1976). unpublished
    observations.
24. Marsh WL, Clark R, Klebanoff SJ (1976) unpublished
    observations
25. Marsh WL, Nichols ME, Øyen R, Thayer R, Deere WL,
    Freed PJ, Schmelter SE (in press). Naturally
    occurring anti-Kell stimulated by E. coli entero-
    colitis in a 20 day old child. Transfusion.
26. Marsh WL, Allen FH, Øyen R, Mandel G, Kroovand S,
    Shepherd S (in preparation).
27. Miller LH, Mason SJ, Clyde DF, McGinnis MII (1976).
    The resistance factor to plasmodium vivax in blacks.
    New Eng J of Med 295:302.

28. Quie PG, White JG, Homes B, Good RA (1967). *In Vitro*
    bactericidal activity of human polymorphonuclear
    leukocytes: diminished activity in chronic granulo-
    matous disease of childhood. J Clin Invest 46:668.
29. Race RR (1971). Is the Xg blood group locus subject
    to inactivation? Proc 4th Int Cong Hum Genet
    "Excerpta Medica," Amsterdam, p. 311.
30. Race RR, Sanger R (1975). "Blood Groups in Man"
    6th ed. Oxford: Blackwell, p. 15.
31. Race RR, Sanger R (1975). "Blood Groups in Man"
    6th ed. Oxford, Blackwell, p. 302.
32. Race RR, Sanger R (1975). "Blood Groups in Man"
    6th ed. Oxford, Blackwell, p. 588.
33. Race RR, Sanger R (1975). "Blood Groups in Man"
    6th ed. Oxford, Blackwell, p. 603.
34. Segal AW, Peters TJ (1976). Characterization of the
    enzyme defect in chronic granulomatous disease.
    Lancet i:1363.
35. Seidl S. Spielman W, Martin H. (1972). Two siblings
    with Rh_{null} disease. Vox Sang 23:182.
36. Shepherd S, Marsh WL (1975) unpublished observations.
37. Sturgeon P (1970). Hematologic observations on the
    anemia associated with blood type Rh_{null}. 36:310.
38. Swanson J, Park B, McCullough J (1972). Kell phenotypes
    in families of patients with X-linked chronic granu-
    lomatous disease. Abstract XII Cong "Int Soc
    Blood Transfusion," Washington, p.26.
39. Taswell HF, Lewis JC, Marsh WL, Wimer BM, Pineda AA,
    Brzica SM (1977). Erythrocyte morphology in
    genetic defects of the Rh and Kell blood group
    systems. Mayo Clin Proc 52:157.
40. Toivanen P, Hirvonen T. (1973). Antigens Duffy, Kell,
    Kidd, Lutheran, and Xg^a on fetal red cells.
    Vox Sang 24:372.
41. Wimer BM, Marsh WL, Taswell HF, Galey WR (1977).
    Haematological changes associated with the McLeod
    phenotype of the Kell blood group system. Brit
    J Haematol 36:219.
42. Windhorst DB, Holmes D, Good RA (1967). Newly
    defined X-linked trait in man with demonstration
    of the Lyon effect in carrier females. Lancet i:737.

DISCUSSION

Dr. Roses: That's an extremely elegant study, both genetically and clinically. As a muscular dystrophy doctor, I've been impressed with the linkage of the Xg locus with Becker's muscular dystrophy, although not with the Duchenne type. Perhaps this locus is on the other side of it. Has this in any way been tested for linkage with X-linked muscular dystrophy?

Dr. Marsh: No, this has not been studied. We have already had some correspondence about following through on this.

Dr. Roses: Yes, is Xg on the short arm or the long arm?

Dr. Marsh: Well, the evidence is that Xg is on the short arm, but there is not very good evidence.

Dr. Schoomaker: Is the Kell antigen also expressed on fetal fibroblasts so that amniocentesis for prenatal diagnosis is possible?

Dr. Marsh: That's another thing we're looking into at the moment. The interesting thing about the linkage work, of course, is that Xg^a is expressed on fetal cells, and, as you know, on fibroblasts. In terms of genetic counseling we think that perhaps the most exciting thing about this is that if you Xg^a type fetal cells, with linkage as close as this, we've got, for genetic counseling purposes, a test where forty-five percent of mothers will be heterozygous at the Xg locus and therefore informative. You can then do genetic counseling by testing fetal cells, and get firm information.

Dr. Freedman: It's interesting to me that there are many, many clinical syndromes that cause acanthocytosis, among them many types of liver diseases. One disease of unknown etiology in newborns is infantile acanthocytosis. Now, the smear looks exactly like that you've shown us, the same as, for example, Kx deficiency. So my question is have you looked at a possible association here.

Dr. Marsh: No, we haven't. There are a lot of things to be done. We have, of course, for the moment been concentrating on the relationship I have described.We wanted to make abso-

The Red Cell, pages 509—511

lutely sure that we had a relationship that was totally
convincing, but there are a number of collaborative studies
goin on in different areas. The newborn syndrome we had not
thought of, but that would be an interesting study. We feel
perhaps that what is interesting is that the Kx work directs
attention to the blood groups; they have to do something
functional. They give me employment and the chance to come
and talk, but, nature had something else in mind. You know
the Rh story, that a deficiency of Rh protein causes red cell
membrane abnormalities. And we are hunting for other associations. We have an ongoing program in which young children who have anemia of unknown etiology associated with abnormal morphology are tested extensively for a wide range
of blood group antigens. We already have evidence that some
of the other blood groups may be involved in somewhat similar
membrane changes.

Dr. Forman: We're obviously all struck by the association
which you describe. However, during your talk, you referred
many times to the antigen as cause for the defect in granulocyte function. I wasn't sure I really saw that in your
presentation. I can see there's a marker but it's hard to
understand the marker as a cause of abnormal function. I
wonder if you could expand on this?

Dr. Marsh: This is a very real qeustion. Are we looking at
a secondary effect of the disease, an antigen change that is
caused by the defect in cell function, or is lack of Kx a
primary causation? The evidence, we think, is that it is a
primary defect. First of all, we know that Kx synthesis
is X-linked; the McLeod phenotype is inherited as an X-linked
characteristic. This puts a very close association at the
gene level. The female carriers, we think, are the most
significant feature. If Kx deficiency were a secondary
change of the disease, then one would expect to find absence
of the antigen in affected boys but not in the carrier mothers, who themselves are healthy. The fact that the carrier
mothers have a double population of Kx positive and negative
leukocytes and red cells we think is pretty good evidence
that we are looking at a primary genetic involvement.

Dr. Forman: But looking from a functional basis, are you
implying that the antigen that is expressed on the white
cell membrane and the enzyme that may be located on the white
cell membrane are linked? Is that what you're saying?

Dr. Marsh: Yes, that's what we think. We think that we are
looking at a marker on a functional structure. Segal and
Peters, for example, concluded that the abnormality in CGD
is a defect in activation of an NADH-dehydrogenase on the
leukocyte plasma membrane. There is a failure of the
enzyme trigger mechanism. Now, we don't understand the
biochemical nature of Kx and we don't know the exact nature
of the biochemical lesion **on the** cell but we think that
Kx is involved in the trigger mechanism of enzyme activation.

Dr. Forman: So, I may have missed it in your paper, but would
the implication of that be, then, that it would not be possible to have white cells with the antigen present but with
the bactericidal defect present?

Dr. Marsh: Not in this particular disease. Every case we see
is leukocyte Kx negative. The easy way to diagnose the disease
is to test for this antigen. The sad thing is that the antibody supply is very limited, because the only source of antibody is immunized McLeod boys. We've been attacking rabbits
to try and persuade them to make anti-Kx, so far without success. Once we can get a large amount of antibody, Kx typing
is a simple diagnostic test. Tests for bactericidal functional
activity of leukocytes are difficult, but they have to be
done at the moment.

Dr. Chilcote: I don't think any of the evidence that you've
presented so far would exclude the hypothesis that the activation of NADH dehydrogenase might not be involved in the
synthesis of the antigen itself. There is, perhaps, some post-
translational change that takes place with the antigen, and
since you don't know the structure of the antigen, that's still
a possibility.

Dr. Marsh: Yes, absolutely. We wouldn't disagree with you.
We need to know the structure to understand the relationship.

TRACE METALS AND THE RED CELL

Chairman: A. Prasad

DEOXYTHYMIDINE KINASE ACTIVITY, TOTAL COLLAGEN AND PROTEIN
IN THE SPONGE CONNECTIVE TISSUE OF SICKLE CELL ANEMIA SUBJECTS

Ananda S. Prasad, Felix Fernandez-Madrid and
James R. Ryan

Department of Medicine, Veterans Administration
Hospital, Allen Park, Michigan and Departments
of Medicine and Orthopedic Surgery, Wayne State
University School of Medicine, Detroit, Michigan

INTRODUCTION

Chronic leg ulcers and impaired wound healing in sickle
cell anemia (SCA) subjects is a well known clinical entity
(Wintrobe, 1974). However, as yet, studies related to protein
and collagen synthesis in SCA patients have not been reported
in the literature.

Our previous studies indicate that zinc plays an important role in deoxyribonucleic acid (DNA), collagen and protein
synthesis (Fernandez-Madrid et al, 1973 and Prasad et al,1974)
and that a deficiency of zinc may be a complicating factor in
SCA subjects (Prasad et al, 1975 and Prasad et al, 1976).
Thus it was considered desirable to investigate nucleic acid
metabolism, total protein and collagen content of the sponge
connective tissue of patients with SCA.

In this paper, we wish to: 1) summarize the role of zinc
in nucleic acid metabolism and collagen synthesis, 2) present
evidences supporting the occurrence of zinc deficiency in SCA
patients, and finally, 3) present our recent data with respect
to nucleic acid metabolism, and total protein and collagen
content of sponge connective tissue of the SCA patients.

The Red Cell, pages 515–535

1. Role of Zinc in Nucleic Acid Metabolism, and Protein and Collagen Synthesis

A beneficial effect of oral zinc administration on wound healing in man was reported by Pories et al (1967). Miller et al (1965) reported a retardation in the rate of healing of surgically excised wounds in zinc deficient cattle. Sandstead and Shepard (1968) found that the tensile strength of a healing surgical incision in the skin of zinc deficient rats was significantly decreased 12 days after surgery as compared to the tensile strength of wounds in the pair-fed rats. This was confirmed by Oberleas and co-workers (1971). In these pair-feeding experiments, it was shown that the differences in tensile strength were due to Zn deficiency and not to differences in caloric intake. It has also been reported that zinc deficient chickens and rats develop abnormalities in the epiphyseal plate region of growing bones (Westmoreland, 1971).

Several investigators have suggested that zinc plays a fundamental role in protein biosynthesis. Since collagen is the main fibrous protein of the connective tissue and is largely responsible for the development of tensile strength in the healing wound, biochemical studies have been focused to answer the question whether or not there is a specific effect of zinc deficiency on collagen synthesis, hydroxylation, conversion of procollagen to collagen, or some other aspect of its metabolism. Indeed, in our study a significant reduction in total collagen in sponge connective tissue of zinc deficient rats was found as compared to pair-fed controls (Table 1). However, in the same study there was a reduction in the total dry weight of the sponge connective tissue and of the non-collagenous protein content in the zinc deficient tissue as compared with the pair-fed controls. Moreover, the ribonucleic acid (RNA)/DNA ratio was significantly lower in zinc deficient connective tissue and in more severe deficient states there was also depletion of polyribosomes and a significant reduction of RNA as compared with the connective tissue of pair-fed rats (Tables 1, 2, 3 and Fig. 1). These data clearly indicate that the effect of zinc deficiency on collagen deposition was a generalized effect on protein synthesis and nucleic acid metabolism, rather than a specific effect on collagen synthesis. In fact, no differences were found with respect to level of hydroxylation, ultra-centrifugation, chromatography in CM-cellulose columns, or disc gel electrophoresis between highly purified collagen from zinc deficient animals and pair-fed rats (Fernandez-Madrid et al, 1973).

Table 1. Final body weight of rats, connective tissue weight, and content of zinc, RNA, and DNA of sponge connective tissue (SCT)

Experiment	Final body weight (Gm.)	SCT per rat (mg.)	Total SCT zinc per rat (μg)	SCT DNA (μg/mg.T)	SCT RNA (μg/mg.T)	RNA/DNA
Six day:						
A. Zinc deficient	143 ± 3.0*†	180 ± 19	8.2 ± 1.8	14.2 ± 1.95	20.1 ± 2.7	1.4 ± 0.07
B. P-F	162 ± 2.0	263 ± 19	18.5 ± 2.3	10.2 ± 1.08	21.1 ± 1.7	2.1 ± 0.26
p Value						
A vs. B	< 0.001	< 0.025	< 0.025	NS	NS	< 0.05
Ten day:						
A. Zinc deficient	110 ± 2	260.1 ± 10.7	34.5 ± 8.7	8.9 ± 0.89	7.4 ± 0.62	0.87 ± 0.12
B. P-F	132 ± 5	479.1 ± 29.1	57.3 ± 2.8	9.6 ± 0.79	13.4 ± 0.54	1.42 ± 0.14
C. Ad lib	321 ± 7	601.3 ± 42.8	92.8 ± 19.4	10.6 ± 0.80	15.4 ± 0.55	1.47 ± 0.08
p Value						
A vs. B	< 0.005	< 0.001	< 0.05	NS	< 0.001	< 0.025
A vs. C	< 0.001	< 0.001	< 0.05	NS	< 0.001	< 0.005
B vs. C	< 0.001	< 0.05	NS	NS	< 0.01	NS

P-F = Pair-fed control animals.
Ad lib = Ad libitum-fed control animals.
SCT = Sponge cornective tissue.
T = Tissue.
NS = Not significant.
*Mean ± standard error.
†Eight animals per observations.

Table 2. Protein and collagen content of sponge connective tissue (SCT)

Experiment	Total SCT protein per rat (mg.)	Total SCT collagen per rat (mg.)
Six day:		
A. Zinc deficient	98.31 ± 14.62*†	10.15 ± 1.62
B. P-F	195.1 ± 18.29	21.53 ± 1.62
p Value		
A vs. B	< 0.01	< 0.001
Ten day:		
A. Zinc deficiency	188.6 ± 12.3	27.6 ± 2.78
B. P-F	337.9 ± 39.4	50.1 ± 5.73
C. Ad lib	425.2 ± 29.3	43.9 ± 3.04
p Value		
A vs. B	< 0.025	< 0.01
A vs. C	< 0.001	< 0.005
B vs. C	NS	NS

P-F = Pair-fed control animals.
Ad lib = Ad libitum-fed control animals.
SCT = Sponge connective tissue.
NS = Not significant.
*Mean ± standard error.
†Eight animals per observation.

Table 3. In vitro incorporation of ^{14}C-thymidine into DNA
(10 days SCT)

	Counts/min./mg of DNA
Zinc deficient	$(1.4 \pm 0.36) \times 10^3$
Pair-fed controls	$(7.8 \pm 2.0) \times 10^3$

P < .001

Other studies have also attempted to answer the same
questions.   The work of Hsu et al (1968) revealed that zinc
deficiency drastically reduced the incorporation of labeled
glycine, proline and lysine into rat skin.   This study also
showed that there were no marked changes in the uptake of
these amino acids into liver, kidney, testes, or muscle protein.   Since collagen is unusually rich in these amino acids
it was suggested that perhaps zinc could be more important
in the metabolism of skin collagen than in the metabolism of
other proteins.   McClain et al (1973) have tried to further
elucidate the role of zinc in collagen metabolism.   They
found a decrease in the salt soluble fraction obtained from
zinc deficient animals which was thought to be due to a reduction in protein synthesis.   In support of that conclusion,
they found a reduction in the incorporation of labeled glycine into α_1 and α_2 chains of salt soluble rat skin collagen.
They did not find a significant reduction in the incorporation of labeled leucine into muscle polyribosomes but there
was an overall reduction of the polysome yield in the zinc
deficient animals.   These data, in agreement with the above
mentioned work suggested that total collagen is reduced in
the zinc deficient state as a part of a generalized impairment in protein synthesis.

Early studies of developing sponge connective tissue
have shown that a spurt of DNA synthesis precedes the increase
in the deposition of collagen (Kulonen, 1970).   Indeed, at

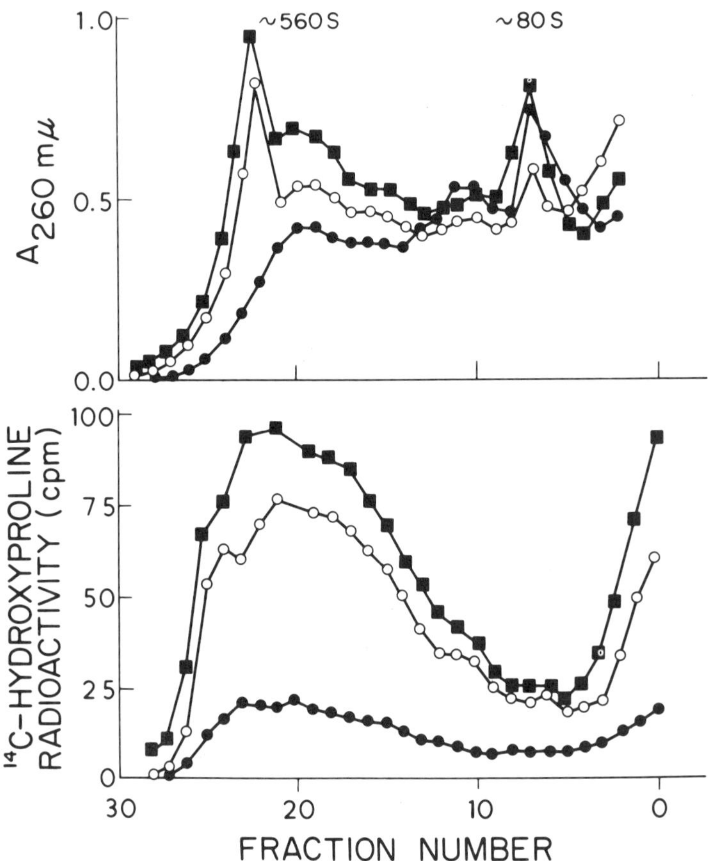

Fig. 1. Zone centrifugation through 15 to 60 per cent linear sucrose gradients of polyvinyl sponge connective tissue polyribosomes. The capsules from polyvinyl sponges removed 10 days after implantation from zinc-deficient, pair-fed, and ad libitum-fed rats were incubated in vitro with ^{14}C-proline for 30 minutes, and the ribosomal suspensions were prepared as indicated in Methods. The suspensions were centrifuged for 3 hours at 20,000 R.P.M. in the SW 25.1 rotor of the Spinco Model L ultracentrifuge. Absorbancy was monitored at 260 mμ and total and ^{14}C-hydroxyproline radioactivity were determined in the individual fractions as indicated in Methods. ■—■, ad libitum-fed control animals; o—o, pair-fed control animals; and ●—●, Zn-deficient animals. (Fernandez-Madrid et al, J Lab Clin Med 82: 951, 1973)

the time when fibroblast proliferation as expressed by DNA
synthesis is very active, there is very little accumulation
of fibrous collagen in the sponge. It seems that this initial
period of cell division preceding collagen deposition is a
common denominator of developing connective tissue in most
circumstances. It is therefore clear that any interference
with the synthesis of DNA and fibroblast proliferation will
profoundly influence the overall deposition of fibrous collagen in the developing connective tissue.

There are numerous studies showing that zinc deficiency
in animals impairs the incorporation of labeled thymidine
into DNA (Fujioka et al, 1964; Sandstead et al, 1969; and
Rubin et al, 1973). This effect has been detected within a
few days after the feeding of the zinc deficient diet was
begun. Williams and Chester (1970) observed a progressive
fall in the thymidine incorporation into DNA of liver, kidney
and spleen within 5 days after the zinc deficient diet was
fed to rats. Thus dietary zinc deficiency may result in an
immediate impairment of DNA biosynthesis. Prasad and Oberleas
(1974) provided evidence that decreased activity of thymidine
kinase may be responsible for this early reduction in DNA
synthesis and may ultimately relate to growth retardation
(Tables 4,5 & 6). The activity of thymidine kinase, an enzyme essential for DNA synthesis, was reduced in rapidly regenerating connective tissue of zinc deficient rats compared
to pair-fed controls as early as 6 days after the animals were
placed on the dietary treatment. These results have been confirmed recently by Dreosti and Hurley (1975). The activity
of thymidine kinase in 12-day fetuses taken from females exposed to a dietary zinc deficiency during pregnancy was significantly lower than in ad libitum and restricted-fed controls.
Activity of the enzyme was not restored by in vitro addition
of zinc whereas addition of copper severely affected the
enzyme activity adversely. In conclusion, the fibroblast
proliferation is impaired as a result of decreased DNA synthesis and this defect is a major contributing factor to the
abnormalities in wound healing found in the zinc deficient
state.

2. <u>Zinc Deficiency in Sickle Cell Anemia Patients</u>

Certain clinical features are common to some SCA patients
and zinc deficient patients, the latter as reported from the
Middle East (Prasad et al, 1975; Prasad et al, 1976). These

Table 4. Thymidine kinase activity in regenerating tissue* (nanomoles TMP formed per hour per milligram of protein).

	Deficient (A)	Restricted-fed (B)	Ad libitum (C)
6 Day	1.04 ± 0.14 (12)	3.57 ± 0.36 (13)	3.37 ± 0.36 (12)
13 Day	0.58 ± 0.02 (6)	2.40 ± 0.59 (5)	1.65 ± 0.12 (5)
17 Day	None (5)	2.70 ± 0.6 (5)	2.68 ± 0.7 (5)

*Mean ± S.E.
 Six day: deficient vs. either control, p < 0.001.
 Thirteen day: deficient vs. either control, p 0.025.

Table 5. ^{14}C-thymidine incorporation into DNA (6-day experiment) (DPM/mg. of DNA)

	Deficient	Restricted-fed	τ†
Experiment I	18.0 ± 5.7 x 10^3* (4)	136.2 ± 15.2 x 10^3 (4)	7.24+
Experiment II	14.4 ± 2.9 x 10^3 (6)	54.7 ± 7.5 x 10^3 (5)	4.99+

*Mean ± standard error.
†p < 0.001.

Table 6. Gain in body weight of rats, sponge connective tissue weight, and concentration of DNA, RNA, protein, and zinc in sponge connective tissue in 6-day experiments.

	Total gain in body wt. (Gm.)	SCT dry wt.(mg.)	DNA (µg) per mg.T	RNA (µg) per mg.T	Protein (mg.) per mg.T	Zn (µg) per mg.T
Zn-deficient	18±1.6* (24)	117.8±10.6 (16)	6.2 ±0.39 (12)	11.3±0.39 (12)	0.54±0.03 (12)	0.10±0.008 (12)
Restricted-fed control animals	14±1.2 (24)	153.3±16.2 (15)	7.54±0.37 (12)	13.4±1.0 (12)	0.56±0.02 (12)	0.14±0.007 (12)
Ad libitum-fed control animals	53±2.0 (24)	176.5±17.7 (15)	6.6 ±0.26 (12)	14.6±1.5 (12)	0.52±0.03 (12)	0.12±0.19 (12)
p value						
Zn-deficient vs. restricted-fed animals	0.05	NS	0.025	NS	NS	0.005
Zn-deficient vs. Ad libitum-fed animals	0.001	0.01	NS	NS	NS	NS
Restricted-fed vs. Ad libitum-fed animals	0.001	NS	NS	NS	NS	NS

SCT - sponge connective tissue.
T - tissue.
Number in parenthesis indicates number of rats.
*Mean ± S.E.

symptoms include delayed onset of puberty and hypogonadism in the males, characterized by decreased facial, pubic, and axillary hair, short stature and low body weight, rough skin, and poor appetite. Inasmuch as zinc is an important constituent of erythrocytes, it appeared possible that long continued hemolysis in patients with SCA might lead to a zinc-deficient state, which could account for some of the clinical manifestations mentioned above. Delayed healing of leg ulcer and the reported beneficial effect of zinc therapy on leg ulcers in SCA patients would also appear to be consistent with the above hypothesis.

We have previously reported the results of our study in detail elsewhere (Prasad et al, 1975; Prasad et al, 1976), and as such only a summary will be provided here. Out of 84 adult subjects with SCA, growth stature was retarded (below 3 S.D. from the normal mean) in 6 males and 5 females. Eighty per cent of the SCA patients in our study were below the 50th percentile from the normal mean for weight. Twenty-eight adult males (out of 38) showed a lack of facial and body hair, and 5 additional subjects showed only scanty facial hair. Eight females gave history of delayed menarche and irregular menstrual cycle. Chronically active leg ulcers were present in 7 patients.

Zinc in plasma, red blood cells and hair (Table 7) was significantly decreased in SCA patients as compared to the controls. The excretion of zinc in urine was high in SCA patients as compared to the controls, suggesting that increased loss of zinc may be one of the mechanisms by which these patients become zinc deficient. This is further supported by a significant negative correlation between values for 24-h urinary zinc excretion and erythrocyte zinc (Fig. 2).

Inspite of tissue zinc depletion in SCA patients, the observed hyperzincuria may suggest that this was a result of increased filtration of zinc by the glomeruli, owing to continued hemolysis, or there may have been a defect in tubular reabsorption of zinc somehow related to SCA. Whether or not zinc loss in urine was solely responsible for zinc depletion in SCA, cannot be settled at present. Additional factors such as predominant dietary use of cereal protein and other nutritional factors that affect zinc availability adversely, must be investigated in the future in order to account for zinc deficiency in SCA.

Table 7. Zinc in sickle cell disease patients and controls.

	Zinc (Mean ± S.D.)					
	Plasma µg%	RBC µg/g Hb	Hair µg/g	Urine µg/24 hr.	Urine µg/g creatinine	Plasma* RNase ΔA/min per ml
SCD	104 ± 10.5 (84)	34.0 ± 7.0 (84)	121.0 ± 30.0 (43)	759 -182 (21)	897 ± 590 (13)	0.435 ± .002 (16)
Controls	113 ± 13.6 (70)	40.0 ± 4.0 (61)	190.0 ± 17.0 (24)	633 ± 158 (20)	495 ± 113 (10)	0.310 ± .001 (16)
P	< .001	< .001	< .001	< .025	< .05	< .001

*Mean ± Standard Error.
Numbers in parenthesis are number of subjects. At least three 24-h urines were collected for each subject.

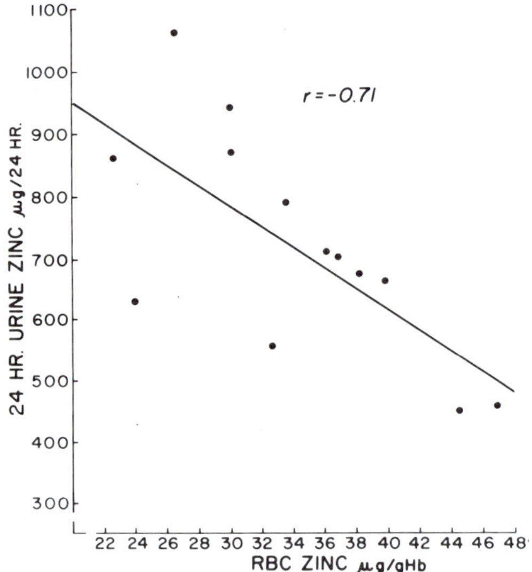

Fig. 2. Twenty-four-hour urinary zinc excretion compared with erythrocyte zinc content of sickle cell disease patients. (Prasad et al, Clin Chem 21: 582, 1975)

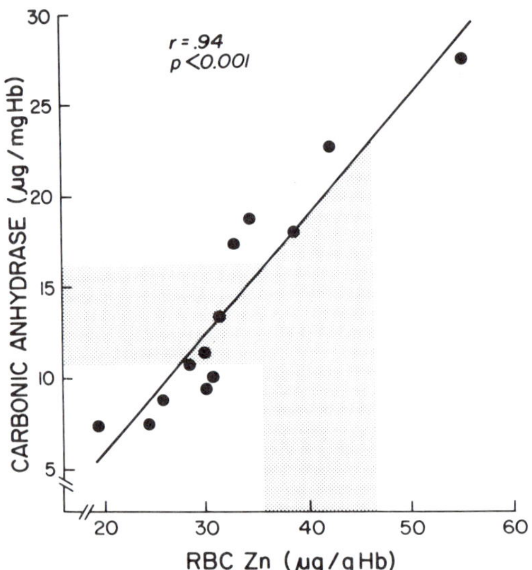

Fig. 3. Carbonic anhydrase protein and zinc content of erythrocytes in sickle cell disease patients.
Shaded areas indicate mean ± SD for erythrocyte zinc (vertical) and erythrocyte carbonic anhydrase protein (horizontal). (Prasad et al, Clin Chem 21: 582, 1975)

Carbonic anhydrase is a zinc metalloenzyme. Fig. 3 shows results of carbonic anhydrase determinations in relation to erythrocyte zinc concentration in SCA patients. The values correlated closely (γ = 0.96, P <.001). Another plasma enzyme, the activity of which is regulated by zinc, is RNase. Zinc is an inhibitor of this enzyme, as such in zinc deficiency its activity is expected to be increased. Indeed in our studies, the activity of plasma RNase was increased in comparison to the controls (Table 7).

Thus on the basis of decreased levels of zinc in the plasma, red cells and hair and changes in the activities of zinc dependent enzymes such as carbonic anhydrase and RNase, we concluded that adult SCA subjects were zinc deficient, although the degree of deficiency varied greatly from one subject to another.

Hypogonadal features in SCA patients were more common in males as compared to the females. This is consistent with our previous observation that testes are more susceptible to a lack of zinc as compared to the ovaries (Prasad, 1966). Our recent studies indicate that androgen deficiency is SCA subjects was related to a primary testicular failure (Abbasi et al, 1976). Besides abnormal steroidogenesis in the Leydig cells, spermatogenesis also appears to be affected in SCA. These effects are very similar to those we have reported in experimental animals, as a result of zinc deficiency (Prasad, 1966; Prasad, 1976).

We have used zinc supplementation in a limited number of subjects with SCA. Seven men and two women with SCA were orally administered zinc sulfate, 660 µg daily for varying lengths of time (Prasad et al, 1975). Two males 17 years old, gained 5 cm and 7 cm in height following 49 and 92 weeks of supplementation respectively. Changes in secondary sexual characteristics and external genitalia were also observed in these two subjects. Eight subjects gained weight and majority showed some changes in body hair growth.

Thus our results of limited uncontrolled trial with zinc therapy revealed beneficial effects of zinc on growth, and development of primary and secondary sexual characteristics in male subjects with SCA. These observations further support our biochemical data that deficiency of zinc was a complicating factor in our SCA patients.

Serjeant et al (1970) from Jamaica and Karayalcin et al (1974) from New York have also reported a decrease in plasma zinc level in SCA patients and a beneficial effect of zinc supplementation on leg ulcers was observed by Serjeant et al (1970) in their group of patients. A recent report by Butler et al (1977), however, failed to observe a decrease in plasma zinc level. It should be emphasized that hemolysis in vivo or in vitro is likely to give spuriously high levels of zinc in the plasma and it appears that this may have been a factor in the studies reported by Butler et al (1977). In very carefully monitored unhemolyzed samples of plasma, Brewer (1977) observed the mean plasma zinc level in SCA patients to be 66 µg%. His values in SCA patients were significantly lower (P <.01) than the controls (mean - 96 µg%).

With respect to red cell zinc determination, it is important to express the values in terms of per g hemoglobin rather than per ml red cells, inasmuch as gelling of the sickle hemoglobin at room temperature introduces significant error in accurate pipetting of one ml red cells. Perhaps this may have been a factor accounting for the results of Butler et al (1977) who did not observe any difference in the red cell zinc level of SCA patients and controls.

Measurement of zinc dependent enzymes in the plasma is also likely to give erroneous activity if the sample is hemolyzed inasmuch as several elements that are released from the red cells as a result of hemolysis, may activate or inhibit the enzyme activity (Vallee et al, 1959). It is clear, therefore, that one has to exercise extreme care and precaution in collection of plasma samples for measurement of zinc and the activity of zinc dependent enzymes. The concentration of copper in the red cells is in the same order of magnitude as the plasma, therefore hemolysis does not interfere with its measurement in the plasma. It is therefore not surprising that with respect to plasma copper levels, the results of Butler et al (1977) agree with ours (Prasad et al, 1976). We have interpreted our data of increased plasma copper in SCA patients to be related to a mild zinc deficient state since a reciprocal relationship between zinc and copper levels in tissues of experimental animals is a well recognized phenomenon (Prasad, 1966; Prasad, 1976).

Plasma zinc has also been measured in SCA patients in Nigeria (Kapu et al, 1976). Whereas the SCA patients in Nigeria had significantly decreased plasma zinc level in

comparison to Nigerian elites and Europeans, the values were
not significantly different from those of Nigerian non-elites
(Kapu et al, 1976). Since no nutritional data are available,
it is difficult to interpret the low plasma zinc levels of
non-elite Nigerians but it is likely that their decreased
plasma zinc levels were probably due to nutritional factors.
A high cereal protein intake such as may be prevalent in
Nigeria, is likely to affect the availability of zinc adversely due to high phytate and fiber content of the diet
(Reinhold et al, 1976).

We would thus like to conclude that zinc deficiency does
appear to be a complicating factor in patients with SCA, although the mechanism responsible for this phenomenon is not
well understood at present.

3. Deoxythymidine Kinase Activity, RNA/DNA, Total Collagen
    and Protein in the Sponge Connective Tissue of SCA
    Subjects

Inasmuch as zinc deficiency in experimental animals is
known to affect adversely the activity of deoxythymidine
kinase and protein and collagen synthesis (Fernandez-Madrid
et al, 1973; Prasad et al, 1974), and since zinc deficiency
may complicate SCA (Prasad et al, 1975; Prasad et al, 1976),
it was considered desirable to determine RNA/DNA, deoxythymidine kinase activity, total protein and total collagen
content of the sponge connective tissue of patients with
SCA. For comparison, two types of controls were used: 1)
Normal volunteers and 2) Human volunteers who consumed a
synthetic soybean protein base diet of low zinc content
(2.5 mg daily intake) for 6 months, followed by identical
dietary intake with 30 mg of zinc supplementation for 3
months. In the latter groups of subjects, the sponge connective tissue samples were obtained twice, once during zinc
depletion phase and again following zinc repletion.

Four patients from the Detroit Medical Center Sickle
Cell Adult Clinic and 5 normal adult volunteers (medical
personnel) volunteered for this study. Informed consent was
obtained from every subject in this study after the nature
of all procedures had been fully explained.

Following local anesthesia one polyvinyl sponge measuring approximately 4 cm by 3 cm by 3 mm was implanted subcutaneously under the rib in human subjects. Twenty-one days after implantation the sponges were isolated by blunt dissection and the capsules surrounding the sponges were collected for study. In preliminary experiments in human subjects, it was found that the optimal time for harvesting the sponge connective tissue was 21 days after sponge implantation.

Mild deficiency of zinc was induced by dietary means in two adult male volunteers aged 53 and 56 years, respectively (Prasad et al, 1976). The former had a history of benign hypertension but requiring no medication and mild diabetes which was controlled by diet alone. The latter had degenerative osteoarthritis and allergic rhinitis. Both subjects were normal with respect to zinc status as judged by zinc levels in the plasma, red cells, hair and urine.

The daily intake of zinc was only 2.5 mg during zinc depletion phase which lasted for 6 months. RDA* for zinc is 15 mg. At the end of this period, a sponge was implanted under the rib and connective tissue was harvested for studies. Following this, these subjects received the same diet but zinc (30 mg as zinc acetate) was supplemented, daily. After three months of supplementation, another sponge was implanted and connective tissue obtained for repeat studies.

For the determination of zinc, protein, and nucleic acids, the sponges were removed by blunt dissection and quickly frozen in dry ice, lyophilized, and then weighed. The sponge wetted with 1 or 2 ml of deionized water following which the connective tissue was easily removed and teased out. The sponge was again lyophilized and weighed in order to determine the weight of the connective tissue by difference. RNA and DNA were determined in the connective tissue by the Schmidt-Thannhauser method as modified by Munro and Fleck (1966). Protein was determined by a method reported by Inchiosa (1964). Deoxythymidine kinase activity and total collagen were measured by methods reported previously (Fernandez-Madrid et al, 1973; Prasad et al, 1974).

Table 8 shows the data for total protein, total collagen, RNA/DNA and deoxythymidine kinase activity in the human sponge connective tissue. As compared to the controls, the

*Recommended Dietary Allowance

Table 8. Total protein, total collagen, RNA/DNA and deoxythymidine kinase activity sponge connective tissue (SCT)

Subjects	Total Protein mg	Total Collagen mg	RNA/DNA	Deoxythymidine Kinase* Units per mg Protein
Controls				
K. H.	124.3	86.2	1.00	0.49
T. J.	161.0	51.8	0.87	0.62
S. B.	57.4	17.0	1.30	0.48
B. D.	82.6	17.4	1.00	0.34
M. D.	160.7	40.3	0.87	0.57
Mean ± S.D.	117.4 ± 46.28	42.5 ±28.6	1.01 ± .17	0.511 ± .087
SCA				
B. P.	71.0	8.60	0.40	N.D.
M. S.	50.1	0.03	0.60	N.D.
G. H.	63.8	0.01	0.59	N.D.
G. C.	56.8	N.D.	0.63	N.D.
Mean ± S.D.	60.4 ± 9.0	2.88 ±4.95	0.55 ± .105	
P	< .05	< .02	< .005	

*Unit is nanomoles of thymidine monophosphate generated per mg of protein per hour.
 SCA - Patients with sickle cell anemia.
 N.D. - Non detected.

SCA patients showed a marked decrease in the content of total protein and total collagen in the sponge connective tissue. Total collagen in terms of per mg protein and RNA/DNA were significantly (P < .001) reduced in the SCA patients. The activity of deoxythymidine kinase (mean ± S.D.) in the sponge connective tissue of normal volunteers was 0.511 ± .087 units per mg of protein, but in the case of SCA patients, we were unable to detect any activity by our technique.

Table 9 presents our data in two human volunteers who were on low zinc (2.5 mg daily intake) diet for 6 months, followed by zinc repletion (30 mg of zinc daily intake) for 3 months. A marked increase in the content of total protein and total collagen following repletion with zinc was evident. Similarly RNA/DNA and the activity of deoxythymidine kinase were also increased following repletion with zinc. Changes in plasma and red cell zinc were consistent with zinc depletion and repletion phases in these volunteers.

Our results in the present studies indicate that deoxythymidine kinase in human connective tissue is also zinc dependent and that deficiency of zinc may lead to decreased activity of deoxythymidine kinase and collagen synthesis in human subjects. Thus our studies provide a probable biochemical explanation for impaired collagen synthesis and wound healing in SCA patients. Our previous studies have shown that the effect of zinc deficiency on collagen synthesis is not due to inter or intra molecular cross linkage defect, rather it is related to the generalized effect on nucleic acids and protein synthesis (Fernandez-Madrid et al, 1973).

SUMMARY

Our studies indicate that in sickle cell anemia patients, impaired wound healing is due to a defective collagen synthesis. Deficiency of zinc was a complicating feature in this disease in our study and the activity of deoxythymidine kinase, an enzyme known to be zinc dependent and essential for DNA synthesis, was markedly decreased in SCA subjects. This biochemical defect is believed to result in the impairment of fibroblastic proliferation and collagen synthesis.

Table 9. Total protein, total collagen, RNA/DNA and deoxythymidine kinase activity of sponge connective tissue (SCT) of two subjects during zinc depletion phase and following repletion with zinc.

		Total Protein mg	Total Collagen mg	RNA/DNA	Deoxythymidine Kinase* units/mg protein	Plasma Zn µg %
1.	Depletion	108	29.3	0.69	N.D.	64
	Repletion	226	58.4	0.82	0.385	122
2.	Depletion	94	.013	0.71	N.D.	64
	Repletion	240	121.2	0.95	0.321	110

*Unit is nanomoles of thymidine monophosphate generated per mg of protein per hour.

ACKNOWLEDGEMENTS

Supported by a Contract and a Sickle Cell Center Grant from the National Heart and Lung Institute, Sickle Cell Disease Branch, NIH, Bethesda; Food and Drug Administration Contract, Washington, D.C.; Veterans Administration Hospital Medical Research Service, Allen Park, Michigan; and Meyer Laboratories, Inc., Ft. Lauderdale, Florida.

REFERENCES

Abbasi AA, Prasad AS, Ortega J, et al (1976). Gonadal function abnormalities in sickle cell anemia: Studies in adult male patients. Ann Int Med 85: 601.

Brewer GJ (1977). Personal communication.

Butler LC, Taylor ML, McCurdy PR, et al (1977). Zinc status in adult sickle cell anemia patients. Fed Proc 36: 1139.

Dreosti IE, Hurley LS (1975). Depressed thymidine kinase activity in zinc deficient rat embryos. Proc Soc Exp Biol Med 150: 161.

Fernandez-Madrid F, Prasad AS, Oberleas D (1973). Effect of zinc deficiency on nucleic acids, collagen and noncollagenous protein of the connective tissue. J Lab Clin Med 82: 951.

Fujioka M, Lieberman I (1964). A Zn^{++} requirement for synthesis of deoxyribonucleic acid by rat liver. J Biol Chem 239: 1164.

Hus JM, Anthony WL, Buchanan PJ (1968). Incorporation of glycine-1-^{14}C into liver glutathione in zinc deficient rats. Proc Soc Exp Biol Med 127: 1048.

Inchiosa MA (1964). Direct biuret determination of total protein in tissue homogenates. J Lab Clin Med 63: 319.

Kapu MM, Fleming AF, Ezem BU (1976). Plasma zinc in sickle cell anemia. Lancet 1: 920.

Karayalcin G, Rosner F, Kim KY, et al (1974). Letter: Plasma zinc in sickle cell anaemia. Lancet 1: 217.

Kulonen E (1970). Studies on experimental granuloma. In Balezs EA (ed): "Chemistry and Molecular Biology of the Intracellular Matrix", vol 3, New York: Academic Press, p 1811.

McClain PE, Wiley ER, Beecher GR, et al (1973). Influence of zinc deficiency on synthesis and cross-linking of rat-skin collagen. Biochim Biophys Acta 304: 457.

Miller WJ, Morton JD, Pitts WJ, et al (1965). Effect of zinc deficiency and restricted feeding on wound healing in the bovine. Proc Soc Exp Biol Med 118: 427.

Munro HW, Fleck A (1966). In Glick D (ed): "Methods of Biochemical Analysis", vol 14, New York: Interscience Pub-
lishers, Inc., p 113.

Oberleas D, Seymour JK, Lenaghan R, et al (1971). Effect of
zinc deficiency on wound healing in the rat. Am J Surg 121:
566.

Pories WJ, Henzel JH, Rob CG, et al (1967). Acceleration of
wound healing in man with zinc sulfate given by mouth.
Lancet 1: 121.

Prasad AS (1966). Metabolism of zinc and its deficiency in
human subjects. In Prasad AS (ed): "Zinc Metabolism",
Springfield: Charles C. Thomas, p 250.

Prasad AS (1974). Thymidine kinase activity and incorporation
of thymidine into DNA in zinc-deficient tissues. J Lab Clin
Med 83: 634.

Prasad AS, Schoomaker EB, Ortega J, et al (1975). Zinc deficiency in sickle cell disease. Clin Chem 21: 582.

Prasad AS, Ortega J, Brewer GJ, Oberleas D (1976). Trace
elements in sickle cell disease. JAMA 235: 2306.

Prasad AS (1976). Deficiency of zinc in man and its toxicity.
In Prasad AS (ed). "Trace Elements in Human Health and
Disease", New York: Academic Press, p 1.

Prasad AS, Abbasi A, Oberleas D, et al (1976): Experimental
production of zinc deficiency in man. Fed Proc 35: 658.

Reinhold JG, Faradji B, Abadi P, et al (1976). Binding of
zinc to fiber and other solids of wholemeal bread. In
Prasad AS (ed): "Trace Elements in Human Health and Disease",
New York: Academic Press, p 163.

Rubin H, Korde T (1973). Inhibition of DNA synthesis in chick
embryo cultures by deprivation of either serum or zinc.
J Cell Biol 56: 777.

Sandstead HH, Shepard GH (1968). The effect of zinc deficiency
on the tensile strength of healing surgical incisions in
the integument of the rat. Proc Soc Exp Biol Med 128: 687.

Sandstead HH, Rinaldi RA (1969). Impairment of deoxyribonucleic acid synthesis by dietary zinc deficiency in the rat.
J Cell Physiol 73: 81.

Serjeant GR, Galloway RE, Gueri MC (1970). Oral zinc sulfate
in sickle cell ulcers. Lancet 2: 891.

Vallee BL (1959). Biochemistry. Physiology and pathology of
zinc. Physiol Rev 39: 443.

Westmoreland N (1971). Connective tissue alterations in
zinc deficiency. Fed Proc 30: 1001.

Williams RB, Chesters JK (1970). The effect of early zinc
deficiency on DNA and protein synthesis in the rat.
Brit J Nutr 24: 1053.

Wintrobe MM (1974). "Clinical Hematology". Philadelphia:
Lea & Febiger, 7th ed, p 842.

DISCUSSION

Dr. Cameron: Could you tell us something about the clinical status of patients who participated in this study with respect to leg ulcers?

Dr. Prasad: We included those patients who volunteered for this study and they did not have leg ulcers.

Dr. Serjeant: I would certainly agree that there is an increased prevalence of leg ulceration and a very slow rate of healing of these lesions, but you also mentioned delayed wound healing in patients with SS disease. To my knowledge there is no published evidence of this. Can you enlighten me?

Dr. Prasad: Well, actually what I meant was that in spite of all the therapeutic measures we undertake, the ulcers do not heal properly, and it takes a long time to heal if it does heal.

Dr. Serjeant: So you have no evidence in fact that there is delayed healing of wounds in any other site than at the lower end of the leg?

Dr. Prasad: That's correct.

Dr. Segjeant: So this might be explainable in physical or vascular terms. You have no evidence that wound healing following surgery at other sites is followed by delayed wound healing?

Dr. Prasad: Well, there has been no study to my knowledge in which the tensile strength of the surgical incision has been measured. I believe, such a measurement may indeed show a difference between sickle cell patients and controls on the basis of zinc deficiency.

The Red Cell, page 537
© 1978 Alan R. Liss, Inc., New York, New York

EVIDENCE FOR AN IRON CARRIER SUBSTANCE IN COPPER-DEFICIENT
MITOCHONDRIA

DM Williams, AJ Barbuto, CL Atkin and GR Lee

Departments of Medicine, Biochemistry and
Pathology
University of Utah, Salt Lake City, Utah 84132

The anemia of copper deficiency is explained in part
by defective mobilization of iron from cellular storage
sites to plasma, a consequence of the lack of ceruloplasmin (Lee *et al*, 1968). However, there is considerable
evidence for an additional intracellular defect in iron
metabolism. This evidence includes: the microcytosis and
hypochromia of the erythrocytes, increased numbers of bone
marrow sideroblasts, reticulocytopenia, hyperferremia
during the late stages of the anemia (Lee *et al*, 1968), and
impaired erythrocyte iron uptake and heme synthesis
(Williams *et al*, 1976).

In recent studies, we showed that ferric iron can be
made available for heme synthesis by normal mitochondria
when it is reduced to the ferrous form by electrons contributed from a functioning electron transport system
(Williams *et al*, 1976). Heme synthesis by copper-deficient
mitochondria was diminished as were the copper content,
cytochrome oxidase activity and heme *a* content of these
organelles.

Our studies indicated that the intracellular defect
could be ascribed to impaired ability of the mitochondrion
to acquire iron and incorporate it into the heme molecule.
These studies and those of others, (Romslo and Flatmark,
1973; Llambias, 1976) demonstrated that an intact electron
transport system is required for the uptake and utilization of iron. The electron transport system is impaired
in copper deficiency as a result of decreased cytochrome
oxidase. However, the exact role of cytochrome oxidase

The Red Cell, pages 539—545

and the electron transport system in heme synthesis
requires further delineation. Thus, they may contribute
energy to an energy-dependent uptake process, provide
reducing equivalents for the reduction of iron in preparation for its insertion into heme, or maintain an anaerobic
environment within the mitochondrion to prevent the auto-
oxidation of iron that has been transported into that
compartment. To investigate these possibilities, heme
synthesis in normal and copper deficient mitochondria was
studied by a pyridine mesohemochrome method (Porra, 1975).

MATERIALS AND METHODS

      Copper-deficient swine were raised as described
previously (Roeser *et al*, 1970). Mitochondria from the
livers of exsanguinated animals were prepared in 0.25M
sucrose containing 0.002M HEPES, pH 7.4, (Romslo and Flatmark, 1973). Respiratory control was measured with a
Clark oxygen electrode (Grav *et al*, 1970). Only mitochondria with a respiratory control ratio greater than 2.5
(in the presence of ADP) were used. Mitochondria were
incubated in Thunberg vessels containing 3 mg/ml mitochondrial protein, 0.04mM mesoporphyrin, 0.08M potassium
succinate, and 8.1mM HEPES, pH 8.2 in a total volume of
2.5 ml. The reaction was started by adding the mitochondrial suspension from the sidearm. In some experiments,
200 nmoles of $FeCl_3$ was added. The resultant mesoheme
synthesized was considered to be total mesoheme synthesis.
In other experiments, no iron was added and the resultant
mesoheme synthesized was considered as mesoheme synthesis
from intrinsic iron. The incremental difference of these
two values from matched experiments was considered to be
mesoheme synthesis from extrinsic iron. In some experiments, the vessel remained open to the atmosphere. In
others, the vessel was evacuated 3 times and refilled with
chemically-pure nitrogen which had been bubbled through an
alkaline pyrogallol solution. The vessels were then
sealed under slightly negative pressure. The mitochondrial
suspension was incubated at $37^{O}C$ in the dark for 30 minutes, and the reaction was terminated by the addition of
0.3ml of 0.4 M iodoacetamide. Mesoheme was then determined by the method of Porra (1975). Protein was measured
by the method of Lowry *et al*.(1951).

RESULTS

Under anaerobic conditions and in the presence of
added iron, mesoheme was synthesized by both normal and
copper deficient mitochondria (Table 1). Heme synthesis
was enhanced when succinate was added to the mitochondrial
suspension.

Table 1

Mesoheme Synthesis by Isolated Hepatic
Mitochondria in Aerobic and Anaerobic Atmospheres

Mitochondria	Atmosphere	Succinate	From Intrinsic Fe	Mesoheme Synthesis (nmoles/mg protein/hr) From Extrinsic Fe	Total
Control N = 5	Anaerobic	0	0	6.4+1.36	6.4+1.36
		+	0	7.2+1.10	7.2+1.10
	Aerobic	0	0	0	0
		+	0	3.9+0.80	3.9+0.80
Copper Deficient N = 4	Anaerobic	0	4.2+0.98	2.0+0.82	6.2+1.52
		+	5.8+2.07	3.6+0.54	9.4+2.58
	Aerobic	0	0	0	0
		+	3.2+0.40	2.4+0.71	5.6+0.70

*Values refer to mean ± SE

When no iron was added to an anaerobic system, normal mitochondria failed to synthesize mesoheme whether or not succinate was added. In contrast, copper deficient mitochondria synthesized substantial amounts of mesoheme in the absence of iron. Heme synthesis from extrinsic iron was less in copper deficient mitochondria than in normal.

Under aerobic conditions in the presence of added iron, virtually no mesoheme was synthesized by either normal or copper-deficient mitochondria in the absence of succinate. However, the addition of succinate resulted in increased heme synthesis by both normal and copper-deficient mito-chondria.

As in the anaerobic system, normal mitochondria failed to synthesize heme when no iron was added to the system, whether or not succinate was present. In contrast, copper-deficient mitochondria synthesized heme in the absence of added iron but only if succinate was present.

Heme synthesis from extrinsic iron was less in copper-deficient than in normal mitochondria.

DISCUSSION

These studies have demonstrated that heme synthesis occurs in the absence of added iron in copper-deficient mitochondria but not in control mitochondria. This obser-vation suggests that in copper deficiency an iron-contain-ing substance is contained in or attached to mitochondria. This substance can be utilized for the synthesis of heme under anaerobic conditions and also under aerobic cond-itions if succinate is supplied. The fact that the iron substrate accumulates in copper deficiency but not in controls suggests that copper is required for its utiliza-tion. Other workers have also suggested the existence of a mitochondrial iron substrate (Ponka and Neuwirt, 1970; Flatmark and Romslo, 1975; Fielding and Speyer, 1974). However, the relationship of these iron substrates with that identified in copper deficiency remains to be invest-igated. Furthermore, the location of the iron substrate identified in copper deficiency remains to be established. Thus, it may be bound to the outer membrane receptor sites identified by Romslo and Flatmark (1973), or it may be in the intermembranous space or matrix-bound. The last possibility seems unlikely in view of the electron photo-micrographic studies of Goodman and Dallman (1969). In these studies, iron accumulated within the mitochondria of normoblasts and reticulocytes from animals treated with lead, but accumulated outside of mitochondria in the cytosol of cells from lead-treated, copper-deficient animals. It is also possible, however, that electron microscopy is insufficiently sensitive to detect the amounts or chemical forms of iron that accumulate in copper deficiency.

The metabolic requirements for utilization of the iron suggest that the iron must be reduced before it can be utilized for heme synthesis. Other workers have shown that artificial iron substrates, to be available for heme synthesis, require reducing equivalents provided by a functional electron transport system. Anaerobiosis and reduction, *per se*, do not appear to be essential since rate of heme synthesis does not increase with onset of anaerobic conditions, and reducing agents such as reduced glutathione cannot be substituted (Koller, *et al*, 1976). Thus, it may be that in copper deficiency, the iron accumulates because it is in the ferric form *in vivo* and cannot be properly reduced by a defective electron transport system. Alternatively, the iron may become oxidized as an artifact of mitochondrial preparation. Subsequent reduction may occur more efficiently in normal than in copper-deficient mitochondria, resulting in an apparent difference in iron content. This explanation seems less likely, but at the present time cannot be excluded.

These studies also demonstrate that mesoheme synthesis from added iron is diminished in copper deficiency. This is in good agreement with our previous studies in which heme synthesis was measured by the incorporation of radio-iron (Williams *et al*, 1976). The observation that total heme synthesis was not diminished *in vitro* does not invalidate the conclusion that heme synthesis is impaired in copper deficiency. In fact, accumulation of iron in copper deficiency supports such a conclusion. Total heme synthesis may appear normal because the conditions for assay enhance the utilization of such a substrate. As yet we have no information as to the utilization of this iron substrate by normal mitochondria or the relative rates of utilization as compared with artificial iron substrates such as $FeCl_3$ and ferric sucrose.

SUMMARY

Previous studies have shown that iron uptake and heme
synthesis are defective in copper-deficient erythrocyte
precursors. In this study, we have shown that copper
deficiency results in accumulation of an iron substrate
that can be utilized by intact mitochondria for heme synthesis and that its utilization depends upon anaerobic
conditions or the addition of electron transport substrates. Studies are presently underway to define the
nature and intracellular localization of this substrate.

ACKNOWLEDGEMENTS

Supported by NIH Research Grant AM-04495. We thank
Mrs. Alice Tustison for her technical assistance.

REFERENCES

Fielding J and Speyer BE (1974). Iron transport inter-
    mediates in human reticulocytes and the membrane binding
    site of iron-transferrin. Biochim Biophys Acta 363:387.
Flatmark T and Romslo I (1975). VI. Requirement for re-
    ducing equivalents and evidence for a unidirectional flux
    of Fe(II) across the inner membrane. J Biol Chem
    250:6433.
Goodman JG and Dallman PR (1969). Role of copper in iron
    localization in developing erythrocytes. Blood 34:747.
Grav HJ, Pederson JI and Christiansen EN (1970). Condi-
    tions *in vitro* which affect respiratory control and
    capacity for respiration-linked phosphorylation in brown
    adipose tissue mitochondria. Europ J Biochem 12:11.
Koller M-E, Romslo I and Flatmark T (1976). Studies in the
    ferrochelatase activity of isolated rat liver mitochond-
    ria with special reference to the effect of oxidizable
    substrates and oxygen concentration. Biochim Biophys
    Acta 449:480.
Lee GR, Nacht S, Lukens JN and Cartwright GE (1968). Iron
    metabolism in copper deficient swine. J Clin Invest
    47:2058.
Llambias EBC (1976). The enzymic conversion of mesopor-
    phyrin to mesohaem. Int J Biochem 7:33.

Lowry OH, Rosebrough NJ, Farr AL and Randall RJ (1951).
  Protein measurement with the Folin phenol reagent. J
  Biol Chem 193:265.
Ponka P and Neuwirt J (1970). The use of reticulocytes
  with high non-haem iron pool for studies of regulation
  of haem synthesis. Brit J Haematol 19:593.
Porra RJ (1975). A rapid spectrophotometric assay for
  ferrochelatase activity in preparations containing much
  endogenous hemoglobin and its application to soybean
  root-nodule preparations. Analyt Biochem 68:289.
Roeser HP, Lee GR, Nacht S and Cartwright GE (1970). The
  role of ceruloplasmin in iron metabolism. J Clin Invest
  49:2408.
Romslo I and Flatmark T (1973). Energy-dependent accumulation of iron by isolated rat liver mitochondria I.
  General features. Biochim Biophys Acta 305:29.
Williams DM, Loukopoulos D, Lee GR and Cartwright GE (1976).
  Role of copper in mitochondrial iron metabolism.
  Blood 48:77.

DISCUSSION

Dr. Kreimer-Birnbaum: Two questions: did you use a hemochromogen technique instead of radio iron incorporation to measure
ferrochelatase activity?

Dr. Williams: Yes.

Dr. Kreimer-Birnbaum: Could you elaborate on that? Because
most of the assays we are dealing with have been done with
radio iron and those have many problems.

Dr. Williams: The problem with the ferrochelatase assay using
radio iron is that the size of the unlabelled iron pool is
likely to be variable. To try to get around that, we have
substituted a method described by Porra which is based upon
the appearance of heme measured as a pyridine hemochromogen.
We use mesoporphyrin as substrate because 1) it is artificial
and 2) it is quite stable in contrast to protoporphyrin and
3) there are good peaks which one can see in the presence of
excess amounts of protoheme. At the end of the reaction, the
reaction is terminated with iodoacetamide and solubilized in
pyridine.

Dr. Kreimer-Birnbaum: And you are satisfied with your controls?
The second question is: have you had a chance to look at
some humans with a genetic deficiency of copper?

Dr. Williams: No, and that is something that we have wanted
to do very much. Unfortunately we do not have our methods
worked out for reticulocyte and leukocyte mitochondria as well
as we would like, but we want to do precisely that.

Dr. Winterbourn: Could the fact that the superoxide dismutase is
a copper-containing enzyme be relevant? I know there are two
dismutases, the cytoplasmic one which contains copper, and a
mitochondrial one which does not. Have you any information
of whether the copper enzyme is present, or on the levels of
the manganese enzyme in the mitochondria?

Dr. Williams: We were very interested in that question early
on. In terms of superoxide dismutase levels in the mitochondrial fraction, all I can tell you is that we have the
measured activity in normal and copper deficient preparations
and they don't appear to be appreciably different. In contrast,

The Red Cell, pages 547—549

when you look at the cytosol copper enzyme it falls off as
these animals develop their anemia. Even there, cytosol superoxide dismutase falls off only very late in the course of the
disease, and it remains high enough to dismutate generated superoxide.

Dr. Winterbourn: I was thinking possibly along other lines;
as a long shot, whether a deficiency of the copper enzyme
could stimulate production of the manganese enzyme, and
there could in fact be too much superoxide dismutase. But this
does not appear to be the case.

Dr. Williams: No.

Dr. Cameron: Asking out of my own ignorance, can you take
these animals and correct the copper dificiency, and if you
do so, what is the course of events in the reappearance of
reticulocytes, and do these first reticulocytes show any
abnormalities of heme synthesis?

Dr. Williams: We have not really done that. You can correct
the deficiency although you cannot correct all the copper
associated defects.

Dr. Surgenor: I couldn't help but wonder as you talked
whether the iron transferrin complex was active in your
system. Wouldn't that be an attractive way to study the iron
effect because free iron is so difficult to work with? I
don't know how many people remember but transferrin is a
very good copper binding protein. It also binds zinc quite
well.

Dr. Williams: Well, we are very excited by that notion. All
I can do is tell you is that the iron material does not
seem to be transferrin. As you know, there are very many
people now writing about the actual penetration of the
transferrin iron complex into the red cell. We've added
transferrin iron to our system and we simply can't get the
iron off, at least with the conditions that we have used.
We cannot identify the material as transferrin, and we
cannot identify it is ferritin by radioimmunoassay.

Dr. Brewer: We have given zinc to sickle cell anemia patients.
Dr. Prasad and I have been inducing copper deficiency in
such patients and we don't really know why this is happening.
We are using the same total daily dose that others have

used, except that we divide that dose up into every four hour
aliquots, and of course the patients do have sickle cell anemia. Perhaps that increased the utilization, or possibly
the fact that we give the zinc without food means that it is
more effective. The problem, as I understand it, is zinc
copper competition for absorption sites. What is puzzling
is that the first patient in whom we induced copper deficiency
developed a hypochromic microcytic red cell picture, but
also granulocytopenia. This is apparently true in the animal
literature as well, in copper deficiency, that is both
hypochromic microcytic anemia and leukopenia. Why should the
granulocytes be so sensitive to copper deficiency? Is it
because they are turning over rapidly, or for some other special reason?

Dr. Williams: I wish I knew the answer to that. My own personal bias is that granulocytopenia is related to a deficiency of cytochrome oxydase and decreased mitochondrial function
in rapidly dividing cells, but I don't have any data on it.
As far as I know, nobody else does either. Granulocytopenia
certainly is a feature of copper deficiency that has been for
the most part ignored, and a defect that has really only come
to light since recent observations in patients with hyperali-
mentation.

Dr. Prasad: Do you have a lot of accumulation of iron in
sideroblastic anemias? Does anybody know if cytochrome
oxidase activity is affected and whether or not copper could
be an agent to mobilize iron?

Dr. Williams: So far as I know, nobody has looked at this.

MECHANISMS OF Li$^+$ TRANSPORT ACROSS THE HUMAN ERYTHROCYTE MEMBRANE

Jochen Duhm and Bernhard F. Becker

Physiologisches Institut der Universität
Pettenkoferstr. 12
D-8000 München 2, Germany

INTRODUCTION

The biological significance of Li$^+$ is unknown and no enzyme has been discovered yet which needs Li$^+$ as an essential constituent or activator. In 1948, the therapeutical action of Li$^+$ in treatment of acute manias was discovered by J.F.J. Cade in Australia (3), but only since 1954 has the effectivity of treatment of affective disorders with Li$^+$ salts been generally recognized, mainly due to the work of M. Skou in Denmark (33). Today, Li$^+$ is frequently and successfully applied in treatment of acute manias and in the prophylactic maintenance therapy of manic depressive disease, the doses necessary to maintain plasma Li$^+$ concentrations of about 1 mM being interindividually different (range 10 to 80 mmoles Li$^+$ per day).

The mechanisms of Li$^+$ action on the mood of patients suffering from affective disorders is not known despite extensive research. The possibilities being pursued include the action of Li$^+$ on the Na$^+$-K$^+$ pump, the cellular Na$^+$ and K$^+$ contents and the membrane potential. Other investigations center on interactions of Li$^+$ with Mg^{++} or Ca^{++} in modulating allosteric protein function. Several groups study effects of Li$^+$ on various endocrinal systems. Further work deals with the influence of Li$^+$ on synaptic transmission and the metabolism of catecholamines and related neurotransmitters, as well as with Li$^+$ effects on the function of microtubules and neurites. This survey is by no means complete and the reader is referred to recent publications covering most aspects of Li$^+$ action in biological systems (2,19,24,25,33).

The Red Cell, pages 551—570

Interestingly, not much attention has been paid to the problem how Li^+ itself is transported across cell membranes. In all tissues, including nerve, muscle and erythrocytes, the steady-state Li^+ concentration is much lower than to be expected from a passive distribution of Li^+ in the intra- and extracellular water phase. It was established that the passive transport of Li^+ and Na^+ proceeds at comparable rates, and that Li^+ can traverse the specific Na^+ channel in nerve and muscle cells and the amiloride-sensitive pathway of some epithelia. Furthermore, evidence was collected indicating that Li^+ is not transported effectively by the Na^+-K^+ pump under physiological conditions. However, the mechanism by which Li^+ is continuously extruded from the cells against an electrochemical potential gradient could not be resolved.

To investigate the basic mechanisms of Li^+ transport across cell membranes we chose the human red blood cell as a model. In addition to its well known experimental advantages, the red cell seemed to be a promising model, because interindividual differences in the steady-state Li^+ distribution between red cells and plasma have been reported (21,26,27,28, 29). These differences have been related to the effectivity of Li^+ therapy (5,13,14,29) and to the individually different Li^+ toxicity (34,39). Moreover, it appears as though the Li^+ distribution ratio may be genetically determined (6). Independently, the same approach to the problem has been applied by D.C. Tosteson and coworkers (23,32,35).

In this paper an attempt is made to summarize the recent progress made in the knowledge of Li^+ transport across the human erythrocyte membrane and to focus onto those factors which contribute to the establishment of the Li^+ distribution between red cells and plasma.

THE FOUR Li^+ TRANSPORT PATHWAYS

From studies of Tosteson and coworkers (23,32,35), of Funder and Wieth (18,37), and of our group (7,8,9,10,11,20, 21), the existence of at least four pathways of Li^+ transport across the human red cell membrane is now well established. Some of their properties are listed in Table 1.

The Na^+-dependent Li^+ countertransport system, together with the inwardly directed Na^+ gradient, is responsible for the lower than plasma red cell Li^+ levels in vivo. The system

Table 1: Pathways of Li$^+$ transport across the human erythrocyte membrane

---

1) <u>Na$^+$-Li$^+$ countertransport</u>
    insensitive to ouabain (7,23) and ATP depletion (7,35)
    high affinity for Li$^+$ (K$_m \approx$ 1.5 mM) (10,35)
    low affinity for Na$^+$ (K$_m \approx$ 50 mM) (10,35)
    completely inhibited by
        phloretin (0.2 mM) (10,11,32,35)
        phlorobenzophenone (0.5 mM) (11)
        NEM (0.5 mM) (10,11)
    not affected by K$^+$, Mg^{++}, Ca^{++} and choline$^+$ (7,8,35)

2) <u>Li$^+$ downhill transport stimulated by bicarbonate (carbonate)</u>
    completely inhibited by
        SITS (0.2 mM) (8,11)
        phloretin and phlorizin (0.2 mM) (8,11,35)
        dipyridamole (0.05 mM) (8,9,11)
        phenopyrazone (1 mM) (8)
        ethacrynic acid (0.5 mM) (11)
        furosemide (0.5 mM) (11)

3) <u>Na$^+$-K$^+$ pump</u> (ouabain-sensitive)
    inward Li$^+$ transport at the K$^+$-site (8,35)
    outward transport at the Na$^+$-site (12)

4) <u>Leak pathway</u>
    partly inhibited by
        dipyridamole (0.05 mM) (8,11)
        phlorobenzophenone (2 mM) (11)
        phloretin (0.2 mM) (11)

---

can mediate Li$^+$ uphill or downhill transport across the red
cell membrane in both directions, depending on the distribution of Li$^+$ and Na$^+$ on the two sides of the membrane. This
has been shown for both intact erythrocytes (7,23) and for
ghost membranes (7).

A second, purely passive pathway is observed in the presence of bicarbonate. This pathway was first described by
Wieth (18).

Two further modes of Li$^+$ transport are via the Na$^+$-K$^+$

pump and a Li$^+$ leak (see Table 1).

Some of the properties of three out of four pathways can be resolved from the data given in Figure 1. In these experiments, the dependency of Li$^+$ uptake on external Li$^+$ concentration was studied in the absence (control) and in the presence of ouabain. Clearly, ouabain inhibited Li$^+$ uptake from choline$^+$ media. Li$^+$ uptake increased in a curvilinear manner, both in the absence as well as in the presence of ouabain, without showing any tendency for saturation. In contrast, ouabain-sensitive Li$^+$ transport (i.e., the difference between the uptakes determined in the absence and presence of ouabain) tended to saturate at high Li$^+$ concentrations.

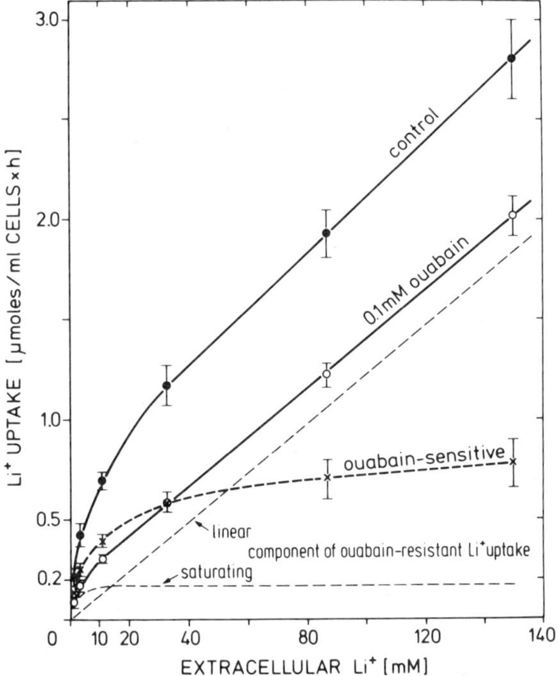

Figure 1: Dependency of Li$^+$ transport by pathways 1), 3) and 4) (see Table 1) on external Li$^+$ concentration (external choline$^+$ replaced by Li$^+$, 150 mM Cl$_e^-$, 10 mM Na$_e^+$, < 0.3 mM K$_e^+$, pH 7.4, 37°C, hematocrit 10%). The ouabain concentration was 0.1 mM. The values are means ± 1 S.D. of three experiments with erythrocytes of the donor G.B. For explanation of the broken lines see text.

Ouabain-sensitive Li$^+$ uptake is mediated by the <u>Na$^+$-K$^+$ pump.</u> This type of transport is also inhibited by oligomycin and ethacrynic acid (8) as well as by ATP-depletion and by external K$^+$ and Na$^+$ (8,35). It can occur against an electrochemical gradient of Li$^+$ under suitable experimental conditions (8). Dunham and Senyk recently reported that the pump can also extrude Li$^+$ from the cells at its Na$^+$-site, provided intracellular Na$^+$ and K$^+$ are absent (12).

The uptake determined in the presence of ouabain (ouabain-resistant Li$^+$ uptake in Figure 1) can be resolved graphically into two components: one saturating component and another which increases linearly with rising Li$^+$ concentration.

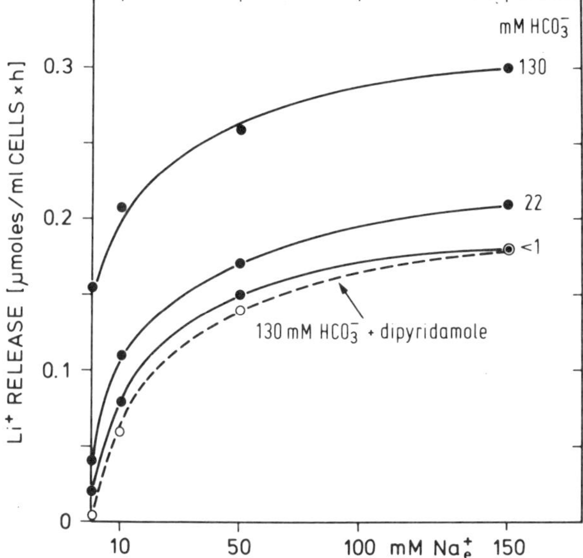

Figure 2: Dependence of Li$^+$ release on external Na$^+$ and bicarbonate.
Red cells preloaded to contain 1.8 µmoles Li$^+$/ml were pre-equilibrated for 5 min in the respective media (choline$^+$ was replaced by Na$^+$ and the chloride by bicarbonate, the pH being maintained at 7.4 by CO$_2$). One hour Li$^+$ net-release was estimated from the red cell Li$^+$ contents determined after 5, 35, 65 and 125 min of incubation and is corrected to a hemoglobin content of 5.2 µmoles/ml cells. Experimental conditions otherwise as described in the legend of Figure 1. Single experiment, donor B.R.D. Dotted line: 130 mM bicarbonate, 0.05 mM dipyridamole added after 4.5 min of preequilibration.

Operationally, the linear component can be ascribed to a leak. About 50% of this leak are inhibited by 0.05 mM dipyridamole. The apparent K_m value for this type of inhibitory effect of dipyridamole in saline solutions (hematocrit 2%) is about 2 µM and thus similar to the apparent K_m value determined for its inhibition of the bicarbonate effect (unpublished results). Phloretin and phlorobenzophenone seem also to inhibit the leak, but to a lesser extent (11).

The saturating component of ouabain-resistant Li^+ uptake in Figure 1 can be ascribed to Li^+ transport by the Na^+-dependent Li^+ countertransport system.

Data on Li^+ release mediated by the countertransport system are given in Figure 2. This Figure shows the dependency of Li^+ release from cells loaded with 1.8 µmoles Li^+/ml on the concentration of external Na^+. First, the data determined in the absence of added bicarbonate are considered. Under these conditions, Li^+ release depends almost entirely on the action of the countertransport system and thus proceeds slowly in Na^+-free media. The rate increases with rising external Na^+ due to the Na^+-induced stimulation of the countertransport system, and saturates at 150 mM external Na^+. This Na^+-dependent Li^+ release can be blocked by the inhibitors of the countertransport system summarized in Table 1.

As furthermore shown in Figure 2, bicarbonate enhances Li^+ release at all Na^+ concentrations. The magnitude of this effect is determined alone by the bicarbonate concentration employed. The Na^+-induced stimulation of Li^+ release is not essentially altered by bicarbonate. The additive component of Li^+ release is mediated by the bicarbonate-stimulated pathway. It is eliminated by a number of inhibitors of anion transfer across the red cell membrane (see Table 1). Dipyridamole, for instance, decreased Li^+ release in the presence of 130 mM bicarbonate towards the values determined in the absence of added bicarbonate (broken curve in Figure 2). In fact, Li^+ release proceeded slightly slower than in media nominally free of bicarbonate, because dipyridamole inhibits not only the bicarbonate-stimulated pathway, but also part of the leak (see above).

THE BICARBONATE-STIMULATED PATHWAY

The bicarbonate effect on transport of monovalent cations was first observed by Wieth and Funder in 1965 (38). They reported that bicarbonate accelerates passive movements of Na$^+$, but not of K$^+$ (15,16,17,36). In 1970 Wieth showed Li$^+$ transport to be enhanced, too, this effect being about 4 times greater than the acceleration of Na$^+$ transport (37).

The bicarbonate effect increases linearly with rising bicarbonate and Li$^+$ (or Na$^+$) concentration (8,11,37, compare Figure 2). At pH 7.4 and 37°C, bicarbonate accelerates Li$^+$ and Na$^+$ transport by about 0.8 and 0.2 nmoles/ml cells and h per 1 mM bicarbonate and 1 mM concentration difference of the transported cation (8,9,11,37). Bicarbonate affects Li$^+$ uptake and release to the same extent, provided the Donnan distribution of the bicarbonate anion and the pH difference across the red cell membrane are considered (11). Among the inhibitors of bicarbonate-stimulated transport summarized in Table 1, SITS is regarded as being a highly specific inhibitor of the anion exchange pathway.

Like bicarbonate, a number of divalent anions increase passive Li$^+$ and Na$^+$ transport, without affecting K$^+$ transfer (oxalate, phosphite, sulfite), the ratio of Li$^+$ over Na$^+$ selectivity decreasing in the order oxalate (79)$>$ phosphite (26) $>$ sulfite (6.4)$>$ bicarbonate (4.4). Maleate and phthalate stimulate not only Li$^+$ and Na$^+$, but also K$^+$ transport (1a, 11). The oxalate effect on Li$^+$ transport shows a pH dependency similar to that observed for the self exchange of Cl$^-$ or I$^-$. SITS-sensitive transfer of Li$^+$ is not induced by monovalent anions, divalent anions with an intercharge distance exceeding 5 Å, divalent but potentially trivalent anions, and trivalent anions (11).

The effect of bicarbonate is attributed to the presence of the divalent carbonate anion in solutions containing bicarbonate (1a,8,11,37). Carbonate and the other effective divalent anions are thought to form monovalent negatively charged ion pairs with the respective cations. These ion pairs apparently are capable of traversing the red cell membrane by means of the anion exchange mechanism. This mechanism can be blocked by all of the inhibitors of the bicarbonate effect listed in Table 1. Evidence for ion pair formation has been gained from ^{31}P-NMR studies on the Li$^+$-phosphite ion pair (11). In resin-competition experiments a binding constant of the Li^+-carbonate ion pair of about 3 l/mole (pertaining to physiological conditions) has been determined (Becker and Duhm, unpublished results).

INTERINDIVIDUAL DIFFERENCES IN Na^+-Li^+ COUNTERTRANSPORT AMONG HEALTHY DONORS

The Na^+-dependent Li^+ countertransport system can be assessed by several experimental approaches:
1) Measurement of the dependence of Li^+ release on internal Li^+ concentration (at a fixed external Na^+ concentration) or on external Na^+ (at fixed internal Li^+) (see Figures 2 and 3).
2) Determination of Li^+ uptake at low Li^+ concentrations in choline$^+$, K^+ or Mg^{++} chloride media containing ouabain (to inhibit the pump) and dipyridamole (to partly inhibit the Li^+ leak). When the external Li^+ concentration is kept below 4 mM, the Li^+ uptake determined under these conditions is a reliable measure of the countertransport system, because the residual Li^+ leak is small compared to the activity of the countertransport system in most red cell specimens (see Figures 1, 4 and 5). In such experiments, the red cell Na^+ content needs to be determined, since Li^+ uptake by the countertransport system strongly depends on the cellular Na^+ concentration.
3) Determination of the inhibitory effect of phloretin, phlorobenzophenone or NEM on Na^+-dependent Li^+ release or uptake (10,11,32,35, compare Fig. 6).
4) Determination of the effect of Li^+ on tracer fluxes of Na^+ (35).
5) Determination of the in vitro or in vivo steady-state Li^+ distribution ratio (10,11,20,21,35).

Data bearing on the first three methods are presented in the following. For these studies four donors were selected on the basis of their markedly different steady-state in vitro Li^+ distribution ratios.

Figure 3 shows the dependence of Li^+ release from their erythrocytes on internal Li^+ concentration. Release increased in a curvilinear manner with internal Li^+ in each case. However, the absolute rates varied considerably among the four, due to the differences in the activity of the Na^+-dependent Li^+ countertransport system.

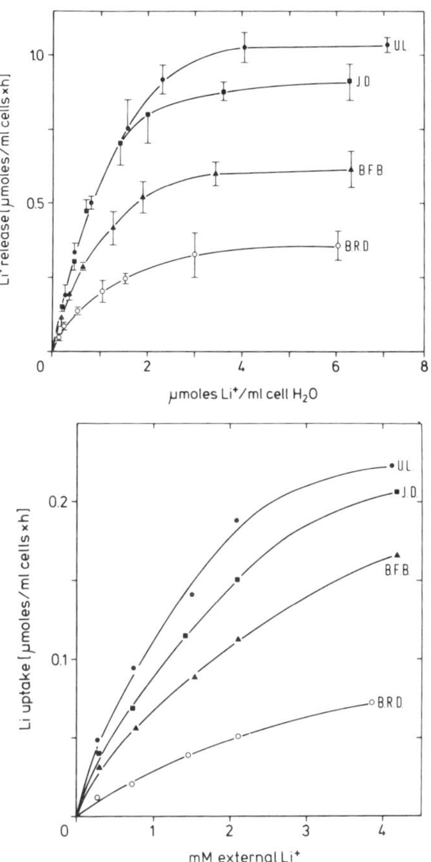

Figure 3: Dependence of Li$^+$ release on internal Li$^+$ concentration, determined at the fixed external Na$^+$ concentration of 150 mM.
The cells of the four donors were preloaded with Li$^+$ to contain the initial concentrations indicated. Li$^+$ release was initiated by adding the loaded cells to the prewarmed incubation media (pH 7.4, 37°C, hematocrit 2%, 0.1 mM ouabain, 0.05 mM dipyridamole). The values are means ± 1 S.D. from three experiments, corrected to a hemoglobin content of 5.2 μmoles/ml cells.

Figure 4: Dependence of Li$^+$ uptake on external Li$^+$ concentration.
The media contained 150 mM choline chloride and 10 mM NaCl. Experimental conditions otherwise as described in the legend of Figure 3. Single experiments.

Corresponding results were obtained in measurements of
Li^+ uptake as affected by external Li^+ (Figure 4). Again,
the maximal transport capacities of the Na^+-Li^+ countertransport system differed by a factor of about three among the
donors, whereas the apparent K_m was close to 1.5 mM Li^+ in
all four cases (10 mM external Na^+). This value is identical
to the apparent K_m for internal Li^+, indicating that the system may be symmetrical with respect to Li^+ (10).

In Figure 5, data on the activity of the countertransport system are given for 39 male members of our Department
of Physiology in Munich. The system was assessed by measurements of Li^+ uptake at 2 mM external Li^+. As in the experi-

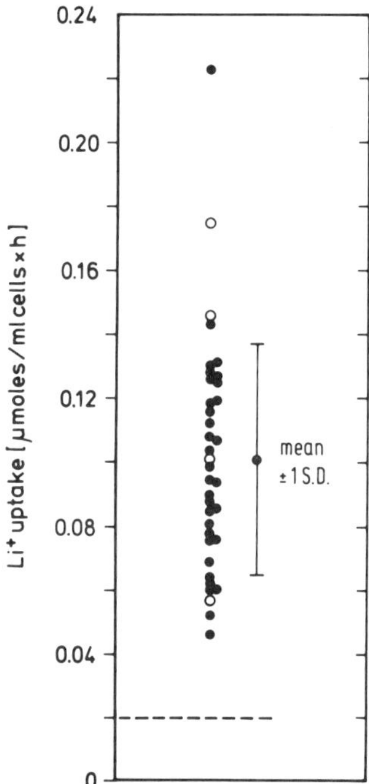

Figure 5: Interindividual differences in Li^+ uptake by the
Na^+-dependent Li^+ countertransport system. The four donors
studied in Figures 3 and 4 are indicated by open symbols.
The media contained 150 mM choline chloride, 10 mM NaCl,
2 mM LiCl, 0.1 mM ouabain, 0.05 mM dipyridamole (pH 7.4,
37°C, hematocrit 2%). All values are corrected to a hemoglobin content of 5.2 µmoles/ml cells.

ments shown in Figure 4, the choline chloride media contained ouabain and dipyridamole. Zero activity of the countertransport system would be expected at the one hour uptake of about 0.02 μmoles Li$^+$/ml cells under these conditions, the residual uptake proceeding through the dipyridamole-insensitive part of the leak (see dotted line in Figure 5). If this residual leak is taken into account, the data demonstrate that the activity of the system can vary by a factor of about 7 among apparently healthy donors. The red cell Na$^+$ content was similar among the donors (range 5.9 to 10.6 μmoles/ml cells, mean ± 1 S.D.= 8.3 ± 1.1). The variations in the Na$^+$ content did not correlate with Li$^+$ uptake. Hence, the differences in Li$^+$ uptake shown in Figure 5 can be attributed almost exclusively to variations in the activity of the Na$^+$-Li$^+$ countertransport system.

INHIBITION OF THE COUNTERTRANSPORT SYSTEM BY NEM

Recently, we have demonstrated that the Na$^+$-Li$^+$ counter-transport system of human erythrocytes is inhibited by N-ethylmaleimide (NEM), but not by the other SH- or amino-reactive agents PCMB, PCMBS, 2,4-DNFB, DTNB and SITS (10,11). Figure 6 deals with the reversibility of the NEM effect. For these experiments, the erythrocytes of the donor U.L. with their highly effective countertransport system were selected (see Figures 3, 4 and 5). To avoid NEM-induced volume changes consecutive to K$^+$ loss, the cells were suspended in KCl media. The closed circles connected by solid lines show the control uptake. Addition of NEM inhibited the countertransport system (broken lines in Figure 6). The action of NEM seems to be instantaneous. Its addition, subsequent to 31 min of incubation, immediately caused the rate of Li$^+$ uptake to fall to the lower value. As to be expected, when the NEM-trapping agent mercaptoethanol was added in a fourfold excess prior to NEM, the NEM effect was completely abolished (open circles in Figure 6). Addition of mercaptoethanol (or dithiothreitol), not prior, but 31 min after NEM, had no effect (see Figure 6).

The inhibition of the countertransport system may therefore result from an irreversible reaction of NEM with SH-(or amino-)groups within the membrane. However, we observed that the seemingly irreversible effect found in K$^+$/Li$^+$ media could not be detected on cells preincubated with NEM in Li$^+$-free choline or potassium chloride media and subsequently

washed with NEM-free medium. After four washings in a 20-fold
excess of medium, the activity of the countertransport system
recovered completely and renewed addition of NEM inhibited
the countertransport system in the cells pretreated with NEM
to the same extent as in fresh cells.

In contrast, when the cells were preincubated with NEM
in media containing 150 mM NaCl or 5 mM LiCl, these cation
concentrations being equivalent with respect to their affinity to the countertransport system (see Table 1), the NEM-in-
hibition could not be removed by washing or by adding mercaptoethanol.   Maximal inhibition was achieved already after

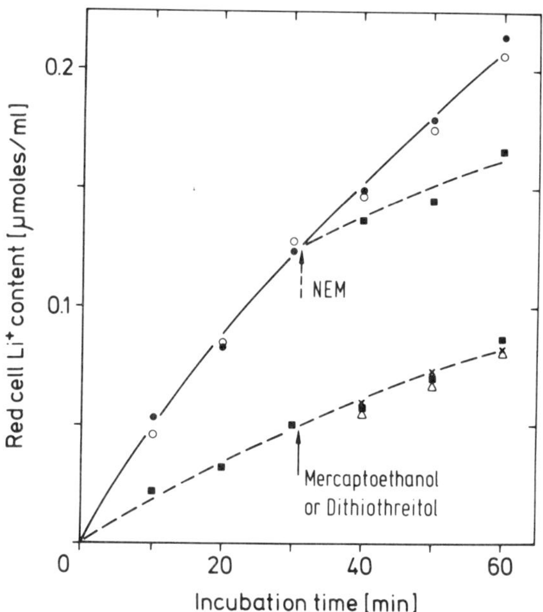

Figure 6: Effect of NEM and of the NEM-trapping agents mercaptoethanol and DL-dithiothreitol on Li$^+$ uptake. The media
contained 150 mM KCl, 2 mM Li$^+$ and 0.1 mM ouabain (pH 7.4,
37°C, hematocrit 2%, values corrected to a hemoglobin content of 5.2 μmoles/ ml cells). One of two experiments with
erythrocytes of the donor U.L. The arrows indicate time of
addition of the reagents. o control; ▪ 0.5 mM NEM; ● 2 mM
mercaptoethanol prior to NEM; x NEM 31 min prior to 2 mM
mercaptoethanol; △ NEM 31 min prior to 2 mM dithiothreitol.

3 min of incubation with NEM in 150 mM NaCl media (unpublished results).

These findings indicate that irreversible binding of NEM to the countertransport system depends on the cation composition of the medium. An appealing interpretation would be that binding of Na$^+$ or Li$^+$ to the system induces conformational changes which allow NEM to react with otherwise shielded sites. This observation may be useful in attempts to identify the protein which probably mediates the Na$^+$-Li$^+$ countertransport.

COMMON PROPERTIES OF Na$^+$-Li$^+$ AND OUABAIN-RESISTANT Na$^+$-Na$^+$ EXCHANGE

Figure 7 shows lineweaver-Burk plots of the dependence of Li$^+$ uptake by the Na$^+$-Li$^+$ countertransport system on external Li$^+$ concentration, determined at the two external Na$^+$ concentrations of 10 and 150 mM, respectively. The two straight lines have a common intercept at the ordinate, indicating that Na$^+$ competes with Li$^+$ for the external site of the countertransport system (10,35). From the insert in the Figure, an apparent inhibitory constant for external Na$^+$ of about 30 mM can be calculated, a value close to the apparent K_m of external Na$^+$ determined in experiments of Li$^+$ release (see Table 1). This observation is one first argument favouring the idea that Na$^+$-Li$^+$ countertransport is mediated by the ouabain-resistant Na$^+$-Na$^+$ exchange system.

Some common properties of ouabain-resistant Na$^+$-Na$^+$ and Na$^+$-Li$^+$ exchange in human erythrocytes are:
    Michaelis-Menten kinetics (10,35)
    one-to-one exchange (10,18,35)
    low affinity for external Na$^+$ (10,30,31,35)
    inhibition by NEM but not by PCMBS (10,11,31)
    identical pH dependency (11).

These similarities, and the observation that Na$^+$ and Li$^+$ compete with one another, led us to conclude that Na$^+$-dependent Li$^+$ countertransport is mediated by the ouabain-insensitive Na$^+$-Na$^+$ exchange system (10,11). Recent results of Tosteson (35) and of Funder and Wieth (18) also support the idea of the identity of the two systems. It is to be noted, however, that the human red cell possibly possesses two ouabain-resistant Na$^+$-Na$^+$ exchange systems which are distinguished by

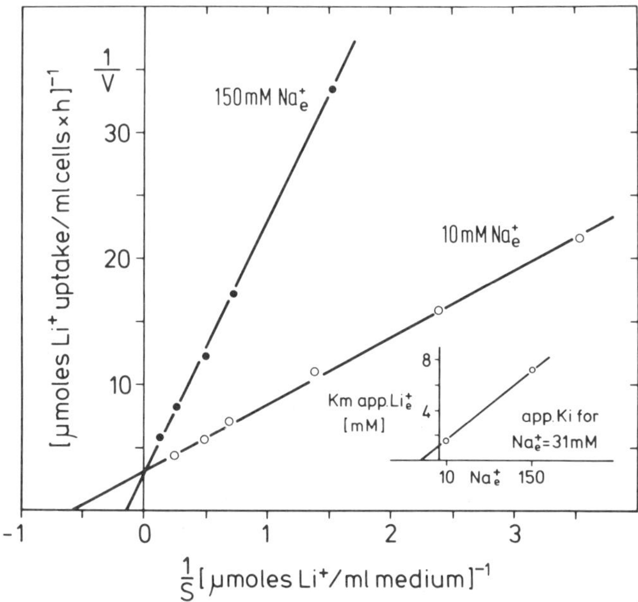

Figure 7: Competition between Na⁺ and Li⁺ for the external
site of the Na⁺-Li⁺ countertransport system.
Double reciprocal plots of Li⁺ uptake versus external Li⁺
concentration are shown, determined at 10 and 150 mM external Na⁺ (Na⁺ replaced by choline⁺, 0.1 mM ouabain, 0.05 mM dipyridamole, pH 7.4, 37°C, hematocrit 2%). Single experiments
with erythrocytes of the donor U.L.

their sensitivity towards NEM (31) or phloretin (35).

THE Li⁺ DISTRIBUTION RATIO

Principally, all of the four Li⁺ transport pathways discussed above can contribute to the establishment of the steady-state Li⁺ distribution between red cells and plasma. However, Li⁺ transport into or out of the cells at the K⁺- and
Na⁺ site of the Na⁺-K⁺ pump, respectively, appears to be unimportant for the human red cell in vivo, since these potential transport properties are almost completely blocked at
the physiological plasma and red cell cation concentrations
(8,12).

If the countertransport system were inactive, Li$^+$ would be passively distributed in the steady-state, the distribution ratio between red cells and plasma being determined by the Donnan potential across the red cell membrane. At a plasma pH of 7.4, the distribution ratio of external to internal Li$^+$ (Li$_e^+$/Li$_i^+$) would be about 1 or 0.65, depending on whether the values refer to red cell Li$^+$ content (μmoles Li$^+$/ml cells) or Li$^+$ concentration in the red cell water. If, conversely, only the countertransport system were operating and no downhill transport along the Li$^+$ gradient established by the system were to occur, the Li$^+$ ratio would attain the value of the Na$^+$ ratio Na$_e^+$/Na$_i^+$, which ranges between 15 and 20 in normal human blood (Na$_i^+$=red cell Na$^+$ content). In terms of the inverse ratio Li$_i^+$/Li$_e^+$ used by most clinicians, the expected ratio would thus lie between 0.05 and 0.07.

The ratios Li$_i^+$/Li$_e^+$ actually found in vivo or in vitro in the steady-state are much higher, ranging between 0.12 (10) and 0.8 (20,35). This is due to the fact that the Li$^+$ leak and the bicarbonate-stimulated pathway are not inactive, but rather mediate Li$^+$ downhill transport at a rate of about 0.016 and 0.019 μmoles/ml cells x h, respectively. These data refer to an 1 mM Li$^+$ concentration difference between plasma and red cell water and to a plasma bicarbonate concentration of 24 mM, respectively (pH 7.4, 37°C). Accordingly, the Li$^+$ ratio finally established depends on both the countertransport system and the "leak pathways". In previous studies we have demonstrated that the leak does not vary considerably among donors, whereas the countertransport system shows individually different maximal transport capacities (10, compare Figures 3 and 4). The same result was obtained with red cells of patients suffering from affective disorders (20). Hence, the individually different Li$^+$ distribution ratios arise almost exclusively from different activities of the Na$^+$-Li$^+$ countertransport system. In comparison, the variations in the ratio resulting from differences in the transmembrane Na$^+$ gradient are small.

From the data on the activity of the leak pathway and the bicarbonate-stimulated pathway given in the previous paragraph, it is immediately apparent that variations in the plasma bicarbonate concentration can induce variations in the Li$^+$ ratio within individuals. As has been discussed in detail earlier, bicarbonate, in addition to accelerating Li$^+$ downhill transport, exerts a second effect on the Li$^+$ ratio through its action on downhill Na$^+$ transport (9). The cellular Na$^+$ content increases with rising bicarbonate concentration (9,16,17), thus aggravating the change in the Li$^+$ ratio (resulting from the accelerated downhill transport of Li$^+$-carbonate ion pairs) through a decrease of the Na$^+$ gradient and the driving force for Li$^+$ countertransport, respectively.

ON THE GENERAL PHYSIOLOGICAL SIGNIFICANCE OF Na$^+$-Li$^+$ COUNTERTRANSPORT

Many tissues, including brain and muscle, exhibit an ouabain-resistant Na$^+$-Na$^+$ exchange with properties similar to the system of human and beef erythrocytes (30,31). Since Na$^+$-Li$^+$ countertransport in the human red cell is certainly mediated by an ouabain-resistant Na$^+$-Na$^+$ exchange system (see above), it is tempting to conclude that a Na$^+$-Na$^+$ exchange system of other organs also mediates Na$^+$-Li$^+$ exchange. If this were so, then Li$^+$ countertransport driven by the Na$^+$ gradient could be responsible for the yet unexplained low cellular Li$^+$ levels in all tissues.

Theoretically, individually different activities of the Na$^+$-Li$^+$ countertransport system of all (or certain) tissues could account for the interindividual differences of the apparent Li$^+$ distribution volume in the body, of the biological t 1/2 of Li$^+$ in the plasma, of the Li$^+$ clearance and in the daily therapeutic Li$^+$ dosis (1).

It has been proposed that differences in cell membrane functioning may be related to the varying effectivity of Li$^+$ in treatment of manic depressive disease and other affective disorders (29). The large variations we observed among erythrocytes of apparently healthy donors seem to indicate that no relationship exists between the activity of the red cell countertransport and affective disorders. However, whether the activity of the system varies in brain and other organs to the same extent as in human erythrocytes, remains to be investigated.

ACKNOWLEDGEMENTS

The authors are indebted to Mrs. Jutta Kronauer for her skillful and expert technical assistance. The work was supported in part by the Wilhelm Sander-Stiftung.

REFERENCES

1) Amdisen A (1977). Serum level monitoring and clinical pharmacokinetics of lithium. Clin Pharmacokin 2:73

1a)Becker BF, Duhm J (1977). Effect of oxyanions on passive Li$^+$ transport across the human red cell membrane. Pflügers Arch 368:R 20

2) Bunney WE,Jr, Murphy DL (1976). "The Neurobiology of Lithium" Neurosc Res Prog Bull 14/2

3) Cade JFJ (1949). Lithium salts in the treatment of psychotic excitement. Med J Austr 2:349

4) Callahan TJ, Goldstein DA (1972). Selective passive cation transport in the human red cell membrane. Fed Proc 31: 845 Abs.

5) Cazzullo CL, Smeraldi E, Sacchetti E (1975). Intracellular lithium concentration and clinical response. Br J Psychiat 126:298

6) Dorus E, Pandey GN, Frazer A, Mendels J (1974). Genetic determinant of lithium ion distribution. I. An in vitro monozygotic-dizygotic twin study. Arch Gen Psychiat 31: 463

7) Duhm J, Eisenried F, Becker BF, Greil W (1976). Studies on the lithium transport across the red cell membrane. I. Li$^+$ uphill transport by the Na$^+$-dependent Li$^+$ countertransport system. Pflügers Arch 364:147

8) Duhm J, Becker BF (1977). Studies on the lithium transport across the red cell membrane. II. Characterization of the ouabain-sensitive and ouabain-insensitive Li$^+$ transport. Effects of bicarbonate and dipyridamole. Pflügers Arch 367:211

9) Duhm J, Becker BF (1977). Studies on the lithium transport across the red cell membrane. III. Factors contributing to the intraindividual variability of the in vitro Li$^+$ distribution across the human red cell membrane. Pflügers Arch 368:203

10) Duhm J, Becker BF (1977). Studies on the lithium transport across the red cell membrane. IV. Interindividual variations in the Na$^+$-dependent Li$^+$ countertransport system. Pflügers Arch 370:211

11) Duhm J, Becker BF (in the press). Studies on Na$^+$-dependent Li$^+$ countertransport and bicarbonate-stimulated Li$^+$ transport in human erythrocytes. In Bolis L, Hoffman JF, Straub R (eds): "Drugs, Hormones and Membranes. International Conference on Biological Membranes" Crans-sur-Sierre (Switzerland), June 12-17, 1977. New York:Raven Press

12) Dunham PB, Senyk O (1977). Lithium efflux through the
    Na/K pump in human erythrocytes. Proc Natl Acad Sci
    USA 74:3099
13) Elizur A, Shopsin B, Gershon S, Ehlenberger A (1972).
    Intra-extracellular lithium ratios and clinical course
    in affective states. Clin Pharmacol Ther 13:947
14) Frazer A, Mendels J, Sekunda SK, Cochrane CM, Bianchi CP
    (1973). The prediction of brain lithium concentration
    from plasma or erythrocyte measures. J Psychiat Res
    10:1
15) Funder J, Wieth JO(1967). Effect of some monovalent
    anions on fluxes of Na and K, and on glucose metabo-
    lism of ouabain treated human red cells. Acta Physiol
    Scand 71:168
16) Funder J, Wieth JO(1974). Human red cell sodium and po-
    tassium in metabolic alkalosis. Scand J Clin Lab Invest
    34:49
17) Funder J, Wieth JO(1974). Combined effect of digitalis
    therapy and of plasma bicarbonate on human red cell
    sodium and potassium. Scand J Clin Invest 34:153
18) Funder J, Wieth JO(in the press). Coupled lithium-sodium
    exchange in bovine red blood cells. In Bolis L,
    Hoffman JF, Straub R (eds): "Drugs, Hormones and Mem-
    branes. International Conference on Biological Mem-
    branes" Crans-sur-Sierre (Switzerland), June 12-17,1977
    New York: Raven Press
19) Gershon S, Shopsin B (1973). "Lithium. Its Role in Psy-
    chiatric Research and Treatment" New York-London:
    Plenum Press (scnd ed 1976)
20) Greil W, Eisenried F, Becker BF, Duhm J (1977). Inter-
    individual differences of the Na^+-dependent Li^+ coun-
    tertransport system and of the Li^+ distribution ratio
    across the red cell membrane among Li^+ treated patients.
    Psychopharmacol 53:19
21) Greil W, Eisenried F, Duhm J (1976). Über die Verteilung
    von Lithium zwischen Erythrocyten und Plasma: In-vitro-
    Untersuchungen zum Transport von Lithium an menschli-
    chen Erythrocyten. Arzneimittel Forsch (Drug Res) 26:
    1147
22) Greil W, Schnelle K, Seibold S (1974). Intra/extra-zel-
    luläres Lithiumverhältnis. Klinische und experimentel-
    le Befunde an Thrombocyten und Erythrocyten. Arznei-
    mittel Forsch (Drug Res) 24:1079
23) Haas M, Schooler J, Tosteson DC (1975).Coupling of li-
    thium to sodium transport in human red cells. Nature
    258:425

24) Johnson FN (1975). "Lithium Research and Therapy" London-New York-San Francisco: Academic Press

25) Johnson FN (in the press). "Lithium in Medical Practice" Proceedings of the First British Lithium Congress, Lancaster, July 15-19, 1977. Lancaster:ATP Press Ltd.

26) Lyttkens L, Söderberg U, Wetterberg L (1973). Increased lithium erythrocyte/plasma ratio in manic depressive psychosis. Lancet 1:40

27) Lyttkens L, Söderberg U, Wetterberg L (1976). Relation between erythrocyte and plasma lithium concentration as an index in psychiatric disease. Uppsala J Med Sci 81:123

28) Mallinger AG, Kupfer DJ, Poust RI, Hanin I (1975). In vitro and in vivo transport of lithium by human erythrocytes. Clin Pharmacol Ther 18:467

29) Mendels J, Frazer A (1973). Intracellular lithium and clinical response. Towards a membrane theory of depression. J Psychiat Res 10:9

30) Motais R (1973). Sodium movements in high-sodium beef red cells: Porperties of a ouabain-insensitive exchange diffusion. J Physiol (Lond) 233:395

31) Motais R, Sola F (1973). Characteristics of a sulphydryl group essential for sodium exchange diffusion in beef erythrocytes. J Physiol (Lond) 233:423

32) Pandey GN, Javaid JJ, Davis JM, Tosteson DC (1976). Mechanism of lithium transport in red blood cells. The Physiologist 19:321 abs.

33) Schou M (1976). Pharmacology and toxicology of lithium. Ann Rev Pharmacol Toxicol 16:231

34) Shopsin B, Johnson G, Gershon S (1970). Neurotoxicity with lithium: Differential drug responsiveness. Int Pharmacopsychiat 5:170

35) Tosteson DC (in the press). Lithium transport in human red cells. In Bolis L, Hoffman JF, Straub R (eds): "Drugs, Hormones and Membranes. International Conference on Biological Membranes" Crans-sur-Sierre (Switzerland), June 12-17, 1977. New York:Raven Press

36) Wieth JO (1969). Effects of bicarbonate and thiocyanate on fluxes of Na and K, and on glucose metabolism of actively transporting human red cells. Acta Physiol Scand 75:313

37) Wieth JO (1970). Effects of monovalent cations on sodium permeability of human red cells. Acta Physiol Scand 79:76

38) Wieth JO, Funder J (1965). An effect of anions on transfer of sodium through the human red cell membrane.

Scand J Clin Invest 17:399
39) Zakowska-Dabrowska T, Rybakowski J (1973). Lithium-induced
     EEG changes. Relation to lithium level in serum and red
     blood cells. Acta Psychiat Scand 49:457

DISCUSSION

<u>Dr. Brewer</u>: If I understood what you were saying about the
manic depressive relationships, there is a possibility that
the individual variations you're seeing in the counter-transport system are related to the development of the disease?

<u>Dr. Duhm</u>: The situation is the following: Mendels and
Frazer proposed that there exists or may exist a relation
between the steady state Li+ distribution between red cells
and plasma on the one hand and the response to Li+ therapy
on the other hand. These authors put forward a membrane
theory of depression that's the subtitle of one of their
papers. We now know that the inter-individual differences
in the Li+ ratio are caused by differences of the sodium-
dependent Li+ counter-transport system. However, the
variability in the activity of the counter-transport system
observed in patients suffering from affective disorders and
in apparently healthy donors is similar or - at least - not
grossly different. The statistical work remains to be done
on that because the relation between the Li+ ratio and the
activity of the counter-transport system and affective
disorders is not clear.

<u>Dr. Brewer</u>: Secondly, as I understand it, there is a vari-
ation in response to administered lithium in manic depressive
patients; that is, some patients are greatly improved and
others are not. Have you looked at whether the individual
differences in this transport system might account for the
differences in response to lithium as a drug?

<u>Dr. Duhm</u>: We are studying this problem in collaboration with
the department of psychiatry at the University of Munich.
The results obtained so far show no consistent relationship.
At the moment, we question this hypothesis, although we
cannot definitely disprove it.

<u>Dr. Brewer</u>: A final question.   Are these inter-individual
differences genetically determined?

<u>Dr. Duhm</u>: There are some studies on twins in the literature
indicating that the distribution ratio may be genetically
determined. We performed a longitudinal study on four
apparently healthy donors with extremely different transport
rates and have shown that the transport system remains unchanged over a period of about ten months, that is, over

The Red Cell, pages 571—573
© **1978 Alan R. Liss, Inc., New York, New York**

more than two red cell life spans. This result is consistent
with the concept that the activity of the system is genetically
determined in some way. The type of inheritance is not known
yet.

<u>Dr. Kraus</u>: In connection with the individuality of the lithi-
um transport, there also appears to be an individuality in
response to the toxicity of the ion. If I could have a
slide, briefly, to show you our studies. We compared lithium
and sodium cations and the anions carbamyl phosphate and
chloride. We were using thirteen millimoles per kilogram
per day of lithium or sodium and in studying the survival
of mice in this way, we found some interesting things. In
this study, which was of three weeks' duration, for the
lithium salts, six out of fifteen animals survived in the
lithium chloride group, and eight out of fifteen in the lithium carbamyl phosphate group whereas when we used sodium
salts of these two compounds, fourteen of fifteen survived in
the carbamyl phosphate group and fifteen of fifteen survived
in the chloride group so that the toxicity resided in the
lithium cation. In the whole blood of these animals at the
time of death, our lithium levels in millimoles per liter
or milliequivalents per liter were almost the levels that
you used in your incubation experiments, 1.4 to 1.9. At
this whole blood level there is a marked depression of white
cells, approximately half of that found at the beginning of
the study. I'm wondering if you looked at white cells, and
if you can explain this, and if there is an correlation
between these data and the red cell parameters that you have
been looking at?

<u>Dr. Duhm</u>: I cannot comment on your data, but only answer
your question concerning the white cell counts. When going
over the literature, you only find comments that in patients
treated with lithium salts, there is sometimes a leukocytosis.
In the last issue of the New England Journal of Medicine you
will find a report on alternation of chemotherapy-induced
neutropenia by lithium. I do not remember any report on
opacity of the lens or retrolental fibrosis being a side effect
of Li+ therapy. Dr. Greil from the Department of Psychiatry
of the University of Munich told me that he observed worsening of glaucoma in one patient which disappeared upon dis-
continuing maintenance Li+ therapy

<u>Dr. L. Kraus</u>: We were aware of the use of lithium to increase
the white cell count, and were therefore very surprised by

this decrease of the white cell count by one half in this three-week period in these animals. Thank you.

Dr. Morse: Do you have any evidence about how lithium is distributed inside the red blood cells, that is, is it pooled or is it just passively distributed throughout the interior of the cell?

Dr. Duhm: That's a difficult question. I have no idea. I do not know whether there exists any protein or cell constituent which specifically binds lithium. If we assume that there exists no protein which does, then I would guess that lithium is homogeneously distributed in the water phase of the red cell. Certainly, Li+ may be bound to the countertransport system within the membrane.

Dr. Smith: The monofunctional maleimide, NEM, is going to bind to several subcompartments within the red cell. My question is, at the 0.5 mM concentration you used, did you measure glutathione levlls, nonspecific membrane permeability, or other parameters and might they have artificially done something to the system?

Dr. Duhm: Glutathione is zero at 0.5 mM NEM and a hematociit of 2%. If you increase the NEM concentration above that level, then you have an increased leakage for all monovalent cations and when you decrease the NEM concentration below 0.5 mM then the inhibition of the countertransport system tends to disappear. Glycolysis is completely inhibited by the NEM concentration applied and red cell ATP levels decrease continuously with time. The deterioration of metabolism, however, should be not harmful for the countertransport system because the system has been shown to be fully active in cells depleted of ATP by substrate-free incubation or in ATP-free ghost preparations.

EFFECTS OF VITAMIN E DEFICIENCY AND LEAD TOXICITY ON THE FILTERABILITY OF RAT ERYTHROCYTES

Orville A. Levander, Virginia C. Morris, and Renato J. Ferretti

Nutrition Institute
Agricultural Research Center
Beltsville, Maryland   20705

INTRODUCTION

Previous work from this laboratory has shown that lead poisoning causes a more severe anemia and splenomegaly in vitamin E-deficient rats than in vitamin E-supplemented rats (Levander et al., 1975). This increased anemia was accompanied by marked reticulocytosis and elevated red cell mechanical fragility which suggested impaired red cell survival rather than impaired red cell production. Lead poisoning also decreased the osmotic and peroxidative fragilities of red cells from vitamin E-deficient rats (Levander et al., 1977a). Such changes in erythrocyte fragility could result from a "tanning" reaction of lead with the red cell membrane thereby making the membrane "tougher" but also more "brittle". Since the mechanical fragility test is rather cumbersome and gave somewhat inconsistent results in our hands (Levander et al., 1978a), we sought an alternate technique for determining the effects of lead on the red cell membrane. If lead reacted with the red cell membrane, it could affect the deformability of the red blood cell. Therefore, we measured erythrocyte filterability as an index of erythrocyte deformability in lead-poisoned and non-poisoned rats fed diets deficient in or supplemented with vitamin E.

The Red Cell, pages 575—590

EXPERIMENTAL

The experimental procedures used in the studies reported here are documented in detail elsewhere (Levander et al., 1975 and 1977b). Weanling male rats were fed a vitamin E-deficient basal diet either with or without 100 ppm vitamin E. Rats in each dietary group received either 0, 250, or 1000 ppm lead, as lead acetate, in the drinking water. After 3 months, blood samples were withdrawn from the abdominal aorta under ether anesthesia. A sample equivalent to 1 ml of blood with a hematocrit of 45 was diluted to 50 ml in tris-buffered saline, pH 7.4, which contained 10 mg glucose/100 ml. The red cell suspension was incubated in air at room temperature. At zero time and at designated intervals, the time required for 2 ml of the red cell suspension to pass through a 25 mm polycarbonate ("Nuclepore") filter with a pore size of 3.0μ under a vacuum of 10 cm of water was determined by visual inspection. This "Filtration Time" was taken as an indication of the red cell filterability. Within any given experiment only filters with identical flow rates, as determined by pre-calibration with buffer, were used (Levander et al., 1977b).

RESULTS AND DISCUSSION

Filterability vs. Anemia and Splenomegaly

Poisoning with 1000 ppm lead in the drinking water depressed weight gains, increased spleen weights and decreased hematocrit values in both vitamin E-supplemented and -deficient rats, but these effects were more pronounced in the deficient group (Table 1). Vitamin E deficiency per se had no effect on any of these parameters in non-poisoned rats. However, vitamin E-deficiency alone markedly decreased the filterability of incubated red cells from non-poisoned rats, and lead poisoning accelerated this decline (Table 2). On the other hand, lead poisoning had no effect on the filterability of erythrocytes from vitamin E-supplemented rats.

Table 1

Effects of vitamin E on lead poisoning[1]

Vitamin E added to basal diet	Lead in water	Weight gain	Spleen weight	Hematocrit value
ppm	ppm	g	% of body wt.	% by vol.
100	0	189 ± 0^a	0.19 ± 0.00^a	45 ± 1^a
100	1000	144 ± 3^b	0.28 ± 0.03^b	40 ± 2^b
0	0	183 ± 2^a	0.20 ± 0.01^a	45 ± 0^a
0	1000	128 ± 1^c	0.39 ± 0.05^c	35 ± 1^c

[1]Means of 3 rats $\pm$ S.E.; means in the same column with different superscripts differ significantly at the $P < 0.05$ level (Duncan's multiple range test).

Table 2

Effects of vitamin E and lead on red cell filterability[1]

Vitamin E added to basal diet	Lead in water	Filtration time after incubation for			
		0 hr	2 hr	4 hr	6 hr
ppm	ppm	seconds			
100	0	15 ± 1^a	17 ± 1^a	24 ± 1^a	76 ± 2^a
100	1000	15 ± 1^a	19 ± 1^a	25 ± 1^a	77 ± 5^a
0	0	15 ± 1^a	20 ± 1^a	36 ± 6^a	$>600^b$
0	1000	19 ± 2^b	55 ± 12^b	195 ± 82^b	$>600^b$

[1]Significance of superscripts as in Table 1.

Our observations suggest that decreased red cell filterability is closely related to the increased anemia and splenomegaly of vitamin E-deficient lead-poisoned rats. For example, decreasing the pH of the red cell suspension medium to 6.6, a value typical of the spleen, markedly decreased the filterability of red cells from vitamin E-deficient lead-poisoned rats but had much less effect on the filterability of red cells from E-supplemented non-poisoned rats (Levander et al., 1977b). Apparently the physiological conditions in the spleen are ideal for generating and trapping non-deformable erythrocytes. Also, fractionation of erythrocytes according to cell age revealed that the old cells were mainly responsible for the decreased filterability of blood samples from our E-deficient lead-poisoned rats (Levander et al., 1978b). For deficient poisoned rats, moreover, the decrease in filterability caused by incubation with hydrogen peroxide was much greater for old than for young cells. These findings support the concept that vitamin E deficiency and lead poisoning accelerate aging and decrease deformability of red cells in vivo and that such cells are preferentially removed from the blood stream by the spleen. During in vitro incubation, red cells from E-deficient lead-poisoned rats undergo morphological transition from discocytes to spherocytes or stomatospherocytes which are non-filterable; red cells from E-supplemented non-poisoned rats maintain their discocytic shape and filterability (Figs. 1 and 2; Levander et al., 1977c). This clarifies the role of the spleen as an in vivo filter that recognizes abnormal cells, turns them into spherocytes, traps them, and then destroys them.

But since splenomegaly occurs in the absence of impaired red cell filterability (lead-poisoned vitamin E-supplemented rats) and impaired red cell filterability occurs in the absence of splenomegaly (non-poisoned vitamin E-deficient rats-Tables 1 and 2), it is possible that red cell destruction in the spleens of lead-poisoned E-deficient rats is controlled by at least two factors each of which is mediated independently by lead or vitamin E. We suggest that splenic erythrocytolysis consists of two more or less separate steps, recognition and destruction, and that the former is mediated mainly by lead, whereas the latter is mediated largely by vitamin E (Fig. 3).

Thus, in lead-poisoned vitamin E-supplemented rats the red
cell is recognized by the spleen of these animals as
abnormal but since vitamin E is present to stabilize the
erythrocyte membrane, red cell destruction is limited and
anemia and splenomegaly are mild. In lead-poisoned E-
deficient rats, however, the red cell is not only recognized as abnormal but is also highly vulnerable to
destruction in the spleen and hence anemia and splenomegaly are severe. On the other hand, the red cell in

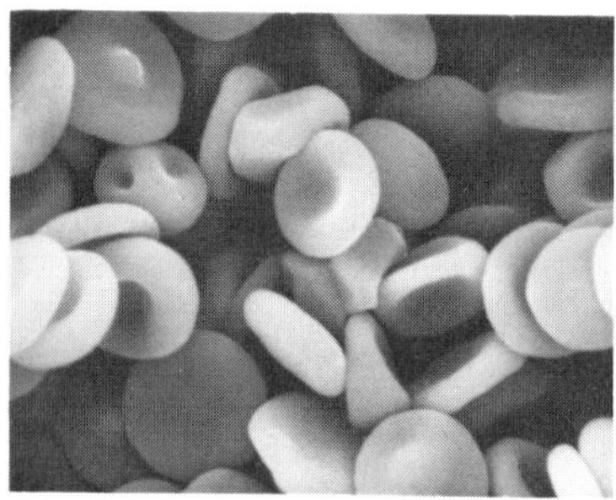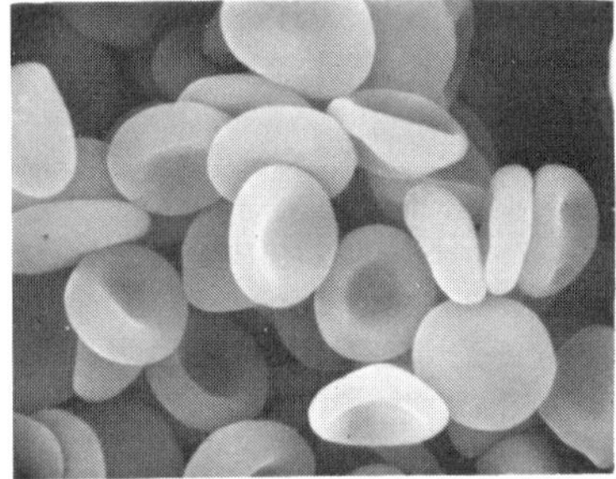

Figure 1. Zero-time samples of erythrocytes from vitamin
E-supplemented non-poisoned (left) and vitamin E-deficient
lead-poisoned (right) rats. Cells suspended in tris-
buffered saline containing 0.25% bovine serum albumin.
From Levander et al.(1977c), with permission.

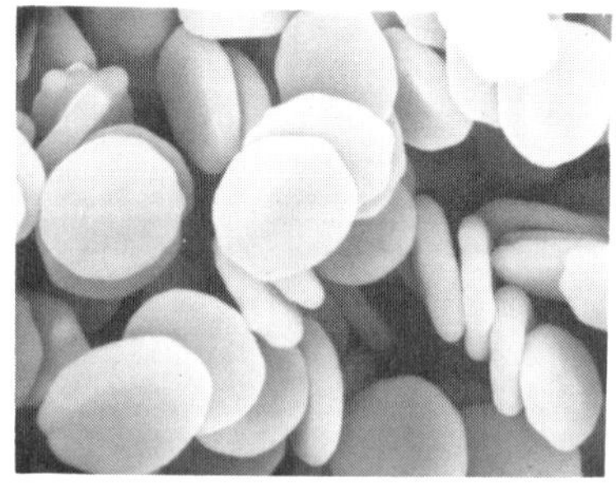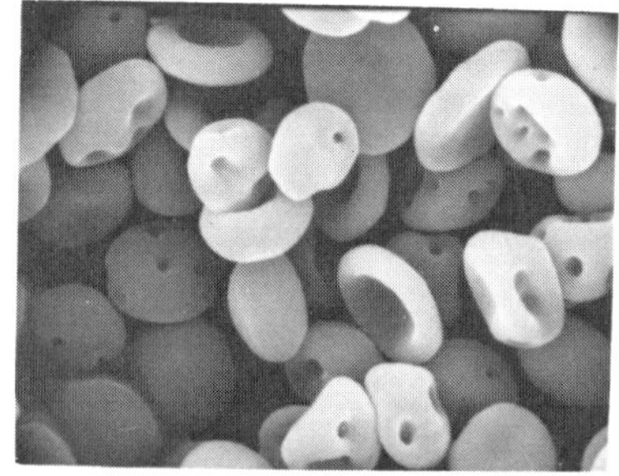

Figure 2. Six-hour samples of erythrocytes as in Fig. 1.

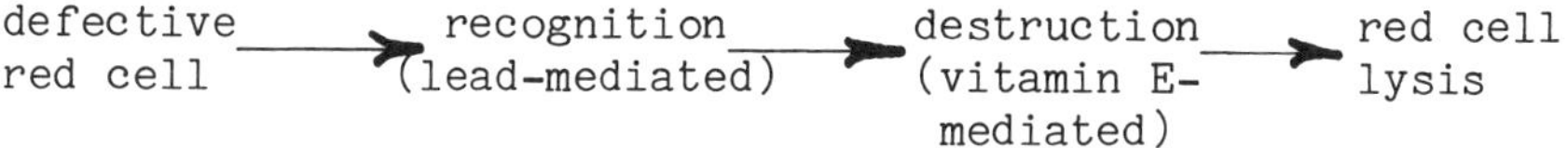

Figure 3. Hypothetical pathway of splenic erythro-cytolysis.

non-poisoned E-deficient rats might not be recognized as abnormal by the spleen so that, in spite of its great vulnerability to destruction, comparatively little hemolysis occurs and the spleen is able to remove any red cell breakdown products efficiently. Under these con-ditions slight, if any, anemia or congestive splenomegaly would be observed.

Vitamin A vs. Vitamin E

Vitamins A and E are fat-soluble and roles have been suggested for both in stabilizing biological membranes (Mack et al., 1972; Lucy, 1972). Moreover, Hodges et al. (1975) hypothesized in an oral report that the simultaneous occurrence of vitamin A deficiency and anemia might be partially explained by decreased stability of erythro-cytes. Therefore, we fed rats the basal diet either deficient in both vitamins A and E or supplemented with either A, E, or both. In this experiment, the poisoned rats received 250 ppm lead in the drinking water and the feeding period was 2 months because of severe weight depression in vitamin A-deficient rats. In this experiment, the filterability of red cells from E-deficient rats tended to decrease after incubation for 6 hours in vitro and concurrent lead poisoning exaggerated this effect (Table 3). On the other hand, acute vitamin A deficiency had no effect on the filterability of red cells from non-poisoned E-supplemented rats and appeared to inhibit the decrease in erythrocyte filterability observed in the non-poisoned E-deficient rats. But vitamin A deficiency shortened the incubation period required to demonstrate a decrease in the filterability of red cells from lead-poisoned vitamin E-deficient rats, so a role for vitamin A in red cell survival under these conditions cannot be ruled out entirely.

Table 3

Effects of lead and vitmins A and E on red cell filterability[1]

| Dietary supplement | | Lead in | Filtration time after incubation for | | |
vit. A	vit. E	water	0 hr	4 hr	6 hr
IU/kg	ppm	ppm		seconds	
10,000	100	0	16 ± 0^a	31 ± 1^a	45 ± 4^a
10,000	0	0	14 ± 2^a	33 ± 4^a	197 ± 35^a
0	100	0	16 ± 1^a	39 ± 3^a	62 ± 11^a
0	0	0	15 ± 1^a	32 ± 2^a	83 ± 15^a
10,000	100	250	15 ± 2^a	29 ± 6^a	39 ± 7^a
10,000	0	250	17 ± 1^a	52 ± 24^a	433 ± 26^b
0	100	250	18 ± 1^a	51 ± 5^a	97 ± 12^a
0	0	250	18 ± 2^a	121 ± 37^b	414 ± 92^b

[1]Means of 3 to 5 rats $\pm$ S.E.; significance of superscripts as in Table 1.

Additional evidence suggesting the specific role of vitamin E in lead poisoning derived from experiments in which excessive levels of selenium, an essential trace mineral metabolically related to vitamin E through its function in the lipid peroxide-destroying enzyme glutathione peroxidase (Hoekstra, 1975), had a relatively minor effect in preventing the decreased filterability of red cells from E-deficient lead-poisoned rats (Levander et al., 1977d). Support for the antioxidant hypothesis of vitamin E action came from studies in which the decreased filterability of incubated erythrocytes from lead-poisoned E-deficient rats was directly related to the extent of red cell lipid peroxidation and this decreased filterability was prevented by feeding the synthetic organic antioxidant N,N'-diphenyl-p-phenylenediamine (DPPD) (Levander et al., 1977b).

Chemical Stress vs. Filterability

Several chemical stress agents were used as probes in an attempt to understand the mechanism by which vitamin E deficiency and lead toxicity decreased erythrocyte filterability. Hydrogen peroxide was tested because of the relationship between decreased filterability and increased lipid peroxidation discussed above. Hydrazines were tried because they decrease filterability (Lubin and Desforges, 1972; Weinstein et al., 1975) and produce superoxide anion after interaction with hemoglobin (Goldberg et al., 1976; Misra and Fridovich, 1976). The aminoquinolines primaquine and chloroquine were compared because the former, but not the latter, puts an oxidative stress on red cells in vivo (Beutler, 1972) and generates hydrogen peroxide in red cells in vitro (Cohen and Hochstein, 1964). When added to red blood cell suspensions in vitro, all compounds tested decreased the filterability of erythrocytes from vitamin E-deficient rats and this effect was intensified by concomitant lead poisoning (Levander et al., 1977e). However, each family of compounds appeared to decrease erythrocyte filterability by a specific mechanism (Table 4). Incubation with hydrogen peroxide, for example, had little or no effect on the production of sulfhemoglobin or on the oxidation of glutathione in red blood cells, but markedly stimulated lipid peroxidation. Therefore, filterability probably decreased because lipid

Table 4

Metabolic effects of chemical stress on erythrocytes from
vitamin E-deficient lead-poisoned rats

Stress agent	Sulfhemoglobin production	Glutathione oxidation	Lipid peroxidation
hydrogen peroxide	0	+	++
phenylhydrazine	++	++	0
primaquine	0	0	0

0 = no effect; + = effect; ++ = strong effect; adapted from
Levander et al. (1977e).

peroxidation induced spherocyte formation as a result of
loss of cell membrane. This mechanism is thought to be
responsible for the decreased filterability of air-
incubated erythrocytes from E-deficient lead-poisoned rats
(Levander et al., 1977b). Phenylhydrazine, on the other
hand, did not increase lipid peroxidation but increased
glutathione oxidation and hemoglobin destruction. Since
hemoglobin degradation products are considered precursors
of Heinz bodies, which impair erythrocyte filterability
(Lubin and Desforges, 1972; Weinstein et al., 1975), Heinz
body formation might be the mechanism by which hydrazines
decreased red cell filterability. However, more recent
work has shown that hemoglobin destruction per se is not a
sufficient condition for decreased red cell filterability,
since methylhydrazine caused similar hemoglobin
destruction in red cells from both E-deficient and
E-supplemented rats, but decreased filterability of red
cells only in E-deficiency (Table 5). Possibly in vitamin
E deficiency the interaction of the hemoglobin degradation
products with the defective cell membrane is actually
responsible for the decreased red cell filterability.

The aminoquinolines differed from the other compounds
tested in that they had no effect on sulfhemoglobin production, glutathione oxidation, or lipid peroxidation.
Also, both chloroquine and primaquine decreased the
filterability of red cells from both vitamin E-supplemented and vitamin E-deficient rats (Levander et al.,
1977e). Those puzzling observations were explained when
it was realized that both of these compounds caused marked
invaginations in the membranes of red cells from deficient
and supplemented rats that led to the formation of non-
deformable stomato-spherocytes (Fig. 4). Others had
reported similar aminoquinoline-induced morphological
changes in normal human erythrocytes (Fugjii et al., 1973;
Trump, 1975). The significance of our work is that such
profound membrane rearrangements can take place, apparently with equal ease, in red cells from rats either
deficient in or supplemented with vitamin E, a nutrient
that is thought to play an important role in membrane
stability (Lucy, 1972).

Table 5

Effect of methylhydrazine on filterability and hemoglobin
destruction in red cells from vitamin E-supplemented and
deficient rats[1]

Vitamin E added to basal diet	Methyl-hydrazine	4 hr filtration time	Hemoglobin	Methemoglobin + sulfhemoglobin
ppm	mM	sec	g/100 ml blood	g/100 ml blood
100	0	24 ± 2^a	10.1 ± 0.3^a	0.22 ± 0.10^a
100	10	28 ± 1^a	8.2 ± 0.0^b	2.23 ± 0.16^b
0	0	53 ± 9^b	10.2 ± 0.2^a	0.27 ± 0.09^a
0	10	$>600^c$	8.2 ± 0.3^b	2.11 ± 0.07^b

[1]Means of 3 rats $\pm$ S.E.; significance of superscripts as in Table 1;
biochemical measurements carried out after 4 hours of incubation.

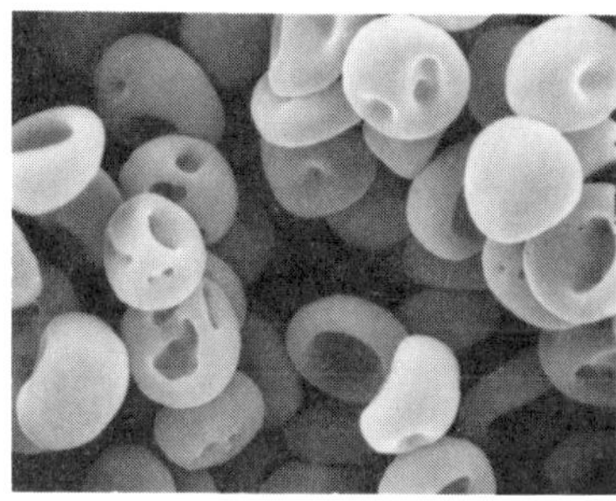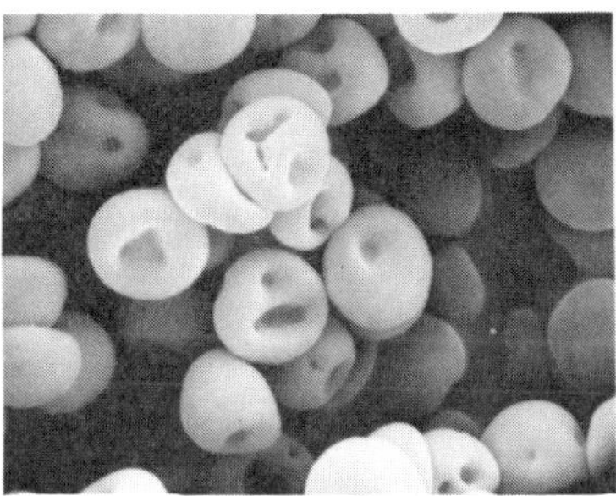

Figure 4. Three-hour samples of erythrocytes from vitamin
E-supplemented (left) and vitamin E-deficient (right)
non-poisoned rats. Cells incubated for 3 hours in tris
buffered-saline containing 10 mM chloroquine. Under these
conditions the red cells from both dietary groups are
essentially non-filterable. From Levander et al.(1977e),
with permission.

It is possible to speculate about the biochemical
mechanisms by which lead may potentiate the effect of
various chemical stress agents in decreasing red cell
filterability. In the case of oxidants, lead might block
the incorporation of iron into hemoglobin (Griggs, 1964),
thereby increasing intracellular levels of non-heme iron
which could then catalyze lipid peroxidation (Smith and
Dunkley, 1962). Lead might increase the effect of
hydrazines by reacting with the hemoglobin and exerting a
destabilizing effect on the molecule. Lead might
accentuate the effect of aminoquinolines by interacting
with the phosphate groups of the phospholipid bilayer of
the cell membrane (Passow, 1971) thus disrupting the
membrane and allowing a more ready penetration by the
aminoquinolines. Needless to say, much additional
biochemical research will be required to sort out and
explain all the effects of lead described above.

Practical Considerations

Elevated levels of Heinz bodies have been reported in children living near lead smelters (Ghelberg et al., 1966) which indicates oxidative stress on their red blood cells. The question that needs to be answered now is whether additional dietary supplements of the antioxidant vitamin E would help those children resist that toxic effect of lead. Also, any future studies that seek to determine the relationship between lead exposure and human disease should take into account the nutritional status of their subjects with regard to vitamin E.

SUMMARY

Vitamin E deficiency worsens the anemia and spleno-megaly caused by lead poisoning in rats. Lead poisoning worsens the decreased filterability of erythrocytes from vitamin E-deficient rats. A two-step model of splenic erythrocytolysis is proposed to relate decreased erythro-cyte filterability to the anemia and splenomegaly observed in vitamin E-deficient lead-poisoned rats. Vitamin E deficiency is quite specific in worsening the response of rats to lead toxicity because neither vitamin A deficiency nor selenium deficiency has similar effects. Lead potentiates the effect of several chemical stress agents in decreasing the filterability of red cells from vitamin E-deficient rats. The multitude of factors that influence the filterability of erythrocytes from vitamin E-deficient lead-poisoned rats suggests many possibilities for hematological research in nutrition, environmental toxicology, occupational hygiene, the physiology of aging, and pharmacology.

REFERENCES

Beutler, E. (1972). Drug-induced anemia. Federation Proc. 31: 141.

Cohen, G., and Hochstein, P. (1964). Generation of hydrogen peroxide in erythrocytes by hemolytic agents. Biochemistry 3: 895.

Fugjii, T., Sato, T., and Nakanishi, K. (1973). In vitro shape changes of human erythrocyte membranes. Physiol. Chem. & Physics 5: 423.

Ghelberg, N. W., Bretter, E., Costin, L., and Chitul, E. (1966). Investigations on the appearance of Heinz bodies under the influence of small lead concentrations in the atmosphere. Igiena 15: 209.

Goldberg, B., Stern, A., and Peisach, J. (1976). The mechanism of superoxide anion generation by the inter- action of phenylhydrazine with hemoglobin. J. Biol. Chem. 251: 3045.

Griggs, R. C. (1964). Lead poisoning: hematologic aspects. Prog. Hematol. 4: 117.

Hodges, R. E., Sauberlich, H. E., Canham, J. E., Mejia, L., Lykke, C., and Wallace, D. C. (1975). Iron deficiency anemia and hypovitaminosis A. Abstracts - 10th International Congress of Nutrition, Kyoto, Japan, 3-9 August 1975, p. 176.

Hoekstra, W. G. (1975). Biochemical function of selenium and its relation to vitamin E. Federation Proc. 34: 2083.

Levander, O. A., Morris, V. C., Higgs, D. J. and Ferretti, R. J. (1975). Lead poisoning in vitamin E-deficient rats. J. Nutrition 105: 1481.

Levander, O. A., Ferretti, R. J., and Morris, V. C. (1977a). Osmotic and peroxidative fragilities of erythrocytes from vitamin E-deficient lead-poisoned rats. J. Nutrition 107: 373.

Levander, O. A., Morris, V. C., and Ferretti, R. J. (1977b). Filterability of erythrocytes from vitamin E-deficient lead-poisoned rats. J. Nutrition 107: 363.

Levander, O. A., Fisher, M., Morris, V. C., and Ferretti, R. J. (1977c). Morphology of erythrocytes from vitamin E-deficient lead-poisoned rats. J. Nutrition, in press.

Levander, O. A., Morris, V. C., and Ferretti, R. J. (1977d). Comparative effects of selenium and vitamin E in lead-poisoned rats. J. Nutrition 107: 378.

Levander, O. A., Morris, V. C., and Ferretti, R. J. (1977e). Effect of oxidants, hydrazines, and amino- quinolines on the filterability of erythrocytes from vitamin E-deficient lead-poisoned rats. J. Nutrition, in press.

Passow, H. (1971). The red blood cell: penetration, distribution and toxic actions of heavy metals. In: Effects of Metals on Cells, Subcellular Elements, and Macromolecules (J. Maniloff, J. R. Coleman, and M. W. Miller, eds.) Charles C. Thomas, Springfield, IL pp. 291-340.

Smith, G. J., and Dunkley, W. L. (1962). Initiation of lipid peroxidation by a reduced metal ion. Archives Biochem. Biophys. 98: 46.

Trump, B. F. (1975). The network of intracellular membranes. In: Cell Membranes: Biochemistry, Cell Biology & Pathology (G. Weismann and R. Claiborne, eds.). H P Publishing Co., Inc., New York, pp. 123-133.

Weinstein, R. S., George, M. E., and Steingart, R. H. (1975). Contribution of Heinz bodies to alterations in red cell deformability. Toxicol. Appl. Pharmacol. 32: 545.

Levander, O. A., Morris, V. C., and Ferretti, R. J. (1978a). Vitamin E deficiency worsens hematological response to lead poisoning. Proceedings of 11th Annual Conference on Trace Substances in Environmental Health, Columbia, MO, 7-9 June 1977, in press.

Levander, O. A., Morris, V. C., and Ferretti, R. J. (1978b). Effect of cell age on the filterability of erythrocytes from vitamin E-deficient lead-poisoned rats. J. Nutrition, in press.

Lubin, A., and Desforges, J. F. (1972). Effect of Heinz bodies on red cell deformability. Blood 39: 658.

Lucy, J. A. (1972). Functional and structural aspects of biological membranes: a suggested structural role for vitamin E in the control of membrane permeability and stability. Ann. NY Acad. Sci. 203: 4.

Mack, J. P., Lui, N. S. T., Roels, O. A., and Anderson, O. R. (1972). The occurrence of vitamin A in biological membranes. Biochim. Biophys. Acta 288: 203.

Misra, H. P., and Fridovich, I. (1976). The oxidation of phenylhydrazine: superoxide and mechanism. Biochemistry 15: 681.

DISCUSSION

<u>Dr. Kreimer-Birnbaum</u>: I have one question: Any direct effect
of the Vitamin E deficiency on the ALA dehydrase? Do you
have data on that?

<u>Dr. Levander</u>: When we originally began these experiments,
we started off by measuring spilling over of ALA into the
urine as a result of possible inhibition of the enzyme either
as a result of the vitamin E deficiency or the lead poisoning, and we had some very promising results early, but then
we couldn't reproduce those results. We don't have any
data on the activity of the enzyme.

<u>Dr. Kreimer-Birnbaum</u>: Because the enzyme is ALA dehydrase,
a sulphydrilic enzyme and a direct effect of reducing agents
on its activity is well known, you could have a direct effect
of the Vitamin E deficiency on the enzyme via oxidants. You
might have two problems: the hemolytic part that you see due
to membrane complications and the direct effect on the heme biosynthetic pathway.

<u>Dr. Levander</u>: Yes.

<u>Dr. Cameron</u>: Do you have some information on heat sensitivi-
ty of these cells or to mechanical and osmotic fragility?
I'd be interested in some of that data.

<u>Dr. Levander</u>: I'm sorry I don't have a slide for that, but
the data that we do have indicate that by incubating the
cells at elevated temperatures either at 37° or 47°, you can
accelerate these filtration changes that I've been showing
you. And this occurs much more profoundly in red cells from
E-deficient animals than in cells from E-supplemented animals.
You can also prevent the changes in the E-deficient cells by
holding the cells at 0°.

<u>Dr. Lubin</u>: Did you try to correlate the filtration changes
you observed with Heinz body formation? The decreased filterability could at least partially be explained by Heinz
body formation, which I'm not sure the scanning EM would
always show.

<u>Dr. Levander</u>: That's right, I don't think it would, and I
must say we haven't done correlations of that kind, although
that would make a very good experiment.

The Red Cell, pages 591—593

Dr. Brewer: The similarity of your results with primaquine
and chloraquine would have suggested to me that this was
not an oxidant effect because only primaquine will cause
hemolysis of the G6PD deficient type. Chloraquine will not.
Thus, these two are different, and the fact that they behaved
similarly in your system suggests that it wasn't an oxidant
effect, and your results are compatible with that, I guess,
since you saw no difference in Vitamin E deficient animals.
Also, primaquine probably needs metabolizing before it is
very effective in producing oxidant-type damage.

Dr. Levander. That's quite so. Originally, we based these
experiments on an observation by others some years ago that
incubation of red cells with some of the oxidant antimalarials
in vitro would cause production of hydrogen peroxide in red
blood cells. You are perfectly correct in saying that there
is a difference in their metabolic behavior. But in vitro,
both these antimalarials cause a decrease in filterability,
both cause the same morphologic changes in the red cells and
both of them do it to the same extent in E-supplemented or
E-deficient groups.

Dr. Morse: Primaquine is one of the techniques used for
inducing inside-outside transitions of erythrocyte membranes,
and I think that this may be done by release of spectrin.
I'm wondering if the sorts of things you are looking at are
affecting the spectrin network that underlies the red blood
cell membrane?

Dr. Levander: I am very interested in that. Deuticke's
earlier work showed that cationic drugs can intercalate in
the inner half of the lipid bilayer, thus causing the invagination of the cell membranes. This may be related to our
explanation for the morphologic changes in our Vitamin E
deficient cells, because we visualize lipid oxidation taking
place preferentially in the inner half of the lipid bilayer,
causing an expansion of that half and the invagination.

Dr. Carrell: I'd like to make the point that I think is
brought out by your experiment with the antimalarials, that
because something occurs in the presence or absence of
Vitamin E does not necessarily mean that it is or is not
associated with an oxidative phenomenon. Antioxidant
activity is very much a localized function, and you may
have an effect in which Vitamin E will inhibit oxidation
at one site but on the other hand, oxidation at another

site even affecting the cell membrane will be unaffected
by the presence of Vitamin E. I just make this as a general
point to the audience, because people sometimes say that
such and such is not occurring in the presence of added
Vitamin E; therefore it's not an oxidative effect.

BLOOD STORAGE

Chairman: D. Surgenor

OXYGEN TRANSPORT FUNCTION OF PRESERVED RED BLOOD CELLS AND
MYOCARDIAL PERFORMANCE

C.R. Valeri,* R.D. Weisel,** R.C. Dennis,*
J.A. Mannick,*** R.L. Berger,** and
H.B. Hechtman***

*Naval Blood Research Laboratory, Boston, MA
**Boston University Medical Center, Boston, MA
***Peter Bent Brigham Hospital, Boston, MA

Most of the blood collected in blood banks throughout
the country is stored at 4 C as liquid red blood cells for
as long as 3 weeks in an anticoagulant such as acid-citrate-
dextrose (ACD) or citrate-phosphate-dextrose (CPD). Liquid
preservation is necessary in the blood banking system
because donors usually are not available to supply fresh
blood when the transfusion is needed. Moreover, physicians
often choose to use red blood cells instead of whole blood
because patients do not always need all the components in
whole blood, i.e., white blood cells, platelets, citrate,
plasma and non-plasma substances. In certain instances,
some of these components may even be harmful to the patient.

Freeze-preservation procedures were developed primarily
to provide a supplemental supply of rare red blood cells and
red blood cells lacking antigens that produce isosensitization.
Freeze-preservation has also been used to stockpile the red
blood cells of certain patients in anticipation of future
autologous transfusions.

Freeze-preserved red blood cells are always washed before
transfusion to remove the cryoprotective agent, glycerol.
Red cell washing has proven to be even more beneficial than
originally thought: significant amounts of isoagglutinins,
plasma protein and non-protein substances, white cells and
platelets are removed, the hepatitis B surface antigen is
reduced, and the citrate used in the anticoagulant medium is
removed (Valeri, 1976). When freeze-preserved red blood cells

The Red Cell, pages 597—614

are washed, the white blood cell and platelet counts are
usually reduced to less than 5%; washing liquid-stored red
blood cells reduces the white cell and platelet counts to
about 15% (Valeri, 1976). The presence of white blood cells
and platelets in transfused blood may sensitize the recipient
to future platelet and granulocyte transfusions, and to
tissue antigens in the kidney, bone marrow, and heart.

Although cryopreservation has been accepted as a means
of stockpiling rare and selected red blood cells and blood
products for autologous transfusion, it is still considered
by many too costly for widespread use, and there is some
concern about a potential risk of contamination during red
cell washing. Some proponents of cryopreservation, on the
other hand, feel that the success of cryopreservation is
being hindered by what is considered to be an unreasonable
and unnecessary restriction, i.e., the 24-hour post-wash
storage limitation. Previously frozen red blood cells have
been stored for as long as 3 days after washing with
satisfactory results (Valeri, 1976).

Restrictions are necessary, and, in fact, standards
should be established with regard to the oxygen transport
function of both liquid-preserved and freeze-preserved red
blood cells. There are restrictions regarding the 24-hour
posttransfusion survival value of preserved red blood cells,
which must be at least 70% at the time of transfusion, but
none for the oxygen transport function, an equally important
function.

Valtis and Kennedy (1954) were the first to describe
the defect in respiratory function of red blood cells
associated with liquid storage, a defect which usually is
repaired within 24 hours after the transfusion. It was later
established that this defect occurred as a result of a
reduction in the level of 2,3 diphosphoglycerate (2,3 DPG)
during storage of red blood cells in a liquid anticoagulant
at 4 C (Benesch and Benesch, 1967; Chanutin and Curnish, 1967).
About 50% of the 2,3 DPG is lost within 48 hours of 4 C
storage in the ACD anticoagulant (Figure 1). CPD provides
better maintenance, and, as a matter of fact, red blood cell
2,3 DPG actually increases slightly during the first 48 hours
of storage in CPD, although the level does fall to about 75%
of normal within 12 days (Figure 1). Red blood cell viability
and function are well maintained at 4 C for as long as 7 days
in CPD or in CPD-with-adenine, but only for about 48 hours in
ACD.

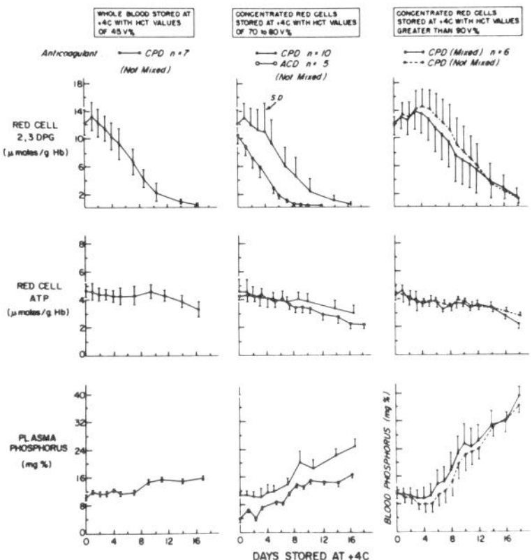

FIGURE 1. Red blood cell 2,3 DPG, ATP, and inorganic
phosphorus levels in red blood cells after storage as whole
blood with a hematocrit value of 45 V% or as concentrated
red blood cells with a hematocrit value of 70 to 80 V% or
of greater than 90 V% in ACD or CPD at 4 C for as long as
17 days. The units of whole blood and the units of red blood
cell concentrates with hematocrit values of 70 to 80 V% were
not subjected to mixing during storage. Each unit of red
blood cell concentrate with a hematocrit value of greater
than 90 V% was separated into two equal parts: one part was
mixed during storage at 4 C and the other was not (From
Valeri, 1976).

     Red blood cells should be frozen when their 2,3 DPG
levels are highest; for ACD-stored red blood cells this is
within 24 hours of collection, and for CPD-stored red blood
cells within 5 days (Figure 1). Red blood cell 2,3 DPG and
ATP levels are not significantly different from pre-freeze
levels after freeze-preservation with 40% W/V glycerol and
storage at -80 C for as long as 10 years (Valeri, 1976).

OXYGEN TRANSPORT FUNCTION OF PRESERVED RED BLOOD CELLS

     Oxygen transport function of red blood cells is impaired
during liquid storage as a result of a reduction in 2,3 DPG,
but the function is restored in vivo (Valtis and Kennedy, 1954;
Valeri and Hirsch, 1969; Beutler and Wood, 1969). When red

blood cells have 2,3 DPG levels of about 10% at the time of
transfusion, the levels increase to about 30% within 4 to 8
hours after transfusion, and to about 50% within 24 hours.
Restoration of the 2,3 DPG level to 25-30% is accompanied by
a reduction in red blood cell affinity for oxygen. In acidotic
and hypercarbic patients in negative phosphorus balance, resynthesis of the reduced red blood cell 2,3 DPG takes longer.
Red cell affinity for oxygen is measured by the P_{50} value,
which is the partial pressure of oxygen in millimeters of
mercury at which 50% of the hemoglobin is saturated.

Oxygen transport function is especially critical during
the 4 to 8 hours after transfusion. An increase in red blood
cell affinity may necessitate an increase in cardiac output,
a decrease in mixed venous oxygen tension, or a combination
of these two in order to provide a stable whole body oxygen
consumption. This control of cardiac output is thought to be
related to tissue oxygen tension (Hechtman, 1976). Further,
several organs such as the heart itself, the brain, and the
retina are especially sensitive to tissue oxygen tension,
which is the primary mechanism regulating the volume of flow
through these tissues. Thus, the heart must have the capacity
of autoregulation of flow if it is to satisfy its oxygen
requirements. Failure of the pump to obtain sufficient
oxygen may limit cardiac output and put the entire body in
jeopardy.

Studies of resuscitation procedures in seriously wounded
but otherwise healthy males with apparently normal cardiovascular systems showed sufficient oxygen delivery to tissue
after two to three blood volume exchanges of low 2,3 DPG red
blood cells (Collins, 1974, 1976; Chance et al, 1969).
Although no impairment in myocardial or cerebral blood flow
was seen in these young men, patients with arteriosclerotic
cardiovascular disease who have compromised flow to the heart
and brain or who have an inability to locally regulate the
distribution of this flow may be adversely affected by the
transfusion of red blood cells with low 2,3 DPG and increased
affinity for oxygen (Valeri, 1976).

RESPIRATORY FUNCTION OF LIQUID-PRESERVED RED BLOOD CELLS WITH
INCREASED AFFINITY FOR OXYGEN IN PATIENTS UNDERGOING ELECTIVE
OR EMERGENCY SURGERY FOR ABDOMINAL ANEURYSM REPAIR

Weisel and associates (unpublished data) transfused large
volumes of liquid-stored red blood cells with reduced 2,3 DPG

levels and increased affinity for oxygen to patients undergoing elective abdominal aortic aneurysm (AAA) surgery or emergency surgery for aneurysm rupture to study the effects of oxygen transport function in acutely ill patients with known arterio-sclerotic disease. Measurements were made of acid-base balance, arterial pO_2, pCO_2, and pH, and mixed venous pO_2, pCO_2, pH, oxygen consumption, and in vitro and in vivo red cell oxygen affinity. A thermister-tipped pulmonary artery catheter was inserted for the thermodilution measure of cardiac output, pulmonary arterial pressure and pulmonary arterial wedge pressure (PAWP). Basal cardiac output and stroke work (stroke volume X arterial pressure - PAWP) was then measured. This was followed by an evaluation of myocardial performance during stress. Patients were volume loaded with 50 to 100 grams of salt-poor albumin or blood over a 15- to 20-minute period. Volume infusion increased the preload (PAWP) and allowed the construction of a Starling myocardial performance curve. This curve relates the rise in left ventricular stroke work to increases in preload. The rise in stroke work is believed to be critically dependent upon myocardial oxygen availability.

The donor red blood cells used in this study had been stored in ACD or CPD at 4 C for about 2 weeks and had impaired oxygen delivering capabilities. The emergency cases received an average of 18 donor units: 12 were infused intraoperatively, and 6 were infused throughout the initial 24-hour postoperative period. Elective patients received 6 donor units: 3 were infused intraoperatively, and 3 units were infused throughout the initial 24-hour postoperative period. The emergency patients with ruptured aneurysm required three times as many red blood cells as the elective patients, and after the trans-fusion their mixed venous pO_2 tension was markedly reduced, red cell affinity for oxygen was markedly increased, and cardiac output was decreased (Figures 2-8). The heart's response to volume loading was also impaired. This, combined with the findings of decreased basal cardiac output and elevated pulmonary artery wedge pressure, indicated an impairment of left ventricular function.

Oxygen consumption was similar in the two groups (Figure 3). The reduced cardiac output in the emergency patients was accompanied by an increase in the systemic arterio-venous difference in oxygen extraction (Figures 3 and 4). There was a marked reduction in mixed venous pO_2 tension, which was a reflection of the decrease in cardiac output, the increase in extraction, and the increase in oxygen affinity

brought about by the transfusion of red blood cells with
decreased 2,3 DPG levels (Figures 6-8). These systemic
adaptations to maintain oxygen consumption in the presence
of reduced flow were not available to the heart where
extraction is usually maximal. Cardiac adaptations to high
red cell affinity states would in theory be coronary vaso-
dilitation and increased flow. The same response would be
expected if oxygen requirements were increased by volume
loading. The aneurysm patients were elderly, many having
coronary artery disease. Under these circumstances, the
response to volume loading in the presence of high affinity
red blood cells was a reduced work capacity. These limited
cardiac reserves prohibited an increase in systemic flow as
one of the adaptive modalities to maintain total body oxygen
consumption. The patients were forced to increase oxygen
extraction. This mechanism is useful but limited, particularly

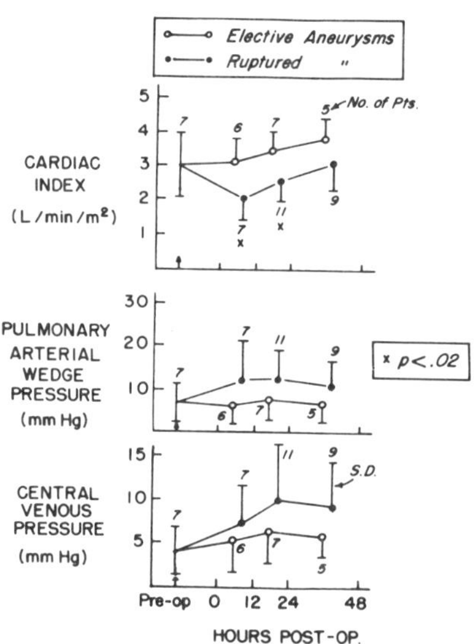

<u>FIGURE 2</u>. Cardiac index, pulmonary artery wedge pressure,
and central venous pressure in patients undergoing elective
and emergency surgery for resection of abdominal aortic
aneurysms. Patients who had elective surgery received 3 units
of 2-week-old liquid-stored ACD or CPD blood intraoperatively
and 3 units of 2-week-old liquid-stored ACD or CPD blood
throughout the 24-hour postoperative period. Patients who had
emergency surgery received 12 units of 2-week-old ACD or CPD
liquid-stored red cells intraoperatively and 6 units of 2-week-
old ACD or CPD liquid-stored red cells throughout the 24-hour
postoperative period.

with high affinity states. Patients who died had in vivo P_{50} values of less than 25 mm Hg and mixed venous pO_2 tensions of less than 25 mm Hg (Figures 6-8).

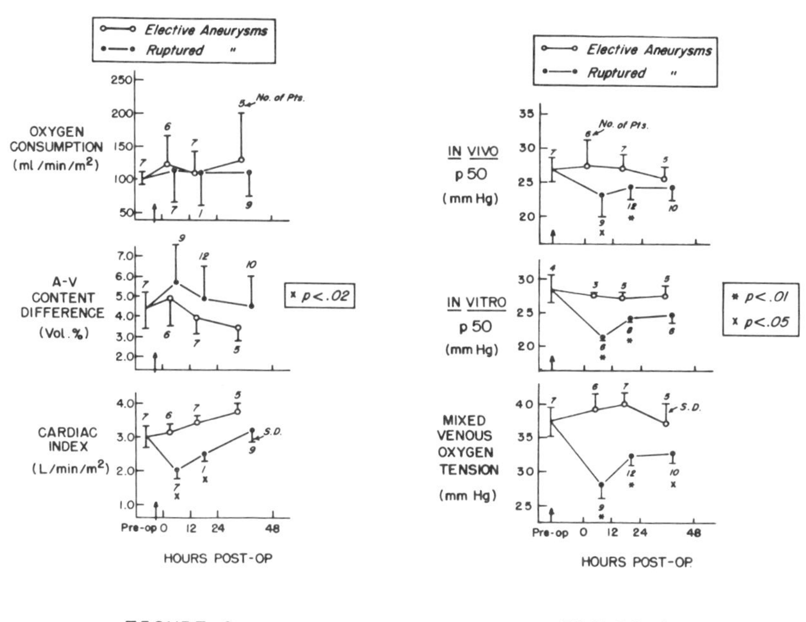

FIGURE 3   FIGURE 4

FIGURE 3. Oxygen consumption, systemic arterio-venous difference in oxygen content, and cardiac index in patients during elective and emergency resection of abdominal aneurysms. The quality and quantity of the blood used was similar to that reported in Figure 2.

FIGURE 4. The in vivo P_{50} value, in vitro P_{50} value, and mixed venous pO_2 tension in patients undergoing elective or emergency surgery for resection of abdominal aneurysms. The quality and quantity of the blood used was similar to that reported in Figure 2.

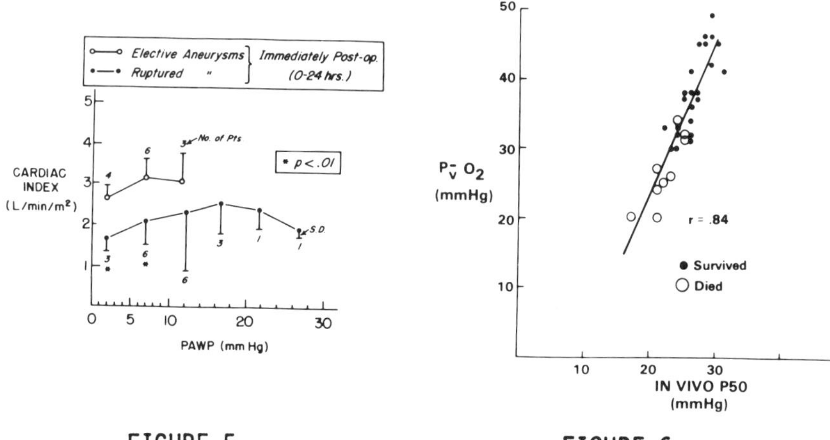

FIGURE 5   FIGURE 6

FIGURE 5. Cardiac output before and after volume loading of
the left ventricle in patients undergoing elective or
emergency surgery for abdominal aneurysm repair. The quality
and quantity of the blood used was similar to that reported
in Figure 2.

FIGURE 6. There was a significant correlation between mixed
venous pO_2 tension and the in vivo P_{50} value during the 24-
hour posttransfusion period. The quality and quantity of the
blood used was similar to that reported in Figure 2. Red
blood cells with increased affinity for oxygen were associated
with decreased mixed venous pO_2 tension. The patients who
died had mixed venous pO_2 tensions of less than 25 mm Hg and
in vivo P_{50} values of less than 25 mm Hg.

INCREASES IN RED BLOOD CELL 2,3 DPG IN VIVO DURING ANEMIC
HYPOXIA (REDUCTION IN NUMBER OF CIRCULATING RED BLOOD CELLS)
AND HYPOXIC HYPOXIA (IMPAIRMENT IN ARTERIAL OXYGENATION OF
THE BLOOD

In patients with anemic hypoxia or hypoxic hypoxia, the
circulating red blood cells develop improved capabilities for
delivering oxygen to tissue at high tissue oxygen tension.
When the reduction in red cell volume-hemoglobin mass is
gradual, patients usually do not exhibit cardiorespiratory
symptoms until the red cell mass is reduced to at least one-

third the normal value. Throughout this period, oxygen
consumption is maintained in a basal condition and blood flow
is not increased. The greater the reduction in red blood
cells, the more efficient the remaining ones become in their
transport of oxygen from the lung to tissue. The circulating
red cells in the body react by increasing the 2,3 DPG levels.
Slightly elevated blood and red blood cell pH, a reduction in
arterial pCO_2, a reduction in the saturation of the venous
blood, and the presence of inorganic phosphorus, all are
involved in increasing the red blood cell 2,3 DPG level in
vivo from 0.8 moles DPG/mole hemoglobin to 1.5 to 2.0 moles
DPG/mole hemoglobin.

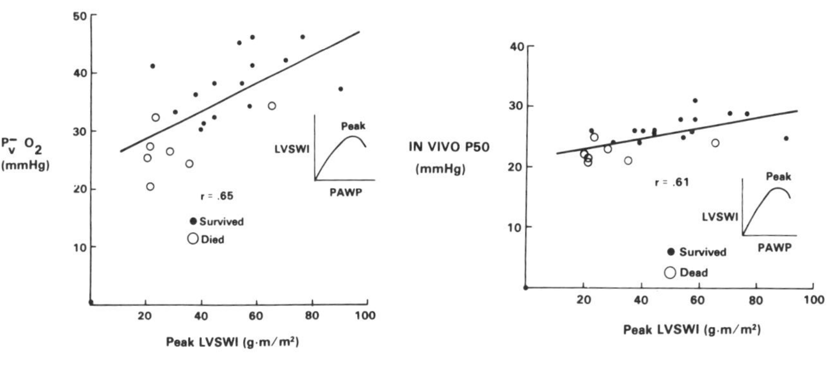

FIGURE 7   FIGURE 8

FIGURE 7. The relation between the mixed venous pO2 tension
and the peak left ventricular stroke work index (LVSWI, g·m/
m²) derived by volume loading during the 24-hour posttransfusion period. The quality and quantity of the blood used
was similar to that reported in Figure 2. Patients who died
had mixed venous pO2 tensions of less than 25 mm Hg and peak
LVSWI of less than 40 g·m/m².

FIGURE 8. During volume loading in the first postoperative
day there was a correlation between the peak left ventricular
stroke work index (g·m/m²) and the in vivo P50 value. The
quality and quantity of the blood used was similar to that
reported in Figure 2.

BIOCHEMICAL MODIFICATION IN VITRO OF HUMAN RED BLOOD CELLS

Solutions containing pyruvate, inosine, glucose, phosphate, and adenine are being used to biochemically modify red blood cells in vitro to increase 2,3 DPG and ATP levels (Table 1). Biochemical modification increases the 2,3 DPG and ATP levels, but it also improves the red blood cell 24-hour posttransfusion survival. When 28-day-old red blood cells were biochemically modified with PIGPA Solution A, the 2,3 DPG and ATP levels after freeze-preservation with 40% W/V glycerol at -80 C for at least 3-1/2 years were similar to pre-freeze values. After washing the red blood cells were stored in sodium chloride-glucose-phosphate solution at 4 C for 3 days, and were perfused through a bubble oxygenator for 3 hours. Posttransfusion survival was acceptable, oxygen transport function was normal or slightly below normal, freeze-thaw-wash in vitro recovery was about 90%, and throughout the process in vitro hemolysis was not excessive.

RESPIRATORY FUNCTION OF PRESERVED RED BLOOD CELLS WITH NORMAL OR DECREASED AFFINITY FOR OXYGEN

During extracorporeal bypass for coronary artery bypass surgery, one group of patients received either fresh blood or packed red blood cells that had been stored in CPD at 4 C for 3 to 5 days and had 70% of normal 2,3 DPG levels and normal affinity for oxygen (control group), and another group received previously frozen red blood cells with 1-1/2 times normal 2,3 DPG levels and decreased affinity for oxygen. The high glycerol method of freeze-preservation was used (40% W/V glycerol at -80 C). During the immediate postoperative period, myocardial function was significantly better in the high 2,3 DPG group than in the control group (Dennis et al, 1975).

Baseline preoperative volume loading with crystalloids was performed, and myocardial performance curves of the heart were obtained. The patients were studied immediately after coming off cardiopulmonary bypass, at which time red blood cells were used to volume load the left ventricle. Twenty-four hours after bypass, albumin was used as the volume load. The response of the heart to volume loading with crystalloid before surgery was similar in the two groups (Figure 9). Cardiac output immediately after bypass was significantly improved in the patients who received high 2,3 DPG red blood cells. At a filling pressure of 10 mm Hg, cardiac output was 2.0 liters/min·m² in the control group, and 3.0 liters/min·m² in the high 2,3 DPG group. The difference in volume loading response of the heart between the two groups could be due to several factors, e.g., differences in red cell 2,3 DPG levels, the fact that citrate was infused with CPD-stored red blood cells but not with previously frozen washed red blood cells, and possibly the presence of other obscure vasoactive agents.

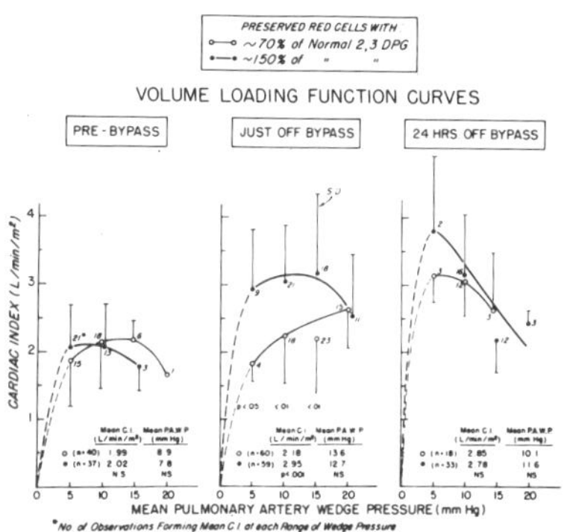

FIGURE 9. Volume loading of the left ventricle was done to increase pulmonary arterial wedge pressure (PAWP) and measure cardiac output response in patients before and immediately after cardiopulmonary bypass, and 24 hours after the surgical procedure. Patients received red blood cells with 70% of normal 2,3 DPG levels and normal affinity for oxygen, or 1-1/2 times normal 2,3 DPG levels and decreased affinity for oxygen. Volume loading curves before bypass with crystalloid, just off bypass with blood, and 24 hours after bypass with colloid were analyzed in a similar manner. Just off bypass, the cardiac indices in the lower three ranges of filling pressure were significantly higher in patients who had received red blood cells with 1-1/2 times normal 2,3 DPG (From Valeri, 1976).

TABLE 1

SOLUTIONS USED TO BIOCHEMICALLY MODIFY RED BLOOD CELLS
AFTER STORAGE IN ACD OR CPD AT 4 C FOR AS LONG
AS 4 WEEKS

PIGPA-SOLUTION A

Pyruvate	50 mmoles/liter
Inosine	50 mmoles/liter
Glucose	100 mmoles/liter
Na_2HPO_4	50 mmoles/liter
Adenine	5 mmoles/liter
NaCl	9 grams/liter
mOsm/kg	650
pH	7.2

PIGPA-SOLUTION B (MODIFIED)

Pyruvate	100 mmoles/liter
Inosine	100 mmoles/liter
Glucose	100 mmoles/liter
Na_2HPO_4	100 mmoles/liter
Adenine	5 mmoles/liter
mOsm/kg	550
pH	7.2

A 50 ml aliquot of the rejuvenation solution was added to a
unit of whole blood or a unit of concentrated red blood cells
and incubated at 37 C for 1 hour prior to glycerolization and
freezing.

In both groups, the donor red blood cells accounted for approximately 40% of the total red blood cells after transfusion. The mean 2,3 DPG level in the high 2,3 DPG group was about 12.5 umoles/g Hb, and in the control group it was 10.0 umoles/g Hb (Figure 10). The red blood cell affinity for oxygen in vivo was 3 mm Hg higher in the high 2,3 DPG group. Cardiac output after bypass was 35% higher in the high 2,3 DPG group at the same filling pressure of the heart. Synthesis of red blood cell 2,3 DPG occurred in both groups during the 24-hour postoperative period. Oxygen delivery to the heart was better in the high 2,3 DPG group.

Does improved oxygen delivery mean anything in terms of morbidity and mortality? In the control group, 5 patients required inotropic agents, and 2 patients required intraaortic balloon assistance. In the high 2,3 DPG group, there was no morbidity, and use of inotropic agents and intraaortic balloon assistance was negligible.

When the red cell 2,3 DPG level was increased 15 to 20%, there was a 3 mm change in the red cell P_{50} value; cardiac output was about 35% greater after transfusion of red blood cells with 1-1/2 times normal 2,3 DPG than after transfusion of red blood cells with 70% of normal 2,3 DPG.

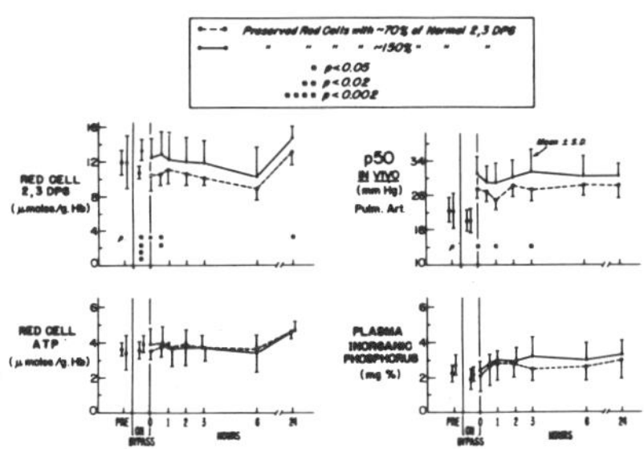

FIGURE 10. In vivo P_{50}, red blood cell 2,3 DPG and ATP levels, and plasma inorganic phosphorus levels for 11 patients who received red blood cells with 150% of normal 2,3 DPG levels during and after cardiopulmonary bypass (solid lines) and for 11 matched patients who received red blood cells with 70% of normal 2,3 DPG levels (dashed lines).

When intermittent perfusion of the coronary circulation
is performed during hypothermia, red blood cells with
increased 2,3 DPG levels help to lessen the increase in red
blood cell affinity associated with this treatment (Vecchione
et al, unpublished data). As oxygen delivery improves, oxygen
tension of the myocardium increases, and the ischemic damage
that occurs with hypothermia and during the surgical procedure
is reduced.

Biochemically modified red blood cells need not
necessarily be frozen, but they must be washed before transfusion. Washing reduces the levels of inosine and adenine
which may produce hyperuricemia and 2,8 dioxyadenine in the
recipients when infused in large quantities.

Questions have been raised regarding the risk of
contamination during biochemical modification of red blood
cells, but sterility has been maintained throughout biochemical modification, freeze-preservation, washing, and post-
wash storage (Ellis et al, unpublished data).

The Naval Blood Research Laboratory, Boston, MA, has
modified the high glycerol freeze-preservation method so that
red blood cells can be kept in the original collection plastic
bag throughout the biochemical modification and freeze-
preservation procedures. This not only simplifies the process
but reduces cost significantly (Figure 11). The polyvinyl
chloride plastic bag used with this modified method cannot be
used with the low glycerol method (20% W/V glycerol at -150 C).

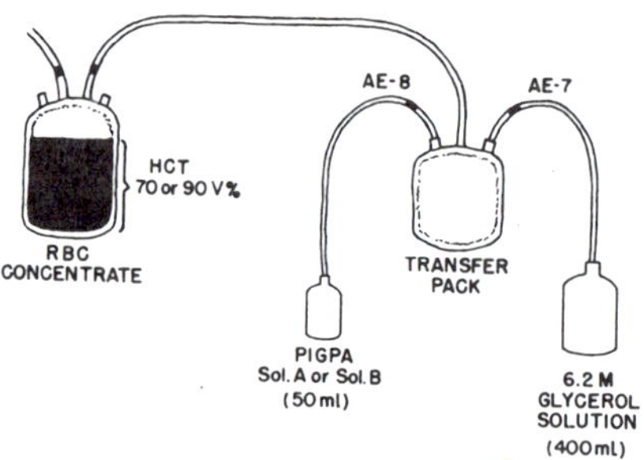

FIGURE 11. Diagram describes biochemical modification of red
blood cell concentrates prior to freeze-preservation with 40%
W/V glycerol at -80 C in the original polyvinyl chloride
plastic collection bag (From Valeri et al, to be published).

The red cells are washed with 1.5 liters of a solution
containing a 50 ml volume of 12% sodium chloride and 1.5
liters of 0.9% sodium chloride-glucose-phosphate solution
(Figure 12).

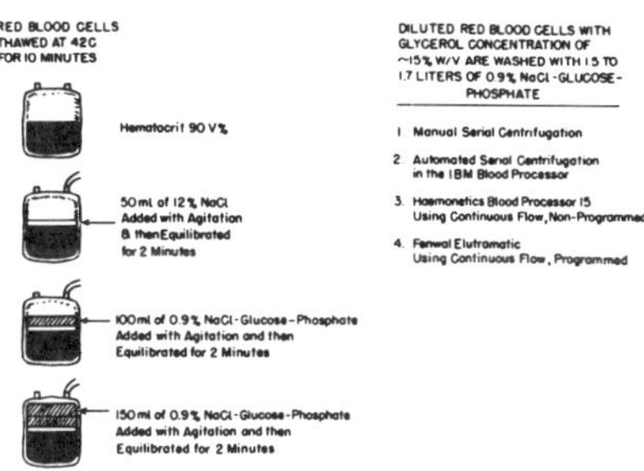

FIGURE 12. Diagram describes thawing and washing of red
blood cell concentrates freeze-preserved with 40% W/V
glycerol at -80 C in the original polyvinyl chloride plastic
collection bag (From Valeri et al, to be published).

The studies reported here show the value of biochemically modifying red blood cells to restore or increase
their 2,3 DPG and ATP levels and thus improve the transport
of oxygen to tissue. Biochemically modified red blood cells
can be freeze-preserved or not as the situation demands.
Obviously, the cost of the blood product is increased when
these procedures are used, but it is a superior product
(Table 2). Moreover, when considered on a wider scope, the
cost per unit would probably be reduced if outdated red
blood cells were restored by biochemical modification and
freeze-preserved for future use. The amount of waste
associated with the present system could be reduced
significantly, the acute blood shortages could be eliminated,
and the patients would be receiving a healthier blood
product.

TABLE 2

JUSTIFICATION OF WASHED FREEZE-PRESERVED RED BLOOD CELLS

1. Rare and selected red cells.

2. Autologous transfusion.

3. Red cells low in white blood cells and platelets for transplant recipients.

4. Reduction in HB_sAg antigen and other viral agents.

5. Salvaging universal donor red blood cells (rejuvenation of outdated red blood cells) for freeze-preservation.

6. Red blood cells with 1-1/2 to 3 times normal 2,3 DPG levels and with decreased affinity for oxygen (rejuvenation of indated and outdated red blood cells) for freeze-preservation.

7. Reduction in plasma protein (IGG, IGA, and IGM).

8. Removal of vasoactive substances (angiotensin, serotonin, and bradykinin).

SUMMARY

Preserved red cells are transfused to increase red cell volume and to improve the delivery of oxygen to tissue, and in order to do this the red cells must circulate properly. We know that the oxygen transport function of preserved red cells is important, but just how important is not really clear. Red cells stored at 4 C for 3 weeks have similar 24-hour post-transfusion survival values whether acid-citrate-dextrose (ACD) or citrate-phosphate-dextrose (CPD) is used as the preservative. In ACD-preserved red cells, the oxygen transport function deteriorates during the first week of storage at 4 C, whereas deterioration occurs within 2 weeks of storage in CPD-stored red cells. Thus, while red blood cells can be stored for 3 weeks at 4 C and still have satisfactory posttransfusion survival, the oxygen transport function, and thus the ability to deliver oxygen to tissue at normal tissue oxygen tension, is impaired. When oxygen delivery is impaired, a reduction in tissue oxygen tension is necessary for the release of oxygen to tissue.

The defect in oxygen delivery occurs as a result of a loss of red cell 2,3 diphosphoglycerate (2,3 DPG). A defect in the respiratory function of liquid-stored red cells was reported by Valtis and Kennedy in 1954. The reduced 2,3 DPG level of donor red cells is usually resynthesized within 24 to 48 hours after transfusion: in slightly alkalotic, hypocarbic patients with normal blood inorganic phosphorus levels, about 30% are resynthesized within 4 to 8 hours after transfusion, and about 50% are resynthesized in about 24 hours. The rate of resynthesis is retarded in patients with acidosis, hypercarbia, and decreased blood inorganic phosphorus levels, and the patient must compensate by increasing cardiac output or decreasing tissue oxygen tension, or a combination of these two. When red cells with reduced oxygen delivery are transfused to anemic patients with coronary artery disease or cerebrovascular disease, the heart and brain are placed in jeopardy during the acute posttransfusion period.

Liquid-stored red cells can be biochemically modified with a solution of pyruvate, inosine, glucose, phosphate, and adenine to restore or increase the 2,3 DPG levels. Red cells with high 2,3 DPG levels have decreased oxygen affinity. Biochemically modified red blood cells have been freeze-preserved and have been found to have acceptable posttransfusion survival and improved oxygen releasing capacity.

Preserved red cells with increased affinity for oxygen may be harmful in certain patients in whom the accompanying demand for increased blood flow cannot be met, and the venous-capillary oxygen tension may fall to critical levels. Red cells with 1-1/2 to 2 times normal 2,3 DPG levels should be used for patients in hemorrhagic or septic shock, those subjected to extracorporeal circulation during cardiac surgery, and anemic patients with myocardial or cerebrovascular insufficiency.

ACKNOWLEDGMENT

This work was supported by the U. S. Navy (Naval Medical Research and Development Command Research Task Nos. MOO95-PN.001-0011 and MOO95-PN.001-0012), the U. S. Army (Army Medical Research and Development Command Contract No. DA17-76-C-6034), and the National Institutes of General Medical Sciences (Grant No. GM24891-01).

The opinions or assertions contained herein are those of the authors, and are not to be construed as official or reflecting the views of the Navy and Army Departments or the Naval and Army Services at large.

The authors acknowledge the excellent assistance of Marilyn E. Sullivan in the preparation of this manuscript.

REFERENCES

Benesch R, Benesch RE (1967). The effect of organic phosphates from the human erythrocyte on the allosteric properties of hemoglobin. Biochem Biophys Res Commun 26:162.

Beutler E, Wood L (1969). The in vivo regeneration of red cell-diphosphoglyceric acid (DPG) after transfusion of stored blood. J Lab Clin Med 74:300.

Chance B, Thurman R, Gosalvez M (1969). Oxygen affinities of cellular respiration. Forsvarsmedicin 5:235.

Chanutin A, Curnish RR (1967). Effect of organic and inorganic phosphates on the oxygen equilibrium of human erythrocytes. Arch Biochem Biophys 121:96.

Collins JA (1974). Problems associated with the massive transfusion of stored blood. Surgery 75:274.

Collins JA (1976). Massive blood transfusion. Clinics in Haematology 5:201.

Dennis RC, Vito L, Weisel RD, Valeri CR, Berger RL, and Hechtman HB (1975). Improved myocardial performance following high 2,3 diphosphoglycerate red cell transfusion. Surgery 77:741.

Hechtman HB (1976). Adequate circulatory response or cardiovascular failure. Surg Clin N Amer 56:929.

Valeri CR (1974). Metabolic regeneration of depleted erythrocytes and their frozen storage. In Greenwalt TJ, Jamieson GA (eds): "The Human Red Cell In Vitro," New York and London: Grune & Stratton, p 281.

Valeri CR (1976). "Blood Banking and the Use of Frozen Blood Products." Cleveland: Chemical Rubber Company Press, Inc.

Valeri CR, Hirsch NM (1969). Restoration in vivo of erythrocyte adenosine triphosphate, 2,3 diphosphoglycerate, potassium ion, and sodium ion concentrations following the transfusion of acid-citrate-dextrose-stored human red blood cells. J Lab Clin Med 73:722.

Valtis DJ, Kennedy AC (1954). Defective gas transport function of stored red blood cells. Lancet 1:119.

DISCUSSION

<u>Dr. Mansouri</u>: My comment pertains to the first part of your
study. I agree that DPG is very important, but I cannot
help saying that in the first part of your study you compared groups of patients that were not comparable. Obviously, the patient who has ruptured his aortic abdominal aneurysm
is much sicker than the patient who had elective surgery for
repair of an aortic abdominal aneurysm; patients with ruptured aortic abdominal aneurysms needed more blood, were
sicker, and most of them died. Your study was not randomized.

<u>Dr. Valeri</u>: I agree with your concern that this study was
not randomized. We are now performing a randomized study
on patients undergoing emergency surgery for ruptured aortic
abdominal aneurysms. In the current study patients with
ruptured aortic abdominal aneurysms receive either red cell
concentrates with low 2,3 DPG levels and increased affinity
for oxygen or previously frozen washed red blood cells with
1-1/2 times normal 2,3 DPG levels and decreased affinity
for oxygen. The liquid-stored red blood cell concentrates
are prepared by centrifugation of blood after storage at
4°C in CPD for 2 weeks. All the visible plasma is removed
and the red blood cells are diluted with 35 ml of 0.9% NaCl
to adjust the hematocrit to about 75 V%. The previously
frozen washed red blood cells with 1-1/2 times normal 2,3
DPG levels are concentrated to hematocrits of 75 V%. This
study will compare nonwashed red blood cells with low 2,3
DPG levels and increased affinity for oxygen and washed red
blood cells with 1-1/2 times normal 2,3 DPG levels and
decreased affinity for oxygen. Red blood cells with elevated
2,3 DPG levels have normal or improved capacity to release
oxygen and they should maintain or increase the mixed venous
pO_2 tension. The maintenance of mixed venous pO_2 tension
should improve myocardial performance, and may reduce the
mortality associated with ruptured abdominal aneurysm surgery.

<u>Dr. Chilcote</u>: I had a question about the relevance of the
mixed venous oxygen tension. If you're trying, as I understand it, to measure the extracted oxygen, could you comment
on whether the oxygen saturation of the mixed venous blood
is more discriminating index rather than the mixed venous
pO_2?

<u>Dr. Valeri</u>: Our data suggest that per cent saturation of the

The Red Cell, pages 615—616

mixed venous blood is not as critical as the mixed venous
pO_2 tension, and that when the per cent saturation is reduced,
the mixed venous pO_2 tension may be increased, normal, or
decreased, depending on the red cell affinity for oxygen.
A reduction in mixed venous pO_2 tension was associated with
a reduction in the oxygen saturation of the blood and a
reduction in myocardial function in patients undergoing surgery for ruptured aortic abdominal aneurysms.

Dr. Chilcote: Right, When you are on the steep part of the
oxyhemoglobin dissociation curve, there are so many variables
involved in what saturation you might have given the mixed
venous pO_2 tension. You could probably get a better measure
of the oxygen extracted by looking at the per cent saturation.

Dr. Valeri: The relation between mixed venous pO_2 tension
and the in vivo P_{50} demonstrated that the low mixed venous
oxygen tension occurred when red blood cell affinity for
oxygen was increased in patients who are unable to increase
their cardiac output. Mixed venous pO_2 tension and red cell
affinity for oxygen appeared to influence myocardial performance. Transfusions of large volumes of stored blood appear
to reduce both the in vivo P_{50} value and the mixed venous oxygen tension. When patients undergoing abdominal aortic aneurysm surgery were given red blood cells with increased affinity for oxygen they did not compensate by increasing cardiac output because myocardial performance was impaired.

Dr. Rosa: Yes, just a short comment. I don't think that
2,3 DPG is as important as you believe, and my proof is
that we have must described a patient, I don't say a patient
but a propositus who has zero 2,3 DPG in his red cells, and
he has a very good health.

Dr. Valeri: I cannot see a relation between your observations
and those from our laboratory. Apparently, a mechanism
independent of 2,3 DPG allowed your patient to supply his
oxygen requirements.

Dr. Rosa: So, I would say that preserved red cells with low
2,3 DPG may not be detrimental to patients because absence
per se of 2,3 DPG is not so bad.

Dr. Valeri: Your observation may be valid. However, the 2,3
DPG in normal red blood cells does influence oxygen transport
function. Thus, in the preservation of normal red blood cells,
the 2,3 DPG level is important to ensure satisfactory function.

THE AGE AND HEMATOCRIT OF STORED BLOOD IN DETERMINING THE
SURVIVAL OF RATS AFTER EXCHANGE TRANSFUSION AND HEMORRHAGE*

John A. Collins, M.D.

Stanford University Medical School

Department of Surgery, Stanford University
Medical Center, Stanford, California 94305

Red blood cells stored in the liquid state in citrate
undergo a diminution in the content of 2,3-DPG and an increase in the affinity of hemoglobin for oxygen.[2] This
decreases the efficiency of hemoglobin as an oxygen-delivering
agent at physiological gas tensions.[11] At least several hours
are required for the restoration of 2,3-DPG levels toward
normal after the cells are transfused. The massively transfused patient will undergo nearly complete replacement of red
cell mass with stored red cells before significant restoration can occur. This replacement occurs at a time of life-
threatening impairment of the oxygen-delivering system. Thus,
there has been serious concern about the efficacy of stored
blood as treatment for exsanguinating hemorrhage.

While red cells depleted of 2,3-DPG are theoretically
significantly less effective in delivering oxygen in vivo,
clinically or physiologically significant impairment has
been difficult to demonstrate in patients or animals.

<u>Materials and Methods</u>. White male Wistar rats obtained
from the same supplier, about 350 grams, were allowed to
spend at least two weeks in a room at 22-24° C and 40-60%
relative humidity, with free access to Purina rat chow and
tap water. On the day of study, they were lightly anesthe-
tized with intraperitoneal pentobarbital, and a femoral artery
and vein were cannulated with fine plastic catheters. Hep-
arin, 2000 units per kilogram body weight, was given intravenously. Exchange transfusion was carried out in increments

*This work has been submitted for publication elsewhere.[5]

The Red Cell, pages 617—624
© 1978 Alan R. Liss, Inc., New York, New York

of 1.2 mls per 100 grams body weight, approximately 20% of
the estimated blood volume. The subject's blood was withdrawn from the arterial catheter, and an equal amount of
citrated blood + 15% (1.38 mls per 100 grams body weight)
was infused intravenously over a ten minute period. The
extra 15% was intended to make up for the dilution of the
donor blood with citrate anticoagulant. This exchange was
repeated nine times, so that about two blood volumes were
exchanged, which should have left less than 10% of the original red cells in the subject animal. After a 30 minute
rest, the animals were challenged with a modification of a
previously devised model for hemorrhagic shock:[3] 2.25 mls
per 100 grams body weight were removed from the arterial
line. After 20 minutes, an additional 0.9 mls per 100 grams
body weight were removed. Ten minutes after completing the
last hemorrhage, the animal was treated with the test blood
in a volume 1.15 times the volume of shed blood. The wounds
were closed and the animals returned to their cages and
allowed free access to food and water. Wounds were clean
but not sterile. All animals which died, died within 24
hours except for one that died at three days after treatment.
Three rats at autopsy showed significant hemorrhages into the
wounds or into the peritoneal cavity and were discarded from
the series.

The blood used for exchange transfusion and for treatment was obtained from similar rats handled in a similar
manner. The blood was allowed to flow freely from the femoral artery into a plastic syringe containing a pre-set amount
of anticoagulant, ACD, NIH solution A (Fenwal). Terminal
blood was not collected. Additional ACD was added to bring
the final collection to the usual proportions used in clinical blood banking (450:67.5). Any excess air was expelled,
and the syringe was either capped with a sterile needle and
needle carrier, or was transferred via a sterile 3-way stop-
cock to a larger syringe and pooled with the blood from
several donors. The blood was stored at 4° C and was mixed
and warmed in a 38° C water bath before transfusion. No
testing for compatibility was attempted. Hematocrit was
varied by allowing similarly collected red cells to settle,
then injecting off plasma and using it for dilution.

For measurement of oxygen-hemoglobin dissociation curves
and 2,3-diphosphoglycine acid (2,3-DPG) in red cells, animals
were prepared and exchange-transfused as above, then exsanguinated through the arterial catheter at the time when

hemorrhage would have started. One rat supplied blood for a single oxyhemoglobin dissociation curve (OCD) and duplicate measurements of 2,3-DPG. The ODC was measured by tonometry in sequence in an Instrumentation Laboratories (IL) tonometer with six different gases of known composition. Oxygen saturation was measured on an IL Cooximeter and pH on an IL Model 213 Blood Gas Analyzer. PO_2 was periodically checked on the blood samples. The best fit on the six point curve was used to estimate P_{50}. 2,3-DPG was measured on a well mixed aliquot of the same sample taken just before determination of the ODC, using the enzymatic method in kit form (Sigma Chem. Corp.). Both ODC and 2,3-DPG were measured promptly after the samples were obtained from the subject rats.

Results. Rats exchange-transfused with fresh blood had 2,3-DPG of 15.3μ Moles/Gram Hgb and P_{50} of 34.5 mm Hg (N=10). Rats exchange-transfused with old blood had 2,3-DPG of 2.5μ Moles/Gram Hgb and P_{50} of 23.5 mm Hg (N=10).

The first set of experiments involved exchange transfusion and treatment after hemorrhage with the same category of blood. Blood was either fresh (same day) or old (14-21 days in storage), each at three different hematocrits, 35%, 25%, and 18%. Six groups were thus exchange-transfused and treated. The results are given in Table 1. Body weights and hematocrits were not different between survivors and non-survivors within groups, or between fresh and old blood groups at respective ranges of hematocrit. Since the same kind of blood was used for both exchange and treatment, death during hemorrhage can be included in the total mortality when comparing groups, although the results are given as death before treatment and death after treatment. There were only two deaths during exchange transfusion and these rats were excluded from the series.

Two facts are notable. There was no change in mortality as hematocrit was decreased when fresh blood was used, but there was a doubling in mortality when hematocrit was decreased to 25% when old blood was used. By chi square analysis, the mortality between fresh and old blood is statistically significant (P=.05) at hematocrits of 25%, but at neither of the higher hematocrits. The other noteworthy result is that old blood at normal hematocrits gave the same results as fresh blood at all hematocrits (surviving ratio .57 versus .59, .65, and .63).

In order to heighten the differences due to age and hematocrit of the blood used for treatment, a second set of experiments was carried out in which all the animals were exchange-transfused with old blood at low hematocrits and then hemorrhaged, thus creating the most disadvantageous circumstances for survival. Treatment after hemorrhage consisted of fresh or old blood, each at high (55%) or low (20%) hematocrits. The results (Table 2) should now be considered only for death after treatment when comparing the efficacy of hematocrit versus age of blood, as all groups had the same kind of blood used for exchange.

As in the first group of experiments, there is little difference for fresh blood between a high and low hematocrit, whereas with old blood, reducing the hematocrit to half normal nearly doubles the mortality (.28 versus .50). Also again, there is little difference between old blood at high hematocrits and fresh blood at high or low hematocrit, although in this experiment there is a suggestion of greater efficacy when both hematocrit and age of storage are optimal. Even this is somewhat qualified, however, by the fact that there was no difference between fresh and old blood at high hematocrits except for one sub-group of animals, the only ones studied during summer time. In this sub-group, there was a very high mortality both before and after treatment in the group with old blood at high hematocrit. These results were very atypical, but are included.

Discussion.

The physiologic effects of a marked shift in the affinity of hemoglobin for oxygen have been debated. Theoretically, there should be a significant effect,[11] but such has been difficult to demonstrate clinically or experimentally. For one of the most worrisome situations, that of massive transfusion with stored blood, little data are available.

Animals with red cells depleted of 2,3-DPG have lower mixed venous oxygen tensions and occasionally higher cardiac outputs.[10] Oski et al[8] demonstrated a striking difference in the hemodynamic response to exercise in anemic patients with widely differing P_{50}, favoring the patient with the right-shifted ODC. Huggins et al[7] reported increased survival of rats with red cells normal in 2,3-DPG compared to those depleted of 2,3-DPG when exchange-transfused to severe anemia with dextran. Dennis et al[6] reported improved sur-

Table 1

Hematocrit after Exchange	Old Blood			Fresh Blood		
	Alive	Died after Treatment	Died before Treatment	Alive	Died after Treatment	Died before Treatment
38%	8	2	4	10	1	6
31%	9	4	6	11	3	3
25%	5	5	11	10	1	5

Table 2

Hematocrit after Treatment	Old Blood			Fresh Blood		
	Alive	Died after Treatment	Died before Treatment	Alive	Died after Treatment	Died before Treatment
50%	18	7	20	19	2	14
26%	12	12	13	15	5	12

vival and fewer complications after cardiopulmonary bypass
in the patients given red cells augmented in 2,3-DPG compared to those given cells with normal levels, but there
were several uncontrolled variables, and the differences
were so great as to be difficult to attribute to the small
difference in P_{50}.

There have been a number of studies seeming to indicate
little physiologic effect from depletion of 2,3-DPB. Wranne
and associates found little impairment of aerobic work capacity in rats[12] or in man[13] following exchange transfusion
with depleted red cells. Rand and Norton[9] found no effect
on the ability of rabbits to withstand hypoxia. Arturson
and Westman[1] exchange-transfused rats with red cells high or
low in 2,3-DPG and hemodiluted them to lethally anemic levels.
There was no difference in survival between the groups.

It is noteworthy that most of the studies cited that
demonstrated a favorable effect of a higher 2,3-DPG were
carried out in anemic subjects,[6,7,8] while most of those
(but not all[1]) showing no benefit were performed at normal
hematocrits.[9,12,13]

The current studies contrasted hematocrit with 2,3-DPG
as variables determining the survival of rats after hemorrhage. An interesting pattern is evident. At normal hematocrits there was little effect of depletion of 2,3-DPG. With
hemodilution to half-normal hematocrits, however, there was
significantly poorer survival after hemorrhage in the animals
given red cells depleted of 2,3-DPG. Looked at from the age
of the blood, dilution to half-normal hematocrits produces
no impairment of survival after hemorrhage when fresh blood
was used, but caused a higher mortality when old, 2,3-DPG-
depleted blood was used. These observations were confirmed
by testing hematocrit and age of storage for the ability to
rescue rats from the lethal combination of anemia, red cells
poor in 2,3-DPG, and severe hemorrhage. Both sets of conclusions are consistent with an interpretation that oxygen
delivery is not the survival-limiting factor after treatment
for hemorrhage in this model unless either the mass or the
functional quality of hemoglobin are reduced by half. This
is not surprising in view of the repeatedly demonstrated
efficacy of non-red cell replacement regimens for hemorrhages
up to one-half the blood volume, and of the remarkable efficacy of blood stored in ACD as treatment for exsanguinating
injuries in Vietnam, with rapid restoration of aerobic metabolism.[4]

The potentially clinically important implications of these studies are that even extensive exchange-transfusion with stored red cells depleted of 2,3-DPG is acceptable treatment for hemorrhage if anemia is avoided. Conversely, the combination of anemia and depletion of 2,3-DPG should be avoided, especially if subsequent hemorrhage is likely. It must be emphasized that these were healthy subjects and that such conditions as coronary arteriosclerosis might well change the results.

(Supported by Contract DADA 17-68-C-8006, US Army Medical Research and Development Command)

<u>REFERENCES</u>

1. Arturson G, Westman M (1975). Survival of rats subjected to acute anemia at different levels of erythrocyte 2,3-diphosphoglycerate. Scand J Clin Lab Invest 35: 745.

2. Bunn HF, May MH, Kocholaty WF, Shields CE (1969). Hemoglobin function of stored blood. J Clin Inv 48:311.

3. Collins JA, Braitberg A, Butcher HR (1973). Changes in lung and body weight and lung water content in rats treated for hemorrhage with various fluids. Surg 73: 401.

4. Collins JA, Simmons RL, James PM, Bredenberg CE, Anderson RW, Heisterkamp CA (1971). Acid-base status of seriously wounded combat casualties. II Resuscitation with stored blood. Ann Surg 173:6.

5. Collins JA, Stechenberg L (Submitted for publication). The effects of the concentration and function of hemoglobin on the survival of rats after hemorrhage.

6. Dennis RC, Vito L, Weisel RD, Valeri CR, Berger RL, Hechtman HL (1975). Improved myocardial performance following high 2,3-DPG red cell transfusion. Surg 77:741.

7. Huggins CE, Suzuki H, Grove-Rasmussen M (1971). "Life Support by Liquid and Frozen Blood." Presented at the 24th Annual Meeting, Am Assoc Blood Banks, Chicago.

8. Oski FA, Marshall BE, Cohen PJ, Sugerman HJ, Miller LJ (1971). Exercise with anemia: the role of the left-shifted or right-shifted oxygen-hemoglobin equilibrium curve. Ann Int Med 74:44.

9. Rand PW, Norton JM, Barker ND, Lovell MD, Austin WH (1973). Responses to graded hypoxia at high and low 2,3-diphosphoglycerate concentrations. J Appl Physiol 34:827.

10. Riggs TH, Shafer AW, Guenter CA (1973). Acute changes
    in oxyhemoglobin affinity. Effects on oxygen trans-
    port and utilization. J Clin Invest 52:2660.
11. Valeri CR (1971). Viability and function of preserved
    red cells. New Engl J Med 284:81.
12. Woodson RD, Wranne B, Detter JC (1973). Effect of in-
    creased blood oxygen affinity on work performance of
    rats. J Clin Inv 52:2717.
13. Wranne B, Nordgren L, Woodson RD (1974). Increased
    blood oxygen affinity and physical work capacity in
    man. Scand J Clin Lab Invest 33:347.

DISCUSSION

[Question not recorded.]

<u>Dr. Collins</u>: I strongly suspect, on the basis of work of
other people, that optimal survival occurs at near normal
hematocrits. I suspect though that hemorrheology is vastly
more complicated than we've given it credit for. For example, the Fahraeus-Lindqvist effect, showing that the change
in viscosity due to hematocrit is much less when you study
it in a series of branching tubes of decreasing diameter. This
is really the geometry we have in the circulation and indicates that the specifics under which rheology is studied are
very important. The philosophy that I usually apply is that
Mother Nature may be a bitch, but she's not a fool. Some of
the studies indicating that the optimal hematocrit for survival is about half-normal, I suspect, are a little bit over-
drawn on the basis of in vitro studies of hemorrheology. to
get more specifically to your question, there was an element
of control in here, in that the old and fresh blood animals
have the same hematocrits, but it's not complete control.

<u>Dr. Duhm</u>: I would just add one paper more which you may have
missed, the authors being Eaton, Skelton, and Berger which
demonstrated that the rats subjected to severe hypoxia survived better when they had a left-shifted curve.

One point I missed, you certainly know, is that the
situation may be different when you have people with lung
disease and restricted oxygen diffusion or patients with a
right-left shunt. Then, a left-hand shift of the curve might
be advantageous due to the increased arterial oxygenation
and arterial pO_2, especially where only unloading in the
peripheral circulation is to be considered.

<u>Dr. Collins</u>: Yes, that's quite right, in fact it's been
shown both theoretically and in certain models (the one you
referred to is by Bakker) that with severe ventilatory hypoxia, there may be an advantage to a left shift. I think
nature herself showed that because yaks and llamas, in fact,
most high altitude species have left-shifted curves, presumably because they survived better at altitude with the left-
shifted curves. To extrapolate that to patients with pulmonary disease, though, I think is very tricky. Patients with
ventilatory disease rarely have inspiratory hypoxia; it's
not the same as high altitude. What's happening is that a
fraction of the blood is going through the lungs normally
ventilated, equilibrated with a normal oxygen tension, and a

The Red Cell, pages 625—626

fraction of the blood is never seeing the alveolar gas so it
is in essence shunted. The resulting arterial hypoxia results
from a mixing of blood that hasn't been ventilated at all
with blood that's been normally ventilated. As long as part
of that blood is seeing normal alveolar gas, then the advantage of the right-shifted curve should still persist because it's being loaded with oxygen at a tension that's up
in a range that should produce the beneficial effect. I
think high altitude is a different situation. So, I think
if you're bleeding during your mountain climbing expedition
to Everest, you may be better off with left-shifted hemoglobin.

BLOOD PRESERVATIVES AND HEMOGLOBIN OXYGEN AFFINITY XXX:
2,3-DPG AND ITS MAINTENANCE BY ASCORBATE

R. B. Dawson, M. Dabezies, R. T. Hershey, C. S.
Myers, S. Holmes, L. D. Sisk and R. M. Miller
Blood Research Lab, Dept. of Pathology, Univ. of
Md., School of Medicine
22 S. Greene Street, Baltimore, Maryland 21201

We are all aware that Greenwalt (1925) described the
presence of 2,3-DPG (2,3-diphosphoglycerate) in mammalian
red cells and that Rapoport and Luebering (1950) described
the enzymic activities responsible for maintaining the high
concentrations in the rabbit red cells. Some of us may
have forgotten that Grant Bartlett (1960) first reported
decreases in 2,3-DPG as well as ATP (adenosine triphosphate)
with increasing inorganic phosphate during human blood storage at 4°. Two years before that, Berry and Chanutin (1958)
had reported disappearance of their Tiselius electrophoretic "component B" under similar conditions of blood storage.

Then Sugita and Chanutin (1963) reported an increase
in the electrophoretic hemoglobin "component B" with 2,3-
DPG and ATP added to hemolysates. They also observed increases in "component B" with adenosine diphosphate and
3-phosphoglycerate added to red cells. Thus, 2,3-DPG maintenance was being achieved 15 years ago. However, the possible clinical importance of these findings to transfusion
therapy wasn't obvious until Chanutin (1966), Chanutin and
Curnish (1967) and Benesch and Benesch (1967) reported the
reciprocal effect of 2,3-DPG on human hemoglobin oxygen
affinity. Akerbloom (1968) correctly concluded that changes
in the oxygen dissociation curve of red cells in stored
blood are due to depletion of 2,3-DPG. He also showed that

The Red Cell, pages 627—648

this change could be reversed by incubating the red cells
with inosine. Bunn confirmed both of these observations
(1969) and in the same year, (at Bunn's suggestion) Dawson
(1969) compared the blood preservatives ACD and CPD, showing that the new preservative, CPD (citrate-phosphate-
dextrose) maintained p50 and DPG levels better than the
older, standard ACD (acid-citrate-dextrose) solution.

The development of these blood preservatives is of
some interest as it represents the parallel development of
another aspect of this field during the same period of time
that hemoglobin function was being explored. Rous and Turner added dextrose to citrate anticoagulants in 1916 to
retard the progression of hemolysis. In 1943, Loutit, Mollison, and Young, using a low pH (the acid effect) showed
that blood collected into an acid-citrate-dextrose solution
should survive storage for 3 weeks. However, it remained
for Ross and Finch (1947) to demonstrate the beneficial
effects of a cold storage temperature. It is important to
note that this 1947 issue of the Jour. of Clin. Invest.has
15 articles on blood preservation and that year corresponds
in time with the establishment of blood banks in many hos-
pitals in the U.S. In 1948 the American Association of
Blood Banks was founded, providing a professional and scientific forum for workers in the field.

The other important piece of this puzzle is Valtis and
Kennedy's description (1953, 1954) of increased oxygen
affinity in vitro during blood storage and in patients
transfused with stored blood. Their ability to correct
what they referred to as a "gas transport defect" with
chloride salts demonstrated an ionic or charge-mediated
effect which we were later to see demonstrated as an allosteric mechanism for 2,3-DPG. At the First International
Conference on Red Cell Metabolism and Function, I reviewed
how Taylor and Hastings (1942) and Rossi-Fanelli (1961)
showed similar salt or chloride effects on hemoglobin solutions and reported increases of p50 with urea and the acetate salts of sodium and potassium (Dawson 1970).

Salt effects became of interest again when it was found
that several hours were required for regeneration of 2,3-
DPG by the recipient after transfusion (Beutler and Wood,
Valeri and Hirsch 1969). Dawson (1970a) confirmed Valtis
and Kennedy's observation that salt treated red cells would
immediately have their oxygen transport function restored.

This, of course, was Valtis and Kennedy's suggestion of the usefulness of the salts. It still seems to be an impractical approach since salts would readily diffuse out of the red cell upon transfusion. However, the paper by Shappell (1970) seemed to document a new rapid type of adaptation to hypoxia which was observed during angina pectoris. The observations of Shappell suggested a possible role for the "salt effect" (Dawson, 1970b) which needs to be explored.

In salt experiments it is important that the pH is controlled. Adolph and Ferry in 1921 reviewed the work of Barcroft and Roberts (1909) on salt effects and made their own observations on alkaline effects and electrolytes. They may be credited with dialyzing hemoglobin, decreasing oxygen affinity with neutral salts, and showing that the hemoglobin oxygen equilibrium is a function of the relation between hemoglobin and electrolytes. It is of note that this work was done before the concept of pH had been established.

With NaCl a salt effect is difficult to demonstrate with a near normal concentration of 2,3-DPG, using either red cells (Dawson 1972), or dilute hemoglobin solutions (Benesch, et al 1969).

Effects of sulfhydryl groups on affinity of hemoglobin for oxygen have been studied by a number of laboratories, but the work of Horejski (1970) reviewed at the First International Symposium suggested that SH effects of glutathione and related substances were independent of pH. In this author's laboratory, the glutathione effect was demonstrated to be dependent on the pH changes produced by glutathione addition (Dawson, 1972a).

Maintenance of red cell ATP by adenine and 2,3-DPG by inosine during storage at 4° C has been reviewed by this author (Dawson, 1972b). The metabolic mechanisms were discussed and presented in diagramatic form in the proceedings of the Second International Conference on Red Cell Metabolism and Function. The decision to license a CPD-adenine preservative for five week 4° storage of whole blood and packed cells was made at a combined NIH-FDA meeting in Oct. 1976. The summary of this meeting (Simon, 1976) and the in vivo survival study which supported it (Zuck, et al 1977) will be useful references for students of this subject.

Inosine was used for a few years in two blood centers in Germany as an ACD-inosine-adenine-guanosine preservative until it was realized that an accumulation of uric acid, a metabolite of inosine could be toxic (Seidl, 1976). Although inosine may be useful in rejuvenation systems or other special storage systems in which the supernatant is removed after incubation, in ordinary blood storage situations other sources of 5 carbon sugars are now being investigated. Preliminary studies with ribose and xylose have been carried out (Dawson, et al 1977).

Besides 5 carbon sugars, six carbon sugars such as fructose and mannose are being reevaluated as an alternative to glucose. Dihydroxyacetone (DHA) may help to raise levels of 2,3-DPG. The red cell can use it as a 3 carbon sugar (Fig. 1). A triokinase has been characterized as assisting the red cell in DHA metabolism (Beutler and Guinto, 1973). I have pictured glycerol metabolism here to show that DHA is a natural biologic compound.

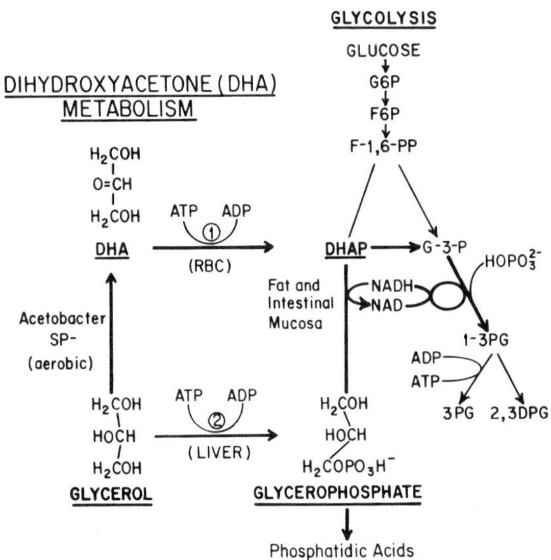

Fig. 1 Dihydroxyacetone (DHA) metabolism.

Pyruvate is useful as a metabolic regulator (McManus, et al 1957). When added to the red cell, (Fig. 2), it oxidizes NADH to NAD. This mechanism is analogous to the effect of a methylene blue (MB) prototype red-ox compound which mainly oxidizes NADPH to NADP. NAD is needed as shown in the glyceraldehyde 3-phosphate dehydrogenase reaction which becomes inhibited during storage, partially blocking glycolysis just above the Rapoport-Luebering (2,3-DPG) shunt. Pyruvate provides NAD to overcome this inhibition, resulting in increased 2,3-DPG. It is of interest and some importance that the oxidation/reduction electrode voltage potential for pyruvate/lactate (-0.19) is less than MB (0.01), which is less than ascorbate (0.18).

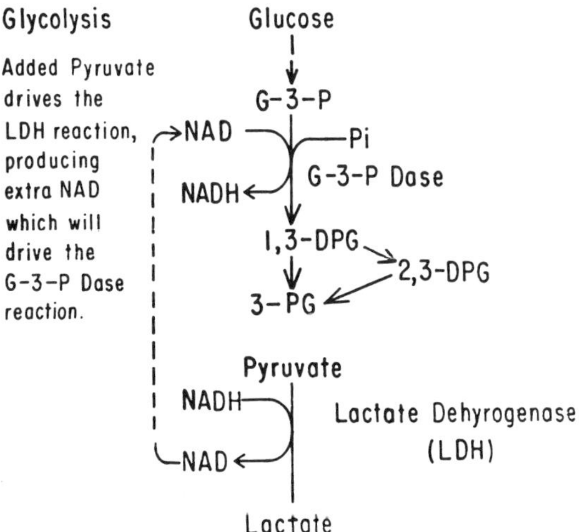

Fig. 2 Pyruvate effect on red cell 2,3-DPG.

Ascorbic acid is probably a metabolic regulator because of its favorable red-ox potential, but there is some evidence for its being metabolized (Dawson, 1977a)(Fig. 3). Thus, Vitamin C (VC) may help the red cell maintain 2,3-DPG during storage by several possible mechanisms. The suggestion of a nutritional metabolic mechanism will be discussed here for the first time. Concerning regulatory metabolic mechanisms, Jacob and Jandl (1966) showed increased hexose monophosphate shunt activity with ascorbate which implies oxidation of NADPH to NADP. Oxidation of NADH to NAD by ascorbate, favoring formation of 1,3-diphosphoglycerate was suggested by data of Wood & Beutler (1973). We have reported that the red cell does not distinguish between the natural L-form and the unnatural D-isomer in maintaining 2,3-DPG (Dabezies and Dawson 1975). Other studies have been carried out with glutathione (GSH), N-ethylmaleimide (NEM) and iodoacetate (IA) to further characterize the mechanisms and are reported here.

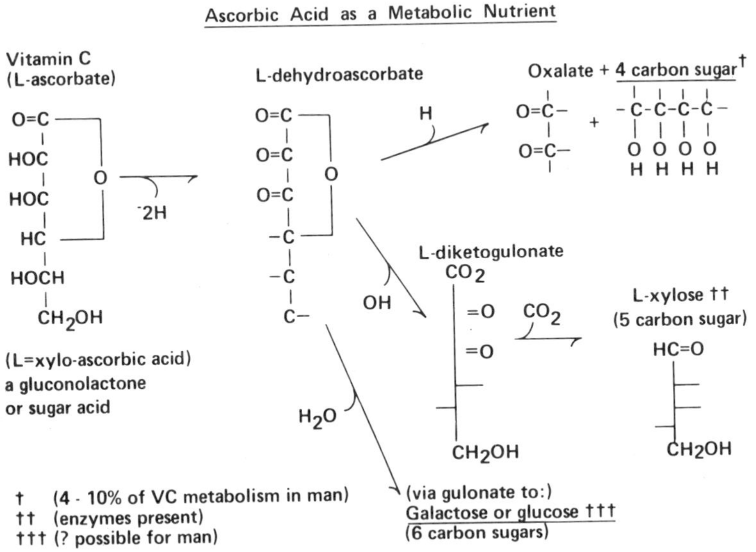

Fig. 3 Possible pathways for ascorbic acid metabolism in the red cell.

MATERIALS AND METHODS

Units of blood from healthy donors were split during donation so that for each donor 100 mls were collected into each of six transfer packs containing 14 ml of CPD-adenine (0.25 mM) and other chemicals as indicated. Except for the volume of blood drawn, recognized standards and methods of the American Association of Blood Banks were followed throughout donor selection, blood collection, and storage.

CPD was obtained from Fenwal (Deerfield, Ill.) full unit blood packs; transfer packs of 150 ml size were made of Fenwal's PL-146. Recrystalized adenine, obtained from Grant Bartlett, PhD, Laboratory of Comparative Biochemistry, San Diego, Calif. was added to give a final concentration of 0.25 mM in the blood preservative mixture. Following the addition of other chemicals to a CPD-adenine solution, the pH was adjusted to 5.5 and the solutions were sterilized by millipore filtration (0.22 micron pore). After collection, on days 0, 3, 7, 10, 14 and at weekly intervals thereafter for a total of 42 days, aliquots were removed aseptically and anaerobically for analysis of pH (measured anaerobically at 37° C), ATP, and 2,3-DPG concentrations. Analysis of ATP and 2,3-DPG was carried out by methods previously described by this laboratory (Dawson et al, 1972c).

RESULTS

Fig. 4 shows in the upper graph equal maintenance of 2,3-DPG by D and L isomers of VC during five weeks of storage. 10 mM VC is apparently slightly better than 5 mM for both D and L forms. In the bottom graph ATP maintenance is hindered by the presence of VC, however, it appears that the unnatural, D isomer has a greater effect in lowering ATP values.

Although the evidence of the D isomer having a greater inhibitory effect on ATP is preliminary, this form was chosen for further studies because of the slight difference and because the red cell does not seem to distinguish between it and the natural form in 2,3-DPG maintenance.

Maintenance of 2,3-DPG and ATP is shown in Fig. 5 with VC and glutathione (GSH). The highest 2,3-DPG levels are with VC alone and the lowest are with GSH alone. GSH

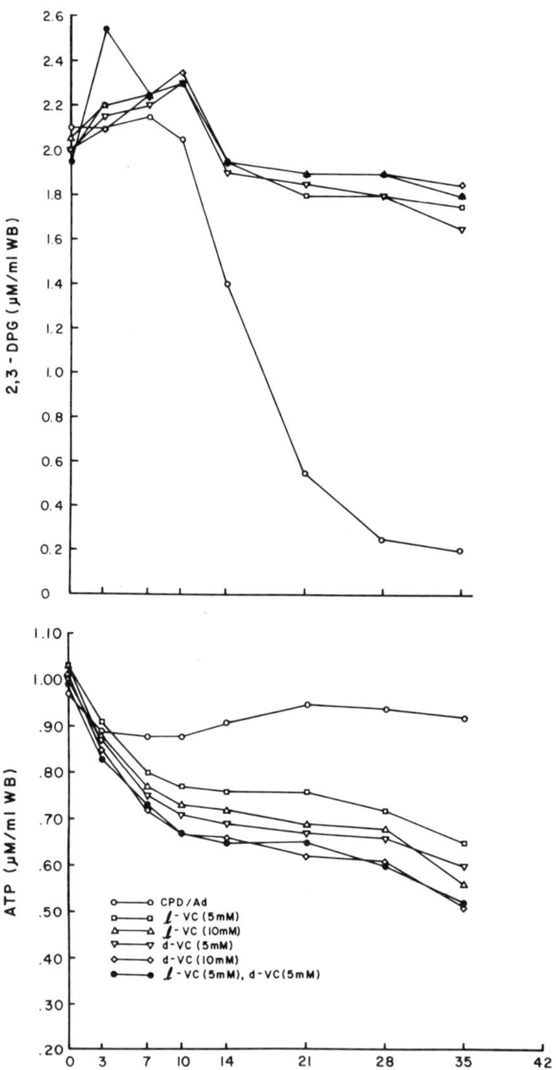

Fig. 4 2,3-DPG and ATP levels in blood with D and L ascorbic acid (VC).

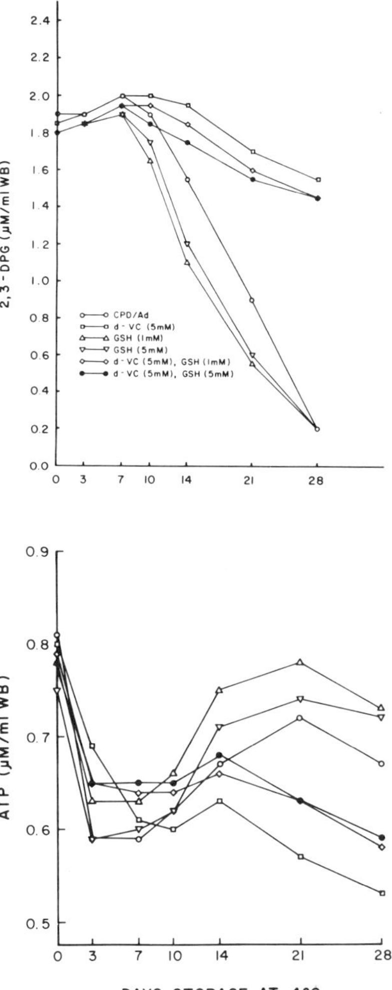

Fig. 5 2,3-DPG and ATP levels in blood stored with D ascorbic acid and GSH.

depresses 2,3-DPG values after 7 days whereas in the control
CPD-adenine preservative, 2,3-DPG levels do not decrease
rapidly until after 10 days. This data is certainly very
tenuous as the origins are not equal for the experimental
preservatives; however, glutathione appears also to depress
2,3-DPG levels in the presence of VC. **GSH in the**
presence of VC produces ATP levels that are higher than
those in the preservative with VC but without GSH. As with
the DPG values these changes become obvious only after 10
days of storage.

Fig. 6 shows DPG and ATP values during 6 weeks of
storage with VC, GSH, NEM, and IA. By 10 days the 3 preservatives containing VC show better maintenance of 2,3-DPG,
and by 21 days the 2,3-DPG levels in preservatives without
VC are quite low and apparently uneffected by the other
additives. However, ATP values in this experiment show
the worst maintenance in the 3 preservatives containing VC
and GSH. Further, NEM appears not to have an effect by
itself and the effect of IA if any is slight.

In Fig. 7 and Fig. 8, 2,3-DPG and ATP values are shown
with D-VC and L-VC, respectively. In both experiments,
2,3-DPG is better maintained when VC is present. Also, in
both experiments NEM and IA further enhance the 2,3-DPG
maintenance already improved by VC. In both experiments
initial ATP maintenance during the first 3 weeks is better
with the VC preservative that does not contain either NEM
or IA.

DISCUSSION

The literature on vitamin C as it may relate to red
cell metabolism during blood storage seems to span nearly
50 years, from the work of Szent-Gyorgyi (1931), in which
the vitamin was posited in electron transport reactions,
to the continuing work of Linus Pauling who reports (1977)
that some 68% of ingested ascorbate is converted into unidentified substances that have not been traced in the human body.

For those who are anxious for specific references to
ascorbate and red cell storage there are only a few. Wood
and Beutler (1973, 1974) first demonstrated the very great
effect of ascorbate on the maintenance of 2,3-diphosphogly-

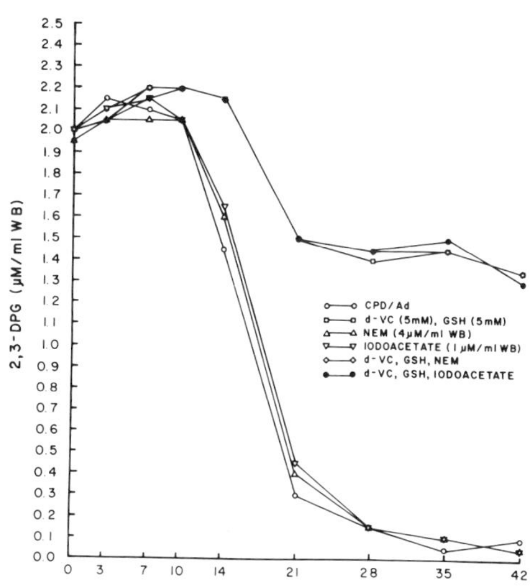

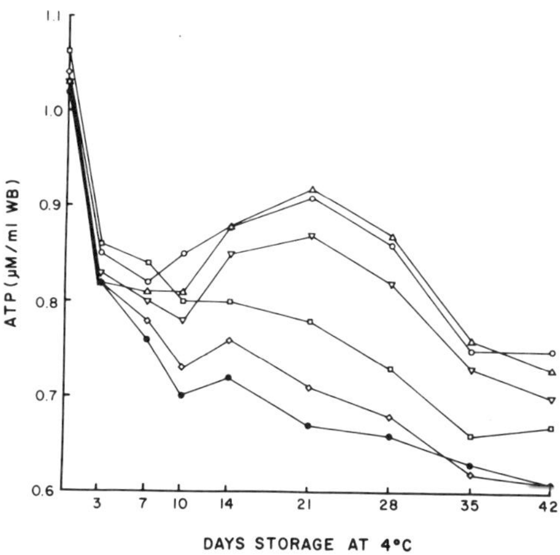

Fig. 6 2,3-DPG and ATP levels in blood stored with D
ascorbic acid, GSH, NEM and IA.

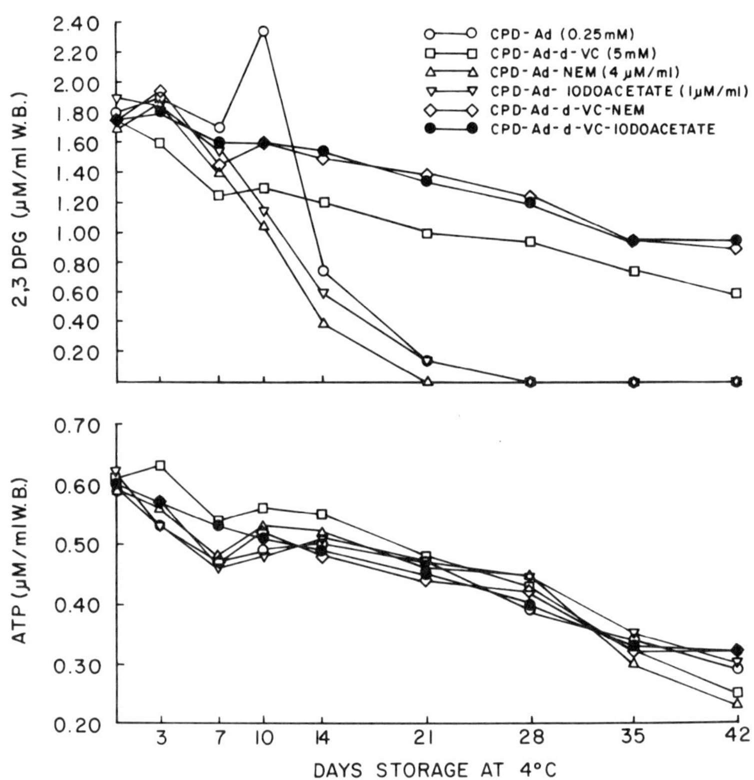

Fig. 7 2,3-DPG and ATP levels in blood stored with D ascorbic acid, NEM and IA.

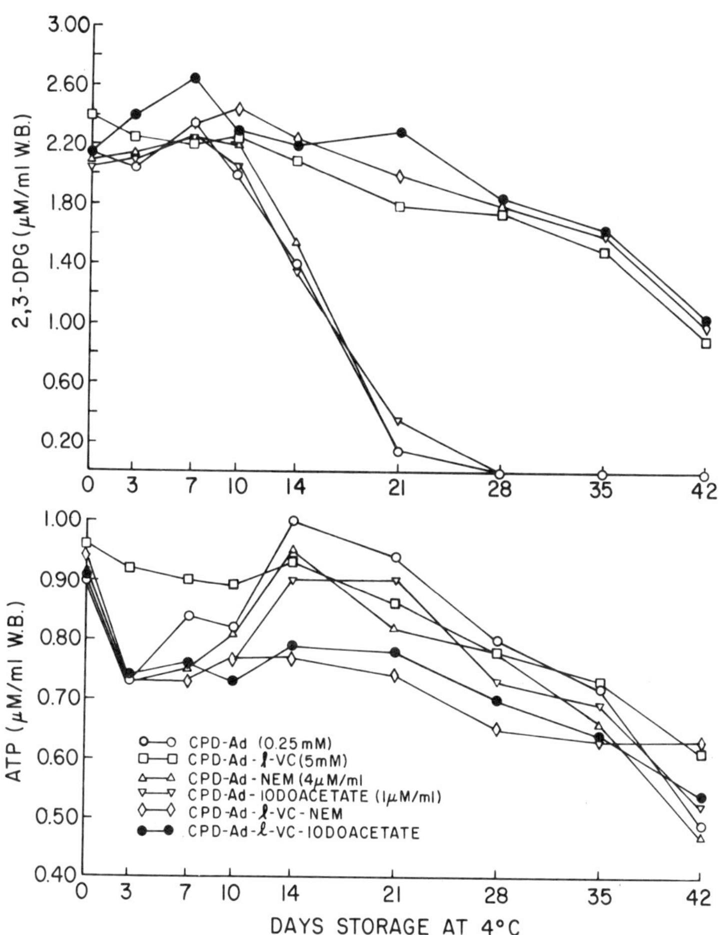

Fig. 8 2,3-DPG and ATP levels in blood stored with L ascorbic acid, NEM and IA.

cerate (2,3-DPG) during liquid blood storage and showed the effect of dihydroxyacetone when used with ascorbate. In canine blood storage, ascorbic acid was shown to improve 2,3-DPG and have an adverse effect on ATP (Eisenbrandt and Smith, 1973), findings which our results support in human red cells. Subsequently, it was shown that the unnatural D-isomer maintained 2,3-DPG as well as the natural L form (Dabezies and Dawson, 1975), and further studies with ascorbate, DHA, and pyruvate were published (Dawson, 1977b). A third laboratory, concerned about the relative instability of ordinary forms of ascorbic acid, has shown that trisodium ascorbate phosphate, a stabilized form, is as effective in maintaining 2,3-DPG as the usual so-called "unstable" form (Bensinger and Zuck, 1976).

It has long been known that higher mammals including man are unable to synthesize vitamin C. Since something may be learned about the metabolism of vitamin C and its functions in the cell by reviewing the evolution of synthetic capabilities, a brief summary is given here. The ability to synthesize vitamin C is absent in insects, invertebrates, and fish. The biosynthetic capacities evolved in the kidney of amphibians, remains in the kidneys of reptiles, became transferred to the liver of mammals, and finally disappeared from the guinea pig, the flying mammals, monkey and man. A similar transition of biosynthetic ability occurred in the branched evolution of birds from reptiles.

Although the major metabolite of parenterally administered ^{14}C vitamin C in monkeys is $^{14}CO_2$ (Baker 1975), less than 2% of Vitamin C carbon is converted to CO_2 in man as compared to 20-30% in the guinea pig. Thus, it would be hard to conceive of vitamin C as being degraded for useful purposes in man (Brin, 1977). This "standard literature" on metabolism of ascorbate in man contrasts with the report from Pauling above noting 68% conversion into unidentified substances. It should be noted that Pauling's data was derived after an intake of 200 mg ascorbate per day. He explains this observation by the assumption that an increased intake of ascorbate induces formation of enzymes that catalize its conversion to other substances.

The major known function of vitamin C in humans is to detoxify histamine, (Chatterjee, 1975), perhaps by the formation of hydroxylysine and/or hydroxyproline (Brin, 1977).

Ascorbic acid has been found to be involved in a variety of
metabolic processes such as collagen biosynthesis, steroid
metabolism, electron transport processes, and cholesterol
metabolism (see Chatterjee).

Of perhaps greater interest for us is the degradation
of L-ascorbic acid. Nearly 20 years ago it was proved that
L-ascorbic acid can be metabolized back to glucose and that
degradation can take place to form L-xylose (Chan, 1958).
Whereas a DPN (NAD) L-gulonate dehydrogenase participates
in the decomposition of L-ascorbic acid and its metabolism
to D-glucose, (Shimazono, 1961), the NAD dehydrogenase produces L-xylulose and D-ribulose, respectively depending on
whether it is acting on L-gulonate or D-gluconate. These
reactions which have been observed in the rat and guinea
pig are of interest to us because of the demonstration in
the human red cell of ascorbate's activity as an oxidant
of NADH (Wood & Beutler, 1973) and of NADPH (Jacob & Jandl,
1966). Staudinger (1961) had previously shown NADH oxidation by ascorbate in mammalian adrenal microsomes.

However, it is the NADPH oxidation studies of Jacob
and Jandl to which I will direct your immediate attention
as it seems most important to an understanding of the
studies reported here with GSH and SH inhibitors. Jacob
and Jandl showed that oxidation of glutathione (GSH) is
involved in the hexose monophosphate shunt activity of
red cells. Further, they showed an increase of HMP activity with ascorbic acid and then proved a 75% inhibition
of this VC enhanced activity by N-ethylmaleimide (NEM).
Their studies substantiated the existance of the glutathione peroxidase mechanism in human red cells proposed by
Mills (1957). Besides demonstrating inhibition of ascorbate stimulated HMP activity, Jacob and Jandl also demonstrated NEM blockage of the unstimulated GSH component of
HMP activity.

Before attempting an interpretation of our ascorbic
acid studies with GSH and inhibition by NEM and IA (iodoacetate) it may be useful to see if anything can be learned
from the current status of our knowledge of another metabolic regulator of the hexose monophosphate shunt, methylene blue. Jacob and Jandl showed 53% inhibition of glucose utilization via the hexose monophosphate shunt with
NEM alone compared with 75% in the presence of ascorbic
acid and only 8% with methylene blue. Stimulation rather

than inhibition of HMP activity was regularly seen when GSH
blockade was partial and the stimulatory effect was exaggerated when the NEM treated cells were "exposed to H_2O_2
by treatment with ascorbic acid". It is important that
hemolysates which were pretreated with NEM and therefore
devoid of free GSH did not catalyze the oxidation of NADPH,
even with H_2O_2 present; they did catalyze oxidation, however, when GSH was added. In studies which Jacob and Jandl
did not present, they noted that oxidation of NADPH by
molecular oxygen in the presence of methylene blue occurred
at undiminished rates with GSH blockaded.

Mills (1969) published his review and studies, sum-
marizing data showing that methylene blue facilitates a
non-enzymic oxidation of NADH to NAD and of NADPH to NADP.
In addition, work from this laboratory was published in
1972d showing a definite although small positive effect of
methylene blue on 2,3-DPG maintenance during blood storage.
Since then Metz (1976) has shown that stimulation of the
HMP by methylene blue may occur by more than one mechanism
in which the presence of oxygen is not required. Thus, a
methylene blue mechanism not utilizing glutathione to stimulate the HMP is suggested and of course raises the same
possibility for a mechanism of ascorbic acid HMP stimulation.

It was noted by Staudinger in 1961 that microsomal
NADH oxidation occurs with the unnatural D-isomer of VC,
although with a distinctly lower activity than oxidation
with the L-isomer; however, dehydroascorbic acid cannot
be substituted. On the other hand, red cells have shown
oxidation of NADPH by dehydroascorbate (Stankova, et al
1975).

What then is the mechanism of ascorbic acid utilization in the red cell? Some of the published reports and
unpublished data may help clarify the red cell mechanisms.
Although our Fig. 4 shows no differential effect of L versus D forms of ascorbic acid on 2,3-DPG, ATP maintenance
is disfavored by the D form in both 5 and 10 mM concentrations. Since the redox mechanisms proposed for NADH or
NADPH oxidation are thought not to be enzymic--or so our
biochemical dogma tells us--a redox mechanism would thus
be favored in our experiments because of the equal effect
of L and D forms. A predominately enzymic mechanism, as in
nutrient metabolism, would likely show a greater difference

between effects of D and L forms.

A study by Jacob and Jandl showed a greater inhibition of hexosemonophosphate shunt glucose utilization by NEM in the presence of ascorbate than in control or methylene blue treated cells. Our Fig. 6 shows that both NEM and IA, which are sulfydryl inhibitors, enhance the suppressive effect of D ascorbate on ATP maintenance. Further, in Fig. 7 the improved 2,3-DPG maintenance by D ascorbate is intensified by NEM and IA. Thus, sulfydryl inhibition enhances the two observed effects of D ascorbate; that is, to inhibit ATP maintenance and to favor 2,3-DPG maintenance.

The effect of added glutathione with and without D ascorbate was seen in our Fig. 5 to enhance ATP maintenance and suppress 2,3-DPG maintenance. Thus, in this latter experiment glutathione has no effect on the two (ATP and 2,3-DPG) ascorbate effects. In the former experiments, inhibition of sulfydryl groups with added glutathione enhances the suppressive effect of ascorbate on ATP maintenance; the 2,3-DPG effect is enhanced by NEM and IA without added glutathione. These results indicate that the glutathione system is not involved in the ascorbate 2,3-DPG maintenance but is utilized in the suppressive effect of ascorbate on ATP maintenance.

Our proposed mechanism is that ascorbate assists the red cell in 2,3-DPG maintenance by oxidation of NADH which is not dependent on the sulfydryl or glutathione systems. Ascorbate has an adverse effect on ATP maintenance which is dependent on the red cell's sulfhydryl system. GSH is related to the hexose monophosphate shunt and depends on continued oxidation of NADPH. ATP would be used for each glucose entering the HMP as a result of NADPH oxidation. Thus, ATP decreases as the HMP is stimulated.

Further evidence for an oxidation mechanism for ascorbic acid is afforded in Fig. 8. The natural L-ascorbic acid is seen to be affected by NEM and IA in a manner similar to the studies with D-ascorbic acid. Both studies show an enhancement of the 2,3-DPG effect which is not dependent on sulfydryl systems, and enhancement of the suppressive effect on ATP.

Finally, there is evidence in these studies for a metabolic role of ascorbic acid in addition to the above

discussed regulatory mechanisms. Fig. 8 shows improved ATP
maintenance by L-ascorbate during the first 10 days of
storage, whereas D-ascorbate (Fig. 5) shows minimal or no
improvement in ATP maintenance. Also, in data not given,
L-ascorbate in the presence of NEM appears to raise glucose
and pH as well as ATP. If L-ascorbate were contributing a
glucose or related metabolic nutrient, glucose might be
spared, thus raising pH or preventing the usual fall. These
two experiments give evidence for a nutritional role for
ascorbate in red cell metabolism.

In summary, our data indicate that ascorbic acid may
act by 3 different mechanisms in the human red cell during
blood storage. The regulatory mechanisms, oxidation of
NADH and NADPH, have been shown before in the human red cell,
but not under these conditions. Also, it is suggested for
the first time that NADH oxidation is the main mechanism
involved in ascorbate maintenance of 2,3-DPG. Further,
experiments reported here suggest a new, nutritional role
for ascorbate in the human red cell.

REFERENCES

Adolph, EF, Ferry, RM (1921). The oxygen dissociation of
    hemoglobin, and the effect of electrolytes upon it.
    J Biol Chem 47:547.
Akerblom, O et al (1968). Restoration of defective oxygen-
    transport function of stored red blood cells by addition
    of inosine. Scand J Clin and Lab Invest 21:245.
Baker, EM et al (1975). Metabolism of ascorbic acid and
    ascorbic-2-sulfate in man and the subhuman. Ann N Y
    Acad Sci 258:72.
Barcroft, J and Roberts, F (1909). The disscoation curve of
    haemoglobin. J Physiol 39:143.
Bartlett, GR and Barnet, HM (1960). Changes in the phosphate
    compounds of the human red blood cell during blood bank
    storage. J Clin Invest 39:56.
Benesch, R and Benesch, RE (1967). The effect of organic
    phosphates from the human erythrocyte on the allosteric
    properties of hemoglobin. Biochem Biophys Res Commun
    26:162.
Benesch, RE et al (1969). The oxygenation of hemoglobin in
    the presence of 2,3-diphosphoglycerate. Effect of temper-
    ature, pH, ionic strength, and hemoglobin concentration.
    Biochem 8:2567.

Berry, ER and Chanutin, A (1958). Effect of blood storage conditions on the electrophoretic patterns of red cell hemolysates. J Clin Invest 37:974.

Beutler, E and Wood, L (1969). The in vivo regeneration of red cell 2,3-diphosphoglyceric acid (DPG) after transfusion of stored blood. J Lab and Clin Med 74:300.

Beutler, E and Guinto, E (1973). Dihydroxyacetone metabolism by human erythrocytes: Demonstration of triokinase activity and its characterization. Blood 41:559.

Bigley, RH and Stankova, L (1974). Uptake and reduction of oxidized and reduced ascorbate by human leukocytes. Jour of Exp Med 139:1084.

Brin, M (1977). Personal communication.

Bunn, HF et al (1969). Hemoglobin function in stored blood. J Clin Invest 48:311.

Campbell, GD et al (1975). Ascorbic acid-induced hemolysis in G-6-PD deficiency. Ann of Intern Med 82:810.

Chanutin, A (1966). Red blood cell preservation: Effects of organic and inorganic phosphate compounds on the oxygen equilibrium of human hemoglobin. U.S. Army Report R&D Command, Washington, D. C.

Chanutin, A and Curnish RR (1967). Effect of organic and inorganic phosphates on the oxygen equilibrium of human erythrocytes. Arch Biochem Biophys 121:96.

Chatterjee, IB et al (1975). Synthesis and some major functions of vitamin C in animals. Ann of the N Y Acad Sci 258:24.

Cheson, BD et al (1976). The origin of the chemiluminescence of phagocytosing granulocytes. Jour Clin Invest 58:789.

Dabezies, M and Dawson, RB (1975). Hemoglobin function in stored blood: Combining use of metabolic regulators and nutrients: III. Ascorbate and sulfydryl reagents. Clin Res 23:580A.

Dawson, RB (1969). The hemoglobin function of blood stored at 4°C in ACD and CPD. Clin Res 17:323.

Dawson, RB et al (1970). The control of hemoglobin function during storage of blood at 4 C. G. Brewer (eds),"Red Cell Metabolism and Function", p. 305.

Dawson, RB et al (1970a). Hemoglobin function and 2,3-DPG levels of blood stored at 4 C in ACD and CPD pH effect. Transf 10:299.

Dawson, RB (1970b). Rapid adaptation to hypoxia. (Letter), New Eng J Med 283:265.

Dawson, RB (1972). Hemoglobin function VII. Effects of salts and glutathione. Vox Sang 22:26.

Dawson, RB, Loken, MR and Crater, DH (1972a). Hemoglobin function in stored blood: IX. A modified preservative with pH to maintain red cell 2,3-DPG (function) and ATP (viability). Transf 12:46.

Dawson, RB and Kocholaty, WF (1972b). Hemoglobin function during blood storage XV. Effects of metabolic additives inosine and methylene blue on p50 and 2,3-DPG. G. J. Brewer (eds) "Hemoglobin and Red Cell Structure and Function", p. 495.

Dawson, RB (1976). Blood storage XXV. Ascorbic acid (vitamin C) and dihydroxyacetone (DHA) maintenance of 2,3-DPG for six weeks in CPD-adenine. Transf 17:248.

Dawson, RB et al (1977). Blood preservation XXVII. Fructose and mannose maintain ATP and 2,3-DPG. Transf in press.

Dawson, RB (1977a). Red cell metabolism: GSH, NEM and IA with ascorbate. Intern Soc of Hem Euro & Afri Div 4th meeting, Istanbul, Sept.

Dawson, RB (1977c). Blood storage XXV: Ascorbic acid (vitamin C) and dihydroxyacetone (DHA) maintenance of 2,3-DPG for six weeks of CPD-adenine. Transf 17:248.

DeChatelet, LR (1971). Stimulation of the hexose monophosphate shunt in human neutrophils by ascorbic acid: mechanism of action. Antimicrobial agents and chemotherapy, 1:12.

Eisenbrandt, DL and Smith, JE (1973). Use of biochemical measures to estimate the viability of red blood cells in canine blood stored in ACD solution with and without added ascorbic acid. J Am Vet Med Assoc 163:984.

Greenwalt, I (1925). A new type of phosphoric acid compound isolated from blood with some remarks on the effect of substitution on the rotation of L-glyceric acid. J Biol Chem 63:339.

Gulbring, B and Strom, G (1956). Changes in oxygen-carrying function of human hemoglobin during storage in cold acid-citrate-dextrose solution. Acta Med Scand 115:413.

Horejski, J (1970). Effect of glutathione and some other substances on the oxygen dissociation curve of hemoglobin and experimental therapy of hemorrhagic shock with solutions enriched with glutathione. G. Brewer (eds) "Red Cell Metabolism and Function", (Op cit).

Jacob, HS and Jandl, JH (1966). Effect of sulfydryl inhibition on red blood cells. II. Glutathione IX the regulation of the hexose monophosphate pathway. Jour Biol Chem 18:4243.

Loutit, JF, Mollison, PL and Young, IM (1943). Citric acid-
    sodium citrate-glucose mixtures for blood storage; report
    to Medical Research Council from Southwest London Blood
    Supply Depot. Q J Exp Physiol 32:183.
McCall, CE (1971). The effects of ascorbic acid on bacteri-
    dal mechanisms of neutrophils. J Infect Dises 124:194.
McCallister, J et al (1977). Alteration of microtubule
    function in glutathione peroxidase deficient polymorpho-
    nuclear leukocytes. Clin Res 25:381a.
McManus, TJ, Rees, JS and Gibson, JG (1957). Effect of
    purine ribosides on glucose and pyruvate metabolism of
    human erythrocytes. Fed Proc 16:220.
McManus, TJ (1974). Alternate pathways for metabolism in,
    TJ Greenwalt & G Jamieson (eds), "The Human Red Cell in
    Vitro", Gruhn & Stratton, N Y p. 51.
Metz, EN, Balcerzak, SP and Sagone, AL (1976). Mechanisms
    of methylene blue stimulation of the hexose monophosphate
    shunt in erythrocytes. J Clin Invest 58:797.
Mills, GC (1969). The physiologic regulation of erythrocyte
    metabolism. Tex Rep Biol Med 27:773.
Paulin, L (1977). Personal communication.
Rapoport, S and Luebering, J (1950). The formation of 2,3-
    diphosphoglycerate in rabbit erythrocytes: The existence
    of a diphosphoglycerate mutase. J Biol Chem 183:507.
Ross, JF et al (1947). The in vitro preservation and post-
    transfusion survival of stored blood. J Clin Invest
    26:687.
Ross-Fanelli, et al (1961). Studies on the relations between
    molecular and functional properties of hemoglobin II.
    The effects of salts on the oxygen equilibrium of human
    hemoglobin. J Biol Chem 236:397.
Rous, P and Turner, JF (1916). The preservation of living
    red blood cells in vitro. I. Methods of preservation.
    II. The transfusion of kept cells. J Exp Med 23:219.
Scrivastava, SK et al (1977). Use of hydroperoxides in the
    metabolism of glutathione in red cells. Am Soc Hemat
    Ann Meeting, p. 41.
Seidel, S (1976). Personal communication.
Shappell, SD, et al (1970). Acute change in hemoglobin
    affinity for oxygen during angina pectoris. N Engl J
    Med 282:1219.
Simon, ER (1976) (eds) Workshop on Adenine. Transcript of
    B.O.B., F.D.A., H.E.W. Oct 1-2, Bethesda, Md.
Smith, WB et al (1975). Alteration in human granulocyte
    function after in vitro incubation with L-ascorbic acid.
    N Y Acad Sci 258:329.

Stankova, L et al (1975). Dehydroascorbate uptake and reduction by human blood neutrophils, erythrocytes, and lymphocytes. N Y Acad Sci 258:238.

Staudinger, HJ et al (1961). Role of ascorbic acid in microsomal electron transport and the possible relationship to hydroxylation reactions. Ann N Y Acad Sci 92:195.

Sugerman, HJ et al (1972). Experimentally induced alterations in affinity of hemoglobin for oxygen. II. In vivo effect of inosine pyruvate and phosphate on oxygen-hemoglobin affinity in Rhesus monkey. Blood 39:525.

Sugita, Y and Chanutin, A (1963). Electrophoretic studies on red cell hemolysates supplemented with phosphorylated carbohydrate intermediates. Proc Soc Exp Biol 112:72.

Szent-Gyorgyi, A (1931). On the function of hexoronic acid in the respiration of the cabbage leaf. J Biol Chem 90:385.

Taylor, JF and Hastings, AB (1942). The equilibrium between oxygen and hemoglobin in concentrated urea solution. J. Biol. Chem. 114:1.

Taylor, TV (1974). Ascorbic acid supplementation in the treatment of pressure-sores. Lancet, 544.

Udomratn, T et al (1977). Effects of ascorbic acid on glucose-6-phosphate dehydrogenase-deficient erythrocytes: Studies in an animal model. Blood 49:471.

Valeri, CR and Hirsch, NM (1969). Restoration in vivo of erythrocyte adenosine triphosphate, 2,3-diphosphoglycerate, potassium ion, and sodium ion concentrations following the transfusion of acid-citrate-dextrose-stored human red blood cells. J Lab Clin Med 73:722.

Valtis, DJ and Kennedy, AC (1953). The causes and prevention of defective function of stored red blood cells after transfusion. Glasg Med J 34:521.

Valtis, DJ and Kennedy, AC (1954). Defective gas transport function of stored red blood cells. Lancet 1:119.

Vanderbilt, BL et al (1977). Effects of ascorbic acid on polymorphonuclear microtubule function and on polymerization of ixolated bovine brain tumor. Clin Res 25:481A.

Wood, LA and Beutler E (1973). The effect of ascorbate on the maintenance of 2,3-diphosphoglycerate (2,3-DPG) in stored red cells. Blood 25:611.

Zuck, TF and Bensinger, TA (1976). Trisodium ascorbate phosphate, a stabilized form of ascorbic acid, promotes 2,3-diphosphoglycerate maintenance during blood storage. Transf 16:518.

Zuck, TF et al (1977). The in vivo survival of red blood cells stored in modified CPD with adenine: Report of a multi-institutional cooperative effort. Transf 17:374.

DISCUSSION

<u>Dr. Myerstein</u>: It's not really a question that I want to ask you, but just to report about some studies that we've been running on camel erythrocytes in Beer Sheeva. It has some relevance with the maintenance of ATP level in erythrocytes and its correlation between the ATP level and the shape of the cell. The camel erythrocyte is really famous for having some special characteristics. One, it is oval, and it is unique in being oval and a non-nucleated, mammalian erythrocyte; another thing is that it has a unique stability both in hypotonic and in hypertonic solution, and so we were wondering what would happen to the camel erythrocyte during storage, as compared with the changes that happen to the human erythrocyte during storage. We really expected that, like the human stored erythrocyte, osmotic fragility would increase, ATP would go down, and there would be some morphological changes, but we had our little surprise, that first of all, the ATP level of the camel was a little lower than we expected: It was less than two micromoles of ATP per gram hemoglobin, and with the storage we found some interesting phenomena. ATP went down very, very quickly. It went down after two or three days; it went down to zero level of ATP. At the same time, the oval shape of these cells persisted. There were no morphological changes during storage for at least two months, and only after three months, shape changes occurred. Osmotic fragility did increase, but also very, very late in the storage. So the first change that happened in the stored camel erythrocyte was a decreased ATP level to almost zero after the first three or four days, then a very slight increase in osmotic fragility, and only then, very slight morphological changes in the cells. I still don't know if it has any correlation with the ability to survive; we didn't do any survival studies on this cell.

<u>Dr. Dawson</u>: These are fascinating studies. I know several of us would like to have some camels, although I'm not sure what we'd do with them, in Boston or Baltimore.

<u>Dr. Lehmann</u>: Did you estimate the oxalic acid levels after?

<u>Dr. Dawson</u>: No, sir, I did not.

<u>Dr. Lehmann</u>: May I say, dihydroxyacetone is metabolized by polymerization to hexose with subsequent phosphorylation,

The Red Cell, pages 649–650

but this is a very slow process and for practical purposes,
you may well consider it as a non-metabolite.

Dr. Brewer: Are you thinking of the possibility that this
might be added sometime to clinical use in blood storage?

Dr. Dawson: Very definitely, George, because of two fairly
obvious reasons. Ascorbate maintains 2,3 DPG levels very
nicely during 5 or 6 weeks of storage in CPD as well as
anything which was in our protocol before. The other important reason is that ascorbate may be acceptable to the
FDA and the public as a drug. Inosine has been tried; we've
decided it's not acceptable because its metabolite, hypoxanthine, goes to uric acid, once the blood is transfused,
and high uric acid levels have been seen in patients. And
so, in the countries in which inosine was used for a few
years, they have stopped using it. I think ascorbate has
potential, and that's why I'm studying it.

Dr. Brewer: The one problem I can think of is with G6PD
deficient recipients. I don't know what the total load
would be, but we showed, many years ago, that ascorbate
administered to G6PD deficient people decreased the red cell
survival. I think that Steinberg and others reported a case
of a G6PD deficient patient who took massive doses of Vitamin
C for a cold and expired. So there is some toxicity related
to that type of problem. I suppose that you'd also need to
worry about whether the blood itself that you're storing
with ascorbate was G6PD deficient?

Dr. Dawson: Yes.

Dr. L. Grindlay Moore: We have a paper coming out (Moore,
et al, J. Pharm. Exp. Therap., in press), in which we showed
that oral treatment with reasonably low doses of ascorbate
(2 gms q.i.d.) does not lead to elevation in DPG levels _in
vivo_.

Dr. Surgenor: Any other response, Ben?

Dr. Dawson: If there are any other suggestions for further
tricks I might use in studying these mechanisms, and especially
studying how ascorbate might be metabolized, I'd be grateful
for suggestions.

The Introduction of an Adenine-Supplemented Anticoagulant
Preservative Solution into U. S. Blood Services

Ernest R. Simon, M.D.
Associate Director for Clinical Research
Division of Blood and Blood Products,
Bureau of Biologics, FDA
Bethesda, Maryland

Studies performed in the early 1960's demonstrated that
supplementation of anticoagulant citrate dextrose (ACD)
blood with small amounts of adenine (0.75 $\pm$ 0.25 mM final
concentration, that is 0.75 $\pm$ 0.25 μmole/ml ACD blood)*
could extend red cell shelf life from 21 to at least 35
days.(48-50)
     Since 1965, ACD-adenine preserved blood (adenine, 0.5
mM) has been used routinely in Sweden; by 1976, more than
two million units had been transfused.(21,26,53) West
Germany introduced ACD-adenine into blood banking practice
to a limited extent in about 1967; in 1972, nearly 200,000
ACD-adenine units were collected, accounting for about 10%
of the total.(55) Both countries have continued its use.
     A major portion of the biochemical, pharmacologic, and
posttransfusion survival data underlying the Swedish and
West German usage was accumulated in the U.S. Nevertheless,
adenine-supplemented preservative solutions were not adopted
in the U.S. because several issues remained unsettled.(18)
     Efficacy considerations included: 1) shelf life of
adenine-supplemented red cells when stored as red cell
concentrates, 2) implications of increased oxygen affinity
of the stored red cells, and 3) efficacy (as well as safety)
of components and derivatives prepared from adenine-
supplemented blood. Safety considerations included:

---

*In the remainder of the text the notation mM refers to the
final adenine concentration in the blood-anticoagulant
mixture at the time of collection.

The Red Cell, pages 651—664
© **1978 Alan R. Liss, Inc., New York, New York**

1) toxicity of adenine, and 2) safety of transfusing red
cells stored beyond 21 days in adenine-supplemented
solutions, particularly in regard to compatibility testing.
A further impediment to the introduction of adenine into
U.S. blood services was disagreement regarding the need to
extend the shelf life of liquid-preserved red cells.

Accelerated activity by several groups and individuals
over the last several years has lead to the resolution of
most of these issues. As a result, the introduction of the
first substantially different anticoagulant preservative
solution into U.S. blood banking in 35 years is now being
vigorously pursued.(58) Both whole blood and red cell
concentrates collected into anticoagulant citrate phosphate
dextrose adenine solution (CPDA) (adenine 0.25 mM, glucose
increased 25% over standard CPD) will be expected to have a
permissible shelf life of 35 days.

The impact of this change is uncertain. The intended
effect is to increase flexibility in blood banking by
improving the logistics of supply and reducing wastage due
to outdating of a product for which demand sometimes
exceeds supply. At least as important, the quality of the
red cells which are transfused prior to the outdating limit
may be improved. Evaluation of the impact of this change
will be important.

The purpose of this communication is to review briefly:
1) the biochemical mechanism of action of adenine in red
cell preservation, 2) major issues, now largely resolved,
underlying the introduction of CPDA, and 3) areas in which
additional information is needed.

MECHANISM OF ACTION OF ADENINE IN RED CELL PRESERVATION.

Studies reported by Nakao and his associates in 1959
and 1960 demonstrated that when blood, which had been
stored previously at 4 °C for 8 to 10 weeks in ACD, was
subsequently incubated at 37 °C with both adenine and
inosine, regeneration of adenosine triphosphate (ATP) and
restoration of posttransfusion viability took place. ATP
regeneration did not occur when the incubation medium
contained either adenine or inosine alone.(38-40,62)

These studies indicated that both inosine and adenine
were necessary for the rejuvenation of long-stored red cells.
We reasoned that adenine could act without inosine in
maintaining viability (as opposed to rejuvenation) when it
was present from the beginning of storage, since at the

outset, unlike later in storage, glucose utilization could
yield both energy and a source of pentose for nucleotide
synthesis. Moreover, eliminating inosine would avoid
toxicity from uric acid overload in the blood recipient.
Accordingly, we studied the effect of supplementing the
ACD preservative with adenine alone from the beginning of
storage. The results indicated that small amounts of
adenine (0.75 $\pm$ 0.25 µmole/ml ACD blood), without added
nucleoside, maintained higher ATP and adenine nucleotide
levels and preserved satisfactory viability for at least
five weeks.(48-50,56)

In order to investigate the mechanism by which adenine
affects adenine nucleotide levels, 8-^{14}C-adenine (0.6 µmole
per ml) was added to ACD blood at the outset or after two
weeks of refrigerated storage, and its effect on the concentration and specific radioactivity of purines and purine
nucleotides was determined throughout a six week storage
period.(56) With supplementation at the outset, the initial
adenine concentration decreased rapidly at first, then more
slowly, so that by six weeks, about one-half of the initial
adenine remained. The adenine was incorporated into adenine
nucleotides, resulting in net adenine nucleotide synthesis
and values of ATP and of total adenine nucleotides that
were about 12 and 25% higher, respectively, after 1 to 2
weeks of storage than at the outset. Thereafter, the total
adenine nucleotide concentrations declined but more
gradually than in the ACD controls. This slower decline
could be accounted for by continued incorporation of adenine
into nucleotide rather than by inhibition of nucleotide
breakdown. Adenine supplementation after 2 weeks of storage
appeared slightly less effective in maintaining adenine
nucleotide levels than was supplementation at the outset.
The specific activity of adenine did not change during
storage.

A mechanism whereby stored red cells incorporate
adenine into adenine nucleotides which is consistent with
these results most likely includes the following reaction
sequences:(4,12,13,32-34,39,43,52,56)

$$A + PRPP \rightarrow AMP + PP \qquad [1]$$
$$PP \rightarrow 2\ P_i \qquad [2]$$
$$AMP + ATP \leftrightarrow 2\ ADP \qquad [3]$$
$$Glucose + 2\ ADP + 2\ P_i \rightarrow 2\ lactate + 2\ ATP \qquad [4]$$
$$R\text{-}5\text{-}P + ATP \rightarrow PRPP + AMP \qquad [5]$$
$$Glucose \rightarrow R\text{-}5\text{-}P \qquad [6]$$

Adenine (A) initially reacts with 5-phosphoribosyl-1-pyrophosphate (PRPP) to form adenosine monophosphate (AMP) and pyrophosphate (PP) via adenine phosphoribosyl transferase(6,28,43)(step 1). Removal of pyrophosphate via inorganic pyrophosphatase (step 2) may account for the irreversibility of step 1, a necessary requirement since the specific activity of adenine remained constant throughout the storage period. The increased AMP reacts with ATP via adenylate kinase to form adenosine diphosphate (ADP) (27,59) (step 3). ADP is phosphorylated to ATP via Embden-Meyerhof glycolysis (line 4). PRPP is formed from ribose-5-phosphate (R-5-P) and ATP(28) (step 5). Early in storage, glucose serves as precursor for R-5-P (line 6), partly via reactions catalyzed by the dehydrogenases of the hexose monophosphate shunt, but mostly through the reaction of glyceraldehyde-3-phosphate and fructose-6-phosphate, via transketolase.(33)

Crucial to this mechanism of action is the availability of PRPP (step 1), yet levels of PRPP in freshly collected red cells are negligible.(6) However, early in storage PRPP accumulates(6) making net adenine nucleotide synthesis possible in the presence of free adenine, to replace the adenine nucleotide which is lost irreversibly by deamination during the storage period.

MAJOR ISSUES

Efficacy

Red cells, whether stored as Whole Blood (Human) or as concentrates [Red Blood Cells (Human)], must maintain adequate posttransfusion viability and, preferably, near-normal oxygen affinity throughout the dating period.

Supplementation of ACD or CPD whole blood with adenine (0.25 to 1 mM) provides satisfactory red cell preservation (70% or more of the red cells remain in the circulation 24 hours after the transfusion) for at least 35 days.(35,49,52-54)

Several posttransfusion survival measurements on red cell concentrates have been reported. An early study compared seven units of whole blood in ACD-adenine (0.5 mM) with seven units of red cell concentrates (hematocrit 80 $\pm$ 5%) after six weeks of storage in plastic containers.(47) Posttransfusion survival was 71 $\pm$ 3% for whole blood and 68 $\pm$ 4% for the concentrates. More recently, four units of whole blood collected into CPD-adenine (0.25 mM) were compared with four units of concentrates (hematocrit

85 + 2%)(31) After five weeks of storage in plastic
containers, posttransfusion survival of whole blood was
78.7 + 3.5%, compared to 76.5 + 6.7% for the concentrates.
    A collaborative study involving four laboratories has
just been completed,(68) using plastic containers prefilled
with CPDA. The 24-hour posttransfusion survival of 32 units
of whole blood stored 35 days was 80.5 + 6.5% with 31 units
exceeding 70%. Nineteen units of red cell concentrates,
prepared on the day of collection,(hematocrit 75 + 3.7%)
were also studied after five weeks of storage. Posttransfusion survival was 71.4 + 10.3%, with 12 of the 19 units
exceeding 70%. These studies indicate that red cell
survival in CPD-adenine at 35 days of storage is approximately equivalent to red cell survival in CPD or ACD
(without adenine) at 21 days of storage, although published
data for red cells stored as concentrates in ACD or in
CPD are meager.(15,26,55,63)
    The oxygen affinity of red cells increases during
refrigerated storage in the liquid state(61) owing to
progressive metabolic depletion of red cell 2,3-diphospho-
glycerate (DPG).(14,17,23) While stored red cells
resynthesize DPG in vivo following transfusion, it takes
from a few hours to a day or two for enough DPG regeneration
to restore normal oxygen affinity.(10,60) Theoretically,
DPG-depleted cells should deliver less oxygen than normal
to the tissues at any given partial pressure of oxygen in
the capillaries. Whether infusion of DPG-depleted cells
limits the amount of O_2 delivered to tissues compared with
red cells containing normal DPG and, if so, under what
clinical conditions, has not been established conclusively.(18,19)
This effect is almost certainly unimportant when one or only
a few units of blood are transfused into adults. It may
become important when massive transfusion therapy is required
to obtain immediate improvement in tissue oxygen delivery
as for severe trauma or complex surgery, in patients with
concomitant cardiac or pulmonary decompensation or coronary
artery disease, and in newborns with respiratory distress
syndrome.
    In ACD preserved blood, most of the DPG is depleted by
four to seven days. Red cells stored in CPD maintain normal
or slightly increased DPG levels for about seven days.
Thereafter, DPG decreases, but levels of DPG considered
adequate (i.c., approximately 0.6 μmole/μmole Hgb) are
maintained for 12 to 16 days. DPG loss is slightly more
rapid when adenine is present, in ACD as well as in CPD.
(2,8,9,17,20,45,56) This effect of adenine is dose-dependent;

the higher the adenine concentration, the more rapid the
DPG fall.(2) With CPD-adenine (0.25 - 0.5 mM) adequate
levels of DPG are maintained for 10 to 14 days;(2,35,53)
this interval is only slightly less than with CPD, and
considerably longer than with ACD.

The data on efficacy may be summarized as follows:
Adenine supplementation of ACD and CPD preservative media
permits prolongation of the shelf life of whole blood and
of red cell concentrates to five weeks, and increases the
quality of the stored red cell population with respect to
viability after the first week or ten days of storage.(18,26,
52,68) With respect to red cell survival CPD-adenine is
comparable to ACD-adenine; both are superior to ACD or CPD
after about ten days of storage. With respect to DPG
maintenance only, and hence oxygen unloading, CPD-adenine
is superior to ACD-adenine and to ACD; CPD-adenine may be
slightly inferior to CPD.

Safety

Safety concerns include: toxicity of adenine, safety
of whole blood and red cell concentrates stored with
adenine up to 35 days in transfusion services, and safety
of components and derivatives prepared from adenine-
supplemented blood.

The toxicity of adenine is due to conversion in vivo
of about 5% of infused adenine to 2,8-dioxyadenine (DOA)
which is almost insoluble in neutral aqueous solutions
including plasma and urine.(5,7,22,42,53) Large amounts of
adenine infused into several species of experimental
animals can be nephrotoxic due to precipitation of DOA in
kidney tubules. The pharmacology and toxicology of adenine
in animals and man has been reviewed recently.(64) These
studies indicate that adenine toxicity is probably
negligible in any transfusion episode in which 15 mg/kg or
less of adenine is administered. In a 70 kg individual
this will allow the transfusion of about 60 units of fresh
whole blood collected in CPDA, which contains 0.25 mM
adenine. Since free adenine equilibrates rapidly between
the red cells and plasma,(36,56) about one-half of the free
adenine is removed when red cell concentrates are prepared.
Accordingly, when freshly collected red cell concentrates
are used as many as 120 units per transfusion episode
should be tolerated. If the units of whole blood or red

cells have been stored for several days or weeks before
transfusion, the number of units tolerated should be even
greater because, as indicated previously, adenine is
continously incorporated into intraerythrocytic adenine
mononucleotides throughout storage; in ACD or CPD blood
containing 0.5 mM adenine, 35-50% is metabolized in two
weeks, 40-70% in four, and 60-85% after six weeks.(4,36,56)
With CPD containing 0.25 mM adenine, incorporation of adenine
into nucleotide may be complete by three to five weeks in
whole blood and by two weeks in red cell concentrates.(53)
Finally, if blood is administered while blood loss continues,
some adenine will be lost through hemorrhage.

Clinical experience and observations are consistent
with these considerations.(26,46,55,57) Signs of impaired
kidney function attributable to adenine were not detected:
1) after transfusion of five to 33 units (mean 13) of ACD-
adenine (0.5 mM) blood during extra-corporeal circulatory
bypass;(65) 2) in a prospective, randomized, double-blind
field study of 78 Vietnam combat casualties, 9% of whom
received more than 20 units of ACD-adenine (0.5mM) blood;(53)
or 3) in children exchange transfused one to seven times
with ACD-adenine blood containing about 12 mg of adenine per
kg body weight per exchange transfusion.(29,30)

No DOA deposits were found in the kidneys of 12 patients
post mortem after transfusion episodes containing adenine
in doses up to 15 mg/kg; several patients received substantially larger amounts without DOA crystal formation. Renal
deposits of DOA were present in four patients who received
15, 41, 45 and 95 mg/kg respectively; a relationship
between the deposits and renal impairment could not be
established.(24,66)

With prolongation of shelf life, red cell antigen
reactivity must be preserved to permit compatibility testing
throughout the dating period. Red cell antigens retained
their reactivity on red cells stored as whole blood in
plastic containers and in segmented donor tubing in excess
of six weeks in ACD-adenine (0.5 mM) at 4-6°C.(16) In
another study, red cells stored as whole blood in both ACD
and ACD-adenine (0.5 mM) displayed little loss in specific
hemagglutinability for at least three weeks. Beyond four
weeks for ACD and six weeks for ACD-adenine, a statistically
significant loss of specific hemagglutinability was
observed.(44) This loss appears insufficient to impair
performance of satisfactory compatibility testing.(53)

Clinical transfusion experience is compatible with these results. In studies involving several thousand units of blood, differences in frequency, severity or type of transfusion reactions were not recorded between units stored up to 21 days in ACD versus 21 to 35 days in ACD-adenine(1,53) or CPD-adenine.(31) Difficulty with compatibility testing has not been reported. Unexpected untoward effects have not been encountered with the transfusion or more than two million units of adenine-supplemented blood having a 35 day dating limit.(26,53,55)

The effect of adenine on derivatives and components prepared from blood collected and stored in adenine-supplemented preservatives was examined in a number of studies.(3,25,37,41) The data indicate that adenine supplementation does no harm to blood components and derivatives; however, studies documenting the hemostatic effectiveness of stored platelets harvested from ACD-adenine or CPD-adenine whole blood have not been reported.

ADDITIONAL DATA NEEDED

While the major issues have now been largely resolved, information is needed regarding the hemostatic effectiveness of platelets collected and stored in CPDA.

The optimal concentration for glucose and adenine supplementation, especially of red cells stored as concentrates, should also be established. Because of the potential for toxicity with any additive, the minimum amount necessary to achieve the desired effect with reasonable consistency should be used. The existing data suggest that, for red cell concentrates with hematocrits of 75% or more, the amounts of both adenine and glucose in CPDA (which contains adenine to produce an initial 0.25 mM concentration in the whole blood from which the concentrates are prepared, and glucose at 1.25 times the standard CPD) may be less than optimal to sustain consistent viability in excess of 70% at five weeks of storage. This is especially true when donor variability, breaks in refrigeration, and possibly variations in the amount of leukocyte admixture(3) are considered. Increasing the glucose to 1.5 times the amount present in standard CPD might produce a more acceptable margin of safety and is not likely to be harmful.

In the absence of definitive data, it remains a matter
of opinion whether the slightly greater loss of DPG and
potential toxicity by increasing the amount of adenine out-
weigh the better assurance of efficacy with respect to
viability which a higher concentration is likely to provide.
A level nearer 0.5 mM, for example, 0.4 mM, may turn out to
be preferable because: 1) adenine toxicity is not a significant issue in this concentration range, except in the most
extreme transfusion circumstances; 2) preservation of viability is an absolute requirement, while the necessity for
DPG maintenance remains uncertain; 3) differences in the
rate of DPG loss within the range of 0.25 to 0.5 mM are
probably insignificant.

Finally, additional options such as supplementation
of red cell concentrates after platelet and plasma separation.
with or without artifical media,(67) or fortification with
adenine later in storage, with or without other additives,
should be explored further.(11,26,55)

SUMMARY

Anticoagulant citrate phosphate dextrose adenine solution
(CPDA) extends the shelf life of whole blood and red cell
concentrates from 21 to 35 days. Equally important, the
quality of the red cells with respect to viability during
the permissible shelf life is improved, an effect which
becomes increasingly significant after about ten days of
storage. The mechanism of action involves <u>net</u> synthesis
of adenine nucleotide due to continued incorporation of
adenine into adenine nucleotide throughout the storage
period, which delays the progressive fall in total adenine
nucleotide.

Adenine supplementation has little effect on the
oxygen delivery function of transfused red cells, and is
neither beneficial nor harmful to plasma components and
derivatives. The effect of CPDA on the hemostatic
effectiveness of platelet concentrates has not been reported.

1. Akerblom O, de Verdier C-H, Finnson M, Garby L, Högman CF, Johansson SGO (1967). Further studies on the effect of adenine in blood preservation. Transfusion 7:1.

2. Akerblom O, Kreuger A (1975). Studies on citrate-phosphate dextrose (CPD) blood supplemented with adenine. Vox Sang 29:90.

3. Ambrus JL, Ambrus CM, Okade K, Mink IB, Shields R, Warner W, Bishop C, Tritch GL, Golden G, Mittelman A (1975). Clinical and experimental studies on adenine, various nucleosides and their analogs in hematology. Ann New York Acad Sci 255:435.

4. Bartlett GR (1972). Effects of adenine on stored human red cells. Adv Exp Med Biol 28:479.

5. Bartlett GR (1972). In vivo metabolism of exogenous adenine in rabbit and man. In VI International Symposium über Struktur und Funktion der Erythrocyten. Berlin, Akademie-Verlag, p. 355.

6. Bartlett GR (1977). Biology of free and combined adenine; Distribution and metabolism. Transfusion 17:339.

7. Bartlett GR (1977). Metabolism in man of intravenously administered adenine. Transfusion 17:367.

8. Bensinger TA, Metro J, Beutler E (1975). In vitro metabolism of packed erythrocytes stored in CPD adenine. Transfusion 15:135.

9. Bessis M, Mohandis N (1975). Measurement of red cell deformability: Its utility in clinical medicine. Schweiz Med Wochenschr 105:1568.

10. Beutler E, Wood L (1969). The in vivo regeneration of red cell 2,3-diphosphoglyceric acid (DPG) after transfusion of stored blood. J Lab Clin Med 74:300.

11. Beutler E (1974). Experimental blood preservatives for liquid storage. In The Human Red Cell In Vitro. TJ Greenwalt and GA Jamieson, Eds. New York, Grune and Stratton Inc, p 189.

12. Bishop C (1960). Purine metabolism in human and chicken blood, in vitro. J Biol Chem 235:3228.

13. Bishop C (1961). Purine metabolism in human blood studied in vivo by injection of C^{14}-adenine. J Biol Chem 236:1778.

14. Bunn HF, May MH, Kocholaty WF, Shields CF (1969). Hemoglobin function in stored blood. J Clin Invest 48:311.

15. Button LN, Orlina AR, Kevy SV, Josephson AM (1976). The quality of over- and undercollected blood for transfusion. Transfusion 16:148.

16. Camp FR Jr, Shields CE, Kaplan HS, Lawrence, MW, McPeak ME
    (1969). Study of military blood banking and cross
    matching using blood group antigens stored over five
    months in ACD-adenine. Milit Med 134:1317.
17. Chanutin A (1967). The effect of the addition of adenine
    and nucleosides at the beginning of storage on the
    concentrations of phosphates of human erythrocytes during
    storage in acid-citrate-dextrose and citrate-phosphate-
    dextrose. Transfusion 7:120.
18. Chaplin H Jr, Beutler E, Collins JA, Giblett ER, Polesky H
    (1974). Current status of red-cell preservation and
    availability in relation to the developing national blood
    policy. N Engl J Med 291:68.
19. Collins JA (1976). Massive blood transfusion. Clin
    Haematol 5:201.
20. Dawson RB, Ellis TJ (1970). Hemoglobin function of blood
    stored at $4°$ in ACD and CPD with adenine and inosine.
    Transfusion 10:113.
21. de Verdier C-H, Garby L, Hjelm M, Högman C, Eriksson Å (1964).
    Adenine in blood preservation: Posttransfusion viability
    and biochemical changes. Transfusion 4:331.
22. de Verdier C-H, Groth T, Westman M (1974). Adenine
    metabolism in man: Interpretation of excretion data by
    means of a computer simulation model. Acta Universitatis
    Upsaliensis 181.
23. Duhm J, Gerlach E (1974). Metabolism and function of 2,3-
    diphosphoglycerate in red blood cells. In The Human Red
    Cell In Vitro. TJ Greenwalt and GA Jamieson, Eds,
    New York, Grune and Stratton Inc, p 111.
24. Falk JS, Lindblad GTÖ, Westman BJM (1972). Histopathological
    studies on kidneys from patients treated with large
    amounts of blood preserved with ACD-adenine. Transfusion
    12:376.
25. Graybeal FQ Jr, Mooreside DE, Langdell RD (1969). Clotting
    factor activity in cryoprecipitates and supernatant
    plasma prepared from blood collected into ACD, ACD-
    adenine, CPD, and CPD-adenine and from plasma collected
    by plasmapheresis. Transfusion 9:135.
26. Högman CF, Åkerblom O, Arturson G, de Verdier C-H,
    Kreuger A, Westman M (1974). Experience with new
    preservatives: Summary of the experiences in Sweden.
    In The Human Red Cell In Vitro. TJ Greenwalt and
    GA Jamieson, Eds, New York, Grune and Stratton, Inc,
    p 217.

27. Kashket S, Denstedt OF (1958). The metabolism of the erythrocyte. XVI. Adenylate kinase of the erythrocyte. Canad J Biochem 36:1057.

28. Kornberg A, Lieberman I, Simms ES (1955). Enzymatic synthesis of purine nucleotides. J Biol Chem 215:417.

29. Kreuger A (1973). Exchange transfusion with ACD-adenine blood. A follow-up study. Transfusion 13:69.

30. Kreuger A (1976). Adenine metabolism during and after exchange transfusion in newborn infants with CPD-adenine blood. Transfusion 16:249.

31. Kreuger A, Åkerblom O, Högman CF (1975). A clinical evaluation of citrate-phosphate-dextrose-adenine blood. Vox Sang 29:81.

32. Lowy BA, Williams MK, London IM (1962). Enzymatic deficiencies of purine nucleotide synthesis in the human erythrocyte. J Biol Chem 237:1622.

33. Manohar SV, Denstedt, OF, Rubinstein D (1966). The metabolism of the erythrocyte XVI. Incorporation of glucose into adenine nucleotides by human and rabbit erythrocytes. Canad J Biochem 44:59.

34. Manohar SV, Denstedt, OF, Rubinstein D (1967). The metabolism of the erythrocyte, XVII. Mechanism of incorporation of adenine into and resultant elevation of ATP and ADP in human erythrocytes. Canad J Biochem 45:1153.

35. Messeter L, Ugander L, Monti M, Lundh B, Löw B (1977). CPD-Adenine as a blood preservative – studies _in vitro_ and _in vivo_. Transfusion 17:210.

36. Moore GL, Ledford ME (1977). The uptake and egress of adenine from human red blood cells in vitro. Transfusion 17:38.

37. Mooreside DE, Graybeal, FQ, Langdell RD (1969). Effects of adenine on clotting factors in fresh blood, stored blood, and stored fresh frozen plasma. Transfusion 9:191.

38. Nakao M, Nakao T, Arimatsu Y, Yoshikawa H (1960). A new preservative medium maintaining the level of adenosine triphosphate and the osmotic resistance of erythrocytes. Proc Japan Acad 36:43.

39. Nakao M, Nakao T, Tatibana M, Yoshikawa H (1960). Phosphorus metabolism in human erythrocytes. III. Regeneration of adenosine triphosphate in long-stored erythrocytes by incubation with inosine and adenine. J Biochem 47:661.

40. Nakao M, Nakao T, Tatibana M, Yoshikawa H, Abe T (1959). Effect of inosine and adenine on adenosine triphosphate regeneration and shape transformation in long-stored erythrocytes. Biochim Biophys Act 32:564.

41. Ness PM, Pennington RM (1974). The National Blood Resource Program adenine experience. Transfusion 14:530.

42. Peck CC, Bailey FJ, Moore GL (1977). Enhanced solubility of 2,8 dioxyadenine (DOA) in human urine. Transfusion 17:383.

43. Preiss J, Handler P (1957). Enzymatic synthesis of nicotinamide mononucleotide. J Biol Chem 225:759.

44. Rosenfield RE, Berkman EM, Nusbacher J, Hyams L, Dabinsky C, Stux S, Hirsch A, Kochwa S (1971). Specific agglutinability of erythrocytes from whole blood stored at 4 C. Transfusion 11:177.

45. Shafer AW, Tague LL, Welch MH, Guenter CA (1971). 2,3-diphosphoglycerate in red cells stored in acid-citrate-dextrose and citrate-phosphate-dextrose. Implications regarding delivery of oxygen. J Lab Clin Med 77:430.

46. Shields CE, Bunn HF, Litwin SD, Reed LJ, Dauber LG (1969). Clinical evaluation of transfused blood after long-term storage in ACD with adenine. Transfusion 9:246.

47. Shields CE (1971). Effect of plasma removal on blood stored in ACD with adenine. Transfusion 11:134.

48. Simon ER, Chapman RG (1961). A role of adenine in red cell metabolism. Clin Res 9:167.

49. Simon ER, Chapman RG, Finch CA (1962). Adenine in red cell preservation. J Clin Invest 41:351.

50. Simon ER (1962). Red cell preservation: Further studies with adenine. Blood 20:485.

51. Simon ER, Sugita Y (1965). Red cell preservation. Addition of adenine to improve preservation in ACD-solution. Proc 10th Congr Int Soc Blood Transf Stockholm, Basel, Karger, p 607.

52. Simon ER (1967). Adenine and purine nucleosides in human red cell preservation: A review. Transfusion 7:395.

53. Simon ER Ed (1976). Workshop on Adenine and Red Cell Preservation. Transcript of Proceedings. Bureau of Biologics, Food and Drug Administration, Department of Health, Education, and Welfare, October 1-2.

54. Simon ER (1977). Adenine in blood banking. Transfusion 17:317.

55. Spielmann W, Seidl S (1974). Summary of clinical experiences in Germany with preservative-anticoagulant solutions with newer additives. In The Human Red Cell In Vitro. TJ Greenwalt and GA Jamieson, Eds, New York, Grune and Stratton, Inc p 255.

56. Sugita Y, Simon ER (1965). The mechanism of action of
    adenine in red cell preservation. J Clin Invest 44:629.
57. Sussman LN, Camacho D, Rosen E (1971). Use of adenine-ACD
    solution in long term storage of blood. Am J Clin
    Path 55:565.
58. Swisher SN (1977). The introduction of adenine fortified
    blood preservatives: Introduction and an interpretation
    of its history. Transfusion 17:309.
59. Tatibana M, Nakao M, Yoshikawa H (1958). Adenylate kinase
    in human erythrocytes. J Biochem (Tokyo) 45:1037.
60. Valeri CR, Hirsch NM (1969). Restoration in vivo of
    erythrocyte adenosine triphosphate, 2,3-diphosphoglycerate,
    potassium ion, and sodium ion concentrations following
    the transfusion of acid-citrate-dextrose-stored human red
    blood cells. J Lab Clin Med 73:722.
61. Valtis, DJ, Kennedy AC (1954). Defective gas-transport
    function of stored red blood cells. Lancet 1:119.
62. Wada T, Takaku F, Nakao K, Nakao M, Nakao T, Yoshikawa H
    (1960). Posttransfusion survival of the red blood cells
    stored in a medium containing adenine and inosine.
    Proc Japan Acad 36:618.
63. Warner WL (1970). Red cell preservation and survival
    determinations in anticoagulant systems. In Modern
    Problems of Blood Preservation. W Spielmann and S Seidl,
    Eds, Stuttgart, Gustav Fisher Verlag, p 63.
64. Warner WL (1977). Toxicology and pharmacology of adenine
    in animals and man. Transfusion 17:326.
65. Westman BJM (1972). Serum creatinine and creatinine
    clearance after transfusion with ACD-adenine blood and
    ACD blood. Transfusion 12:371.
66. Westman M (1974). Studies for elevation of blood preser-
    vation procedures with special regard to the oxygen
    release function and toxicity of adenine. Acta
    Universitatis Upsaliensis 181.
67. Wood L, Beutler E (1971). Storage of erythrocytes in
    artifical media. Transfusion 11:123.
68. Zuck TF, Bensinger TA, Peck CC, Chillar RK, Beutler E,
    Button LN, McCurdy PR, Josephson AM, Greenwalt TJ (1977).
    The in vivo survival of red cells stored in modified
    CPD with adenine: Report of a multi-institutional
    cooperative effort. Transfusion 17:374.

DISCUSSION

<u>Dr. Surgenor</u>: Ernie, I think we are all impressed by the careful approach that you have taken in this analysis of all the factors, and I just had one very small question. Is there any evidence on what adenine is going to do to the platelets and, further still, you didn't mention granulocytes and we are all beginning to get into them now--do you have any information on that front?

<u>Dr. Simon</u>: Let me take the granulocyte issue first. I would not envision that granulocyte separation would take place from blood collected into CPD adenine. Granulocytes would almost certainly be collected and separated immediately. I therefore don't see a practical need for studying the effect of CPD-adenine on granulocytes, and I'm not aware of any studies.

Many of the studies dealing with adenine and platelets were done in the late 60's. Adenine produced neither benefit nor harm. But at that time no studies were done regarding hemostatic effectiveness. Furthermore, most of the studies were done in ACD. Now ACD and CPD become virtually equivalent within a few days of storage. But on immediate collection and at the time the platelets are separated these are not equivalent solutions and I think we should require proof that these platelets in fact work. We feel that specific data on hemostatic effectiveness, i.e., correction of bleeding time and elevation of platelet count in hypoproliferative thrombocytopenic patients should be demonstrated.

<u>Dr. Brewer</u>: Is there any reason that if one wanted to rejuvenate these red cells after a period of time that they could not be frozen as Dr. Valeri described for blood collected in CPD itself?

<u>Dr. Simon</u>: No, no reason that I can see.

HYPOXIA, HYPEROXIA, AND OXIDANT STRESS

Chairman: R. Carrell

MECHANISMS OF COPPER TOXICITY IN RED CELLS

Paul Hochstein, K. Sree Kumar and Stephen J.
Forman
Department of Pharmacology
University of Southern California, School of
Medicine
Los Angeles, California   90033

It is well known that the acute toxicity of ingested
copper salts is often associated with hemolytic anemia. However, it is generally less widely recognized that disturbances
in the binding and distribution of endogenous copper, such
as take place in patients with Wilson's Disease may also be
manifested by altered erythrocyte survival. Recent reports
note that in these patients, who are deficient in ceruloplasmin, there is a spectrum of damage ranging from mild to ful-
minant intravascular hemolysis with a rapidly fatal course
(Iser, et al., 1974). One theory holds that after a prolonged stage of copper accumulation in the liver there is
cell necrosis and subsequent release of copper (Roche-Sicot
and Benhamou, 1977). The high levels of serum copper attained in such episodes would presumably have direct "oxidant"
effects on circulating erythrocytes which lead to their hemolysis.

The exact mechanisms of copper toxicity vis-à-vis the
red cell are not known. In many respects the hemolysis induced by copper in normal red cells appears to have the
features common to the acute hemolytic episodes associated
with the administration of "oxidant" drugs in individuals
with a deficiency of glucose-6-phosphate dehydrogenase
(G-6-PD deficiency). In these latter instances, we have
previously described the generation of hydrogen peroxide
from the so-called "oxidant" drugs (Cohen and Hochstein,
1964; Cohen and Hochstein, 1965; Hochstein, 1971) and the
role of G-6-PD in the detoxification of hydrogen peroxide
(Cohen and Hochstein, 1961). It has therefore been of special
interest to us that Metz and Sagone (1972) have reported that

The Red Cell, pages 669–681

hydrogen peroxide may also be generated as a consequence of the interaction of copper with normal human erythrocytes.

For many years most investigators believed that hydrogen peroxide was not a very interesting biological intermediate. However, in the years since the discovery of glutathione peroxidase (Mills, 1957) and the illucidation of the role of this enzyme in peroxide detoxification (Cohen and Hochstein, 1963) it has become clear that a major adaptation to aerobic life has involved the development of systems for dealing with this product of the two electron reduction of oxygen.

The existing literature on copper has made it seem likely that its deleterious effects in erythrocytes was related primarily to the toxicity of hydrogen peroxide not because of a special sensitivity to peroxide, as in the case of G-6-PD deficient cells, but rather because of the formation of peroxide in amounts that are excessive for even the detoxification mechanisms of normal cells.

In this paper, we describe some new experiments on the action of copper on red cell membranes. These experiments suggest that the metal may initiate the formation of hydrogen peroxide and the peroxidation of lipids through its interaction with membrane sulfhydryl groups. Our current view is that such peroxidation reactions, which lead to the formation of fluorescent polymers, are intimately associated with the hemolytic toxicity of copper.

RESULTS AND DISCUSSION

The elegant investigations of Rifkind (1974) and of Winterbourn and Carrell (1977) have made it abundantly clear that a primary source of peroxide generation in red cells treated with copper is through the acceleration of the autoxidation of hemoglobin to form methemoglobin and superoxide anions. This latter species may undergo either spontaneous or enzymatic dismutation to form hydrogen peroxide. Peroxide formed by such a mechanism might well account for the deleterious effects of copper on erythrocytes. For example, Boulard and his colleagues (1972) have reported that incubation of normal red cells with copper caused a dramatic inhibition of various glycolytic enzymes including hexokinase. Implicit in such findings is the view that in the absence of glycolysis, red cell ATP levels will fall, osmotic equilibrium will not

be maintained by active extrusion of sodium ions, and cells
will attain their critical hemolytic volume.

We too have investigated the inhibitory effects of
copper on red cell glycolytic enzymes and the results of these
experiments are shown in Table 1.

TABLE 1. The effect of $CuSO_4$ (0.2 mM) on the hexokinase activity of human erythrocytes after incubation
under either aerobic or anaerobic (argon) conditions
and in the presence of methemoglobin. Glucose, when
added, was at a final concentration of 5.0 mM. Incubations were carried out at 37° C. for 60 minutes.

Additions	Hexokinase Activity* (nmoles NADPH/min/mg Hb)		
	Aerobic	Anaerobic	$HbFe^{+3}$
1. None	0.47	0.48	0.29
2. $CuSO_4$	0.0 (100%)	0.37 (23%)	0.22 (24%)
3. Glucose	0.47	0.62	0.44
4. Glucose + $CuSO_4$	0.33 (30%)	0.59 (5%)	0.44 (0%)

* The figures in brackets are percentage inhibition

It may be seen in this Table that as a consequence of the
incubation of erythrocytes, under aerobic conditions, with
copper at a concentration of 0.2 mM there is complete inhibition of hexokinase activity. However, if the incubation
flasks are flushed with argon to remove oxygen prior to the
addition of the copper the inhibition of hexokinase is much
reduced. Not only is the inhibition of hexokinase more
marked in the presence of oxygen, but additionally, there is
a requirement for the presence of ferrous hemoglobin. This
may also be seen in the data of Table 1. When the cells are
pretreated with sodium nitrite, in order to convert ferrous
to ferric hemoglobin, and then incubated with copper, the
inhibition of hexokinase activity is again diminished. We
have also found that the addition of copper to crystalline
hexokinase does not result in inhibition of the enzyme unless
ferrous hemoglobin is included in the reaction mixture. It
is of interest that the hexokinase activity of nitrite-
treated cells is less than that of untreated cells (Table 1).
The mechanism of this effect is not clear. However, if not
the consequence of a direct effect of nitrite on hexokinase,

it may be the result of the generation of peroxide during
the interaction of nitrite with oxyhemoglobin in the pretreatment of these cells (Cohen, et al., 1964).

It may be seen in Table 1 that when glucose is included
in the incubation medium the effects of copper on red cell
hexokinase are greatly diminished either aerobically or
anaerobically and in the presence of methemoglobin. Glucose
has stimulatory effects on the hexokinase of anaerobically
incubated cells which are as yet unexplained.

These experiments demonstrate that although copper may
indeed produce inhibition of the glycolytic enzymes such as
hexokinase, as a consequence of its interaction with oxyhemoglobin and the formation of hydrogen peroxide, the
inhibition may be largely prevented if glucose is present in
the incubation medium. Although the data are not shown, with
these concentrations of copper (0.2 mM), cellular glutathione
levels are maintained in the presence of glucose. Apparently
adequate detoxification of hydrogen peroxide takes place
through the glutathione peroxidase pathway.

Despite the protection afforded by glucose against the
copper-induced inhibition of glycolytic enzymes this substrate
does not protect cells against hemolysis! This phenomenon
is illustrated in Table 2.

TABLE 2. The effects of glucose (5.0 mM), BHA (5.0 ug)
and EDTA (5.0 mM) on the hemolysis induced by $CuSO_4$
(1.0 mM) in human erythrocytes incubated at 37° C for
120 minutes.

Additions	Percent Hemolysis
1. None	1
2. $CuSO_4$	10
3. Glucose + $CuSO_4$	10
4. BHA + $CuSO_4$	1
5. EDTA + $CuSO_4$	1

Copper causes hemolysis of about 10% of the red cells during
a two hour incubation period. However, as shown in the Table
glucose has no protective effect on this hemolytic effect of
copper. Hemolysis is prevented by the addition of the lipid

antioxidant butylated hydroxyanisole (BHA) to the cells during
incubation. Of course, hemolysis is also prevented by chelation
of the copper with EDTA. The effect of BHA on copper-induced
hemolysis suggests that the formation of membrane lipid peroxides are associated with cell damage. The hemolytic consequence of the peroxidation of membrane lipids are well
known (Hochstein, 1966).

Because of the dramatic effect of BHA on copper-induced
hemolysis we also investigated the direct effects of copper
on the erythrocyte membrane. It may be noted in Figure 1
that the addition of copper at a concentration of 25 µM to
preparations of erythrocyte ghosts results in a prompt
oxidation of epinephrine to adrenochrome (curve 1) suggesting
the formation of superoxide radicals (McCord and Fridovich,
1969). In the absence of membranes, copper alone causes
some oxidation of epinephrine. This is shown in the curve
marked 3.

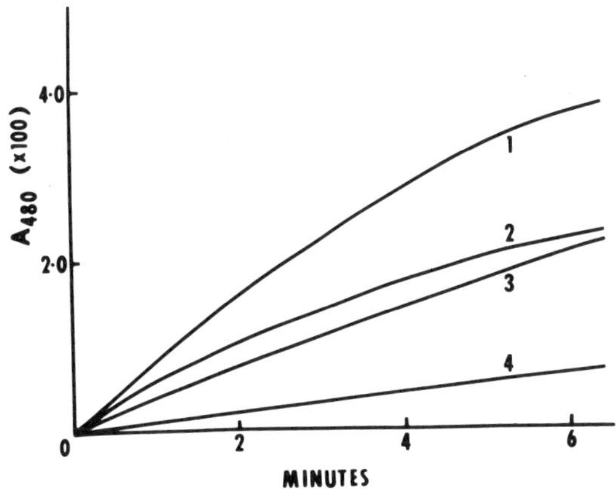

Figure 1.   The oxidation of epinephrine to adrenochrome in erythrocyte ghost preparations in the
presence of $CuSO_4$ (25 µM). The assays were carried
out at 37° C. in borate buffer (10mM), pH 10.1. Each
cuvette contained 0.3 mg of ghost protein. Superoxide
dismutase (10 units) was purified from bovine erythrocytes. See text for description of curves.

In the absence of copper there is little adrenochrome formation
(curve 4). Finally, if superoxide dismutase is included in the
incubation mixture the formation of adrenochrome is suppressed to
to the level seen in the absence of membranes (curve 2).
Parenthically, the generation of superoxide radicals is completely suppressed if the membranes are first treated with
pCMBS to complex SH groups prior to the addition of copper.

Figure 2 shows that the generation of superoxide in
membranes induced by copper is accompanied by the reduction
of cupric copper to the cuprous form. This effect is
illustrated by the upper curve (open squares) in the Figure.
Pretreatment of the cells with 0.1 mM pCMBS largely prevents
the reduction of copper in the presence of the ghosts. This
is illustrated by the curve with open circles in Figure 2.

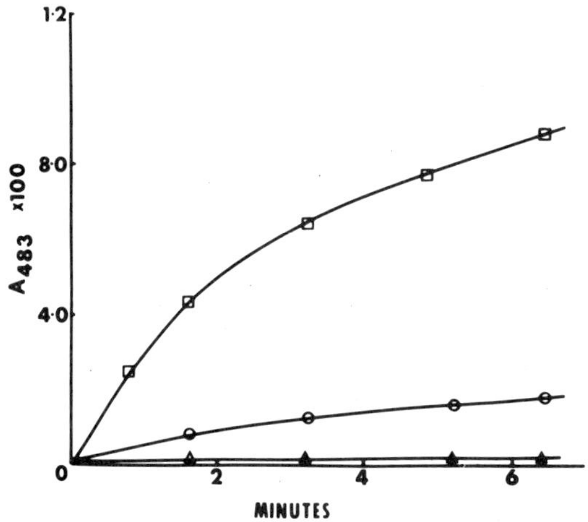

Figure 2. The reduction of Cu^{+2} to Cu^{+} by erythrocyte
ghost preparations. The bathocuproin method of Jensen,
et al., (1964) was utilized. The reactions were carried out at 37° C. in Tris-HCl (10 mM), pH 7.0. Each
cuvette contained 0.3 mg of ghost protein. See text
for description of curves.

In the absence of membranes as shown by the lower curve
(open triangles) in the Figure there is little detectable
formation of cupric copper.

The experiments described above suggest that the interaction of copper with membrane sulfhydryl groups results in
the generation of oxygen radicals which through dismutation
and peroxide formation have the potential to initiate the
peroxidation of endogenous lipids in the red cell membrane
and hemolysis. Thus, we have not been surprised to find the
presence of lipid peroxides in red cell membranes after incubation of the cells with copper. However, in addition to the
formation of lipid peroxides in copper treated cells one may
also observe the accumulation of fluorescent chromolipids.
This is illustrated in Figure 3.

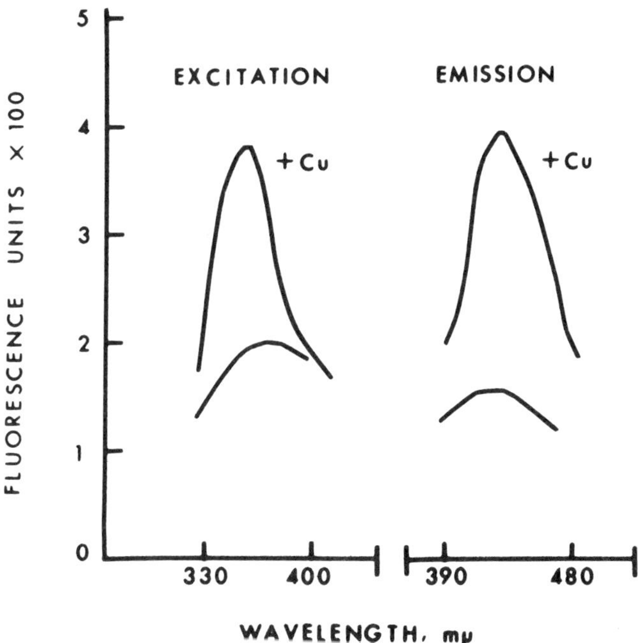

Figure 3. Fluorescent pigment formation in human
erythrocytes treated with $CuSO_4$ (25 mM).   Cells
were incubated for 120 minutes at 37° C. At the termination of the incubation the cells were washed three
times with isotonic saline solutions and the sedimented
cells extracted with isopropanol and chloroform in the
cold. The organic solvent layer was removed and the
fluorescent determined in a Farrand Spectrofluorimeter
standarized with quinine sulfate.

Lipofuscin of chromolipids have been long recognized products of the peroxidation of cellular lipids (Ciaccio, 1915). It has been suggested that their occurence in certain tissues is associated with the aging process (Strehler, et al., 1959). The concept that these fluorescent products are derived from peroxidized lipid is substantiated by the observation that their accumulation in the tissues of experimental animals is markedly reduced after the inclusion of lipid antioxidants in the diet (Tappel, et al., 1973). Presumably, the degradation of peroxidized lipid may lead to the formation of malonyl dialdehyde, an agent which cross-links the amino groups, either of lipids or of proteins, through the formation of Schiff bases (Chio, et al., 1969). Such cross-linked derivatives when formed with malonyl dialdehyde <u>in vitro</u>, have characteristics similar to the fluorescent pigments found <u>in vivo</u> (Chio and Tappel, 1969). Their exact solubility properties and excitation and emission spectra depend on whether they are derived from lipid or protein (DeVard and Tappel, 1973; Bidlack and Tappel, 1973).

The spectral characteristics of the fluorescent product formed after incubation of cells with copper and extraction with organic solvent are shown in Figure 3. The pigment has an excitation maximum at 365 nm and an emission maximum between 430-435 nm. Control cells incubated without copper display diminished and not well defined excitation and emission peaks in these areas. Although not shown in Figure 3, washing the cells with EDTA solutions to remove the copper at the end of the incubation period did not alter the intensity of the fluorescent peaks in these areas. This suggests that the fluorescent material is in fact formed during the incubation of the cells with copper and nor a consequence of the action of copper on the extracted lipids.

On the basis of the experiments described above we visualize effects of copper on the erythrocyte as illustrated in the diagram below.

There seems to be little question that copper has the capacity to accelerate the autoxidation of ferrous hemoglobin to form methemoglobin and superoxide radicals (Reactions A). These radicals may serve as a source of hydrogen peroxide through a dismutation reaction. The possibility must also be considered that copper may enhance the oxidation of glutathione and hydrogen peroxide (Reaction B). Such a reaction would not only form hydrogen peroxide but also deplete the cell of the reduced glutathione necessary for peroxide detoxification.

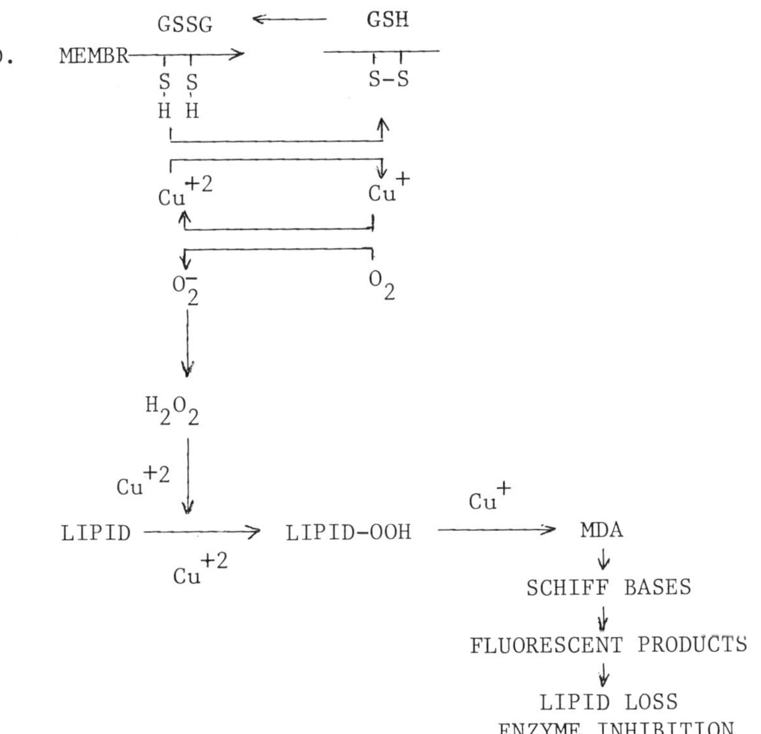

A. $Hb^{+2}-O_2 \longrightarrow Hb^{+3} + O_2^-$ (Cu^{+2})
$2O_2^- + 2H^+ \longrightarrow H_2O_2 + O_2$
B. $2GSH + O_2 \longrightarrow GSSG + H_2O_2$ (Cu^{+2})
C. GLUCOSE $\longrightarrow$ G-6P NADP 2GSH H$_2$O$_2$
6-PG NADPH GSSG H$_2$O
D. MEMBR GSSG GSH
S S S-S
H H
Cu^{+2} Cu$^+$
O$_2^-$ O$_2$
H$_2$O$_2$
Cu^{+2}
LIPID $\longrightarrow$ LIPID-OOH $\longrightarrow$ MDA
Cu^{+2} Cu$^+$
SCHIFF BASES
FLUORESCENT PRODUCTS
LIPID LOSS
ENZYME INHIBITION

Since we have found that at copper concentrations less than
one millimolar glucose is able to prevent the loss of glutathione and to protect glycolytic enzymes such as hexokinase
against inactivation but not prevent hemolysis, we assume that
peroxide generated by these intracellular mechanisms does not
play a major role in the ultimate hemolysis caused by copper.
Of course, at higher concentrations of copper the capacity of
the glutathione peroxidase system to detoxify peroxide and of
glucose to regenerate reduced glutathione (Reactions C) may
be compromised or overwhelmed.

We visualize a primary effect of copper to be on the
oxidation of membrane (pCMBS-sensitive) sulfhydryl groups to
form disulfides (Reactions D). This oxidation is accompanied
by the formation of cuprous copper which may oxidize with
molecular oxygen to generate superoxide anions. Since neither
glucose nor ethanol which act as scavengers of hydroxy radicals
prevent red cell lysis we presume that hydrogen peroxide formed
by dismutation of the superoxide within the membrane acts to
initiate the peroxidation of membrane lipids. It is possible
that copper participates in the breakdown of hydrogen peroxide
to yield initiating radicals not scavenged by glucose (or
ethanol). The direct participation of copper in an initiating
reaction by electron abstraction from unsaturated fatty acid
is also not excluded by the current experiments. We believe
it reasonable to posit that the membrane disulfides formed in
the presence of copper may be in equilibrium with intracellular
reduced glutathione, and hence they may be readily regenerated
so that a cyclic system for the reduction of large amounts of
membrane associated cupric ions through a smaller pool of
membrane sulfhydryl groups may function.

The formation of **lipid** peroxides in **itself** may be suffi-
cient cause for the disruption of membranes and hemolysis
through the loss of phospholipids (Jacobs and Lux, 1968).
Additionally, the finding of fluorescent pigments in copper
treated cells suggests that the lipid peroxides may be undergoing degradation to form malonyl dialdehyde (MDA) which has
the capacity to cross-link the amino groups of both lipids
and proteins through Schiff base formation. It is of interest
that we have previously shown that cuprous salts may accelerate
the breakdown of peroxidized lipids in hepatic microsomal
systems (Hochstein and Ernster, 1963) to form a variety of
short chain hydrocarbons which include ethane, ethylene as
well as malonyl dialdehyde (Lieberman and Hochstein, 1966).

Although the experiments described in this paper demonstrate the formation of fluorescent pigments in the material extracted from cells with organic solvents, it seems reasonable to assume that such products are also formed from proteins and would appear in aqueous extracts. In the former event, the formation of lipid polymers may enhance membrane lipid loss and cell damage. In the latter event, they may represent cross-linked and inactivated enzymes which are essential for the integrity of the erythrocyte and its membrane.

SUMMARY

The presence of serum copper in excess of the availability of ceruloplasmin leads to severe hemolytic disease. Hemolysis is apparently associated with the formation of hydrogen peroxide. The experiments reported in this paper indicate that peroxide generated intracellularly by low (less than 1.0 mM) copper concentrations is adequately detoxified in the presence of glucose via the glutathione peroxidase system. However, erythrocytes continue to hemolyze in the presence of glucose. For this reason, it is suggested that the primary cytotoxic effects of copper result from its interaction with membrane sulfhydryl groups. Such interaction leads to the formation of cuprous ions which may react with oxygen to form superoxide. Hydrogen peroxide generated within the plasma membrane by the dismutation of superoxide may participate in the initiation of lipid peroxidation, membrane damage and hemolysis. Hemolysis is prevented in the presence of lipid antioxidants such as butylated hydroxyanisole. The peroxidation of membrane lipids has been found to be associated with the accumulation of fluorescent pigments whose formation may further compromise the structure and function of the plasma membrane. In addition to its interaction with membrane sulfhydryl groups it is possible that copper also participates directly in the initiation of membrane lipid peroxidation and the formation of fluorescent products. It seems obvious that these complex actions of copper may have relevence to its toxicity in tissues other than the erythron.

ACKNOWLEDGEMENTS

This work was supported in part by grants from the National Institute of Health (HD-08159 and CA-05297).

REFERENCES

Bidlack, W.R., and Tappel, A. (1973). Fluorescent products of phospholipids during lipid peroxidation. Lipids 8(4):203.

Boulard, M., Blume, K.G., and Beutler, E. (1972). The effect of copper on red cell enzyme activities. J. Clin. Inves. 51:459.

Chio, K.S., Reiss, V., Fletcher, B., and Tappel, A. (1969). Peroxidation of subcellular organelles: Formation of lipofuscinlike fluorescent pigments. Science 166:1535.

Chio, K.S., and Tappel, A.L. (1969). Synthesis and characterization of the fluorescent products derived from malonaldehyde and amino acids. Biichem. 8:2821.

Ciaccio, C. (1915). Untersuchungen über die Autoxydation der Lipoidstoffe und Beitrag zur Kenntnis einiger Pigmente (Chromolipoide) und Pigmentkomplexe. Biochem. Z. 69:313.

Cohen, G., and Hochstein, P. (1961). Glucose-6-phosphate dehydrogenase and the detoxification of hydrogen peroxide in human erythrocytes. Science 134:1574.

Cohen, G., and Hochstein, P. (1963). Glutathione peroxidase: The major pathway of peroxide detoxification of erythrocytes. Biochem. 2:1420.

Cohen, G., and Hochstein, P. (1964). Generation of hydrogen peroxide in erythrocytes by hemolytic agents. Biochem. 3:895.

Cohen, G., Martinez, M., and Hochstein, P. (1964). Generation of hydrogen peroxide during the reaction of nitrite with oxyhemoglobin. Biochem. 3:901.

Cohen, G., and Hochstein, P. (1965). In vivo generation of hydrogen peroxide in mouse erythrocytes by hemolytic agents. J. Pharm. Exp. Therap. 147:139.

Dillard, C.J., and Tappel, A. (1973). Fluorescent products from reaction of peroxidizing polyunsaturated fatty acids with phosphatidyl ethanolamine and phenylalanine. Lipids 8:183.

Hochstein, P., and Ernster, L. (1964). Microsomal peroxidation of Lipids and its possible role in cellular injury. Ciba Foundation Sym. on Cellular Injury, 123.

Hochstein, P. (1966). Antioxidant mechanisms associated with lipid peroxidation. Proc. III Intern. Conf. Hyperbaric Oxygen, Publ. No. 1404, National Academy of Sciences.

Hochstein, P. (1971). Glucose-6-phosphate dehydrogenase deficiency: Mechanisms of drug-induced hemolysis. Exp. Eye Res. 11:389.

Iser, J.H., Stevens, B.J., Stening, G.F., Hurley, T.H., and
    Smallwood, R.A. (1974). Hemolytic anemia of Wilson's
    Disease. Gastroenterology 67:290.
Jacob, H.S., and Lux, S.E. (1968).Peroxidation of membrane
    phospholipids and thiols in peroxide hemolysis: Studies
    in vitamin E deficiency. Blood 32:549.
McCord, J.M., and Fridovich, I. (1969). Superoxide Dismutase:
    An enzymatic function for erythrocuprein. J. Biol. Chem.
    244:6049.
Metz, E.N., and Sagone, A.L. (1969). The effect of copper
    on the erythrocyte hexose monophosphate shunt pathway.
    J. Lab Clin. Med. 80:405.
Mills, G.C. (1957). Hemoglobin catabolism, Part I. Gluta-
    thione peroxidase, an erythrocyte enzyme which protects
    hemoglobin from oxidative breakdown. J. Biol. Chem. 229:189.
Rifkind, J.M. (1974). Copper and the autoxidation of
    hemoglobin. Biochem. 13:2475.
Roche-Sicot, J., and Benhamou, J.P. (1977). Acute intravascular
    hemolysis and acute liver failure associated as a first man-
    ifestation of Wilson's Disease. Ann. Intern. Med. 86:301.
Strehler, B.L., Mark, D.D., Mildwan, A.S., and Gee, M.V.
    (1959). Rate and magnitude of age pigment accumulation
    in the human myocardium. J. Geront. 14:430.
Tappel, A., Fletcher, B., and Deamer, D. (1973). Effects
    of antioxidants and nutrients on lipid peroxidation,
    fluorescent products and aging parameters in the mouse.
    J. Geront. 28:415.
Winterbourn, C.C., and Carrell, R.W. (1977). Oxidation of
    hemoglobin by copper: Mechanism and suggested role of
    thiol group of residue β93. Biochem. J. 165:141.

DISCUSSION

Dr. Jacob: I think it should be pointed out that patients
with Wilson's disease rarely hemolyze, although there are
scattered case reports of such occurring. In this regard
you might be interested in studies we performed some time
ago in which we generated superoxide or hydrogen peroxide
about red cells using xanthine/ xanthine-oxidase or glucose/
glucose-oxidase, respectively. We obtained no detectable
hemolysis unless the red cells came from vitamin E deficient
animals. Therefore, I wonder about the vitamin E status
of your donors. I also wonder whether the rare patients
with Wilson's disease who evidently do hemolyze may, in
fact, be in poor nutritional balance and thus be deficient
in this important lipid anti-oxidant.

Dr. Hochstein: I wonder if I can refer that question to my
colleague, Dr. Forman , who has followed several patients
that we've seen at USC and perhaps can comment more directly than I about the importance of anemia in Wilson's disease.
I think he may disagree with you.

Dr. Forman: I think the first statement you made about hemolysis being rare in Wilson's disease is probably true and
I think that's probably true because of several things that
we noted in reviewing both the literature and our patients
in Los Angeles with Wilson's disease. One of the things
that was noted about these patients was that hemolytic anemia
was a problem only on presentation of Wilson's disease. You
will never find anybody who's been treated for Wilson's
disease having hemolysis, the thought being that untreated
Wilson's disease represents a problem in copper accumulation
in the tissues, and that at a certain point in time a lot
of copper is released from the liver. Characteristically,
in people with Wilson's disease, you will find in the blood
a low ceruloplasmin and a low serum copper. In contrast,
patients with hemolysis in Wilson's disease tend to have
low ceruloplasmins and elevated coppers. Obviously with
no ceruloplasmins, since that is the major copper binding
protein, most of this copper will be relatively free and,
we think, act as an oxidant stress. Several years ago
Dr. Dice in Salt Lake reported a woman who had Wilson's
disease and was treated with penicillamine, the standard
of treatment as it presently stands. Because she desired
to become pregnant and the effects of penicillamine not
being known on the fetus, the medicine was discontinued.

The Red Cell, pages 683—686

Obviously when one discontinues the penicillamine the state of
copper accumulation begins, and in fact, nine months later she
developed hemolysis. Now, she represents one case that was
fairly well studied of that nature. On the other hand, when
patients present with hemolysis with Wilson's disease they
are generally sicker than ordinary patients who present
with Wilson's disease. The amount of hepatic necrosis and
ongoing active active disease is usually more significant so
that it's conceivable that from a dietary point of view they
would be like any other hepatic patient. To what extent
their vitamin E may be low and contributing therefore to
ongoing nonprotection of oxidant stress of copper may in
fact be a factor but it's never been measured. But I think
the important thing to remember about hemolysis in Wilson's
disease is that it only occurs at presentation and is always
associated with at least normal or elevated serum coppers
which is a direct distinction to the ordinary circumstance
of Wilson's disease which is obviously a condition of trapped
copper within the tissues.

Dr. Hutquist: Do you see any room for the so-called "NADH-
cytochrome reductase" (that is on the inside of red cell
membranes) playing a role either in the copper-induced
peroxide formation or in the case where you saw production
of cuprous ion from cupric ion? Perhaps a small amount of
membrane-bound NADH is present.

Dr. Hochstein: Since finding some years ago that hepatic
endoplasmic reticulum contains an NADPH-dependent system
for inducing the formation of lipid peroxides, we have been
continually interested in the possibility that it also exists
in the red cell and is dependent on metals such as iron and
copper. We've found no evidence for the presence of such
a system. It would be attractive if there were an NADH or
NADPH metal-requiring lipid-peroxidizing system that used
the cytochrome B5 of the red cell to produce lipid peroxides.

Dr. Brewer: I was wondering why the glucose dosen't protect
against the membrane sulfhydryl damage as opposed to the
enzyme hexokinase protection. Does that infer that the
GSH system in the cytosol is not available, that these
sulfhydryl groups of the membrane are not available to the
GSH of the cytosol?

Dr. Hochstein: I presume that glucose protects against
glycolytic inhibition through its maintenance of reduced

glutathione in the cell and consequent peroxide detoxification. On the other hand, the generation of peroxide or
radicals within the membrane may make them unavailable to
intracellular glutathione peroxidase. This may account for
the peroxidation in the membranes which is not prevented
by glucose under conditions in which enzyme inhibition is
prevented.

Dr. Brewer: People have said, at least I have tended to say,
that intracellular glutathione protects the membrane sulfhydryl groups, the enzyme sulfhydryl groups, and the hemoglobin sulfhydryl groups. This suggests that not all the
membrane sulfhydryl groups are available.

Dr. Hochstein: Yes, presumably there are membrane SH groups
not available to intracellular glutathione. It is also possible that copper induces cell damage by initiating electron
abstraction from unsaturated fatty acids and directly causing lipid peroxidation. Such a mechanism would not involve
SH groups. I'm willing to leave open the question of what
the effect of copper is. I think it may turn out, when
the story is all told, that we have a variety of things going
on at the same time, all contributing to cell damage. Perhaps we should not look for a single mechanism for the
copper effect.

Dr. Winterbourn: Concerning the last question about membrane
sulfhydryl groups, in the mechanism you propose, the membrane
sulfhydryl groups are oxidized by reaction with copper, and
a product of the reaction goes on to give lipid peroxidation.
Even if the membrane disulfides produced were accessible to
the intracellular glutathione system, and could be reduced,
this would not prevent the membrane damage. The other question I would like to ask is do you have any evidence that the
membrane sulfhydryl groups are more reactive towards copper
than say reduced glutathione or other sulfhydryl compounds?
Do you think there is a very specific copper binding site?

Dr. Hochstein: No, we have not studied the reactivity of
membrane SH groups versus that of either glutathione or
protein SH groups.

Dr. Orringer: Dr. Hochstein, have you had a chance to
examine G6PD-deficient patients and the effect of copper on
them? Also have you looked at the rate of the hexosemonophosphate shunt pathway as a function of the copper concentration?

<u>Dr. Hochstein:</u> No, we have not. But Metz and Sagone have carried out such experiments (J. Lab Clin. Med. 80:405, 1972).

HEMOGLOBIN AUTOXIDATION: THE RISK TO THE RED CELL
AND THE CONTRIBUTION OF COPPER

R.W. Carrell[1], R. Krishnamoorthy[2], and C.C. Winterbourn[3].

1. Dept. of Clinical Biochemistry,
   University of Cambridge, Cambridge

2. Institut de Pathologie Moléculaire,
   Université de Paris, Paris.

3. Pathology Dept,, Christchurch Hospital,,
   Christchurch, New Zealand.

INTRODUCTION

There is good evidence to support the proposition that
hemoglobin is a modified oxygenase or oxidase. The prime
mechanism of these enzymes is an activation of oxygen which
occurs by electron transfer to the oxygen from the heme. This
process has been modified in the hemoglobin molecule by the
evolution of the globin to enclose the heme in an environment of low dielectric constant. This allows the process to
be reversible; the gain and loss of oxygen being accompanied
by the transfer of negative charge backwards and forwards
between the oxygen and the heme group.

Oxyhemoglobin can therefore be regarded as a ferric
superoxide (Collman et al, 1976). This was predicted by Weiss
(1964) who pointed out that the spontaneous formation of
methemoglobin should be accompanied by the release of superoxide. (O_2^-) i.e.

$$Hb\ Fe^{3+}O_2^- \rightarrow HbFe^{3+} + O_2^- \qquad 1$$

This has been subsequently confirmed experimentally by Misra
and Fridovich (1972) and others.

It follows that the red cell will be exposed to a continuous production of O_2^- even under physiological conditions.
Fluctuations in the conformation of the globin will, from
time to time, allow the displacement of O_2^- , the methaemoglobin formed being reduced again to the ferrous form by the
NADH-diaphorase system.

The Red Cell, pages 687—695

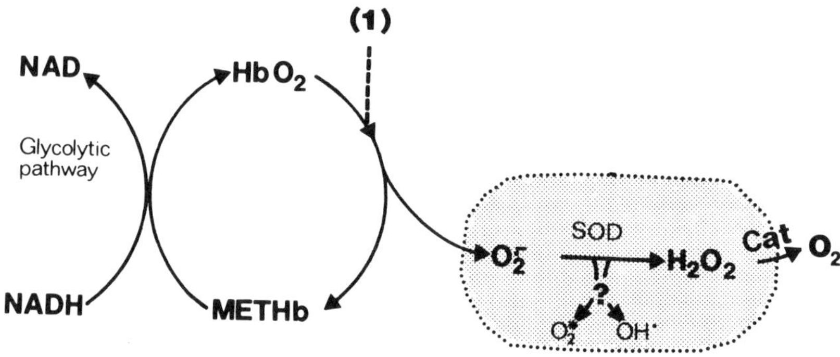

Figure 1. A continuous cycle of activated oxygen production exists as shown, which will be amplified by factors giving an increased formation of methemoglobin by an. O$_2^-$ displacement mechanism (1). (SOD superoxide dismutase; Cat. catalase).

Just how significant this production is and to what extent it poses a threat to the red cell is not clear as yet. Two particular questions to be answered are; what proportion of methemoglobin formation in the red cell is coupled to superoxide release and what damage does this produce ?

TOXICITY OF SUPEROXIDE

The universal presence of superoxide dismutase in aerobic cells provides inferential evidence of the toxicity of O$_2^-$. In the red cell the dismutase is present in a concentration equivalent to that of catalase, there being one dismutase and catalase molecule for each thousand of hemoglobin. However, the study of the action of O$_2^-$ in isolated systems indicate that it is relatively benign in itself. It reacts with hemoglobin to give, as a preferential reaction, oxidation to methemoglobin and with methemoglobin to give reduction to oxyhemoglobin, i.e. the reverse of equation 1 (Sutton, Roberts and Winterbourn 1976).

Work we have done (with J.K. French) demonstrated that in some circumstances O$_2^-$ may even have a protective function as in the reaction of acetylphenylhydrazine with oxyhemoglobin (Fig. 2). Here the O$_2^-$ produced in the reaction is apparently acting as a scavenger of other free radicals. Its removal with superoxide dismutase increased the rate of loss of oxyhemoglobin whereas additional production of O$_2^-$ from xanthine and xanthine oxidase, decreased the rate of loss.

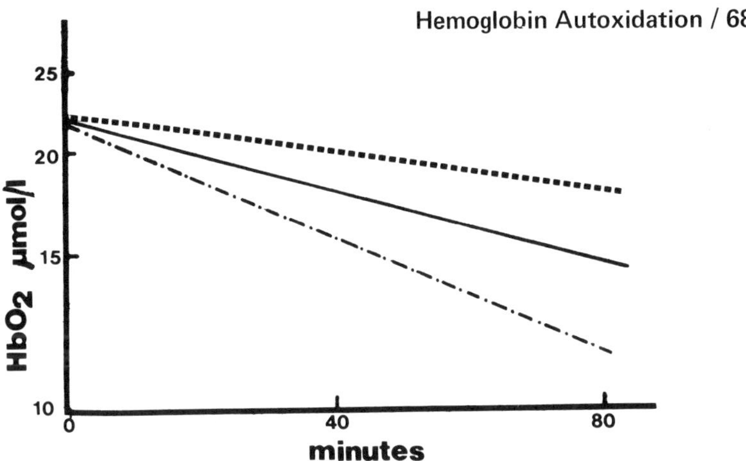

Figure 2. A semi-log plot of the rate of oxidation of oxy-hemoglobin by acetylphenylhydrazine. Initial concentrations of oxyhemoglobin and acetylphenylhydrazine were 20μM. All solutions contained catalase.——, no other additions;—·—, plus superoxide dismutase;····, plus xanthine and xanthine oxidase.

These findings in isolated systems are supported by red cell experiments in which hemolysis is induced by ultra-violet radiation (Michelson & Durosay, 1977). Although O_2^- was the major product, it was shown that it was not directly involved in the membrane lysis. Goldberg and Stern (1977) using large external production of O_2^- were able to produce membrane lysis which was associated with attachment of denatured hemo-globin to the cell membrane. This reinforces the view that it is not superoxide itself that is directly the damaging species but a product, such as the hydroxyl radical, formed by inter-action with Fe(II) ions and hydrogen peroxide. An intriguing alternative is the interaction with hemoglobin itself to give direct catalysis of membrane oxidation (Carrell, French and Winterbourn, 1977).

FORMATION OF METHEMOGLOBIN

An estimated 3% of the red cell hemoglobin undergoes autoxidation to methemoglobin each day. We have studied the factors contributing to *in vitro* autoxidation using isolated hemoglobin (Winterbourn, McGrath and Carrell, 1976, Winter-bourn and Carrell, 1977). The most important factor is the presence of copper ions. Addition of 0.9μM $CuSO_4$ to 28μM oxyhemoglobin (i.e. one Cu(II) ion per 120 heme groups) gave a fourfold increase in the rate of autoxidation. Fe(II) or Fe(III) ions also gave increased autoxidation, although with

less than 1% the efficiency of copper. Even at 1:1 concentration with heme groups, Fe(II) and Fe(III) ions only gave a
40-70% increase in rate. Co(II), Pb(II) and Cd(II) ions did
not contribute to autoxidation.

The addition of EDTA abolishes the copper effect. As
Fig. 3 shows, the autoxidation that occurs in the absence of
copper is accompanied by superoxide release.

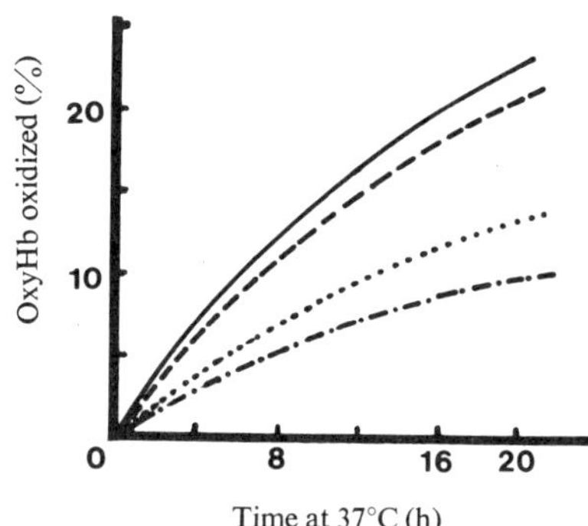

Fig. 3. The autoxidation of oxyhemoglobin in the absence of
copper. Isolated oxyhemoglobin A incubated at 37° in
0.067M phosphate buffer pH 7.4 containing 0.11 M NaCl and
5ᵐᴹEDTA ——, control; ----, +SOD; ·····, + Cat.;-·-·-,+SOD + Cat.

The removal of the hydrogen peroxide by catalase slowed
down the rate of oxidation to about 60% and the dismutation of
O_2^- slows it down further to about 35% of the original rate.
This demonstrates that oxidation is accompanied by the
production of O_2^- which in turn oxidises further hemoglobin
both directly and via consequent peroxide production. The
per cent inhibitions observed are in fair agreement with the
overall stoichiometry

$$4Fe(II)O_2 + 4H^+ \rightarrow 4Fe(III) + 2H_2O \qquad (2)$$

ROLE OF COPPER

The oxidation of hemoglobin by copper has been described
by Rifkind (1974) and colleagues (1976) and Winterbourn and
Carrell (1977). There are four high affinity binding sites
for copper on each hemoglobin (tetramer) molecule. The first
pair of sites are as yet unidentified but the second pair
involve the SH group of the β-93 cysteines. Bonding of

this second pair is accompanied by rapid oxidation of 50% of the hemoglobin to methemoglobin. The evidence supports a mechanism involving direct electron transfer from the β-chain heme iron as below:

$$Cu(II) \quad + \quad Fe(II)\ S^- \quad \rightarrow \quad Cu(I) + Fe(11)S^{\bullet} \quad (3)$$

$$Fe(II)\ S^{\bullet} \quad \rightarrow \quad Fe(III)\ S^- \quad\quad\quad (4)$$

This is a rapid reaction but there is also a slower production of O_2^- due to the oxidation of the cuprous ion by oxygen with subsequent oxidation of more hemoglobin

$$Cu(I) + O_2 \quad \rightarrow Cu(II) \quad + O^-_2 \quad\quad (5)$$

Thus there are two types of oxidation stimulated by copper; a rapid oxidation involving stoichiometric concentrations of copper and a slower, copper catalysed oxidation, taking place at much lower copper concentrations. In both mechanisms the initiating reaction is the direct oxidation of the β-93 cysteine residue.

From the *in vitro* results there is good reason to support the proposition of Rifkind, 1974, that the copper-catalysed reaction may be the prime source of methemoglobin in the red cell. We have examined this possibility by following the formation of oxidation hybrids.

Materials and Methods

Hemoglobin was prepared from human red cells both as standard 5% aqueous hemolysate and in purified form by DEAE Sephadex chromatography. The solutions were diluted with an equal volume of phosphate buffer 0.067 M, pH 7.4; and 50 mM copper sulphate or freshly prepared potassium ferricyanide added to give the required molar ratios. Isoelectric-focusing was carried out on polyacrylamide gel columns containing ampholytes in the range pH 6-8, as described by Drysdale, Righetti and Bunn (1971) and modified by Krishnamoorthy Wajcman and Labie (1977). Samples were usually applied within three minutes of preparation but only minor differences in results were noticed when samples were left to stand for longer periods (up to 1 hour).

Results and Discussion

As Fig. 4 shows, the addition of a 2:1 molar ratio of ferricyanide gives the expected 50% oxidation divided between methemoglobin and two partially oxidised hybrids IBI (αIIβIII) and IBII (αIIIβII); Park,(1973).The addition of copper sulphate in progressively increasing molar ratios from 0.25:1 hemoglobin tetramer up to 2:1 leads to the appearance of a new, as yet unidentified acidic component. After the molar ratio exceeds 2:1 oxidation products begin to appear, being virtually solely confined to the hybrid IBI (i.e. $\alpha II \beta III$) and reaching a maximum at a molar ratio of 4:1 (Fig. 4).

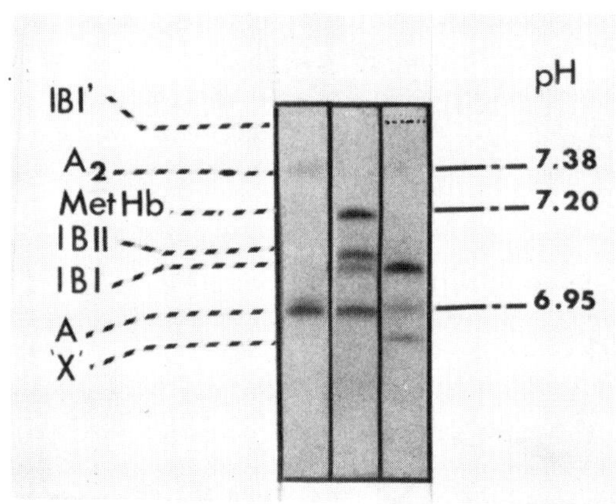

Figure 4.   Isoelectric focusing of (from left to right) normal hemolysate; plus 2:1 ferricyanide; plus 4:1 copper sulphate. The addition of copper has produced a fast 'X' component but otherwise there is almost complete conversion to IBI ($\alpha II \beta III$). Hb A_2 in the same sample has similarely been converted to IBI' ($\alpha II\ \delta III$).

Thus the oxidation of hemoglobin by copper is confined in the first instance to the β-chain, the presence of superoxide dismutase and catalase *in vivo* preventing the non-specific oxidation that follows O_2^- release. Consequently, if copper is contributing significantly to *in vivo* autoxidation a predominance of the β-oxidised hybrid would be expected. Such a predominance is seen in autoxidised (pH 7.5)hemolysates in the absence of EDTA (Bunn and Drysdale, 1971). However, hemolysates which have had EDTA added, give on autoxidation a pattern in which the α-oxidised hybrid predominates. This confirms that the proportion of each hybrid will give an indication as to whether copper catalysed oxidation has occurred.

The test is to examine hemolysates from autoxidised whole cells. These show a predominance of the α-oxidised hybrid. This is seen convincingly in Fig. 5 which shows the electrophoresis of hemolysate obtained from the patients of Mast et al (1976) with an NADH diaphorase deficiency.

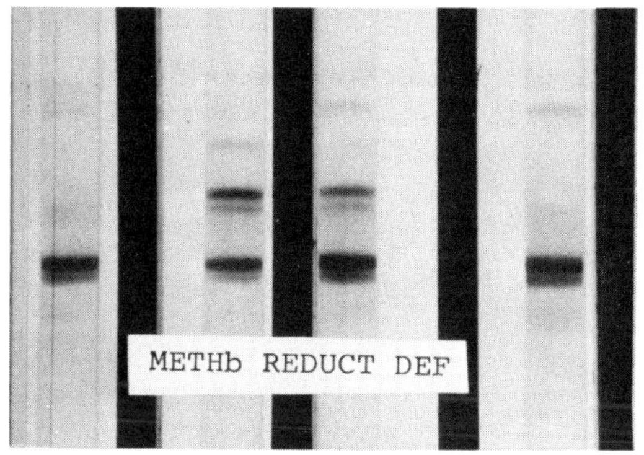

Figure 5.   Isoelectric focusing of hemolysates from NADH-diaphorase deficient brothers(centre marked) compared with unaffected members of the same family. Note the predominance of IBII (αIIIβII) in the affected samples.

Conclusions

These results should be interpreted with caution as allowance has to be made for the pH dependence of the oxidation hybrids (Bunn and Drysdale, 1971) and the results, at this stage, are observational rather than quantitative. Nevertheless, they do provide a strong indication that copper is not a major contributor to the physiological autoxidation of hemoglobin.

SUMMARY

The process of reversible oxygenation involves an activation and deactivation of oxygen with transfer of partial negative charge from the heme to the oxygen. The reversibility of this reaction is dependent on the maintenance of an apolar environment surrounding the heme group. Fluctuations or perturbation of this environment allow displacement of the oxygen as superoxide with the formation of methemoglobin. Two questions follow. What proportion of the methemoglobin formation within the red cell is accompanied by superoxide release and what damage does this superoxide produce ?.

These questions are only partially answered by *in vitro* experiment. There is strong circumstantial evidence that superoxide does result in cell damage but our experimental findings with isolated systems is that, by itself, it is relatively benign and may even act protectively as a free radical scavenger. The danger arises *in vivo* from the interaction of superoxide with free iron or heme groups to give the formation of the hydroxyl free radical or direct function of hemoglobin as an oxidase/oxygenase

The study of autoxidation of *isolated* hemoglobin emphasises the predominant role of copper ions. When copper is removed there is a substantial decrease in oxidation to a base level that appears to be due to a superoxide displacement reaction. The *in vivo* contribution of each of these can be studied by the use of isoelectric focusing. The primary oxidation of hemoglobin by cupric ions is confined to the β-chains and gives solely the hybrid (αIIβIII). However, hemoglobin from autoxidised red cells, or NADH-diaphorase deficient cells, contain predominantly, the other hybrid (αIIIβII). This *indicates* that copper is not a major contributor to the physiological autoxidation of hemoglobin.

ACKNOWLEDGEMENTS

This work was supported by grants and a research fellowship (RWC) from the Institut Nationale de la Santé et la Recherche Médicale of France and in part by a grant from the Medical Research Council of New Zealand.

REFERENCES

Bunn HF and Drysdale JW (1971). The separation of partially oxidised hemoglobins. Biochim Biophys Acta 229:51.

Carrell RW, Winterbourn CC and French JK (1977) Haemoglobin A frustrated oxidase? Implications for red cell metabolism. In Press: Hemoglobin.

Collman, JP, Brauman JI, Halbert TR and Suslick KS (1976). Nature of O_2 and CO binding to metalloporphyrins and heme proteins. Proc. Natl Acad Sci 73:333.

Drysdale JW, Righetti P and Bunn HF (1971). The separation of human and animal hemoglobins by isoelectric focusing in polyacrylamide gel. Biochim biophys Acta 229:42.

Goldberg B and Stern A (1977). The role of superoxide anion as a toxic species in the Erythrocyte. Archives of Biochemistry and Biophysics, 178:218.

Krishnamoorthy R, Wajcman H and Labie D (1976). Isoelectric focusing: A method of multiple applications for hemoglobin studies. Clin Chim Acta 69:203.

Mast A, Milo R, Junien C, Leroux A, Krishnamoorthy R, Wajcman H, Labie D and Kaplan JC (1976) Congenital enzymopenic methaemoglobinaemia. Acta Haematologica 56:174.

Michelson AM and Durosay P (1977). Hemolysis of human erythrocytes by activated oxygen species. Photochemistry and Photobiology 25:55.

Misra HP and Fridovich (1972). Generation of superoxide radical during autoxidation of hemoglobin. Journal of Biological Chemistry 247:6960.

Park CM (1973). Isoelectric focusing and the study of interacting protein systems. Ann. New York Acad Sci 209:237.

Rifkind JM (1974). Copper and the autoxidation of hemoglobin. Biochemistry 13:2475.

Rifkind JM, Lauer LD, Scott C, Chiang C and Norman C Li (1976). Copper and the oxidation of hemoglobin: A comparison of horse and human hemoglobins. Biochemistry 15:5337.

Sutton HC, Roberts PB and Winterbourn CC (1976). The rate reaction of superoxide radical ion with oxyhaemoglobin and methaemoglobin. Biochem J 115:503.

Weiss JJ (1964). Nature of iron-oxygen blood in oxyhaemoglobin. Nature (London) 202:83.

Winterbourn CC, McGrath BM and Carrell RW (1976). Reactions Involving Superoxide and Normal and Unstable Haemoglobins. Biochem J 155:493-502.

Winterbourn CC and Carrell RW (1977). Oxidation of Human Haemoglobin by Copper. Biochem J 165:141-148.

DISCUSSION

Dr. Hochstein: Can you make any comments about the toxicity
of superoxide in the red cell? Isn't is more likely that
other radicals generated by the Haber-Weiss reaction are of
greater importance?

Dr. Carrell: I think this gets back to the point that I
rather skipped over in the talk, and again that was raised
by Dr. Jacob that you can demonstrate that the superoxide
and hydrogen peroxide are being formed by these systems.
You can also demonstrate that damage is occurring, but it's
been a frustrating experience, not merely in the red cells
but also in other cells, that by and large you can't reproduce damage by external stimulation with superoxide and
hydrogen peroxide. There does seem to be another factor.
Possibilities are the interaction with a third body such as
iron to give you the hydroxyl radical or direct catalysis
as occurs with the copper mentioned in your talk. The other
factor is localization and this is a point that Slater from
London makes very strongly, that in fact it's not merely the
species that you're producing but where you're producing it
and to what you're exposing it.
     But I think it likely that damage involves another
free radical, most likely, the hydroxyl radical.

Dr. Mizukami: I'm interested from the practical aspect of
hybrid formation. You mentioned that the hybrid seems to
be reasonably stable in your experiment but you also mentioned that it could be unstable depending upon pH. You
must have meant unstable exchange from alpha to beta oxidation and so on.

Dr. Carrell: Yes, I meant exchange with the other hybrid. But
it is remarkably stable. You can produce a bottle of the
$\alpha_{II}\beta_{III}$ form and leave it in the fridge for two or three days
and come back and refocus it and get basically the same material, although some shift has occurred.

Dr. Mizukami: I think you mentioned during your talk, but I
did not quite get it. That is, in the so-called normal
methemoglobulin reductase deficient patient, the alpha-chain
seems to be the oxidized form.

Dr. Carrell: Yes.

The Red Cell, pages 697—699

<u>Dr. Mizukami</u>: Could you tell me why it was so?

<u>Dr. Carrell</u>: Well, if you remember in the talk of Tucker, which opened this session, it was pointed out that the alpha chain has a water associated with the distal histidine. This would make it just that much more vulnerable to perturbation, so I think from a theoretical or crystallographic point of view, one would predict that the alpha chain would be more liable to autoxidation. This is well documented, in fact Dr. Winterbourn and others have shown that the alpha chain autoxidizes much more readily than does the beta chain.

<u>Dr. Brewer</u>: I'd like to respond to the question, is superoxide dangerous to your health? I think that at least in one situation, G6PD deficiency, we have circumstantial evidence that it is. In a series of studies started several years ago, we, by we I mean Rosanne Leipzig, who's doing her thesis work on this topic, asked the question whether or not the hemolytic drugs cause hemolysis in G6PD deficiency by virtue of superoxide production. I think that to answer the question of damage from superoxide it is not necessary to prove that superoxide is actually the damaging species if one can show that it is the initiating species which then leads to damage. If it is, I think one can conclude that it is damaging to your health. What Rosanne has been able to show is that a number of these drugs, acetylphenylhydrazine and menadione among others, do produce superoxide. Since these early papers she has gone on and done a very nice series of studies. What happens if you expose intact red cells to superoxide-generating systems is, in the case of G6PD deficient red cells, a sequence of events in which the glutathione levels drop, methemoglobin forms, and Heinz bodies develop and there is a little hemolysis. Normal cells are almost completely resistant to this sequence. This is the same sequence, of course, that you see in vivo when you administer hemolytic drugs, first the drop in glutathione, then methemoglobin formation, then Heinz bodies, and then the hemolysis. The work is in vitro, but I'm convinced at least, that superoxide is a species which leads to hemolysis. This may explain something that has been puzzling, why do infections sometimes precipitate hemolysis in G6PD deficiency? Because superoxide is produced.

<u>Dr. Carrell</u>: I completely agree. I agree with your conclusions, too, but I think in talking to Rosanne it isn't a simplistic relationship. In fact rather exasperatingly super-

oxide dismutase doesn't abolish the observed toxicity which
demonstrates that the role of superoxide is indirect in
this system.

Dr. Brewer: This may be because subsequent metabolites cause
the damage.

Dr. Hultquist: Do you get any evidence for the hybrid with
one alpha ferric and one beta ferric or do you get any minor
band where only one of the four hemes would be oxidized?

Dr. Carrell: Hemoglobin can be regarded as being formed of
two alpha-beta dimers. The electrophoretic procedure is
actually focusing the dimers. So, we are really looking
at dimers although they will restabilize to tetramers. Naturally, the tetramers will be made up of symmetrical (or
identically oxidized) dimers so there is no way of telling
whether in fact there is a single oxidized chain in the in
vivo situation. But of course, it is a reasonable assumption that the process occurs through the oxidation of just
one iron in the tetramer.

Dr. Labie: The evidence of the two hybrids was mostly
brought through hemoglobins M. We had M alpha and M beta
hemoglobins and we found only one of the hybrids in each
case. Our M alpha and M beta mutants showed each a single
band on electrofocusing migrating respectively like the
hybrids IB II and IB I.

BACTERIAL SITES OF OXYGEN TOXICITY POTENTIALLY COMMON TO RED
CELLS AND ERYTHROPOIESIS.

Olen R. Brown, Frederick Yein and Daniel Boehme
John M. Dalton Research Center and
Department of Veterinary Microbiology
University of Missouri
Columbia, Missouri 65201

There is abundant evidence that radical species of
oxygen are generated during metabolism, and that these
radicals are toxic at the cellular level for species from
bacteria through man (Haugaard, 1968; Fridovich, 1975).
Enzymes such as superoxide dismutase, catalase and peroxi-
dases, reducing agents and free-radical scavengers play
significant roles in protecting cells from oxidative damage
during metabolism in an air environment. However, elevated
oxygen tensions apparently can overwhelm these systems, and
cellular damage occurs. Erythrocytes, like other cells, are
subject to damage from oxygen toxicity. This has become
of increased significance because of the increased use of
elevated oxygen in therapy, and in the maintenance of
personnel in undersea and outerspace environments.

There is evidence that elevated oxygen tension
(hyperoxia) is toxic for, and causes hemolysis of red cells
especially during vitamin E deficient states (Larkin, Adams,
Williams, and Duncan, 1972; Johnson, Jefferson, and Mengel,
1972; Fee and Teitelbaum, 1972). Superoxide anion has been
incriminated in the mechanism of damage (Goldberg and Stern,
1977) and autoxidation of erythrocyte hemoglobin provides a
continuous source of such radicals in red cells. There is
also considerable evidence that hyperoxia impairs erythropoiesis (Fishman, Leonard, Gorshein, Besa, Jepson, and
Gardner, 1973; Kaplan, Piliero, Gordon, and Meagher, 1977;
Voitkevich, Myasnikov, and Shcherba, 1976; Voitkevich,
Volzhskaya, and Myasnikov, 1976) although contradictory
results have been found (Barkova and Petrov, 1976). The
erythrocytes of the newborn and of premature infants may

The Red Cell, pages 701—714

be particularly susceptible to oxygen toxicity because their
red cells contain less superoxide dismutase (Bonta, Gawron,
and Warshaw, 1977; Legge, Brian, Winterbourn, and Carrell, 1977).

BACKGROUND

Most, if not all, life forms are subject to oxygen
toxicity and microorganisms have been used in our research
as convenient model cells for basic biochemical studies of
cellular and subcellular sites of oxygen damage. We
hypothesize that some fundamental damage sites may be common
to many life forms at the cell level. The damage results
not from molecular oxygen but from radicals which arise because oxygen possesses unpaired electrons and tends to react
by one electron transfer (Fig. 1). In our recent research
the oxygen sensitivities of enzymes and coenzymes in specific biosynthetic pathways have proved to be of special
relevance. The broad objective is to increase understanding
of fundamental sites of oxygen toxicity as a basis for extending the safe utilization of hyperoxia in therapy and in
breathing mixtures for deep-water diving.

FIGURE 1.

OXYGEN REACTS CHEMICALLY BY UNIVALENT REDUCTION

$$O_2 + e^- \longrightarrow O_2^{1-} \text{ (superoxide radical)}$$

$$O_2 + 2e^- + 2H^+ \longrightarrow H_2O_2 \text{ (hydrogen peroxide)}$$

$$O_2 + 3e^- + 3H^+ \longrightarrow H_2O + OH^{\cdot} \text{ (hydroxy radical)}$$

$$O_2 + 4e^- + 4H \longrightarrow 2 H_2O$$

We have previously established several basic sites of
oxygen poisoning in Escherichia coli; some are possibly
involved in oxygen poisoning of cells of higher life forms
including red blood cells. In basal salts plus glucose
medium at 37°C, growth of E. coli stops within 0.05 generations upon pressurization of a stirred liquid culture to
4.2 atm of oxygen (Brown, Yein, Mathis, and Vincent, in
press). Upon reincubation in air, growth is rapidly

restored (Brown, Yein, Mathis, and Vincent, in press; Brown, 1970; Brown, Howitt, Stees and Platner, 1971). The inhibition is not produced by pressure, per se since similar exposures to hyperbaric N_2 or He do not affect the growth rate. The inhibition of growth occurs before inhibition of transport (Brown, Yein, Mathis, and Vincent, in press), respiration (Brown, 1972), fatty acid synthesis (Brown, Howitt, Stees, Platner, 1971; Yein and Brown, 1977), oxidative phosphorylation (Brown, 1971), or decrease in ATP (Brown, Yein, Mathis, and Vincent, in press; and Mathis and Brown, 1976), although all are reduced in intact bacteria after growth stops.

Experiments with various mutants in medium fortified with, or deficient in specific amino acids provide data to support the following sequence of events during oxygen intoxication. Oxygen inhibits biosynthesis of ten identified amino acids (Boehme, Vincent, and Brown, 1976). Valine inhibition appears to be most significant and within less than 5 minutes the intracellular concentration of valine is limiting for protein synthesis. Subsequently 9 other amino acids [tyrosine, isoleucine, tryptophan, leucine, phenylalanine, cysteine, methionine, asparagine, and threonine (listed in order of decreasing order of effect)] become limiting if valine is supplied (Boehme, Vincent, and Brown, 1976).

The simplest interpretation of these data is that hyperbaric oxygen significantly impairs synthesis of the amino acids whose inclusion provide protection. Presumably, oxygen poisons specific enzymes required for synthesis of these amino acids.

Using intermediates of the various suspect pathways, the potentially sensitive enzymes have been reduced to approximately eight (Boehme, Vincent, and Brown, 1976). α-Ketoisovalerate substitutes for leucine indicating that the four enzymes required for converting α-ketoisovalerate to leucine, are functional in oxygen-poisoned cells. In the parallel pathways for biosynthesis of leucine, valine and isoleucine, there is apparently an impairment in oxygen-poisoned cells of acetohydroxy acid synthetase, acetoxy acid reductoisomerase or dihydroxy acid dehydratase, since α-ketobutyrate does not substitute for isoleucine. The presence of valine is most critical for protection from oxygen toxicity. With valine biosynthesis blocked before

α-ketoisovalerate, and no valine in the medium, the cells
not only would lack valine for protein synthesis, but could
not make pantothenate or products from pantothenate such
as coenzyme A. Valine transaminase is not sensitive since
α-ketoisovalerate substitutes for valine. Leucine is the
least critical of the branched-chain amino acids for growth
protection in hyperoxia, perhaps because valine transamina-
tion is reversible and valine in the medium could provide a
source of α-ketoisovalerate for the non-blocked series of
reactions leading to leucine synthesis.

Protection from oxygen toxicity was also provided by
the aromatic amino acids and by certain of their precursors.
Interpretation of protection by these compounds requires
consideration that there are three isozymes for the production of deoxyheptulosonic acid 2-phosphate and two isozymes
for production of prephenic acid, and separate feedback and
repression mechanisms by the three aromatic amino acids of
the isozymes, and of the enzyme which converts chorismate to
anthranilate. To minimize these problems and to induce
permeability to the compounds, bacteria were grown in each
different medium to adapt them before exposure to hyperbaric
oxygen in the same medium.

Deletions of individual aromatic amino acids, with
inclusions of each of four intermediates, suggest several
conclusions (Boehme, Vincent, and Brown, 1976). Deletion
of phenylalanine decreases protection less than deletion of
either tryptophan or tyrosine, suggesting that the enzymes
in the part of the pathway common to the biosynthesis of
all three aromatic amino acids (shikimate kinase,
pyruvylshikimate-phosphate synthase or chorismate synthase)
are less sensitive than one or more enzymes in the branch
pathways from chorismate to tryptophan and tyrosine. There
is no significant inhibition of the series of enzymes required for converting anthranilate to tryptophan.

The synthesis of cysteine from serine is apparently
impaired in hyperbaric oxygen (Boehme, Vincent, and Brown,
1976). Homocysteine substitutes for methionine; hence,
the oxygen sensitive step occurs before homocysteine synthesis and the methyl transferase enzyme appears to be relatively insensitive to hyperbaric oxygen. The sensitive site
in methionine synthesis probably also accounts for the
fact that threonine protects during exposure to hyperbaric
oxygen. Asparagine protects during exposure to hyperbaric

oxygen apparently because of inhibition of asparagine synthetase.

RESULTS AND DISCUSSION

Inhibition of RNA Synthesis by Hyperbaric Oxygen.

Amino acid deprivation would result during oxygen intoxication of E. coli in minimal medium because of the inability to synthesize certain amino acids as explained in the "Background" section. This would result in failure to aminoacylate tRNA. The "unloaded" tRNAs should stimulate the well-known "stringent response" (inhibition of many cell processes known to occur during amino acid starvation via production of the regulatory compounds, pp-guanosine-pp, and ppp-guanosine-pp). Various processes including transport, and synthesis of RNA and lipids are inhibited strongly by these polyguanosine phosphate regulatory compounds. This would effectively stop growth when bacteria are exposed to hyperbaric oxygen in medium without critical amino acids. Preliminary data confirm that the stringent response is, indeed, evoked by hyperoxia. Strains which show the stringent response and "relaxed" strains which do not, were compared for radioactivity incorporated into protein, RNA and DNA in 4.2 atm of oxygen vs. air (Fig. 2). Comparisons were also made (Fig. 2) during protection from inhibition of protein synthesis by inclusion of critical amino acids, and between the effects of hyperbaric oxygen and chloramphenicol (the latter, although it blocks protein synthesis, does not result in unloaded tRNAs and does not produce the stringent response). From these data it appears that: (a) in both stringent and relaxed strains, inhibition of protein synthesis occurs because of inhibition of synthesis of specific amino acids, (b) in the absence of protein synthesis, DNA synthesis continues to completion of the chromosome but new rounds of replication are not initiated, (c) RNA synthesis in hyperoxia does not occur in either stringent or relaxed strains in the absence of protein synthesis, but occurs proportional to protein synthesis, suggesting specific damage within the pathway of RNA synthesis and that protein synthesis permits repair, and thus, (d) the stringent response contributes significantly to the mechanism by which oxygen inhibits growth in minimal medium.

FIGURE 2.
FAILURE OF RNA & PROTEIN SYNTHESIS IN HYPEROXIA IN A
RELAXED STRAIN, AND RESTORATION BY AMINO ACIDS

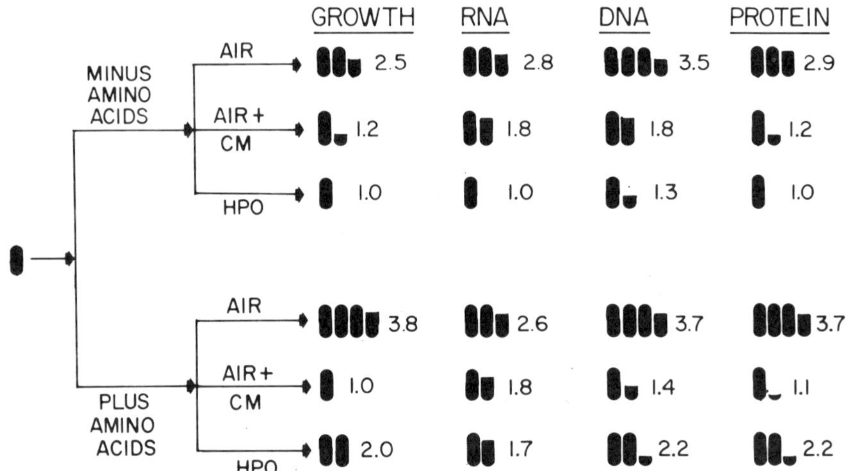

DEPENDENCY OF RNA SYNTHESIS-INHIBITION BY HYPEROXIA ON
PROTEIN SYNTHESIS-INHIBITION IN A STRINGENT STRAIN

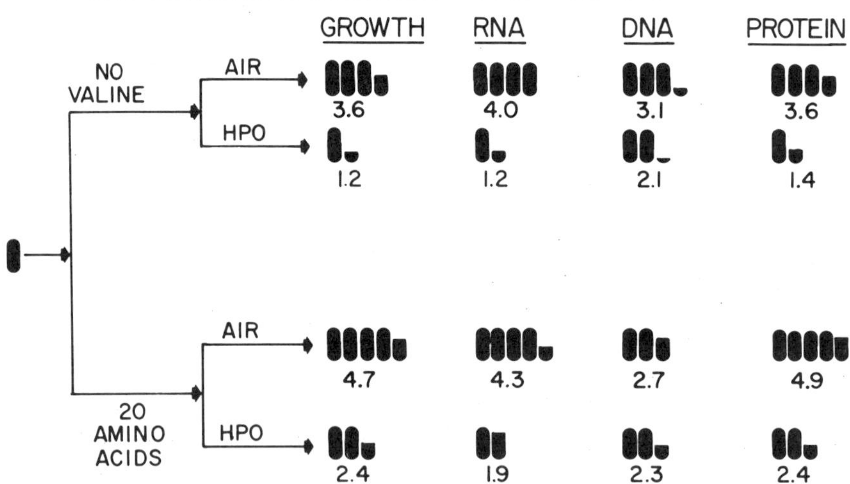

CM = Chloramphenicol; HPO = 4.0 atm O_2 + 1 atm air.

Inhibition of Synthesis of NAD, Thiamine and PRPP.

When the amino acids are supplied, protection from the inhibition of protein synthesis and from the stringent response in hyperoxia would be expected to occur. Indeed bacteria continue to grow for approximately 1 hr in hyperoxia in the presence of amino acids before growth stops. We have found that quinolinate-5-phosphoribosyl transferase (an enzyme required for NAD synthesis), 5-phosphoribose pyrophosphokinase (an enzyme required for synthesis of NAD and of RNA, as well as other cell functions) and possibly an enzyme required for synthesis of thiamine, are oxygen-sensitive. This was determined by measuring the protective effect of various metabolites on the toxicity of oxygen (Fig. 3).

FIGURE 3.

EFFECTS OF VITAMINS ON GROWTH OF E. COLI IN HYPEROXIA

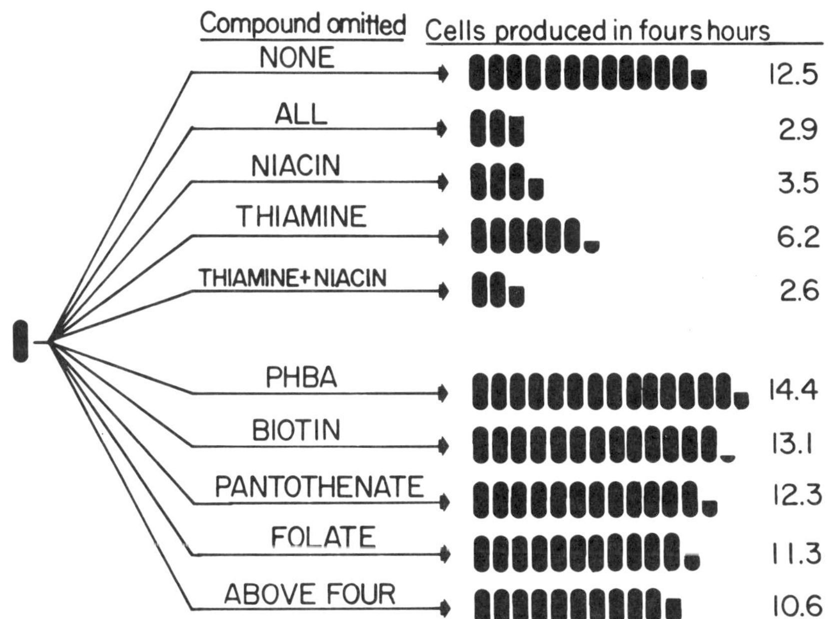

Among sixteen compounds tested, only niacin, and thiamine gave increased growth during exposure to 4.2 atm of oxygen with amino acids supplied to prevent toxicity from failure

of protein synthesis and stringency. For example, the
generation time at 37°C with air as the gas phase is
25 + 0.4 min. In minimal medium without protective amino
acids and vitamins, growth stops in 0.05 generations with a
gas phase of 4.2 atm of oxygen. In 4.2 atm of oxygen, 2.57
generations are completed in the first 2 hrs and 1.80
additional generations are produced over the second 2 hrs in
hyperbaric oxygen in the best protective medium. When
thiamine is deleted from this medium, only 1.90 and 0.74
generations are produced over the first and second 2 hr
intervals, respectively, in hyperbaric oxygen. With deletion
of niacin only 1.61 and 0.21 generations, respectively,
occur. The large impairments in growth during the second
2 hr intervals are particularly suggestive of failure of
synthesis of these vitamins in hyperbaric oxygen.

Both thiamine and niacin are synthesized by man, but in
quantities insufficient for the needs. NAD can be synthesized from niacin (nicotinate) which is in the salvage
pathway (Fig. 4). Deletion of niacin (nicotinate) with
substitution of intermediates in the synthesis and salvage
pathways of NAD, revealed that neither quinolinate nor
quinolinate plus 5-phosphoribosyl-pyrophosphate were
protective but that NMN, NAD, and niacinamide were protective (Fig. 4). This was confirmed using two mutant strains
which grow with quinolinate as a sole carbon source, thus
insuring that quinolinate was transported. However it was
not determined if 5-phosphoribosyl-pyrophosphate was transported. This compound is also relatively unstable. Thus
in the NAD biosynthetic pathway, quinolinate phosphoribosyl-
transferase or 5-phosphoribose pyrophosphokinase are apparently the oxygen-sensitive enzyme(s).

Experiments were done to measure the effect on
quinolinate transferase and 5-phosphoribose pyrophosphokinase, of exposure of bacteria to 4.2 atm of oxygen.
Quinolinate transferase is oxygen sensitive (Table 1). The
loss of enzyme activity was much greater when cells were
incubated in hyperoxia with amino acids present to permit
growth to continue (Table 1). Growth stops almost instantly
in medium without the protective amino acids (Fig. 5) and
apparently continuation of metabolism in hyperoxia produces
higher amounts of superoxide anions and other oxygen radicals, which are the damaging species. 5-Phosphoribose
pyrophosphokinase was also found to be completely inactivated in preliminary experiments. It appears to be more

FIGURE 4.

SITE OF OXYGEN INHIBITION OF NAD BIOSYNTHESIS

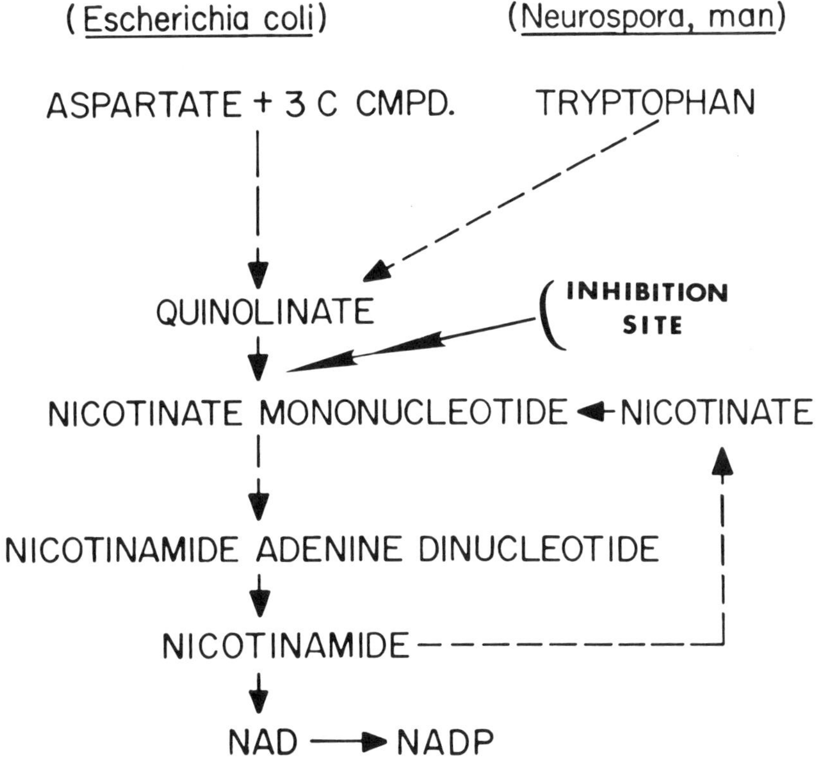

sensitive and is inactivated in bacteria exposed without amino acids. The specific activity of 5-phosphoribose pyrophosphokinase in cells grown with air as the gas phase was 18 + 1 nmoles PRPP per mg protein per hour in crude extracts, and nil in extracts of E. coli exposed to 4.2 atm of oxygen for 30 min. Up to 14 mg protein/assay from oxygen-poisoned cells was used while 4 mg protein/assay was adequate for assays of air-grown cells.

TABLE 1.

Effects of exposure to hyperbaric oxygen on quinolinate transferase activity in _Escherichia coli_.

Condition[b]	Specific Activity (μU/mg)[a]	
	Crude extract	$(NH_4)_2SO_4$ fraction
Air Control without A.A.	41.9 ±2.11(5,20)	43.1 ± 3.43(2,8)
HPO without A.A.	31.5 ± 1.54(2,8)[c]	20.1 ± 1.68(2,8)[c]
HPO with A.A.	3.3 ± 0.31(3,8)[c]	3.2 ± 0.23(2,7)[c]

[a]Average ± 1 S.E.M. for the number of experiments and total determinations shown in parenthesis.

[b]HPO = 1 atm air plus 4 atm oxygen for 1 hr in medium with or without 20 amino acids (A.A.).

[c]Significantly lower ($p \leq 0.001$) compared to air control, using student's t test.

Quinolinate transferase is ubiquitous in both prokaryotic and eukaryotic cells, including human cells, (Fig. 4) and is required for NAD synthesis (Gholson, 1966; Rechsteiner, Hillyard, and Olivera, 1976a; and Rechsteiner, Hillyard, and Olivera, 1976b). NAD, in addition to being an essential coenzyme for more than 200 metabolic reactions, is actively consumed by cell metabolism and recent published data show half-lives of approximately 2 hr in animals, 2 hr in _E. coli_, and 1 hr in a human tissue cell culture (Rechsteiner, Hillyard, and Olivera, 1976b). In hyperbaric oxygen with synthesis of NAD blocked, dilution of the intracellular concentration of this coenzyme occurs due to growth and because of very active catabolic processes. Thus, the concentration of this coenzyme become limiting for growth. Indeed, in earlier work, we had reported a decline in NAD during oxygen poisoning of _E. coli_ (Brunker, and Brown, 1971). The NAD inhibition site may be relevant to

FIGURE 5.

EFFECT OF HYPERBARIC OXYGEN (4.2 ATM) ON SYNTHESIS IN E. COLI

INCORPORATED IN:	CARBON ATOMS (IN BILLIONS)
One generation in air (amt. needed to produce one cell)	**6.42**
Hyperoxia (before growth stops)	**0.27 (4.2%)**

erythropoiesis but probably not to mature red cells since NAD synthesis occurs in the nucleus (Rechsteiner, Hillyard, and Olivera, 1976b). The PRPP inhibition site could be relevant to mature red cells.

Specific reactions affected by a lack of thiamine would include the synthesis of branched-chain amino acids (because of the time-course, this cannot be the sole reason for failure to synthesize branched-chain amino acids in hyperoxia, however); the pentose shunt pathway which provides NADPH needed for reductive biosynthesis, and intermediates for nucleic acid and aromatic amino acid synthesis; and the decarboxylation-dehydration reactions of α-ketoglutarate and pyruvate. Interestingly, the steps catalyzed by the latter complexes have been reported as sites of oxygen inhibition in animal tissues.

Since mature red cells do not have nuclei, and do not grow and multiply it appears that some or all of the biosynthetic inhibitions reported herein may be irrelevant for circulating erythrocytes. However, these inhibition

sites may be critical with respect to limitations of
erythropoiesis in elevated oxygen tensions.

SUMMARY

   Exposure to hyperbaric oxygen produces abrupt inhibition of growth in _Escherichia_ _coli_ in minimal medium with
glucose as the sole carbon source. The growth inhibition
is reversed by incubation in air. Lipid, DNA, and protein
synthesis machinery as well as the enzymes of glycolysis,
Krebs cycle and oxidative phosphorylation, and the transport machinery appear to be relatively resistant and remain
functional for up to 4 generations (the maximum tested to
date). Certain amino acids (principally aromatic and
branched-chain) provide partial protection and growth may
be maintained for approximately one hour. Further supplementation with thiamine and niacin give additional protection and growth, although with a longer generation time,
can be maintained to produce population densities equivalent
to those reached with air as a gas phase. By testing the
protective effects of various intermediates in the amino
acid and NAD biosynthetic pathways, several enzymes appear
to be sites of oxygen poisoning. The effects of exposure of
cells to hyperbaric oxygen, on two suspected sensitive
enzymes have been measured. Both quinolinate transferase
and 5-phosphoribose pyrophosphokinase are very sensitive to
hyperoxia. Niacin and other intermediates beyond quinolinate in the NAD biosynthetic pathway apparently protect
because these two enzymes are poisoned by hyperbaric oxygen.
Phosphoribosyl pyrophosphate (PRPP) is synthesized by
5-phosphoribose pyrophosphokinase and PRPP is needed for
several biosynthetic processes other than NAD synthesis
including synthesis of RNA. This may partially explain why
RNA synthesis fails in hyperbaric oxygen.

   The sequence of events in oxygen poisoning of _E._ _coli_
thus appears to be as follows. There is rapid inactivation
(perhaps within seconds) of certain enzymes required for
biosynthesis of certain amino acids (primarily the
branched-chain and the aromatics). Protein synthesis stops
for lack of amino acids. The lack of amino acids also
triggers the "stringent response" with production of
polyguanosine phosphates which are powerful inhibitors of a
variety of biosynthetic processes. If amino acids are
provided, protein synthesis continues, the biosynthetic

inhibitions of "stringency" are not observed and growth continues until it is limited by the lack of thiamine and niacin. These two vitamins apparently can not be synthesized in adequate amounts in hyperoxia. In the case of niacin, this occurs because two enzymes required for niacin and NAD biosynthesis are oxygen-sensitive. One of these sensitive enzymes is required for synthesis of PRPP which is required for other biosynthetic processes including RNA synthesis. This may explain the failure of RNA synthesis in "relaxed" (non-stringent) mutants.

These events appear to give considerable understanding of oxygen poisoning in E. coli. To the extent that the oxygen-sensitive enzymes are present and essential to functioning in mature red cells or to the erythropoietic system, they would appear to be relevant there as well.

REFERENCES

Barkova EN, Petrov V (1976). Effect of hyperbaric oxygen in the recovery period after hemorrhagic collapse. Bull Exp Biol Med 81:153.
Bonta BW, Gawron ER, Warshaw JB (1977). Neonatal red cell superoxide dismutase enzyme levels: possible role as a cellular defense mechanism against pulmonary oxygen toxicity. Pediat Res 11:754.
Brown OR (1970). Survival of bacterial cells in hyperoxic environments. In "Extreme Environments, Mechanisms of Microbial Adaptation," NASA-Ames Research Center, Moffett Field, California p 50.
Brown OR (1971). Resistance of oxidative phosphorylation in Escherichia coli to hyperoxia. J Bioenerg 2:217.
Brown OR, Howitt HF, Stees JL, Platner W (1971). Effects of hyperoxia on composition and rate of synthesis of fatty acids in Escherichia coli. J Lipid Research 12:692.
Brown OR (1972). Reversible inhibition of respiration in Escherichia coli. Microbios 5:7.
Brown OR, Yein F, Mathis RR, Vincent K (In Press). Oxygen toxicity: comparative sensitivities of membrane transport, bioenergetics and synthesis in Escherichia coli. Microbios.
Brunker RL, Brown OR (1971). Effects of hyperoxia upon oxidized and reduced NAD and NADP concentrations in Escherichia coli. Microbios 4:193.
Boehme DE, Vincent K, Brown OR (1976). Oxygen toxicity: inhibition of amino acid biosynthesis. Nature 262:418.

Fee JA, Teitelbaum HD (1972). Evidence that superoxide dismutase plays a role in protecting red blood cells against peroxidative hemolysis. Biochem Biophys Res Comm 49:150.

Fishman DR, Leonard RA, Gorshein D, Besa EC, Jepson JH, Gardner FH (1973). Stem cell damage induced by hyperoxia. Biomed 19:291.

Fridovich I (1975). Superoxide dismutases. Ann Rev Biochem 44:147.

Gholson RK (1966). The pyrimidine nucleotide cycle. Nature 212:934.

Goldberg B, Stern A (1977). The role of the superoxide anion as a toxic species in the erythrocyte. Arch Biochem Biophys 178:218.

Haugaard N (1968). Cellular mechanisms of oxygen toxicity. Physiol Rev 48:311.

Johnson WP, Jefferson D, Mengel CE (1972). _In vivo_ formation of H_2O_2 in red blood cells during exposure to hyperoxia. J Clin Inv 51:2211.

Kaplan SM, Piliero SJ, Gordon AS, Meager R (1977). Mechanisms underlying the suppression of erythropoiesis by hyperoxia. Am J Med Sci 273:71.

Larkin CE, Adams JD, Williams WT, Duncan DM (1972). Hemotologic responses to hypobaric hyperoxia. Am J Phys 223:431.

Legge M, Brian M, Winterbourn C, Carrell R (1977). Red cell superoxide dismutase activity in the newborn. Aust Paediat J 13:25.

Mathis RR, Brown OR (1976). ATP concentration in _Escherichia coli_ during oxygen toxicity. Biochim et Biophys Acta 440:723.

Rechsteiner M, Hillyard D, Olivera BM (1976a). Turnover of nicotinamide adenine dinucleotide in cultures of human cells. J cell Physiol 88:207.

Rechsteiner M, Hillyard D, Olivera BM (1976b). Magnitude and significance of NAD turnover in human cell line D98/AH2. Nature 259:695.

Voitkevich VI, Myasnikov AP, Shcherba MM (1976). Effect of hyperoxia on rate of restoration of the blood composition after blood loss. Bull Exp Biol Med 82:1477.

Voitkevich VI, Volzhskaya AM, Myasnikov AP (1976). Erythropoietic activity of the blood in man after exposure to hyperbaric hyperoxia. Bull Exp Biol Med 82:1619.

Yein F, Brown OR (1977). Comparative inactivation of yeast fatty acid synthetase component enzymes by 100 atmospheres of oxygen. Biochim et Biophys Acta 486:421.

DISCUSSION

Dr. Rucknagel: You know, we use oxygen a great deal in the management of patients with sickle cell anemia, and for all of the oxygen which is used, I can't say that we've really seen that much benefit. It's occurred to me, as I've listened to the horror story that you've unfolded, that maybe the oxygen is doing more damage than good, by inhibiting protein synthesis and the like. You've used hyperbaric oxygen, I presume, to speed up the process of your experiments. Do these effects on, say, protein synthesis occur pretty much in proportion to the oxygen tension at lower levels?

Dr. Brown: We haven't done a complete study of that relationship, however, the growth and protein synthesis interruption is within 0.05 generation upon exposure of the culture to a gas phase containing 4.2 atm of oxygen. We have measured the actual oxygen concentration dissolved in the liquid phase during the first few minutes, and it's only slightly above one atmosphere when growth and protein synthesis stops.

Dr. Rucknagel: Well, we know that administration of high concentrations of oxygen shuts down the marrow or at least it shuts down erythropoiesis temporarily. I had assumed this was because of the effect on erythropoietin concentration.

Dr. Brown: I think that's very interesting. The literature does indicate that that's the case, but I think studies have not been done to prove whether or not these effects might also be present in the red cell.

Dr. Carrell: Could I just make one comment on that as chairman? If you accept the view that in the unstable hemoglobin hemolytic anemias, there is an oxidative contribution, and that's still a matter of controversy, then I think that you must be prepared to make the same argument in sickle cell disease. We saw yesterday the presence of inclusion bodies, and in particular the presence of a very small amount of membrane attached hemoglobin in the ISC cells. There is just a slight suggestion in my mind that a high oxygen tension might be bad for the sickler.

Dr. Brewer: I am trying to think of occasions where the red

The Red Cell, pages 715–718

cell may have been affected by chronic hyperoxia, and the one
that occurs to me is the anemia that the astronauts get.
As I understand it, they are exposed to a very mild hyperoxia.
I think that the anemia that they get is out of proportion
to what one might expect from greater pO_2 in the arterial
blood. I'm wondering if over a longer period of time, relatively small increases in pO_2 might have some type of damaging effects of the types you're talking about.

Dr. Brown: I think some of the indications of red cell damage in the space program were during the early pre-flight
tests. Unfortunately, in one of those early studies which
showed hemolysis, there was a breakage of a mercury thermom-
eter in the enclosed capsule. There is good evidence that
mercury toxicity contributed to that case. I don't think
that there is any good evidence that the marginal hyperoxic
conditions of the current space program has any detrimental
effect on the red cells of the astronauts. Concerning whether marginally elevated oxygen tensions could be poisonous,
I think that the extreme view held by some people is that
there certainly is toxicity, and that a lifetime of breathing
oxygen represents the toxic limit for twenty per cent oxygen.
The higher the concentration of oxygen you breathe, the faster the toxicity occurs. At hyperbaric pressure, it may occur
within a few minutes.

Dr. Fee: I had a question about the inhibition of the fructose diphosphatase by superoxide. It seemed that you had
incredibly high concentrations of superoxide or was that an
error on the slide?

Dr. Brown: That was measured as the total peroxide anion
that was generated during the exposure of the enzyme. The
superoxide was generated using the xanthine-xanthine oxidase
reaction. The concentration at any given moment was much
less, but the slide showed the total flux of superoxide,
and it was very high.

Dr. Fee: So this would then be integrated over a period of
time. I think your last number was 0.6 millimolar superoxide then that would be integrated over an hour, I guess.
I would like to make a brief comment on superoxide activity.
I've worked in this field for some time now, and greatly
disagree with my friend George Brewer. I don't think that
superoxide really reacts with anything, except itself, and
superoxide dismutases. Certainly, the hypothetical Haber-

Weiss reaction which was debated very vigorously at the
last erythrocyte meeting here has fallen to more careful
experimentation. I had one other comment that has briefly
escaped me, yes, that was with regard to the production of
superoxide by xanthine oxidase. While xanthine oxidase
does in fact produce superoxide, it may produce other compounds which are themselves very toxic, particularly in the
presence of aldehydes. It's very likely that aldehyde derived organic peroxides are being formed and·these of course,
will be toxic. Whether these can react with superoxide
dismutases has yet to be shown. But, certainly, I think
xanthine oxidase should be viewed with some caution as a
source of superoxide.

Dr. Hochstein: With regard to the mechanism of oxygen toxicity, I agree completely with Dr. Fee. It seems to me
that the addition of superoxide dismutase to a reaction
mixture does not demonstrate that superoxide is in fact
the inhibitory species if an inhibitory effect is alleviated.
It only demonstrates that superoxide is no longer around.
As a consequence other radicals may not be formed through
the interaction of hydrogen peroxide and superoxide anions.
Don't you agree?

Dr. Brown: Yes, I agree. I think that the rationale is similar to the rationale given in other published similar uses
of the enzyme. Superoxide dismutase is added with the expectation that if it eliminates a reaction, then this simply
shows that the reaction proceeds by a process that involves
superoxide anion as one of the intermediates.

Dr. Hochstein: Exactly. It does not say that superoxide
is the toxic intermediate.

Dr. Brown: Absolutely, but that could be an academic argument, if it is essential in the pathway of production of
the toxic species.

Dr. Hochstein: Well, if you want to present that argument,
you might as well say that xanthine oxidase is the toxic
substance.

Dr. Brown: Well, I might say in defense that our studies
have been directed not toward the radical species that
are involved, but toward investigations into the sites in
the cells which appear to be first damaged. In this study,

fructose - 1,6-diphosphatase was one such example. Exposure
of the enzyme in vitro to air, or to pure oxygen, does not
produce the inactivation.

ENDOTHELIAL DAMAGE PROVOKED BY TOXIC OXYGEN RADICALS RELEASED
FROM COMPLEMENT-TRIGGERED GRANULOCYTES

T. SACKS, C.F. MOLDOW, P.R. CRADDOCK,
T.K. BOWERS, and H.S. JACOB
Department of Medicine, University of Minnesota
Medical School, Minneapolis, Minnesota   55455

INTRODUCTION

Students of atherosclerosis can recite a long and
widely diverse list of predisposing factors for this disease.
The spectrum ranges from the rare condition of homocysti-
nuria in which a toxic metabolite, homocystine, abnormally
accumulates in the circulation, to more mundane and prevalent conditions such as hypertension. Despite this
diversity, a common thread seems to be emerging that endothelial damage is the common precursor of this condition.
Of particular relevance to the studies to be presented are
recent suggestions, made mainly by British workers (Poston
and Davies, 1974), that immune causes of vascular damage
might be previously-unsuspected, but frequent, initiators
of endothelial damage eventuating in later atherosclerosis.
Two seemingly-unrelated observations have suggested
to us that this hypothesis might be generally sound, and
that activated components of the complement (C) system
might be specifically involved. First, a striking acceleration of atherosclerosis commonly occurs in patients
undergoing chronic hemodialysis (Lindner, 1974); and
second, our laboratory has recently demonstrated that
during this procedure the C cascade is activated by the
cellophane in dialyzers (Craddock et al, 1977a). Thus,
during dialysis, patients are continuously reinfused with
activated C components. Indeed, that one or more of these
reinfused activated components might injure endothelium is
suggested by our findings in dialyzed sheep that protein-
rich edema fluid accumulates in pulmonary interstitial
tissues during the procedure (Craddock et al, 1977b). The

The Red Cell, pages 719—724

activated C component responsible for this disruption in
pulmonary vascular integrity appears to be C5a.

From these observations, we have hypothesized that
repeated C-triggered vascular injury might underlie the
accelerated atherosclerosis seen in chronically hemodialyzed
patients. The present studies in which we have employed
cultured human endothelial cells were devised to investigate
this possibility and to elucidate the mechanism by which
activated complement might injure endothelium. The data
to be presented demonstrates that: a) activated C induces
endothelial damage, but only in the presence of granulocytes;
b) C5a is the major effector of this injury; c) damage is
mainly mediated by granulocyte production of short-lived
toxic oxygen radicals rather than released lysosomal proteases; d) a close proximity between granulocytes and endothelium is required before damage can occur; and e) another
model of vascular injury, shock lung, especially when it is
caused by gram negative endotoxinemia, is probably provoked
by a similar mechanism.

METHODS

Endothelial cells were cultured according to the
method of Jaffee et al (1973) from human umbilical cord veins,
and identified as endothelium by reaction with fluorescienated
anti-Factor VIII antibody. Endothelial cell damage was
assayed by measurement of chromium-51 release from cells
previously treated with radio-labelled sodium chromate
after this assay was independently validated by another
cytoxicity technique--that of fluorochromasia (Celada and
Rotman, 1967). Since each cord yields at least two culture
plates, each experiment was done with an internal control
of spontaneous chromium-51 release from a plate of cells
derived from the same umbilical cord. The leukocytes employed
contained greater than 98% granulocytes after Ficoll-Hypaque
separation, and sera ABO compatible with the endothelial
cells was C-activated by zymosan treatment (Goldstein et al,
1973).

RESULTS AND DISCUSSION

Exposure of cultured endothelial cells to activated C _plus_
granulocytes, but not to either alone, injures these cells.

Thus, the combination of PMNs plus activated C produces
significant (p<.0025) chromium-51 release over that of
simultaneously-incubated, control cells. In contrast, pre-
heating sera to prevent C activation, or deleting the
granulocytes, prevents significant endothelial cell injury.
Because of our previous observations that C5a is a critical
effector of pulmonary vascular damage in hemodialysis, we
investigated its potential role in inducing granulocyte-
mediated damage to endothelial cells in culture. C5a,
purified by Sephadex G-75 chromatography, was resuspended
so as to be equivalent in concentration to that present in
zymosan-activated whole serum. When added to granulocytes
placed on endothelial monolayers, the purified C5a induces
significant (p<.005) endothelial injury, exactly equivalent
to that induced by unfractionated, activated whole serum.
Moreover, this C5a-induced damage is prevented if the C5a
is inactivated by preincubation with anti-C5a antibody.
When these data were first obtained, the most obvious
explanation which surfaced was that endothelial damage was
probably produced by lysosomal proteases released by the C-
activated granulocytes; however, this interpretation is
probably incorrect. That is, although endothelial damage
does accompany exposure of monolayers to granulocytes
phagocytosing C-opsonized particles, which in turn do release significant quantities of myeloperoxidase and other
lysosomal enzymes, such lysosomal release is not a
requirement for endothelial damage. Thus, granulocytes
exposed to soluble activated C components such as zymosan-
treated whole serum or to purified C5a, induce endothelial
damage without releasing their lysosomal proteases to the
environment.

An alternative mechanism for endothelial damage is
suggested from the fact that immune stimuli, including C5a,
cause granulocytes to generate toxic oxygen radicals, such
as superoxide anions (Goldstein et al, 1975), which have
been shown to produce cellular injury in various other
experimental systems. To study the possible deleterious
effects of superoxide on endothelial cell cultures, a well-
established superoxide generating system--that of xanthine
plus xanthine oxidase was employed. This system indeed
induces a greater than 4-fold increase over control in
endothelial release of chromium-51 which is prevented by
simultaneous addition of the free radical scavengers,
superoxide dismutase plus catalase. More interestingly,
superoxide generation by granulocytes is also evidently

critical to C-mediated endothelial damage as well; that is,
damage provoked by C5a plus granulocytes is also markedly
inhibited by addition of superoxide dismutase plus catalase
to the reaction mixture.

Since superoxide and other free radicals are generally
short-lived and rapidly dissipated, it seemed reasonable to
predict that a close apposition of activated granulocytes to
target endothelial cells would be necessary for significant
cellular damage to occur. To test this prediction, we took
advantage of an observation made during other unrelated
studies, that cytochalasin B, a substance which interferes
with microfilament function, diminishes granulocyte motility
and prevents complement-induced spreading of these cells.
Thus, under scanning electron microscopy resting granulocytes
appear approximately spheroidal, with minimal surface
excrescences; however, within 20 seconds after exposure to
activated C, these cells undergo striking surface conformational changes including veil formation, pseudopod generation,
and spreading (Craddock et al, 1977c). This morphology
suggests that such activated cells should be particularly
efficient in attaching to, and intercalating with, various
surfaces, including endothelium. In contrast, cytochalasin
treatment of granulocytes prevents these surface changes, and
cytochalasin-treated granulocytes do not provoke endothelial
injury even though triggered by activated C. This, despite
the fact that others have shown that cytochalasin-treated
cells actually release more proteases and superoxide radicals
than do untreated granulocytes (Goldstein et al, 1975).
These data lead us to hypothesize that untreated granulocytes,
by virtue of their ability to spread and extrude veils and
pseudopods when triggered by activated C, can closely adhere
to target endothelial cells, thus releasing directly there-
upon their damaging free radicals; in contrast, cytochalasin,
by preventing these granulocyte surface alterations, and
thereby inhibiting close physical cellular interaction,
allows much of the injury-mediating substances to be dissipated into the environment.

As already mentioned, one of our earlier findings
which suggested to us that activated C might induce vascular
damage was that hemodialyzed sheep develop protein-rich pulmonary edema. The exudative nature of the edema fluid
suggested that endothelial damage with increased permeability
was being provoked by the infused activated complement
components. A more serious exudative pulmonary edema

characterizes the shock lung syndrome which frequently
accompanies gram negative endotoxinemia--a potentially
C-activating disorder. That, indeed, pulmonary endothelium
might be damaged by endotoxin, which, in turn, might result
in the massive pulmonary fluid exudation of shock lung is
suggested by further studies with cultured endothelial cells.
Thus, endotoxin alone has no evident deleterious effects on
cultured cells, but when granulocytes are also added,
significant cytotoxicity occurs (p<.01) which is further
amplified (p<.001) when a source of activatible C is also
present. The C-induced increment in damage is blocked by
the free radical scavengers, superoxide dismutase plus
catalase, as expected. Of further interest, endothelial
cytotoxicity is also significantly inhibited by hydrocortisone,
added in doses similar to those that have been beneficially
utilized in patients with the shock lung syndrome.

SUMMARY

We have shown that activated C, particularly C5a,
triggers granulocytes to damage endothelial cells, and that
such damage is mediated by toxic oxygen radicals such as
superoxide anion, rather than lysosomal proteases. Furthermore, endotoxin induces vascular damage apparently by this
same mechanism. From these results we suggest that C-mediated
endothelial damage might be the precursor lesion of atherosclerosis, particularly in hemodialyzed patients, and of
shock lung, particularly in patients with gram negative
bacteremias.

REFERENCES

Celada F, Rotman B (1967). A fluorochromatic test for
   immunocytotoxicity against tumor cells and leukocytes in
   agarose plates. Proc Nat Acad Sci USA 57:630.
Craddock PR, Fehr J, Dalmasso AP, Brigham KL, Jacob HS (1977a).
   Pulmonary vascular leukostasis resulting from complement
   activation by dialyzer cellophane membranes. J Clin
   Invest 59:879.
Craddock PR, Fehr J, Brigham KL, Kronenberg RS, Jacob HS
   (1977b). Complement and leukocyte mediated pulmonary
   dysfunction in hemodialysis. New Engl J Med 296:769.
Craddock PR, Hammerschmidt D, White JG, Dalmasso AP, Jacob HS
   (1977c). Complement (C5a)-induced granulocyte aggregation
   in vitro. J Clin Invest 60:260.

Goldstein IM, Brai M, Osler AG, Weissmann G (1973). Lysosomal enzyme release from human leukocytes: mediation by the alternative pathway of complement activation. J Immunol 111:33.

Goldstein IM, Roos D, Kaplan HB, Weissmann G (1975). Complement and immunoglobulins stimulate superoxide production by leukocytes independently of phagocytosis. J Clin Invest 56:1155.

Jaffee EA, Nachman RL, Becker CG, Minick CR (1973). Culture of human endothelial cells derived from umbilical veins. J Clin Invest 52:2745.

Lindner A (1974). Accelerated atherosclerosis in prolonged maintenance hemodialysis. New Engl J Med 290:697.

Poston RN, Davies DF (1974). Immunity and inflammation in the pathogenesis of atherosclerosis. Atherosclerosis 19:353.

DISCUSSION

<u>Dr. Carrell</u>: I wonder if I could start by referring to the last comment concerning arteriosclerosis. Are you prepared to speculate that this might be a wider mechanism, or are you talking about localized arteriosclerosis?

<u>Dr. Jacob</u> :Your British colleagues have made some very interesting speculations in this regard. Two groups in England have discussed in <u>Lancet</u> and other journals, the data demonstrating that patients with severe arteriosclerosis seem to have a higher incidence of antibodies to various common antigens in our environment - for instance,milk antibodies. Also, smokers with, compared to those without, arteriosclerosis, harbor antibodies to tobacco smoke. These observations support speculations that immune mechanisms may be common, previously unsuspected substrates for endothelial damage, lipid inhibition and eventual arteriosclerosis. However, I would doubt that immune damaged endothelium has much to do with arteriosclerosis of hypertension, for instance, although its role in the accelerated vascular disease seen in hemodialyzed patients is suggested.

<u>Dr. Cameron</u>: The pulmonary endothelium has some properties that are thought to be unique to it and I'm wondering if you have any comments on differences between pulmonary and other endothelium. For example, angiotensin converting enzyme is very active in pulmonary endothelium, and you might have some specific symptomatology associated with that. Have you tried some of your assays on cultured endothelium from pulmonary vessels?

<u>Dr. Jacob</u> : No, we haven't done that. Parenthetically, angiotensin converting enzyme is present in all endothelium, not just pulmonary.

<u>Dr. Brewer</u>: I was interested that superoxide dismutase was protective. In the G6PD deficient system that Rosanne Leipzig has worked with, it hasn't been while catalase is, and we have assumed that hydrogen peroxide was then the important mediator of that kind of damage. What species do you think are involved here?

<u>Dr. Jacob</u> : Let me make an important point clear. Superoxide dismutase is not protective alone; catalase must

DISCUSSION

also be added. From such data, I would suggest that activated
hydroxyl radicals are probably importantly involved in producing endothelial damage.

Dr. Carrell: A very brief point -- you mentioned that hydrocortisone gave the same sort of protection. Presumably this
is by a different mechanism?

Dr. Jacob: Yes. This seems very exciting to us. We have
preliminary evidence that hydrocortisone or methyl predniso-
lone in the enormous doses used in shock lung patients do
two potentially additive, beneficial things. They block
complement activation per se and they also "quiet" the
granulocyte membrane.

Dr. Forman: I was wondering what your thoughts were on the
role of alveolar macrophage and its potential interaction with
complement and the cells in this condition. Or do you really think it's really only the granulocytes?

Dr. Jacob: We have preliminarily studied monocytes but not
alveolar macrophages. Monocytes also damage endothelial cells
activated by complement. I suspect alveolar macrophages will
do so, as well, since they are potent superoxide producers
in other systems.

Dr. Forman: I thought I read recently where some people think
that alveolar macrophages are in fact derived ultimately
from bone marrow monocytes and there's a natural link.

A PROTECTIVE ROLE FOR ASCORBATE IN GLUCOSE-6-PHOSPHATE
DEHYDROGENASE DEFICIENCY?

Christine C Winterbourn

Department of Clinical Biochemistry
Christchurch Hospital
Christchurch, New Zealand

INTRODUCTION

Drugs that cause hemolysis in glucose-6-phosphate
dehydrogenase (G6PD) deficiency in general react with
oxyhemoglobin to give oxidation of both the drug and the
hemoglobin, and precipitation of the hemoglobin as Heinz
bodies. Hydrogen peroxide (H_2O_2) and superoxide (O_2^-) are
also reaction products (Cohen & Hochstein 1964; Goldberg &
Stern 1975), and the most frequently given explanation for
hemolysis is that G6PD deficient cells cannot regenerate
sufficient reduced glutathione (GSH) to remove peroxides by
the glutathione peroxidase - catalysed reaction (Mills 1957;
Beutler 1971; Flohé & Günzler 1974). However the exact
mechanism of precipitation and cause of hemolysis are still
debatable (Eaton & Brewer 1974; Carrell et al. 1975; Goldberg
et al. 1976; Itano et al. 1977).

We have recently been investigating the reaction of
purified oxyhemoglobin with acetylphenylhydrazine (APH),
which appears to be typical of this type of drug. The overall
reaction is complex and involves a number of steps (French et
al. 1977; Winterbourn & French 1977). The first step, in
which the hemoglobin - bound oxygen oxidizes both the heme
iron and the APH, is particularly important in influencing
the overall course of the reaction. The oxyhemoglobin can be
regarded as an oxidase (Carrell et al. 1977) and is best
represented as superoxoferrihemoglobin (Collman et al. 1976):

The Red Cell, pages 727–736

$$Hb^{III}O_2^- + RH_2 + H^+ \longrightarrow Hb^{III} + H_2O_2 + RH^\cdot$$

(HbO$_2$)   (APH)

The reaction produces not only H$_2$O$_2$, but also highly reactive
free radicals (RH$^\cdot$). These radicals can react with the heme
and globin of hemoglobin, with O$_2$ to give O$_2^-$, and they have
the potential to react with other red cell constituents, so
must be considered as a threat to the integrity of the cell.
However it appears likely that normal red cells are protected
against damage from these radicals by GSH. GSH, when added to
a mixture of oxyhemoglobin and APH, protects the hemoglobin
against oxidation and precipitation. This protection is
evident in the presence of optimal concentrations of catalase
and superoxide dismutase, so cannot be due to reactions of
GSH with H$_2$O$_2$ or O$_2^-$, but it can be explained by the GSH acting
as a scavenger for the free radicals. The radical scavenging
ability of GSH is well-known (Kosower & Kosower 1974; Slater
1972), but its importance as a red cell protective mechanism
has tended to be overshadowed by the involvement of GSH in
the breakdown of peroxides (Aebi & Suter 1974) and its ability
to undergo exchange with disulfides to regenerate oxidized
sulfhydryl groups (Mannervik & Eriksson 1974). However, our
results imply that GSH plays a much more general role, and
that radical reactions may contribute to red cell hemolysis
in GSH deficiency.

Ascorbate, which is another free radical scavenger
(Slater 1972), was found to have a similar protective effect
to GSH on oxyhemoglobin oxidation (French et al. 1977). This
has led us to speculate that free radical scavengers such as
ascorbate could substitute for GSH in the red cell, and
inhibit the hemoglobin breakdown and hemolysis that occur in
G6PD deficiency. This paper reports the results of some
experiments carried out to examine this hypothesis.

EXPERIMENTAL

The reaction of APH with normal and G6PD deficient red
cells was investigated by incubating the twice-washed cells
in buffered saline (4 parts 0.9% NaCl, 1 part 0.1M phosphate
buffer pH 7.4) at 37°C in a shaking water bath. Glucose (4
mg/ml). ascorbate (0-10mM) and APH (4-30mM) were added as
required to the cell suspension. The amount of oxidation of
oxyhemoglobin was determined by diluting an aliquot of the

cell suspension 1:25 in 5mM phosphate buffer pH 7.4, centrifuging, and calculating the concentrations of oxyhemoglobin, methemoglobin, hemichrome and choleglobin from the absorbances at 700, 630, 577 and 560 nm (French et al. 1977). Heinz body formation was assessed visually on the cells stained with methyl violet. To quantitatively measure the amount of Heinz body formation, the cells were lysed by dilution in an appropriate volume of 5mM phosphate buffer and the turbidity of the solution was determined by measuring the absorbance at 700nm before and after centrifugation.

RESULTS AND DISCUSSION

Incubation of red cells with APH characteristically produces Heinz bodies of variable size and variable number per cell. Although microscopic examination of a stained film gives an overall impression of the extent of Heinz body formation, there are considerable problems in accurately measuring the amount of precipitated material present. An alternative method was therefore developed, based on the turbidity of the solution following lysis of the cells. With cells incubated without APH there was virtually no turbidity, but exposure to APH produced progressively more turbid solutions, as either the APH concentration or the incubation time increased (Fig. 1). Heinz body formation would be expected to increase in a similar manner, and microscopic examination did show that the number and size of the Heinz bodies increased in each case. These results indicate that the turbidity increase parallels Heinz body formation, and appears to be a useful quantitative measure of the process.

As expected, incubation of G6PD deficient cells with APH in the presence of glucose produced more oxyhemoglobin oxidation and Heinz body formation than with normal cells (Table 1). The difference was more marked for Heinz body formation than oxidation, and with the lower APH concentration. Addition of low levels of ascorbate to G6PD deficient cells had a marked inhibitory effect on both the amounts of oxyhemoglobin oxidation and Heinz body formation (Fig. 2). With 1mM ascorbate, Heinz body formation was almost completely prevented, and oxyhemoglobin oxidation reduced to about 20%. A marked diminution in the number of Heinz bodies in the cells was also obvious (Fig. 3). The first step in the overall reaction of oxyhemoglobin with APH is oxidation, and the final step precipitation of the oxidized hemoglobin as Heinz

bodies. A decrease in oxyhemoglobin concentration is therefore
detectable at an earlier stage than precipitation, which is
a measure of all the steps in the sequence. The ability of

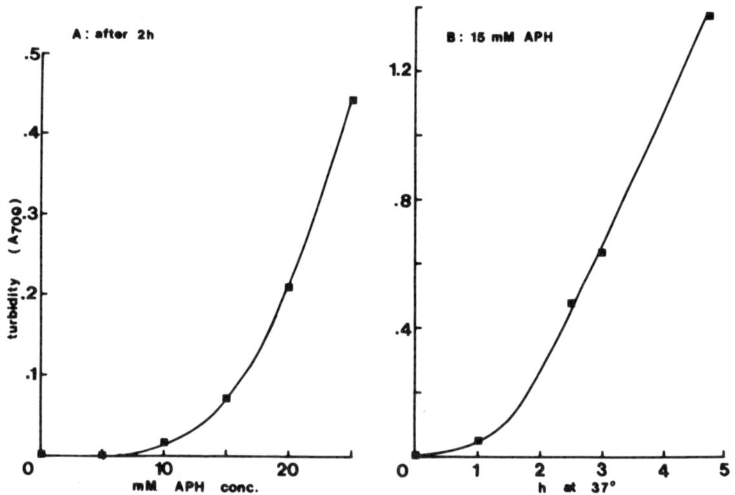

Figure 1: Incubation of red cells with APH: correlation of
the turbidity of the lysed cells with (A) the APH concentration
and (B) the incubation time. The cells were lysed by diluting
the 12.5% suspension 0.2:3 in 5mM phosphate buffer.

Table 1: Oxyhemoglobin oxidation and Heinz body formation in
normal cells compared with G6PD deficient cells incubated
with APH in the presence of glucose.

| Incubation | 4mM APH | | 10mM APH | |
| time (h) | Ratio of Normal : G6PD Deficient Cells | | | |
	oxyHb oxidized	Heinz bodies	oxyHb oxidized	Heinz bodies
2	.48		.82	
3.5				.38
5	.52	.12		.57
7		.20		

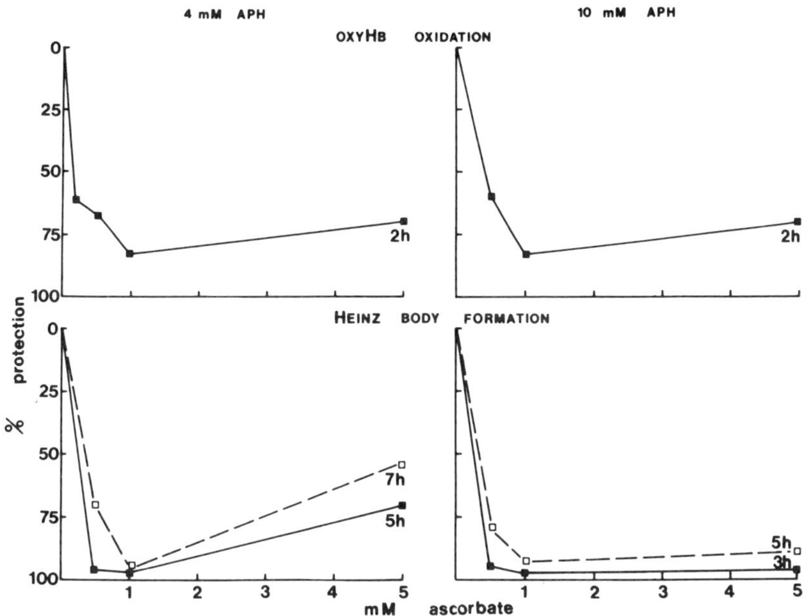

Figure 2: Effect of ascorbate on oxyhemoglobin oxidation and
Heinz body formation in G6PD deficient red cells incubated
with APH in the presence of glucose.

ascorbate to inhibit Heinz body formation more than
oxyhemoglobin oxidation suggests that the oxidation of
oxyhemoglobin is not the only reaction that is inhibited. With
purified oxyhemoglobin, it appears that the APH radicals can
react with sites other than the heme groups, increasing the
rate of precipitation (French et al. 1977). Ascorbate inhibits
these reactions as well as heme oxidation. This mechanism is
also compatible with the results with the intact cells.

It is well known that ascorbate itself can cause oxidative
breakdown of hemoglobin, and it is one of the compounds to
which G6PD deficient cells are sensitive (Udomratn et al. 1977).
It may therefore seem surprising that in the present context
it is being used to prevent oxidation. However the role played
by ascorbate is dependent on its concentration. The concentration that we find gives maximum inhibition is well below
that at which any acceleratory effect of ascorbate alone can
be detected (Table 2) or that at which it starts to make a

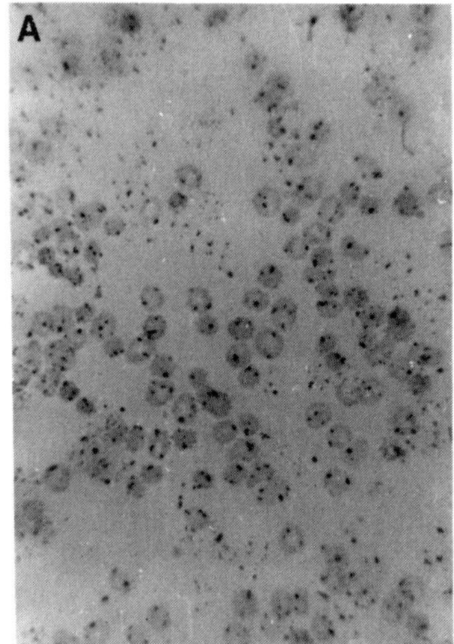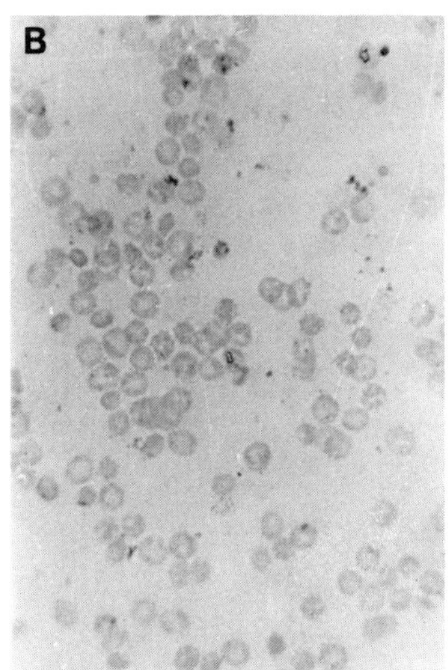

Figure 3: G6PD deficient red cells incubated at 37°C for 4½h with 10mM APH and stained for Heinz bodies with methyl violet. (A) no ascorbate; (B) 1mM ascorbate.

Table 2: Effect of incubating with ascorbate on G6PD deficient red cells.

ascorbate conc (mM)	% of oxyHb oxidized 2h	5h	Heinz body formation A_{700}*/7h
0	0.3	3.0	.007
0.5	0.9	2.0	.007
1	1.3		
5	1.4	8.3	.017

*Measured on 0.2ml of cell suspension diluted to 3ml.

positive contribution to the APH effect (Fig. 2).

    The demonstration that ascorbate can inhibit hemoglobin breakdown in G6PD deficient cells _in vitro_ opens up the

possibility that it could be therapeutically useful in vivo.
Three major questions require answering before this could be
contemplated. (1) Is ascorbate effective against oxidative
drugs in general? (2) Can we be certain that the ascorbate
would have no undesirable effects? (3) Would it be possible
to attain the ascorbate concentrations required to be
effective? So far it is possible to only partially answer
these questions. Firstly, we have not yet studied the effect
of ascorbate with other drugs. However we have investigated
the reactions of hemoglobin with menadione (vitamin K) and
p-hydroxylaminotoluene, which resembles the active metabolites
of a number of drugs that are hemolytic in G6PD deficiency
(French & Winterbourn unpublished observations). Both
mechanisms appear to involve free radical intermediates, so
it is likely that they could be inhibited either by ascorbate,
or possibly another free radical scavenger.

Although the conditions during in vitro incubation are
different from the in vivo situation, such experiments provide
a basis for estimating the likely effect of ascorbate on
circulating red cells exposed to oxidant drugs. The in vivo
situation differs in that the red cell ascorbate concentration
should remain constant, whereas it presumably fell during the
incubation experiments. Also, we have no information as yet
on the ascorbate concentrations actually in the red cells that
were responsible for either protecting against or contributing
to hemoglobin breakdown. Nevertheless, I am reasonably
confident of a positive answer to the second question. With
37.5% suspensions of G6PD deficient cells, incubation with
10mM ascorbate alone caused no detectable Heinz body formation,
and with APH, it still provided maximum protection. This
concentration is about 100 times higher than the normal plasma
level, and almost certainly could not be reached with oral
dosage (Lewin 1976), so hemolysis due to ascorbate seems
unlikely to be a problem. However, a cautionary note must be
given. Until recently, Heinz body formation or hemolysis
caused by ascorbate has not been observed in vivo, but
Campbell et al. (1975) have reported the death of a G6PD
deficient patient following the intravenous administration of
80g of ascorbate. This dose would have produced plasma
ascorbate concentrations so far in excess of the concentration
that would be required for therapeutic use, and many times
what could be obtained by oral dosage, that there should be
no danger of even approaching this level. This group (Udomratn
et al. 1977) have subsequently shown that preincubation with
ascorbate can decrease the survival of G6PD deficient red

cells transfused into rats, but the cells were again exposed
to ascorbate concentrations several fold higher than those
predicted to give protection.

To answer the third question it is necessary to know
what amount of inhibition of the reaction of APH with
hemoglobin in vitro would correspond to a protective role in
vivo. This may be much less than the maximum obtained with
0.5-1mM ascorbate. The amount of oxyhemoglobin oxidation in
normal cells, which are not susceptible to oxidative drugs
in vivo, was about half of that in G6PD deficient cells when
incubated with 4mM APH (Table 1), so less than 50% inhibition
under these conditions may correspond to sufficient protection
in vivo. Inhibition of oxyhemoglobin oxidation by APH was
just detectable when .05mM ascorbate was added to G6PD
deficient cells during incubation. As this is about the
normal plasma level, the concentration of ascorbate that
would be required to protect G6PD deficient red cells against
oxidation by APH in vivo may be only moderately higher than
normal, and attainable by oral dosage. However, before a
reliable estimate of this concentration can be made, more
information is required on how red cell ascorbate concentrations relate to plasma concentrations both in vitro and in
vivo.

Its ability to act as a free radical scavenger is
probably the main property of ascorbate that enables it to
substitute for GSH to protect against hemoglobin breakdown.
It is therefore possible that other scavengers could be as
good as ascorbate, or even better, and their clinical
application should be considered.

I have stressed the importance of GSH in preventing
free radical reactions in the red cell. It is not intended
to suggest this as an alternative to its role in the
elimination of H_2O_2 and peroxides, but rather as an additional
source of protection. There is good evidence that peroxides
are inadequately handled and contribute to hemolysis in GSH
deficient red cells, and in our studies the protection of
of hemoglobin by radical scavengers was additional to that
provided by the removal of H_2O_2. It is important, however,
that the various roles of GSH are considered in the overall
mechanism of hemolysis.

ACKNOWLEDGEMENTS

I am grateful to Dr C. Parr, London Hospital, for
providing the sample of G6PD deficient blood, to the Biology
Department, University of York, where most of this work was
carried out, and to the Medical Research Council of New
Zealand, for financial support.

SUMMARY

The observation that low concentrations of ascorbate
could substitute for glutathione (GSH) and inhibit the
oxidation and precipitation of purified oxyhemoglobin
exposed to acetylphenylhydrazine (APH) has been followed up
with an examination of intact cells. It was found that
addition of ascorbate almost completely prevented the
formation of Heinz bodies when glucose-6-phosphate dehydrogenase deficient red cells were incubated with APH. The ascorbate
concentrations that were effective are only a little higher
than normal blood concentrations, and it may be possible to
elevate the blood ascorbate in GSH deficiency, and thereby
inhibit the reactions responsible for red cell breakdown.

REFERENCES

Aebi H, Suter H (1974). Protective function of reduced
    glutathione against the effect of prooxidative substances
    and of irradiation in the red cell. In Flohé L, Benöhr
    HCh, Sies H, Waller HD, Wendel A (eds): "Glutathione",
    Stüttgart: Georg Thieme, p 192.
Beutler E (1971). Abnormalities of the hexose monophosphate
    shunt. Semin Hematol 8:311.
Campbell GD, Steinberg MH, Bower JD (1975). Ascorbic acid -
    induced hemolysis in G6PD deficiency. Ann Intern Med 82:810.
Carrell RW, Winterbourn CC, Rachmilewitz EA (1975). Activated
    oxygen and hemolysis. Brit J Haematol 30:259.
Carrell RW, Winterbourn CC, French JK (1977). Hemoglobin - a
    frustrated oxidase? Implications for red cell metabolism.
    Hemoglobin (in press).
Cohen G, Hochstein P (1964). Generation of hydrogen peroxide
    in erythrocytes by hemolytic agents. Biochemistry 3:895.
Collman JP, Brauman JI, Halbert TR, Suslick KR (1976).
    Nature of O_2 and CO binding to metalloporphyrins and heme
    proteins. Proc Natl Acad Sci USA 73:3333.

Eaton JW, Brewer GJ (1974). Pentose phosphate metabolism. In Surgenor DM (ed): "The Red Blood Cell" 2nd Edition, New York: Academic Press, p 435.

Flohé L, Günzler WA (1974). Glutathione Peroxidase. In Flohé L, Benöhr HCh, Sies H, Waller HD, Wendel A (eds): "Glutathione", Stüttgart: Georg Thieme, p 132.

French JK, Winterbourn CC, Carrell RW (1977). Mechanism of the reaction of acetylphenylhydrazine with haemoglobin. Biochem J: (submitted for publication).

Goldberg B, Stern A (1975). The generation of O_2^- by the interaction of the hemolytic agent, phenylhydrazine, with human hemoglobin. J Biol Chem 250:2401.

Goldberg B, Stern A, Peisach J (1976). The mechanism of superoxide-anion-generation by the interaction of phenylhydrazine with hemoglobin. J Biol Chem 251:3045.

Itano HA, Hirota K, Vedvick TS (1977). Ligands and oxidants in ferrihemochrome formation and oxidative hemolysis. Proc Natl Acad Sci USA 74:2556.

Kosower NS, Kosower EM (1974). Protection of membranes by glutathione. In Flohé L, Benöhr HCh, Sies H, Waller HD, Wendel A (eds): "Glutathione", Stüttgart: Georg Thieme, p 216.

Lewin S (1976). Vitamin C: Its Molecular Biology and Medical Potential", London: Academic Press, p 151.

Mannervik B. Eriksson SA (1974). Enzymatic reduction of mixed disulfides and thiosulfate esters. In Flohe L, Benöhr HCh, Sies H, Waller HD, Wendel A (eds): "Glutathione", Stüttgart: Georg Thieme, p 120.

Mills GC (1957). Hemoglobin catabolism. I. Glutathione peroxidase, an erythrocyte enzyme which protects hemoglobin from oxidative breakdown. J Biol Chem 229:189.

Slater TF (1972). "Free Radical Mechanisms in Tissue Injury", London: Pion.

Udomratn T, Steinberg MH, Campbell GD, Oelshlegel FJ (1977). Effects of ascorbic acid on glucose-6-phosphate dehydrogenase – deficient erythrocytes: studies in an animal model. Blood 49:471.

Winterbourn CC, French JK (1977). Free radical production from acetylphenylhydrazine and haemoglobin. Biochem Soc Trans 5: 1480.

DISCUSSION

Dr. Brewer: What kind of dose do you think you might have
to give? Do you have any idea?

Dr. Winterbourn: No, not at this stage. I have been trying
to find out from the literature the sort of levels that can
be obtained with high oral doses of ascorbate. Although
the plasma concentration cannot be greatly increased because
the renal threshold is reached, I have not been able to find
out what happens to the red cell concentration.

Dr. Brewer: I might just comment that in studies that I did
about 15 years ago, I think they've only been published in
an abstract, I think the dose was about a gram a day. We did
get about a ten to twenty per cent shortening in the red
cell life span in G6PD deficient people. That is, of course,
rather mild and it may be that if it were in the presence of
a hemolytic drug that the total effect would be beneficial.

Dr. Winterbourn: I think that this is the point. My suggestion is that ascorbate may alleviate a crisis situation
when it's given in combination with a potentially more
hemolytic drug.

Dr. Fung: I would like to know what kind of methemoglobin
you have here. Are all four chains oxidized from oxyhemoglobin or is it like the previous report on copper oxidation,
only αchains, or β chains oxidized?

Dr. Winterbourn: I'm sorry-

Dr. Fung: Is there a hybrid hemoglobin in your case?

Dr. Winterbourn: I don't know.

Dr. Fung: So, your definition of mehemoglobin is by the
presence of methemoglobin feature in the optical spectrum.

Dr. Winterbourn: Yes.

The Red Cell, page 737
© 1978 Alan R. Liss, Inc., New York, New York

UTILIZATION OF HUMANS WITH HIGH OXYGEN AFFINITY HEMOGLOBINS
IN·IDENTIFYING MEDIATORS OF PHYSIOLOGIC RESPONSES TO HYPOXIA

Robert P. Hebbel, M.D., Richard S. Kronenberg, M.D.,
John W. Eaton, Ph.D.
Department of Medicine, University of Minnesota,
Minneapolis, Minnesota   55455

The exposure of humans to an oxygen-poor environment
induces a variety of physiologic responses to hypoxia. Such
responses may be mediated either through a decrement in
arterial oxygen content (CaO2) or tension (paO2). Unfortunately, the position and shape of the normal oxyhemoglobin
dissociation curve are such that CaO2 and paO2 decline
concomitantly under conditions of hypoxia. Thus, it has
been difficult to distinguish between these two factors as
the mediator responsible for any given hypoxic response.

For example, although the ventilatory response to
hypoxia is clearly mediated through the carotid body's
chemoreceptors, it has not yet been shown unequivocally
whether the hypoxic stimulus is a decrement of CaO2 or paO2.
The weight of evidence does favor the latter as the
regulatory factor (Biscoe, 1971; Guz, 1975), but there have
been major difficulties with the experimental models used to
date in the attempt to distinguish the effects of paO2 and
CaO2 on the carotid body (vide infra).

Because individuals with left-shifted oxyhemoglobin
dissociation curves would maintain a higher CaO2 than normals
when confronted with a given decrement in paO2, it occurred
to us that the study of humans with high oxygen affinity
mutant hemoglobins might provide a useful in vivo model in
which to discriminate between paO2 and CaO2 as mediators of
a variety of physiologic responses to hypoxia. Consequently,
we have studied the ventilatory and heart rate responses to
hypoxia in a family with Hb-Andrew Minneapolis, a stable
beta-chain mutant Hb with high oxygen affinity (whole blood

The Red Cell, pages 739—747

P50≈17mmHg) and an oxyhemoglobin dissociation curve of normal
shape (Hill's n=2.4) (Zak et al., 1974).

METHODS

The subjects studied were all healthy non-smoking
adolescents from a family which was large enough so that
high affinity subjects could be paired with age- and sex-
matched normal siblings. Two, a 13-year-old male and a 16-
year-old female, had normal P50s and whole blood hemoglobin
concentrations for age; their affected siblings, a 12-year-
old male and an 18-year-old female, were abnormal in both
respects (Table 1). Pulmonary function of all subjects was
normal (Hebbel et al., 1977).

Table 1. Hematologic parameters of subjects studied.

subject	age yrs	sex	Hb g/dl	P50 mmHg
N1	13	M	13.0	26.9
H1	12	M	16.0	17.0
N2	16	F	13.2	27.0
H2	18	F	16.8	17.2

A detailed description of the method used to evaluate
the ventilatory response to hypoxia has appeared elsewhere
(Kronenberg et al., 1972). Briefly, subjects rebreathed
from a closed system containing a variable CO_2 absorber
bypass and a recording spirometer so that end-tidal gas
tensions (pAO2 and pACO2), tidal volume, and heart rate were
continuously recorded as pAO2 was lowered from 120 to 40mmHg
over 4-5 minutes. pACO2 was kept constant at each subject's
resting level (Table 2). Ventilation was measured by
averaging tidal volume over 5 breaths at each 10mmHg decrement in pAO2. The relationship between incremental ventilation ($\Delta\dot{V}_I$) and pO2 at constant pCO2 is expressed by
$\Delta\dot{V}_I = \Delta\dot{V}_o e^{-(pO2/k)}$, where k is the decrement of pO2 required
to increase ventilation by a factor of e (2.718), and $\Delta\dot{V}_o$ is
the intercept at pO2=0.

During hypoxic response tests, Hb oxygen saturation
(HbO2) was continuously monitored with a standardized
Hewlett Packard 47201A ear oximeter, which we have found
accurately determines the <u>in vivo</u> saturation changes occurring
in these subjects (Hebbel et al., 1977). CaO2 was calculated
from the measured Hb and HbO2, assuming pAO2 to equal paO2.

RESULTS AND DISCUSSION

When plotted as a function of pAO2, individual curves of ventilatory response to isocapnic progressive hypoxia reveal no difference between normal and high affinity subjects (Figure 1). This identity of hypoxic ventilatory response is confirmed mathematically in that there is no difference between subject pairs in the absolute ventilation at pAO2=40mmHg ($\dot{V}_{40}$) or in the decrement in pO2 required to increase ventilation by a factor of 2.718 (k) (Table 2). However, a clear divergence between subject pairs emerges if hypoxic ventilatory response is plotted as a function of HbO2 rather than pAO2 (Figure 2), reflecting a marked difference in the degree of desaturation under hypoxic conditions. Indeed, the arterial oxygen saturation at pAO2=40mmHg (HbO2$_{40}$) of high affinity subjects is 89.5% (mean), while that of normal subjects is only 73% (Table 2).

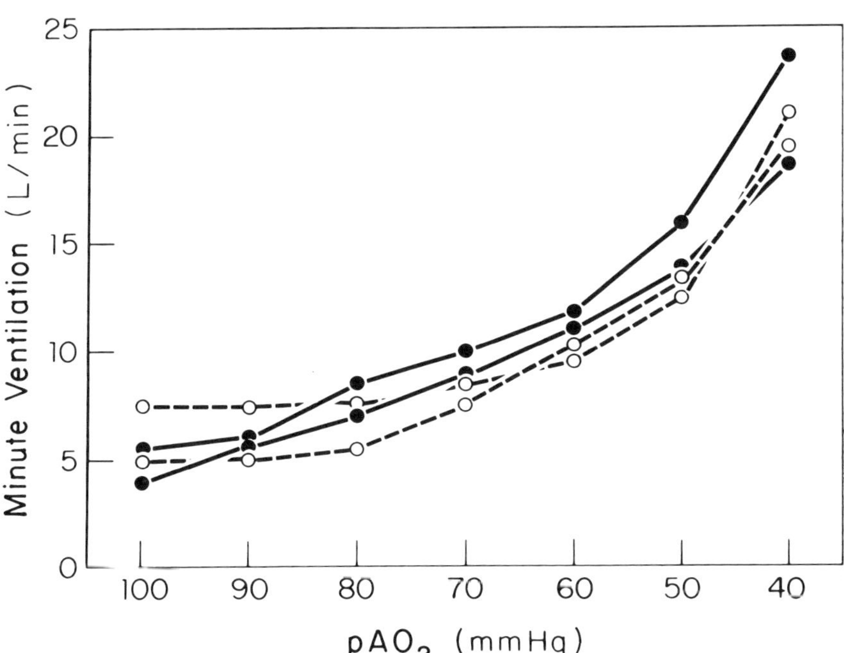

Figure 1. As a function of pAO2, the ventilatory response of high oxygen affinity subjects (●——●) to isocapnic progressive hypoxia is indistinguishable from that of normal subjects (o----o). Correlation coefficients for all curves are 0.9 or greater.

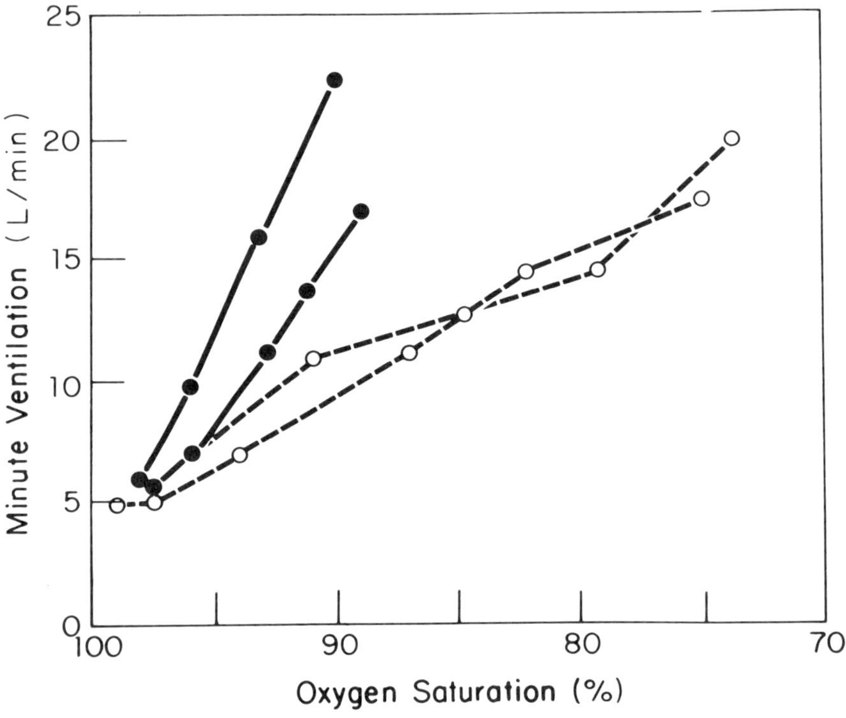

Figure 2. As a function of arterial oxygen saturation, hypoxic ventilatory response of normal (o----o) and high affinity (●——●) subjects diverges, reflecting a marked difference in degree of arterial desaturation during progressive hypoxia.

Table 2. Ventilatory response to isocapnic progressive hypoxia in subjects with normal and high oxygen affinity hemoglobins. (Abbreviations defined in text.)

subject	pACO2	$\dot{V}_{40}$	k	$HbO2_{40}$
	mmHg	1/min	mmHg	%
N1	38	19	24	73
N2	37	21	28	73
H1	39	18	26	89
H2	37	24	27	90

Figure 3 expands upon this apparent difference in oxygen availability and depicts data obtained from the actual dissociation curves of two of the subjects (N1 and H1), as determined by measurement of P50, Hb concentration, and saturation readings obtained by oximeter during progressive hypoxia. While the high affinity subject demonstrates the well-known deficit in oxygen delivery (unloading) under normal conditions (Adamson and Finch, 1975), it is equally apparent that under hypoxic conditions the high affinity subject has a marked oxygen loading advantage--and, therefore, at least a potential advantage in oxygen delivery.

Oxygen delivery is, under the best of circumstances, difficult to determine. Furthermore, in this non-invasive study we were not able to measure a number of critical parameters such as cardiac output or arterio-venous oxygen gradients. However, that actual oxygen delivery does, indeed, differ between subject pairs is suggested by the fact that high affinity subjects manifest significantly lesser heart rate increases as compared to normals during progressive hypoxia (Figure 4). In view of the fact that these high affinity subjects are able to generate the same maximal heart rate as normals if stressed by exercise under hypoxic conditions (Hebbel and Kronenberg, unpublished observation), this implies that during progressive hypoxia there are actual differences in oxygen delivery between subjects--in favor of the high affinity subject under conditions of marked hypoxia.

While a number of significant factors such as cardiac output, arterio-venous oxygen gradients, tissue oxygen tension, CNS acid-base status, and local alterations in blood flow must remain unknown in a study of this nature, we believe that the model employed herein is, nevertheless, subject to fewer potential artifacts than those used in previous investigations of hypoxic ventilatory response. Such investigations have basically attempted to alter the aforementioned relationship between paO2 and CaO2 through the induction of anemia, polycythemia, or carboxyhemoglo-binemia. Unfortunately, each of these manipulations carries as an inherent risk the potential introduction of serious artifacts due to iatrogenic alterations in oxygen delivery and/or chemoreceptor function (reviewed in Hebbel et al., 1977). The model used herein avoids these iatrogenic factors by using unmanipulated subjects in their steady state.

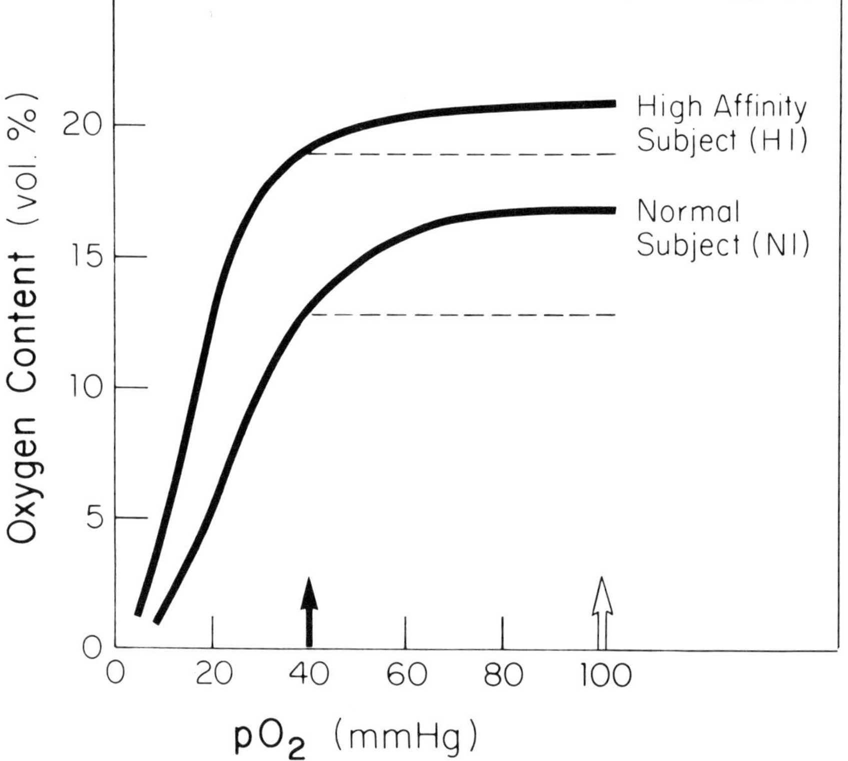

		NORMAL SUBJECT	HIGH AFFINITY SUBJECT
		vol. %	vol. %
HYPOTHETICAL NORMAL CONDITIONS	oxygen loading at pAO₂ = 100 mmHg (⇧)	16.9	21.0
	oxygen unloading at pO₂ = 40 mmHg (↑)	4.1	1.8
HYPOXIA	oxygen loading at pAO₂ = 40 mmHg (↑)	12.8	19.2

Figure 3. Arterial oxygen content and potential oxygen delivery. Under hypothetical normal conditions of paO2=100mmHg (⇧) and end-capillary pO2=40mmHg (↑), the high affinity subject has an oxygen unloading deficit. However, under conditions of marked hypoxia so that paO2=40mmHg (↑), the high affinity subject has much greater oxygen loading and much more oxygen potentially available for tissue delivery.

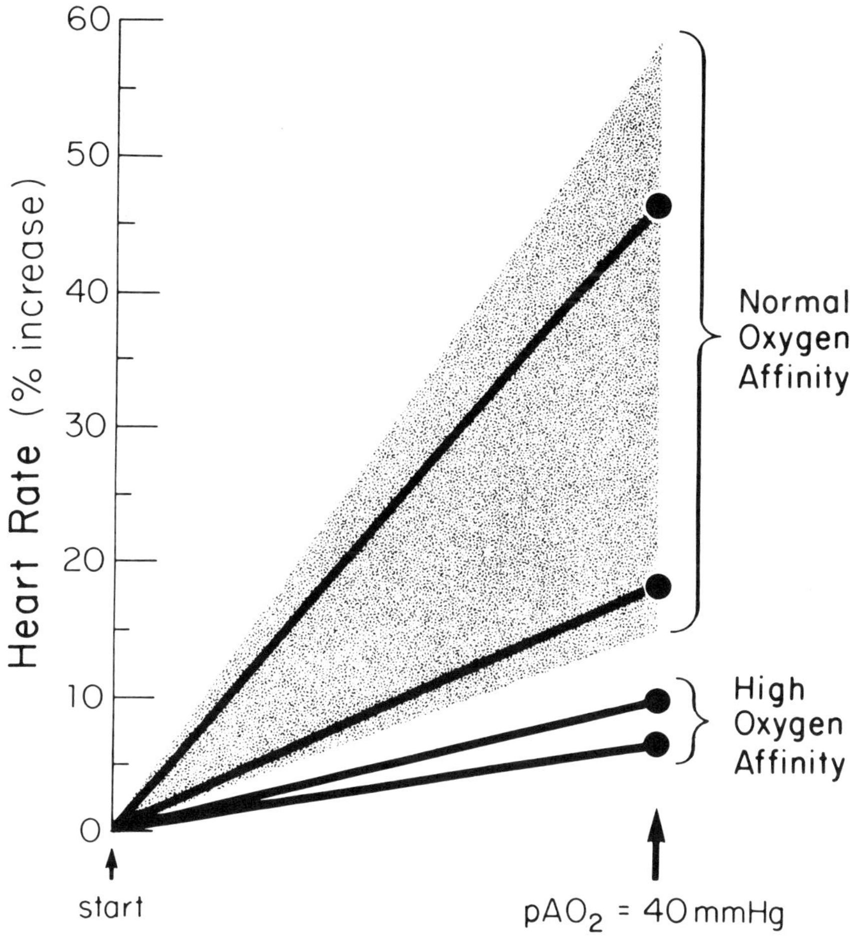

Figure 4. Increase of heart rate during hypoxic response testing, expressed as percentage increase at pAO2=40mmHg over that recorded at pAO2=100mmHg. Subjects reported herein are indicated by closed circles (●). Shaded area indicates range of increase for eight normal young adults previously tested and reported (Kronenberg and Drage, 1973). Average increase of high affinity subjects is 8.5%, while that of normals is 34%. Absolute rates from which this data is derived are reported elsewhere (Hebbel et al., 1977).

CONCLUSIONS

We have demonstrated that the hypoxic ventilatory
response (Figure 1, Table 2) of normal and high affinity
subjects is identical despite marked differences in P50
(Table 1), oxygen carrying capacity (Figure 3), and apparent
oxygen delivery (Figure 4). We conclude that hypoxic
ventilatory response is, indeed, mediated through fluctuations of pa02 rather than Ca02. In addition, we feel that
the study of humans with hemoglobins of varying oxygen
affinities may well provide a useful model in which to
evaluate other physiologic responses to hypoxia. For
example, the increase of erythrocyte 2,3DPG at altitude is
thought to be mediated through a combination of hyperventila-
tion-induced alkalosis and an alteration in the ratio of oxy-
to deoxy-hemoglobin (Lenfant et al., 1971; Brewer et al.,
1970). Since the subjects described herein would all be
expected to hyperventilate to the same degree at altitude,
this factor would be controlled, and the relative contributions of pH and alteration of R:T ratio could be assessed.
In addition, it has been suggested that the right shift of
the oxyhemoglobin dissociation curve that occurs upon
exposure to altitude may actually be a maladaptive rather
than an appropriate physiologic response to hypoxia
(Eaton, 1974). We suggest that the study of oxygen utilization in normal and high affinity humans at different
altitudes may contribute to our understanding of the
appropriateness of our physiologic responses to environmentally
derived hypoxia.

ACKNOWLEDGMENTS

This work was supported by NIH grants HL19725 and
HL16833, the Minnesota Lung Association, and Research Career
Development Award HL70356, training grant HL07062, and the
University of Minnesota. Tables 1 and 2 are presented with
the permission of the <u>Journal</u> <u>of</u> <u>Clinical</u> <u>Investigation</u>.

REFERENCES

Adamson JW, Finch CA (1975). Hemoglobin function, oxygen
    affinity, and erythropoietin. Annu Rev Physiol 37:351.
Biscoe TJ (1971). Carotid body: structure and function.
    Physiol Rev 51:437.

Brewer GJ, Eaton JW, Weil JV, Grover RF (1970). Studies of red cell glycolysis and interactions with carbon monoxide, smoking and altitude. In Brewer GJ (ed): "Red Cell Metabolism and Function," New York: Plenum Press, p. 95.

Eaton JW (1974). Oxygen affinity and environmental adaptation. Ann NY Acad Sci 241:491.

Guz A (1975). Regulation of respiration in man. Annu Rev Physiol 37:303.

Hebbel RP, Kronenberg RS, Eaton JW (1977). Hypoxic ventilatory response in humans with normal and high oxygen affinity hemoglobins. J Clin Invest, in press.

Kronenberg RS, Hamilton FN, Gabel R, Hickey R, Read DJC, Severinghaus J (1972). Comparison of three methods for quantitating respiratory response to hypoxia in man. Respir Physiol 16:109.

Kronenberg RS, Drage CW (1973). Attenuation of the ventilatory and heart rate responses to hypoxia and hypercapnia with aging in normal men. J Clin Invest 52:1812.

Lenfant C, Torrance JD, Reynafarje C (1971). Shift of the O2-Hb dissociation curve at altitude: mechanism and effect. J Appl Physiol 30:625.

Zak SJ, Brimhall B, Jones RT, Kaplan ME (1974). Hemoglobin Andrew-Minneapolis $\alpha_2^A\beta_2^{144}$Lys→Asn: a new high-oxygen-affinity mutant human hemoglobin. Blood 44:543.

DISCUSSION

Dr. Carrell: I wonder if any of the hemoglobins with very minor affinity changes might be an adaptation to high altitude-- the one that comes to mind is Hb D Punjab, but that's really wild speculation.

Dr. Hebbel: This is really very speculative, but there is one report that came out several years ago that intrigues us; it suggests that the Sherpa have a left-shifted curve. There are a lot of problems with that study which I won't go into; but it is at least compatible with such a hypothesis.

Dr. Brewer: All the calculations I've ever done have suggested that at intermediate altitudes, before you get over the shoulder of the dissociation curve, the advantage of the right-shifted curve in terms of unloading is greater than the loss due to less loading. I don't think there's any question that when you go to extreme altitude that lack of loading becomes a dominant feature, first shown by John Eaton with cyanate-treated rats. But I'm a little puzzled by why you think that at intermediate altitudes a left-shifted curve would be advantageous?

Dr. Hebbel: Well, we don't know for sure how the experiment of taking these four subjects to Leadville, Colorado would come out. I think it is clear that at very extreme altitudes a left-shifted curve would be an advantage for the reasons stated. Similarly, considering the mechanism by which humans usually encounter hypoxemia, that is anemias, a right-sided curve should be advantageous. Somewhere in the transition from being a normal or anemic human at sea level to being a hypoxic human at extreme altitudes, a left-shifted dissociation curve becomes advantageous. We just don't know at what altitude this occurs. Whether the change from Minneapolis(which is 834 ft. above sea level) to Leadville (which is 10,150 feet above sea level) is extreme enough to reveal any advantage or disadvantage of curve position remains to be seen. In fact, I think any differences we find will not be large. However, I should like to point out that an intermediate (rather than extreme) altitude is, in fact, probally the ideal situation for testing the hypothesis. The P50 of these individuals and the ambient pO_2 at Leadville are such that the high affinity subjects would show essentially no change in arterial saturation. Thus, in contrast to normal subjects, they should

The Red Cell, pages 749—752

© **1978 Alan R. Liss, Inc., New York, New York**

notice little if any effect of the environmental oxygen
deprivation.

Dr. Brown: Is there any evidence for a shift in the p50 values
in well-conditioned athletes who are conditioned aerobically?
Is there any evidence that they're right-shifted or that this
would be an advantage?

Dr. Hebbel: I believe there is (Rand et al., Am. J. Physiol.
224:1334, 1973). Perhaps Dr. Brewer or John Eaton can address this question more fully.

Dr. Brewer: I believe that the DPG in conditioned athletes
is somewhat increased--not a great deal--so that the curve
is probably slightly right-shifted. Then there is an acute
exercise effect which is another issue. It appears to me
that there is one other difference in what you're talking
about versus acute adaptation to altitude where the curve is
right-shifted. Your patients have lived all their lives
with a left-shifted curve and perhaps during development adjustments take place which make altitude exposure a slightly
different experience for them than in someone who hasn't
had a left-shifted curve all their life.

Dr. Hebbel: That is admittedly a possibility and is something
that we have discussed at length. I did not address this
point because we obviously cannot answer it. Certainly,
there is much evidence that tissue adaptations to altitude
take place. We cannot exclude analogous changes in these
high affinity individuals. We do think this is unlikely,
but we acknowledge that it is a possibility. However, we
feel it is very improbable that these individuals have a polymorphism of other respiratory pigments,a situation which may
be occurring in animal species such as the llama.

Dr. Moore: Of course there are a large number of complicating
factors but just to add a few, Leadville residents with excessive polycythemia(chronic mountain sickness) have left-
shifted oxygen dissociation curves. These individuals are
extremely hypoxic, run high erythropoitin and, consequently
high hematocrit levels that become lethal unless corrected.
This suggests that their left-shifted curves contribute to
hypoxia rather than protect from it. Also, we've done some
work in which we've produced slight curve shifts with phar-
macologic treatment at high altitudes and noted some improve-
ments (decreased erythropoietin levels, increased central

nervous system performance as measured in visual tasks)
which suggest that there is some slight advantage associated
with the slight amount of right-curve shift we were able to
produce.

Dr. Hebbel: Yes, I'm aware of that. However, the people
that you're talking about are largely, although admittedly
not entirely, smokers. And there are further complicating
factors, the most significant of which is probably the extreme
erythrocytosis you have alluded to. Some of these people
have hemoglobins as high as 24 gram percent. I think this
"malignant" degree of erythrocytosis is quite different from
the situation we have been discussing. Hopefully, we can let
you know in the near future.

Dr. Mizukami: Since the tissue extractability of oxygen is
quite different, depending upon whether you're talking about
the brain tissues or heart tissues or skeletal muscle tissues,
even though you may set your experiment at a certain altitude,
you may be experiencing a different kind of benefit to a
different tissue. Would this not be true?

Dr. Hebbel: Yes, I entirely agree. There are numerous parameters that would be interesting and important to evaluate in
an experiment of this nature. Unfortunately, most of these
cannot be measured directly in a non-invasive altitude study.

Dr. Mizukami: One more question. When you talked about changing p50s, you did elaborate to the nature of the curves. Have
you seen any particular difference in the dissociation curve
near the saturation as some people are talking about in hemoglobin Sydney? As far as what we could see from the curve
the sigmoidness was considerably lost and the loss could be
attributed to some kind of nonbenefit rather than benefit.
That is, even though you may start from the exact same
alveolar pO_2, depending upon what kind of nature of curve
you have in higher part of the oxygenation, the extractability
of oxygen might be quite different.

Dr. Hebbel: Are you asking about the rats or the people?

Dr. Mizukami: Well, I'm trying to see the difference between
so-called high affinity and low affinity people when you compare them to the normals.

Dr. Hebbel: The curve shape of these high affinity subjects

is normal.

Dr. Mizukami: In the near high oxygenation level?

Dr. Hebbel: Yes.